FORENSIC PSYCHIATRY AND PSYCHOLOGY

FORENSIC PSYCHIATRY AND PSYCHOLOGY:
PERSPECTIVES AND STANDARDS FOR INTERDISCIPLINARY PRACTICE

WILLIAM J. CURRAN, J.D., LL.M., S.M.Hyg.
FRANCES GLESSNER LEE PROFESSOR OF LEGAL MEDICINE
HARVARD UNIVERSITY
BOSTON, MASSACHUSETTS

A. LOUIS McGARRY, M.D.
PROFESSOR OF CLINICAL PSYCHIATRY
STATE UNIVERSITY OF NEW YORK AT STONY BROOK
MEDICAL DIRECTOR OF FORENSIC SERVICES
NASSAU COUNTY DEPARTMENT OF MENTAL HEALTH
EAST MEADOW, NEW YORK

SALEEM A. SHAH, Ph.D.
CHIEF, CENTER FOR STUDIES OF ANTISOCIAL AND VIOLENT
  BEHAVIOR
NATIONAL INSTITUTE OF MENTAL HEALTH
ROCKVILLE, MARYLAND

 F. A. Davis Company/PHILADELPHIA

Library of Congress Cataloging-in-Publication Data
Main entry under title:

Forensic psychiatry and psychology.

  Includes bibliographies and index.
  1. Forensic psychiatry.   2. Psychology, Forensic.
I. Curran, William J.   II. McGarry, A. Louis (Armand
Louis), 1929-   .   III. Shah, Saleem A. (Saleem Alam), 1931-
RA1151.F656   1986   614.4   85-25398
ISBN 0-8036-2295-3

DEDICATION

Dr. A. Louis McGarry, one of the editors of this text, died in early December of 1985 after all of the editorial work had been completed. The other editors wish to dedicate this text to him. We feel that this work and its multidisciplinary purpose is a fitting memorial to Dr. McGarry as one of the country's leading figures in the field of forensic psychiatry. He was one of the organizers and early supporters of formal training and standards for forensic psychiatry work in the United States. A sensitive and gifted clinician, he was also an imaginative writer and researcher. He was a friend and a colleague of both the other editors for over 20 years, and his loss to them and to the field of mental health and law is a very great one indeed.

CONTRIBUTORS

GENE G. ABEL, M.D.
Professor of Psychiatry
Department of Psychiatry
Emory University School of Medicine at Grady Hospital
Atlanta, Georgia

JUDITH V. BECKER, Ph.D.
Director, Sexual Behavior Clinic
New York State Psychiatric Institute
Associate Professor of Clinical Psychology in Psychiatry
College of Physicians and Surgeons
Columbia University
New York, New York

ELAINE (HILBERMAN) CARMEN, M.D.
Associate Professor of Psychiatry
Assistant Director of Psychiatric Residency Training
University of North Carolina School of Medicine
Chapel Hill, North Carolina

DANIEL J. COX, Ph.D.
Associate Professor of Behavioral Medicine and Psychiatry and of Internal Medicine
School of Medicine
University of Virginia
Charlottesville, Virginia

WILLIAM J. CURRAN, J.D., LL.M., S.M.Hyg.
Frances Glessner Lee Professor of Legal Medicine
Harvard University
Boston, Massachusetts

PARK ELLIOTT DIETZ, M.D., M.P.H., Ph.D.
Associate Professor of Law and of Behavioral Medicine and Psychiatry
Medical Director, Institute of Law, Psychiatry and Public Policy
Schools of Law and Medicine
University of Virginia
Charlottesville, Virginia

SIMON DINITZ, Ph.D.
Professor
Department of Sociology
Ohio State University
Columbus, Ohio

THOMAS GRISSO, Ph.D.
Professor of Psychology
Associate Professor of Psychology in Law
St. Louis University
St. Louis, Missouri

R. KIRKLAND GABLE, Ph.D., J.D.
Professor
Department of Psychology
California Lutheran College
Thousand Oaks, California

WALLACE A. KENNEDY, Ph.D., ABPP
Professor of Psychology
Director of Graduate Studies
Florida State University
Tallahassee, Florida

MICHAEL KINDRED, J.D.
Professor of Law
Ohio State University College of Law
Columbus, Ohio

JOHN R. LION, M.D.
Clinical Professor
Department of Psychiatry
University of Maryland School of Medicine
Baltimore, Maryland

A. LOUIS McGARRY, M.D.*
Professor of Clinical Psychiatry
State University of New York at Stony Brook
Medical Director of Forensic Services
Nassau County Department of Mental Health
East Meadow, New York

HERBERT C. MODLIN, M.D.
Noble Professor of Forensic Psychiatry
Menninger Foundation
Topeka, Kansas

SPYROS J. MONOPOLIS, M.D.
Medical School Assistant Professor
Department of Psychiatry
University of Maryland School of Medicine
Baltimore, Maryland

CAROL C. NADELSON, M.D.
Professor and Vice-Chairman
Director of Training and Education
Department of Psychiatry
Tufts—New England Medical Center Hospital
Boston, Massachusetts

MALKAH T. NOTMAN, M.D.
Clinical Professor of Psychiatry
Director of Psychotherapy Out-Patient Clinic
Department of Psychiatry
Tufts—New England Medical Center Hospital
Boston, Massachusetts

SEYMOUR POLLACK, M.A., M.D.*
Professor of Psychiatry and Director
Institute of Psychiatry, Law and Behavior Science
University of Southern California
Los Angeles, California

JERRY CUNNINGHAM-RATHNER, B.A.
Assistant Instructor of Psychology
Department of Psychiatry
Columbia University
College of Physicians and Surgeons
New York, New York

---

*Deceased

ALAN ROSENBAUM, Ph.D.
Assistant Professor
Department of Psychology
Syracuse University
Syracuse, New York

LOREN H. ROTH, M.D., M.P.H.
Professor of Psychiatry
Chief, Adult Clinical Services
Director, Law and Psychiatry Program
Western Psychiatric Institute and Clinic
University of Pittsburgh School of Medicine
Pittsburgh, Pennsylvania

JOANNE-L. ROULEAU, Ph.D.
Assistant Professor of Psychiatry (Psychology)
Department of Psychiatry
Emory University School of Medicine
Atlanta, Georgia

BRUCE D. SALES, J.D., Ph.D.
Professor of Psychology, Sociology, and Law
University of Arizona
Tucson, Arizona

SALEEM A. SHAH, Ph.D.
Chief, Center for Studies of Antisocial and Violent Behavior
National Institute of Mental Health
Rockville, Maryland

SANDRA K. SEIGEL, B.A.
St. Louis University
St. Louis, Missouri

STEPHEN WEGENER, Ph.D.
Research Assistant
Department of Orthopedics and Rehabilitation and Department of Behavioral Medicine
    and Psychiatry
School of Medicine
University of Virginia
Charlottesville, Virginia

CATHY SPATZ WIDOM, Ph.D.
Professor of Criminal Justice and Psychology (part-time)
Indiana University
Bloomington, Indiana

CONTENTS

INTRODUCTION
William J. Curran, J.D., LL.M., S.M.Hyg.

In this volume we have brought together an unusually broad and gifted group of authors who are experts in training, standard setting, practice, and research in the interdisciplinary fields of forensic psychiatry and forensic psychology. Achieving this degree of cooperation in a single venture among psychiatrists, psychologists, and lawyers is no mean accomplishment. Our main objective, however, throughout this effort has been clear from the beginning: We were seeking improvement in the quality of forensic expert testimony and consultation in psychiatry and psychology in the American judicial and correctional systems. Improving quality in these fields has often proven a deceptively difficult task. The obstacles to improvement and change in the forensic mental health professions have been formidable, deeply entrenched, and often treacherously hidden from the view of the naive reformer.

In the long history of the common law's use of expert consultation, the legal system itself—the consumer and patron of forensic science expertise—has been stubbornly unsupportive of quality standards for forensic psychiatrists and psychologists and for essentially all other forensic specialists. Legal impediments to attracting the best of behavioral scientists to cooperate with the law courts have long existed, and their removal has often met resistance from the bench and bar until very recent times. It is still doubtful that the majority of the legal profession—and the law enforcement and correctional authorities as well—have yet acquired sufficient skills to distinguish between the minimally qualified, ethical practitioners in this field and those who are professionally unqualified and unsuitable for forensic work. Also lacking are the ability and confidence to select the best available forensic experts in their jurisdictional regions of the country to participate in the serious business of the civil and criminal justice systems.

Until quite recent decades, conditions have not been much better on the professional side of psychiatry and psychology. The complexities and demands of interdisciplinary law-related service roles have discouraged and retarded the development of forensic training programs for the field. As a result, standards of professional quality have lagged behind other subspecialties. The busy practitioners, often without formal forensic training, have shaped and dominated the service aspects of the field. Most crucial of all, perhaps, has been the lack of support for research. The urgent demands of service have discouraged attention to research by practitioners. Budgetary constraints have discouraged support by the state and county judicial and penal systems for academically based research and consultation efforts. In large measure, only research grant support at the federal level has kept any degree of interdisciplinary research alive in this vital area of cooperation between our judicial-correctional systems and academic research programs.

This volume is intended to provide a comprehensive review of the current problems of this field, ranging from identifying and encouraging high-quality forensic training programs to supporting more effective and ethically acceptable testimonial, consultative, and treatment services. Throughout the analysis of these practical applications of professional skills and knowledge we will be concerned with calling attention to the research components of the field and the need to apply research findings to improve the effectiveness of service programs and to reform the law, which underlies the interface between the legal system and behavioral science.

The impetus for this collection was the effort of a few of the authors for an earlier volume also published by the F.A. Davis Company. That volume—the first in the United States to bring together contributions from all aspects of legal medicine and forensic science—included important work in forensic psychiatry. We asked a selected group of those authors in the forensic psychiatry section to update their chapters for this new volume. To these contributions we added new chapters by leading authorities providing substantially increased attention to forensic psychology, further contributions from forensic psychiatry, greater attention to interdisciplinary research, and a more comprehensive, in-depth review of legal issues in the field which have become of more serious public and professional concern than they were at the time of the earlier volume.

It should be evident from a perusal of the contributions by this diverse group of authors that no single mode or style of writing was imposed by the editors. The styles of writing related to psychiatry, psychology, sociology, criminology, and law are quite dissimilar. It was our common belief that there is a strength—a richness—in this diversity. The psychiatric writing in the text is predominantly clinical in nature, with an emphasis on new developments in practice such as those occasioned by the adoption of the third edition of the American Psychiatric Association's *Diagnostic and Statistical Manual of Mental Disorders (DSM III)*. The writing of the psychologists, coming in large measure from academic doctoral programs specializing in the psychology-law field, contains a depth of analysis firmly based on empirical research. The criminology and sociology writings are also research oriented, with different approaches identified with each field. Most of the legal developments are integrated into the chapters by the authors themselves or were prepared in collaboration with legal scholars. We should note that the diversity we sought was not always displayed only in disciplinary distinctions; among the chapters contributed by psychiatrists, such as that by Loren Roth, the research bibliography spans over two decades of development in correctional systems and prison-based therapeutic efforts. Among the psychologists, both Thomas Grisso and Wallace Kennedy have written state-of-the-art chapters on the application of psychological assessments and courtroom participation, respectively, that are essentially clinical in both approach and style. In other chapters that are psychology-psychiatry collaborations or mental health–law combinations, a mixture of styles has been encouraged and stimulated by the interdisciplinary backgrounds of the authors.

It is our hope that the emphasis of this text upon improved educational programs, accreditation, standard setting, and high-quality performance based upon clinical excellence and research will justify the publication of a new text in the mental health–law field. Our multidisciplinary approach has been designed to achieve a comprehensiveness in the examination of important issues and problems in the field that cannot be resolved by one discipline alone.

The organization of the book has followed the primary objective of improving professional performance in forensic and legally related work. By "forensic" we mean that part of professional examination and evaluation intended for courtroom application and formal litigation issues. A few chapters also deal with more indirect legal issues, correctional or penal matters, and treatment methodologies that are covered under a broader concept of legal, or legally related, psychiatry and psychology.

We have divided the text into six parts, each dealing with a particular portion of our subject. The opening part examines the major theme of the book: professional standards that are the foundation of ethical, quality performance in the field. The second part contains the core of the skill-building chapters of the text: those dealing with techniques and procedures for psychiatric and psychological assessment and treatment. This is the longest and most detailed part in the book, and it contains the most chapters. The three following sections are quite highly specialized. Part 3 deals with family violence and child abuse, child custody issues in divorce and separation litigation, and juvenile delinquency. Part 4 is a collection of chapters on sexually related conduct. Part 5 examines issues in personality disorder, including antisocial personality problems and the newer classifications of impulse control disorders catalogued under that title in *DSM III*.

The last part of the book presents a review of the changing and growing roles played by mental health professionals in the American court and prison systems. Chapters in this section examine current issues in treatment and rehabilitation in prison mental health programs, as well as the problems facing forensic psychiatrists and psychologists as consultants, evaluators, and expert witnesses in both civil and criminal litigation. In very large measure, this section is intended to bring together and to summarize the issues and problems introduced in other parts of the volume. Recurrent themes from other chapters will reappear in this last part in an analysis of a more generalized nature and with more specific goals addressed to the American system of justice. Of particular significance in this section is the report to the American Bar Association (ABA) on mental health professional participation in the criminal justice system. This report, recently adopted by the highest body of the ABA, was prepared by an interdisciplinary task force and contains many important reforms in the utilization of mental health expertise in evaluation and testimonial roles. The general scope and direction of the report and its recommendations are in accordance with the goals and purposes of this text. This is not surprising, inasmuch as so many of the contributors to this text took part in the deliberations of the ABA group and contributed articles, papers, and reform proposals which were relied upon in the preparation of the report.

As the opening pages of this introduction indicated, our purpose in this text has been to gather in one volume contributions from a wide variety of the leading practitioners and scholars in this field with the objective of improving the quality of forensic services to the American courts and prisons. We have sought to present the most current developments in mental health practice, the findings of significant empirical research, and the impact of new legal reforms and proposals in each subject covered in the text. In most instances, the contemporary issues are placed in historical perspective in terms of practice, research, and jurisprudential influences as a means of indicating the direction and strength of trends in the field. As pointed out earlier, considerable freedom has been given the authors in terms of style and approach according to professional discipline and scholarly interest. It is the editors' hope that this variety of styles in an interdisciplinary effort will add to the utility and attractiveness of the contributed chapters on these important issues confronting mental health and the law.

PART 1

FOUNDATIONS OF FORENSIC PSYCHIATRY AND PSYCHOLOGY

Three of the authors of the chapters in this first section of the text are the editors of the book. The theme of this part is the primary objective of the overall text: improvement in professional performance in forensic practice in psychiatry and psychology.

The underlying basis for improved and enhanced performance must be found in recruiting to the field the best-trained applicants and then in development and enforcement of the highest quality standards of practice. This is the subject of chapter 1 by editors Saleem Shah and A. Louis McGarry. In a comprehensive manner, the authors review the requirements for a career in the specialty areas of forensic psychiatry and forensic psychology. They list the major educational and training programs being offered in various parts of the country and provide details concerning admission requirements and curriculum in these programs.

The history of educational efforts in the forensic field is described to provide perspective for evaluation of the changes in current philosophies of education and training. Along with the two major disciplines, attention is also given to special training in the related fields of clinical social work and psychiatric nursing. An effort is made in this chapter to estimate the needs for forensic services in this field in the future and the level of currently available services. Five types of mental health programs are explored: centralized state security facilities, community and regional forensic programs, law court clinics, correctional institutional services, and community-based correctional programs. Massive data on clinical services now being offered throughout the country were surveyed and are cited on these pages.

Most important, the opening chapter reviews and analyzes accreditation systems for educational and training programs in the field and the development of professional standards for practice. The authors point to several reasons for the support of efforts to establish and to enforce quality standards of practice:

the facilitation of mutual understanding between professionals and users of forensic services, the encouragement of more effective evaluation of quality performance, the development of greater uniformity in legislative and regulatory systems, and provision of a reliable and accepted basis for accreditation procedures for forensic clinical facilities.

Chapter 1 is the first of several throughout the book to call attention to the cooperative efforts of lawyers and mental health professionals in developing the American Bar Association's recently adopted mental health standards for the criminal justice field. These standards, adopted unanimously by the American Bar Association in the summer of 1984, provide outstanding support for improved quality standards of testimony and consultation by psychiatrists and psychologists in criminal trials.

The other two chapters in this part deal with ethical considerations. It is the view of each of the editors of this volume that no issue in this field is of greater significance in the mid-1980s than the ethical climate of testimonial and consultative services in this field. In past decades, forensic work in psychiatry and psychology was under widespread attack as highly suspect not only in quality but in its ethical aspect. The battle of experts disparaged in the courts was exemplified most often as a mental health issue, even though many other areas of scientific and technical knowledge have also been seen in bitter conflict in numerous litigated cases.

The second chapter analyzes the formal codes and standards of psychiatry and psychology in regard to ethical conduct in the forensic area. The scope of practice is reviewed in regard to the courts and the prisons, and the conflicts of values and goals between mental health professionals and judicial and correctional authorities are surveyed.

The theme of the chapter on ethical issues is particularly drawn from the writings of the late Seymour Pollack, who contributed a chapter on this subject to our earlier comprehensive text on legal medicine, psychiatry, and forensic science. Throughout his career, Dr. Pollack was the primary spokesman for the view that forensic mental health specialists should conform in their judicial consultations and testimony to the legal rules prevailing in the jurisdiction and that they could not ethically participate and at the same time covertly attempt to undermine or to corrupt the legal requirements they were presumed to follow in the forensic role. The alternative for Pollack was for forensic specialists to refuse openly to participate in legal issues in which their own consciences and professional standards were in conflict with the legal rules but also to advocate needed legal reform in the field. This objective has been retained in this chapter and in the volume as a whole.

CHAPTER 1

LEGAL PSYCHIATRY AND PSYCHOLOGY: REVIEW OF PROGRAMS, TRAINING, AND QUALIFICATIONS

Saleem A. Shah, Ph.D.
A. Louis McGarry, M.D.

During the past two decades there has been markedly increased interest and involvement of the mental health disciplines in the law and the legal systems of this country. Understandably, such increased involvement has been accompanied by the development of a variety of professional service programs and special training programs for mental health professionals who devote significant portions of their time to this interdisciplinary field. These years have also seen the development of guidelines and standards for professional practice in these and related areas.

As indicated in Professor Curran's chapter (chapter 2), the fields of **legal psychiatry** and **legal psychology** include broad applications of these disciplines to a variety of legal concerns, not only to formal involvement and interactions with the judiciary and the courts. The past decade has also been marked by a tremendous surge in research and related interests on the part of many psychologists in various fields of specialization (for example, child, clinical, experimental, educational, industrial/organizational, school, and social) in various aspects of the law, and numerous publications testify to the range and productivity of these endeavors (see Tapp,[1] Monahan and Loftus,[2] and the many relevant references provided in this chapter).

In the interface between law and the mental health field, the major (although by no means exclusive) involvement has been by psychiatrists and psychologists, hence our focus in this book on these two disciplines. We wish to emphasize, however, that social work and nursing also have important roles in this inherently interdisciplinary field. Clearly, professionals in psychiatric social work and psychiatric nursing play key roles in the various law-related mental health service programs. We shall call attention to some special training developments in these related disciplines.

As the title of the chapter indicates, we shall focus here on three major aspects of legal psychiatry and psychology: a description and discussion of the major types of service programs currently in operation, various kinds of training programs that have been developed, and the adoption of standards and qualifications for persons who wish to specialize in the legal psychiatry and psychology fields.

Several years ago one of the pioneers in the field of law and mental health, Professor Sheldon Glueck,[3] reviewed the relations between psychiatry and law in a series of lectures that later appeared as a book with the interesting title *Law and Psychiatry: Cold War or Entente Cordiale?* In more recent years these relationships have certainly been rather chilly, and there have even been periods (for example, during the major reforms of mental health laws in the late 1960s and 1970s) when many psychiatrists and psychiatric groups have felt beseiged and beleaguered,[4] even "belegalled,"[5] by lawyers; others expressed concern about the "holy legal war" against state hospital psychiatry[6] and the perceived "legal onslaught"[7] against existing mental health laws, policies, and related practices. However, these changes were also seen by some as reflecting an appropriate movement toward shared decision making[8] and even as overdue and "imperative reform."[9] (For a review of some of these major developments in mental health laws during the last two decades, see Shah.[10])

As indicated by the title of Glueck's book, the major tension has involved mainly psychiatry, inasmuch as it has been the dominant mental health discipline involved. However, with the increased social and legal acceptance of the other mental health disciplines (since 1977 certification or licensing laws regulating psychologists have been in existence in every state and the District of Columbia), the range of mental health involvement with legal issues, as well as major research contributions, has increased considerably.

It might be noted that the tensions and problems in the relationship between law and the mental health disciplines do not relate simply to the past few decades or even to particular periods of major social movements and reforms, although such movements do highlight and even heighten the underlying tensions. There is a literature describing the historical nature of some of the philosophical, ideological, and even political dimensions of the differences in regard to the labeling, handling, and care of the mentally ill (see Conrad and Schneider,[11] Fox,[12] Freidson,[13] Rothman,[14] and Scull[15]). Very recently, Fleming[16] described a particular instance of the aforementioned tension in an article with the very catchy (if not elegant) title of "Shrinks vs. Shysters: The (Latest) Battle for Control of the Mentally Ill."

The foregoing problems seem to relate rather fundamentally to the differing values; professional ideologies; governing paradigms; and the particular roles, functions, prerogatives, and power of the various groups involved. Discussions between lawyers and mental health professionals tend to become obstructed by the above differences. Understandably, professionals tend to view things from the perspective of their own fields and in the context of their particular social roles, career and professional contingencies, key concepts, and their special "tools of the trade." Predictably, therefore, legally oriented and mental health oriented perspectives can and often do lead to differing notions about the nature of the perceived problems, the controlling values to be applied, the major interests to be protected, the particular objectives to be sought, and the manner in which the major issues should be formulated, addressed, and resolved.

Moreover, the "reforms" and "solutions" adopted several years ago often result in new problems and dilemmas. Whatever the particular balance that is drawn between competing values and interests in addressing complex social problems, there are inevitable trade-offs involved with respect to the particular types and rates of resulting problems. For example, the emphasis in the past on treatment needs of the mentally ill, on broadly worded commitment laws, and on wide discretion for psychiatrists were associated with easier involuntary hospitalization of the mentally ill and longer periods of confinement. The problems were considerably exacerbated by the poor quality of care likely to be available in many public facilities. Following the reforms of the last two decades and the much greater emphasis on the legal rights and liberty interests of the mentally ill (along with associated "deinstitutionalization" policies and budgetary constraints), civil commitment criteria have become far more stringent and hospital stays much shorter. Many chronically and seriously mentally ill persons cannot now be hospitalized involuntarily. These changes have often resulted in situations in which the care of the chronically mentally ill has been "transferred from a single lousy institution to multiple wretched ones"[17] in the community, and thoughtful individuals have been led to wonder if "back alleys (are) any better than back wards."[18]

The aforementioned differences in governing paradigms and the controlling values and perspectives can also be noted with respect to behavioral and social science research on the validity of various assumptions underlying substantive laws and the manner in which these and related issues are approached and addressed by lawyers and judges (see Haney[19] and Monahan and Loftus[2]).

The involvement of mental health professionals in the operations of the legal system continues to be a subject of much debate and discussion. Some leading psychiatrists, such as Halleck,[20] have spoken out against the involvement of psychiatry in the legal system, except in the traditional therapeutic role. Too often psychiatry and psychology have been perceived and judged by the public in the context of the vexing assessments of criminal responsibility in the trial of some notorious defendant and in the full glare of media attention—for example, the trial of John Hinckley, Jr., who attempted to assassinate President Reagan in March 1981. Many questions and concerns have also been raised in regard to the involvement of mental health professionals in predictions of dangerousness (see Dix,[21] Monahan,[22,23] and Shah[24, 25]).

In these situations there have indeed been many reasons for questioning the proper role and functioning of mental health professionals. The issue of criminal responsibility fundamentally involves questions of moral judgments and related legal and public policy issues—**not** medical, psychiatric, or psychological judgments. Similarly, the prediction of behaviors that have very low frequencies (base rates) is fraught with immense difficulties and very high rates of "false-positive" errors. There are also some crucial value judgments and public policy determinations to be made concerning precisely what kinds of behaviors are officially to be viewed, defined, labeled, and handled as "dangerous." In regard to these problems Morris[26] has observed that whenever the criminal justice (police) power and the mental health power are combined (as in the case of various categories of mentally disordered defendants and offenders), there is great potential for both powers to be mutually corrupted. (See chapter 6, "Predictions of Dangerousness and Implications for Treatment"; chapter 8, "Criminal Responsibility"; and chapter 19, "Correctional Psychiatry.")

LAW AND MENTAL HEALTH SERVICE PROGRAMS

The foregoing dilemmas and concerns notwithstanding, mental health professionals are called upon rather frequently to provide various types of assistance and consultation in the legal process with regard to a wide range of civil, criminal, and administrative proceedings. Pollack[27] had estimated some years ago that the total number of "psychiatric-legal consultations" (including both civil and criminal actions) in the United States would easily exceed one million a year. Although we do not know the precise manner in which Pollack arrived at this estimate, if one considers all forensic mental health screening assessments as well as detailed evaluations at various stages of the criminal process and various civil actions (including emergency admissions and civil commitment of the mentally ill, conservatorship and guardianship cases, domestic relations and juvenile law cases, and various tort actions), Pollack's estimate made 16 years ago is very likely an underestimate. Of course, he was referring only to "psychiatric-legal consultations," and we would include **all** forensic mental health evaluations made by psychiatrists, psychologists, social workers, and psychiatric nurses in order to obtain a rough idea of the total mental health effort and resources devoted to forensic evaluations. In sum, if the range of legal actions noted above are considered (even without including developmental disability and supplemental social security cases involving mental health evaluations), we would estimate that the annual number of all such evaluations—**not** the number of persons evaluated—would approach or even exceed two million. We emphasize, however, that without appropriate records and reliable statistics on the subject, ours is nothing more than a rough estimate.

In a study of mental health examinations in criminal justice settings, Keilitz[28] surveyed 121 forensic screening and evaluation programs. Of the 120 that reported information regarding their organization, administration, caseloads, and activities, the total monthly caseloads for the programs was 17,000. Forensic facilities with large caseflows tended to be located in metropolitan areas, to be housed in local jails or state prisons, and to have as their major purpose screening and classification, treatment, and pretrial diversion. However, the small staff-client ratios suggested that typically only screening and cursory mental health evaluations were undertaken in facilities with large caseflows.

Keilitz described law-related mental health service programs as being found in five types of facilities: (1) centralized state institutions (security hospitals or units); (2) community and regional forensic mental health programs; (3) court clinics; (4) state and local correctional institutions; and (5) community corrections programs.

We shall discuss each of these types of facilities.

Centralized State Security Hospitals and Units

Security mental hospitals and units serve a range of mentally disordered offenders and other mentally ill persons requiring secure confinement; these are the oldest types of programs in the legal or forensic mental health service system. For a fairly long period of time accurate information was not available about the precise number of such facilities; the number of patients served and their diagnostic, legal, and other characteristics; the staffing patterns; and treat-

TABLE 1-1. The Admissions and Average Daily Census of Mentally Disordered Offenders in US Facilities by Legal Status in 1978*

LEGAL STATUS	ADMITTED TO FORENSIC MENTAL HEALTH FACILITIES		AVERAGE DAILY CENSUS IN THE FORENSIC MENTAL HEALTH FACILITIES	
	TOTAL	%	TOTAL	%
Incompetent to stand trial	6,420	32	3,400	24
Not guilty by reason of insanity	1,625	8	3,140	22
Mentally disordered sex offenders	1,203	6	2,442	17
Mentally ill prisoners	10,895	54	5,158	37
Total	20,143	100	14,140	100

Percents may not add up to 100 because of rounding
* *Report to the Nation on Crime and Justice: The Data.* Bureau of Justice Statistics, US Department of Justice, Washington, DC, October 1983.

ment programs. During the past 15 years, however, many surveys of these facilities have been conducted.

In 1969, Scheidemandel and Kanno[29] identified 153 such facilities and reported on the responses to a detailed questionnaire obtained from 98 of the programs. Eckerman[30] conducted a comprehensive national survey that was sponsored and funded by the National Institute of Mental Health. This study used more stringent definitions for the security mental health facilities included in the survey, namely, those that had comprehensive inpatient programs for the care and treatment of mentally disordered offenders. A total of 73 such facilities was identified, and usable survey responses were obtained from 68 sites. In addition to the narrative report,[30] a directory of these facilities was published.[31]

Sheldon and Norman[32] used a telephone survey in July 1976 and compiled an inventory of 48 facilities providing comprehensive treatment programs for mentally disordered offenders.

Under a grant from the National Institute of Justice, Steadman and coworkers[33] undertook a national survey of facilities for mentally disordered offenders as of 1978 (Table 1-1). This study was concerned only with adjudicated persons in the following four categories: (1) persons found to be incompetent to stand trial, (2) persons found not guilty by reason of insanity, (3) mentally disordered sex offenders, and (4) mentally ill prisoners.*

A total of 20,143 **admissions** was received during 1978 in the above four categories by the facilities surveyed. The largest group of patients (54 percent) consisted of transfers from prisons; persons who had been adjudicated incompetent to stand trial (IST) constituted 32 percent, those found not guilty by reason of insanity (NGRI) accounted for 8 percent, and mentally disordered sex offenders (MDSOs) accounted for 6 percent of the admissions.

---

* Because the various studies used somewhat different definitions of the facilities and programs encompassed, and the categories of mentally disordered offenders included, it is very difficult to make ready comparisons or to get accurate trend information concerning variations in the number of admissions over the past several years.

The **average daily census** in 1978 for the above categories of mentally disordered offenders was 14,140. Transfers from prison accounted for 36.5 percent of the census, the IST patients were 24 percent, the NGRI patients were 22 percent, and the MDSO cases constituted 17 percent. Based on the gender information that was available, women accounted for 5.2 percent of the admissions and 6.1 percent of the average daily census figures. In both instances, women were disproportionately higher in the NGRI category.

Two other surveys of security hospitals and units have been completed during 1983. Davis[34] has reported on a survey of forensic mental health programs in the 13 member states of the Western Interstate Commission for Higher Education (WICHE). This survey was conducted during May 1983 and indicates the magnitude of the problems faced by the mental health and corrections personnel and the inadequacies in most states regarding information systems to identify and to track mentally ill offenders in various parts of the system. Very useful information is provided in the WICHE report about such things as the location and administrative structure of the forensic facilities, estimated costs of these services across the various jurisdictions, staffing patterns, number and types of annual admissions, and community-based programs for mentally ill offenders.

The other and more comprehensive nationwide survey of public sector facilities and programs for mentally disordered offenders was funded by the National Institute of Mental Health (NIMH) and was conducted by WESTAT, Inc.[35] The following eight categories of persons were included in the survey:

1. criminal defendants being evaluated for competency to stand trial;
2. persons adjudicated incompetent to stand trial;
3. criminal defendants being evaluated for criminal responsibility;
4. persons adjudicated "not guilty by reason of insanity";
5. mentally ill offenders transferred from prisons;
6. mentally disordered sex offenders (variously designated as "sexual psychopaths," "sexually dangerous persons," and so forth);
7. juveniles convicted of or found to be involved in criminal behavior and committed for treatment of mental illness;
8. offenders adjudicated "guilty but mentally ill."*

Following initial location of a much larger universe of potentially eligible facilities, a total of 168 eligible programs was identified, and detailed survey questionnaires were returned by 127. In addition to the survey the NIMH study also involved legal and library research to identify major statutory and case-law developments that may have affected programs for mentally disordered offenders, and 11 programs were visited on site.

Overall, the 127 responding facilities reported a total resident population of 19,543, of which 88 percent were men and 12 percent were women. In terms of the **organizational auspices** of the facilities and characteristics of their residents, the following was found.

---

*As of the end of 1983 there were 12 states that had enacted "guilty but mentally ill" statutes: Michigan (1975); Indiana (1980); Illinois (1981); Alaska, Delaware, Georgia, Kentucky, and New Mexico (1982); Pennsylvania, South Dakota, Utah, and Vermont (1983).

- The overwhelming majority (121) of the facilities were under state auspices, five were federally administered, and there was only one local facility.
- Sixty-two percent of the facilities (N = 79) were under mental health agencies and housed 70 percent of the mentally disordered offenders. Twenty-four percent of the facilities were under corrections, and 18 percent were under various other auspices, such as social service agencies, youth authorities, or combined mental health/correctional agencies.
- Only 3 percent (4) of the responding facilities were solely for women, although 36 percent (46) admitted persons of both sexes. (This distribution is very similar to that found by Eckerman.[30])
- Only 13 percent (17) of the facilities were solely for juvenile court dispositions, another 9 percent (12) accepted dispositions from both adult and juvenile courts, and 77 percent admitted only adults.

The following are some findings regarding the **crimes for which the persons had been charged or convicted;** only the most serious charges were used in cases where multiple charges were involved.

- The majority of mentally disordered offenders (68 percent) had been charged with crimes against persons, and the single most common offense in this category was homicide (18 percent). Other charges were rape, 11 percent; other sexual offenses, 11 percent; other crimes of violence, 28 percent; various property crimes, 22 percent; and all other offenses accounted for the remaining 9 percent.
- The proportions of homicide charges (18 percent) and all crimes against persons (68 percent) in these facilities were significantly greater than the respective proportions (13 percent and 57 percent) in the general prison population.

With respect to the **treatment programs** in the facilities surveyed, the following was found.

- Over 90 percent reported some form of individual treatment planning, although only 48 percent reported state statutes or regulations requiring this. There were substantial variations in regard to the nature and quality of what was considered to be individual treatment planning.
- Psychotropic medication was the most widely available treatment; it was used in 98 percent of the facilities and administered to a median 61 percent of the residents for crisis intervention, short-term stabilization, or longer-term maintenance.
- Prerelease services were offered by about 90 percent of the facilities that released residents directly to the community and varied from counseling about release to referral to community agencies and negotiating conditions of treatment and follow-up with community agencies.

Among the issues and problems that were found to be of concern to the administrators of the facilities were such things as (1) prevention and management of critical incidents such as suicides, assaults on other patients and/or staff, and escape; (2) control of admission policies in order to reduce overcrowding and to improve patient treatability; (3) staff "burnout" and turnover; and (4) the general problem of trying to balance treatment and security concerns.

Community and Regional Forensic Mental Health Programs

During the past 15 years there has been a strong national trend for moving away from the centralized security hospitals and units (often located in areas somewhat remote from major population centers) and toward the development of regional and even community-based forensic mental health services. These changes appear to have been influenced by a variety of factors; for example, the deinstitutionalization movement in the mental health field more generally, the network of community mental health centers that have been developed over the past 20 years, and the lawsuits that have helped expose the sad and sorry conditions in some of the centralized security hospitals. Yet another factor has been budgetary considerations. It simply does **not** make any sense at all for criminal defendants to be sent routinely to centralized security facilities for forensic evaluations (for example, determination of competency to stand trial), when such screening evaluations could be done locally for a fraction of the cost. What may be disconcerting—although not surprising—is that courts have often disregarded or underutilized the potential for the less restrictive and less costly alternative of local screening evaluations (using mental health consultants paid through court funds) while routinely sending defendants to security hospitals for such evaluations. In these cases, of course, the departments of mental health typically end up assuming the costs. In many of these situations, considerations of using "less restrictive alternatives" and related concerns about the rights of criminal defendants appear to give way to the opportunity and expediency of responding to the fiscal contingencies available in the system.

Several jurisdictions are now routinely using relatively brief outpatient screening examinations conducted in the mental health clinics, cellblocks, or other detention facilities and thereby have considerably reduced reliance on the longer, more restrictive, and more costly inpatient evaluations in security hospitals or units.[28,36-43] In 1971, for example, Ohio established its first community forensic center, following litigation involving Lima State Hospital, the centralized security hospital in the state. By early 1974 the state had six regional forensic centers in operation.[36,37] Similarly, Tennessee has for several years been using specially trained forensic mental health staff (psychiatrists, psychologists, social workers, as well as psychiatric nurses) in several community mental health centers to do forensic screening evaluations.[38,39] Others have reported related developments,[40-43] and Petrilla[44] has described some of the aforementioned developments and the implications for staff training, quality control, and related concerns associated with the decentralization efforts.

Court Clinics

The psychiatric court clinic model that was developed by Healy and Fernald in 1909 proved to be the forerunner of the child guidance clinics.[45] Although a large number of the facilities we shall refer to as court clinics are located physically in courthouses and are administratively under the court system, this rubric will also include clinics that may be under mental health or other auspices but which primarily or exclusively serve the courts and other criminal justice system agencies. Mental health professionals who have worked in court clinics stress the importance of the courthouse location, because much can be accomplished with court personnel, especially probation officers and attorneys, by informal "corridor consultation."

Most court clinics in the United States tend to limit their activities to screening and more detailed forensic evaluations and related consultations for court and other criminal justice system agencies and have only a limited treatment and/or training role. This restrictive approach has the associated risks that the work can become routinized, unrewarding, and even somewhat stultifying. In New York City, where much of the work of court clinics is concerned with examinations on the question of competency or fitness to stand trial, the facilities have been dubbed "fitness factories." However, a few of the clinics of our concern do have fairly active involvement in treatment, training, and related activities.[46]

Most court clinics are located in the larger cities and are associated with felony courts. Their activities usually include examinations to determine competency to stand trial and criminal responsibility and to provide dispositional recommendations associated with evaluations of convicted offenders. Much less frequently, domestic relations, juvenile, and family courts are also served by court clinics which become involved in substantial measure with the difficult challenges of divorce and child custody, child abuse and neglect, and juvenile delinquency matters.

The Medical Service of the Circuit Court for Baltimore City (previously known as the Medical Service of the Supreme Bench of Baltimore) was started in 1920, very possibly making it one of the oldest clinics of its kind in the country. This facility provides a wide range of screening assessments, detailed mental health evaluations, consultations, as well as treatment recommendations and referrals.[28,47]

The court clinic system in Massachusetts traces its roots to a pilot project established in 1948 by the Department of Mental Health, initiated by child psychiatrist Donald Russell and probation officer James Devlin.[48] The major purpose was to provide mental health services to delinquent or alleged delinquent youngsters in the Boston area. The success of this pilot project led to the expansion of the court clinic concept in Massachusetts and resulted in the establishment in 1954 of the Cambridge Court Clinic as a district court demonstration project to serve both adult and juvenile cases. In 1956, a Division of Legal Medicine was established within the commonwealth's Department of Mental Health to facilitate the further development of the court clinic system. In some contrast to court clinics in other jurisdictions, the initial focus in Massachusetts was not on the larger superior courts with felony jurisdiction but, rather, on neighborhood lower courts having misdemeanor jurisdiction and covering geographic areas with populations of roughly 50,000 to 75,000. From the very beginning these court clinics were actively involved in treatment functions, often as alternatives to incarceration, especially for juveniles. In later years the Massachusetts legislature added drug-abuse screening and competency-to-stand-trial evaluations to the responsibilities of the court clinics. By 1977 there were 32 court clinics across Massachusetts, constituting the only statewide system of its kind in the country. As of July 1983 there were 31 court clinics offering a full range of services and an additional 28 offering limited or partial services.*

Although we are not aware of any recent survey of court clinics in the

---

* Information obtained from the Office of Planning and Policy, Massachusetts Department of Mental Health.

country, we estimate that the number easily reaches and most probably exceeds 100.

State and Local Correctional Agencies

The latest published statistics indicate that a total of 598,200 persons (526,408 adults and 71,792 juveniles) is confined in the United States in some type of correctional institution. On June 30, 1982, an estimated 209,582 persons were being held in various local jails.[49] The figure for persons confined in various types of correctional institutions (the total of 598,200) reflects only one quarter of the total number of persons under some type of correctional supervision. Thus, considering all those who are under some type of correctional supervision, especially those in various jails and prisons, and bearing in mind that the prevalence rates for mental disorders have generally been found to be somewhat higher among correctional inmates, it would be safe to say that the vast majority of mentally ill offenders are to be found in the various jails and prisons—rather than in the centralized security hospitals and units discussed earlier.

Inasmuch as there has been much variation in the samples and populations of correctional inmates that have been studied with respect to mental health morbidity, as well as varying definitions and criteria used for this purpose, the ascertained rates of mental disorders have also varied (see Brodsky,[50] Gibbs,[51] Bentz and Noel,[52] and Collins and Schlenger[53]). Even allowing for such variations, we would agree with Collins and Schlenger that the weight of the available evidence indicates that the prevalence of mental disorders is higher among correctional inmates than in the general population. It also appears that morbidity is higher for persons confined in jails than for prison inmates. The comptroller general of the United States, for example, has estimated that from 20 percent to 60 percent of jail inmates on any given day have mental health problems.[54] This report points out that jails typically do not screen and evaluate all inmates who may need mental health services. Even if such screening were to be done and larger numbers of persons were to be identified as needing such services, the required mental health services would simply not be available.

The following appear to be fairly well established.

- The suicide rate among incarcerated correctional populations is much higher than in the general population. Danto and coworkers[55] estimated that the rate of suicide among jail and prison inmates is between 3 and 13 times higher than that for the general population.
- In estimating various **lifetime prevalence*** rates for mental disorder, Collins and Schlenger[53] found that 29 percent of male inmates admitted to North Carolina prisons met the *Diagnostic and Statistical Manual of Mental Disorders, edition 3 (DSM III)*[56] diagnostic criteria for antisocial personality disorder; fully half of the prison inmate sample was diagnosed as being or having been alcohol abusers or dependent on alcohol at some time in their lives; and 21 percent of the inmates were diagnosed as having a sexual dysfunction (based on criteria such as persistent lack

---

* **Lifetime prevalence** refers to the proportion of a group who have ever during their lifetime met the criteria for a particular disorder.

of interest in sex, persistent problems with pain during intercourse, rare or absent orgasms, and lack of pleasure in sex).

- Monahan and Steadman[57] concluded that the weight of the available evidence indicates that the true prevalence rate of psychosis among inmate populations does not exceed the rate among class-matched community populations. We would agree with this conclusion, inasmuch as psychotic persons are very likely to be screened out or transferred to security hospitals. However, this would not be the case for personality and other psychiatric disorders.

Most prisons have some type of mental health or psychological services available, although typically rather limited and inadequate in reference to the needs. As noted above, inmates suffering from acute psychotic disorders are likely to be transferred to security hospitals or units within the jurisdiction. The availability of mental health services in local jails is much more limited, especially for the many small facilities. Morgan[58] surveyed 193 jails identified as having mental health programs and has reported on the responses obtained from 97 of these facilities; several rather interesting and innovative approaches for obtaining and utilizing mental health services for inmates were found. Brodsky[50] has provided some useful suggestions regarding intervention models for mental health services in jails, and McCarty[59] and Morrissey[60] and their associates have recently reported on the findings of their study of the relationships between local jails and the mental health systems. In chapter 19 of this volume Roth provides a wealth of information about mental health problems and needs in correctional institutions and about the specific challenges and dilemmas that commonly confront mental health professionals working in these settings. (Ethical issues particular to these settings are examined in chapters 2 and 3.)

Community Corrections Programs

More than 2.4 million persons in the United States are estimated to be under some form of correctional care, custody, or supervision on any given day; fully three quarters of these (more than 1.8 million) are under community supervision (probation, parole, and other conditional release programs).[49]

Although a few of the larger probation and parole programs have some mental health consultants or staff available (particularly in the very large cities), in the main these community corrections agencies utilize existing community resources and services for the mental health needs of their clients. However, given the general limitation of available services and associated problems (for example, often the poor motivation of the offenders to seek mental health services appears to be matched by similarly poor motivation on the part of service delivery staff for working with these clients), community corrections agencies seem to prefer to obtain services from specialized forensic programs and/or consultants directly available to them.

TRAINING AND QUALIFICATIONS

The past two decades have seen markedly increased interest in the development of formal and systematic training programs for mental health professionals who work in the legal or forensic mental health areas. Similarly, during the last decade there has been a marked surge of interest in the discipline of psychology to develop a variety of graduate programs with research and service specialization in the law-psychology area. This section of the chapter will concentrate on the relevant developments in the disciplines of psychiatry and psychology. We shall also make reference to some of the related developments in the other mental health disciplines of social work and nursing.

Legal Psychiatry

A major landmark in the development of specialized training programs and standards in legal or forensic psychiatry was the establishment in 1969 of the American Academy of Psychiatry and the Law (AAPL). Membership in this organization is limited to psychiatrists who devote a substantial portion of their professional activity to the forensic-legal areas. The current membership of AAPL is 900.

A review of the relevant literature indicates that during the early years of AAPL there was much discussion as to the precise definition, meaning, and scope of the subspecialty area referred to as **forensic psychiatry**.[61-65] This discussion and delineation of the specialty continues.[66] Similar discussions about legal or forensic psychiatry, its interrelationships with other disciplines, and the precise scope and functions of the subspecialty have been underway in Europe.[67,68]

Although the total membership of AAPL has yet to reach 1000, it must be emphasized that many additional psychiatrists have interest and involvement in forensic and legal issues even though they do not devote a substantial proportion of their time to this area and would not identify themselves as specialists in the field. Then, too, there are literally thousands of physicians who are not formally trained in psychiatry but who are involved in the legal system occasionally in such matters as evaluations for emergency psychiatric admissions, civil commitment, conservatorship, and guardianship. They also become involved in competency to stand criminal trial, criminal responsibility, as well as work in jail and prison health and mental health programs. In recent years many physicians have also assisted courts and other civil and criminal justice system agencies in regard to problems of substance abuse.

TRAINING

There has been much discussion and writing about the kinds of training programs, experience, supervision, and relationships with other relevant disciplines that are needed for sound teaching in legal or forensic psychiatry.[69-73] In 1974, Sadoff and coworkers[74] conducted a survey of teaching programs in law and psychiatry and reported on the programs. At that time there were 13 formal training programs in forensic psychiatry in the United States. Although there have been additions and probably some deletions since that time, no newer survey of these programs has been reported.

STANDARDS AND ACCREDITATION

After a number of years of planning, an accreditation system was established for certifying forensic psychiatrists. In 1979, the first 29 psychiatrists were certified by the American Board of Forensic Psychiatry. This board was founded by the American Academy of Psychiatry and the Law. Basic to the subspecialty accreditation in forensic psychiatry is the prior certification in psychiatry by the American Board of Psychiatry and Neurology, the body that is recognized by organized medicine as competent to confer specialty status in general psychiatry, neurology, and child psychiatry. The Forensic Psychiatry Board requires prior board certification in general psychiatry, licensure to practice in the jurisdiction in which the applicant resides, and citizenship in either the United States or Canada. Prior to taking the subspecialty written and oral examination the applicant must also have had five years of "substantial experience" in forensic psychiatry, defined as at least 16 hours per week. As of May 1983, 135 persons out of 289 accepted candidates had been certified (a 46.7 percent rate of success).

At the present time there is no formal system for the accreditation of training programs in forensic or legal psychiatry. However, an impressive beginning has been made by the work of the Joint Committee on Accreditation of Fellowship Programs in Forensic Psychiatry, chaired by Richard Rosner. The standards for fellowship programs were published in the AAPL bulletin in 1982[75] and are reproduced in their entirety as an appendix at the end of this chapter.

The report includes a then current listing of a core library of textbooks and research monographs. Major new publications and related teaching materials would, of course, be added periodically to this core library by the training programs. A review of the publications listed in the core library reflects a major step in formalizing and making more consistent the professional quality of the teaching materials and brings in the contributions of the various behavioral disciplines to the legal process in the last dozen or more years. Compared with the dearth of authoritative texts which existed before 1970, there has been a relative profusion of such materials in recent years. Since 1970, also, the NIMH Center for Studies of Crime and Delinquency (now retitled the Center for Studies of Antisocial and Violent Behavior) has produced a series of monographs in the law and mental health area (for example, Schwitzgebel,[76,77] McGarry and coworkers,[78,79] Stone,[80] Wexler,[81] Frederick,[82] Monahan,[23] and Dunn and Steadman[83]). The monographs by Stone[80] and Monahan[23] won the Manfred Guttmacher Award of the American Psychiatric Association.

The growth of the American Academy of Psychiatry and the Law, most particularly the various professional educational programs sponsored by AAPL and by its various regional affiliates, has been associated with a rich and increasingly sophisticated quality of continuing education for its members as well as for the other mental health professionals who attend these programs.

Legal Psychology

The history of interactions between psychology and law dates back to at least the early part of this century when, in 1908, Hugo Munsterberg (a professor of psychology at Harvard) tried to apply psychology to various legal problems in his book *On the Witness Stand: Essays on Psychology and Crime*.[84] Further historical context for developments at the interface of psychology and law has been provided by Tapp.[1] The relevant history pertains not only to clinical psychological aspects of such interactions but also to contributions from experimental psychological laboratories on such basic subjects as perception, memory, and recall and their relationship to testimonial evidence in courts of law (see Whipple,[85] Hutchins and Slesinger,[86] McCarty,[87] and Burtt[88]). However, it was not until the late 1960s and early 1970s that something considerably more than the sporadic activities at this interface began to increase at a very rapid and productive pace.

It is now about 25 years since the establishment of the American Association of Correctional Psychology and the American Psychology-Law Society. More recently, a division of psychology and law was established within the divisional structure of the American Psychological Association. Even though this division is barely four years old, its membership is rapidly approaching 1000 (current membership is 980). In addition, there are sections in other divisions of the American Psychological Association focusing on correctional psychology and police psychology.

The considerable surge of interest and activities in various aspects of the psychology-law interface has also been reflected during the past two decades in an increasing number of programs on this general topic that have been presented at the annual meetings of the American Psychological Association and of the various regional and state psychological associations. The topic for the Master Lecture Series at the 1982 annual meeting of the American Psychology Association was psychology and the law; the five major lectures given by Bersoff,[89] Diamond,[90] Monahan,[91] Rosenhan,[92] and Sales[93] have recently been published.[94]

Four new journals have appeared in the last decade (*Behavioral Sciences and the Law, Criminal Justice and Behavior, Law and Human Behavior,* and *Law and Psychology Review*), and numerous articles relating to the law-psychology area have appeared and continue to appear in a variety of other psychological journals. For example, *Professional Psychology* 9:3, August 1978 was devoted to law and professional psychology, and a special section of *Journal of Personality and Social Psychology* 36:12, 1978 was devoted to applications of personality and social psychology to criminal justice concerns. In sum, a very sizable and impressive literature has accumulated in the form of literally dozens of books and hundreds of articles and book chapters. These publications cover a wide range of substantive topics in the several specialty areas within the discipline of psychology and include clinical psychology,[95-103] child and developmental psychology,[104-107] experimental psychology,[108-111] and social psychology,[112-118] to mention just the major areas and some of the relevant books. A number of texts and related books have also appeared and cover a variety of research and professional topics.[119-135]

TRAINING

It would be fair to say that the development of graduate training programs in the area of forensic and legal psychology has tended to lag behind the increased professional, research, and related activities. The general topics of crime, delinquency, corrections, and forensic psychology generally have been addressed in a variety of other graduate courses to some degree. Starting about 15 years ago special courses also began to be offered at a few psychology departments; a variety of clinical internship opportunities in the forensic area have been available for much longer.

The markedly increased interest in the psychology-law area during the past 15 years has been associated with the development of more formal graduate training programs and a variety of ideas and proposals have been discussed.[136–141] In the introductory chapter to his very comprehensive and useful *Professional Psychologist's Handbook*, Sales[142] identifies seven areas of knowledge, in addition to the basic substantive psychological knowledge and skills, that form the context of professional psychology and with which all professional psychologists—not just those in the forensic area—should be familiar in order to function effectively. The seven areas are (1) knowledge of standards of professional practice (these are discussed in the next section of this chapter), (2) knowledge of relevant professional organizations, (3) knowledge of the major professional developments (regarding criteria for the accreditation of professional training programs, quality assurance and related peer review procedures), (4) knowledge of the laws affecting professional practice (including laws regulating the business aspects of the delivery of various types of psychological services, laws regulating the profession; for example, certification and licensing statutes and laws regulating the clients likely to be served), (5) knowledge of the managerial and business skills associated with professional practice, (6) knowledge of the values and interests affecting professional decision making, and (7) knowledge of the political and regulatory processes.

With respect to graduate training programs, Levine and coworkers[143] surveyed all 118 APA-approved internship sites and two that were on probation. Of the 85 sites that responded, 55 percent reported having legal/forensic experiences as either a regular or optional aspect of their program. The 47 internship sites that provided such training experiences were listed in the article, and other useful information was also provided about the kinds of experiences available. More recently, Ross and Sales[144] updated the earlier report about internship programs providing legal or forensic training opportunities.

Grisso and others[145] conducted three surveys to determine the extent to which graduate programs in psychology were offering courses, programs, or other opportunities for specialization in the law and psychology area. Information was sought about the types of law-related courses being offered in graduate psychology departments, and questionnaires were sent to 413 academic departments in the United States; an 88 percent response rate was achieved. Twenty-three percent (85) of the departments indicated that they had one or more courses addressing the psychology-law interface and a total of 121 courses were reported. The survey also inquired about formal law-related **programs** within the psychology departments; to qualify as a program there had to be (1) an identified body of graduate students in psychology and the commitment of at least one faculty member in psychology, (2) an identifiable structure and purpose related to the psycholegal interface, (3) at least two law-related psychology courses, and (4) a requirement for some specialized non-classroom experience such as placements in a law-related or criminal justice practicum setting or participation in a law-related psychological research project. Ten of the 14 programs that were reported met the above criteria. Five of these formal programs offered joint degrees (J.D. and Ph.D. or Psy.D.), and the other five offered a specialized Ph.D., M.A., or postdoctoral training in the psychology-law area. An appendix in the Grisso and coworkers[145] article lists the various textbooks and related teaching materials that were being used by the programs surveyed.

Under the auspices of the APA Division of Psychology and Law, Roesch[146] has compiled course outlines and syllabi for various psychology and law courses that are currently being taught. The list is not meant to be complete.

In a recent chapter, Roesch and coworkers[147] provide a very informative description and discussion of various types of training programs in the psychology-law area. These authors report that there are now at least eight universities offering joint degree (J.D. and Ph.D. or Psy.D.) programs in psychology and law. These programs are listed below with the specialization areas in psychology indicated in parentheses.

1. Northwestern University, Evanston, IL (clinical, personality/social)
2. University of Nebraska–Lincoln, Lincoln, NB (developmental, experimental, mental health policy, personality/social)
3. University of Maryland School of Law and Johns Hopkins University (Department of Psychology), Baltimore, MD (experimental/general)
4. Hahnemann University (Department of Psychology) and Villanova University Law School, Philadelphia, PA (clinical)
5. University of Arizona, Tucson, AZ (biological, clinical, cognitive, developmental, environmental, personality/social and psycholegal)
6. University of Denver, Denver, CO (developmental)
7. Stanford University, Stanford, CA (cognitive, personality/social, psychopathology)
8. University of Wisconsin, Madison, WI (clinical, personality/social)

The major objectives and emphases of these joint degree programs vary somewhat. Some programs (for example, those at the University of Arizona, University of Nebraska, Johns Hopkins University–University of Maryland, Stanford University) have as their objective the training of professionals and scientists who can perceive and evaluate various problems of law, the legal system, and legal processes with a behavioral science perspective and who can apply their sophisticated legal and behavioral science research skills to these problems. Other programs (for example, Hahnemann University–Villanova University) emphasize the forensic applications of psychology in legal cases. Completion of the joint degree program requires at least five full years (including some work during the summer), but generally students seem to require almost six years to complete the demanding schedule. And, if the Ph.D. degree involves specialization in clinical psychology, a full year's internship would be added.

There are at least two universities with specialized master's degree programs relevant to our concerns. Stanford University offers graduate students in psychology a one-year training in law resulting in the degree of master of legal studies, and students in law can obtain a one-year M.A. in psychology. The Department of Forensic Psychology at John Jay College of Criminal Justice (City University of New York) offers a master's degree in forensic psychology.

There are at least five universities that offer **Ph.D programs with specialization in the areas of psychology and law, criminal justice, and corrections.** These are listed below.

1. University of Arizona, Tucson, AZ (the specialty is listed as psycholegal studies)
2. University of Alabama, Tuscaloosa, AL (the specialty is listed as forensic psychology and is largely clinical in emphasis)
3. Florida State University, Tallahasse, FL (within the clinical program there is specialization in the criminal justice, corrections, and forensic areas)

4. University of Nebraska, Lincoln, NB (the specialty is listed as forensic psychology and is largely clinical in orientation)
5. University of Virginia, Charlottesville, VA (a developmental specialization is listed as "Psychology, Children, and the Law")

There are also a number of universities and forensic mental health programs that provide **postdoctoral training opportunities** for persons interested in the psychology-law and forensic psychology areas. These are listed below.

1. University of Arizona, Tucson, AZ
2. California School of Professional Psychology, Berkelcy, CA
3. Florida State University, Tallahasse, FL
4. University of Nebraska, Lincoln, NB
5. Center for Forensic Psychiatry, Ann Arbor, MI
6. University of Southern California School of Medicine, Los Angeles, CA
7. Stanford University, Stanford, CA
8. Saint Elizabeths Hospital, Forensic Division, Washington, DC
9. University of Virginia, Charlottesville, VA
10. University of Wisconsin, Madison, WI

As the foregoing information should indicate, there certainly has been considerable interest and associated developments in the development of formal training programs in many graduate programs in psychology. As far as accreditation goes, the various programs are part of graduate psychology departments and internship sites that have been evaluated and approved by the American Psychological Association.

STANDARDS

The American Board of Examiners in Professional Psychology was established in 1946 by the Council of Representatives of the American Psychological Association to evaluate and to certify psychologists in some specialty areas. The name of the board was later changed to the American Board of Professional Psychology (ABPP). To be eligible for candidacy applicants must meet several requirements such as a doctoral degree in psychology from a university with an approved program, at least five years of acceptable postdoctoral qualifying experience, membership in the APA, and certification or licensure in the jurisdiction where the applicant works. Candidates are examined by their peers and, if judged to perform at an advanced level of professional competence, are awarded a diploma by ABPP. Such advanced certification is currently available in five specialty areas: (1) clinical psychology, (2) clinical neuropsychology, (3) counseling psychology, (4) industrial/organizational psychology, and (5) school psychology.

Certification as a diplomate in forensic psychology is provided by the American Board of Forensic Psychology (ABFP), which was established in 1978 by the American Psychology-Law Society. To be eligible for candidacy applicants should, for example, have an earned doctoral degree in psychology from an accredited university; be duly certified or licensed to practice in any state, territory, or province of the United States or Canada; and be members in good standing of the American Psychology-Law Society, the American Psychological Association, or the Canadian Psychological Association. With regard to professional experience and training, applicants must have accumulated at least 1000 hours of experience in forensic psychology over at least a five-year period, and four of those years should have been postdoctoral. Holders of an earned LL.B. or J.D. degree may substitute that degree for two of the required five years of relevant experience; however, the 1000 hours of relevant experience in the area of forensic psychology must still be met. Once the candidacy requirements have been met there is a two-stage examination process: (1) applicants must submit acceptable work samples for evaluation (about 65 percent of the candidates generally pass this stage); and (2) an oral examination is given, and about 65 percent of the candidates successfully pass this stage. Hence, based on the experience to date, of all those who meet candidacy requirements and go through the examination process, about 42 percent are certified as diplomates in forensic psychology.

There is at present no formal relationship between the ABPP and the ABFP. And, unlike the situation in psychiatry, persons do not first have to be certified as diplomates by ABPP prior to taking the examination for certification by the American Board of Forensic Psychology.

Some brief mention needs to be made of developments during the past decade regarding standards for providers of psychological services. A rather significant step was taken ten years ago by the American Psychological Association to develop national standards for providers of psychological services. The goal was to codify "a uniform set of standards for psychological practice that would serve the respective needs of users, providers, and third-party purchasers and sanctioners of psychological services."[148] The first set of standards was proposed in 1974, and after much consultation and revision it was published in 1977 as the Standards for Providers of Psychological Services.[148] In 1980, the APA also adopted specialty guidelines for the delivery of services by clinical, counseling, industrial/organizational, and school psychologists.[149] Similar standards are not presently available for the forensic psychology specialty.

Such standards of practice are important for several reasons: They facilitate mutual understanding between providers and users of services, they facilitate more effective evaluation of the services, they constitute an important step toward greater uniformity in various legislative and regulatory actions involving providers of services, and they provide the basis for development of accreditation procedures for service facilities.[150] In essence, these sets of standards facilitate greater accountability by the professional group. Jacobs[150] has pointed out that

> Unlike its ethical standards, which are limited in their impact to members of APA, the Association's standards of practice represent the most authoritative statement available to the public at large on matters affecting quality control of psychological services. As such, they are addressed to all who are party to them.

Social Work

If one thinks of public sector agencies and programs for the delivery of mental health services to persons involved with the juvenile and criminal justice systems, it is quite evident that the profession of social worker (mainly the specialty of clinical social work) plays a very major role. Reflecting this role and involvement, for at least the past three decades numerous graduate social work training programs have offered concentration or specialization in the area of corrections, juvenile and criminal justice.

Within the last decade several graduate schools of social work have begun to offer more formalized training programs in the forensic/legal areas, and some dual or joint degree (M.S.W./J.D.) programs are also available. Based on information available from the Council of Social Work Education (CSWE),[151] as of 1983 seven schools of social work offer **joint or special degree programs in the area of social work and law.** These programs are

1. School of Applied Social Sciences, Case Western Reserve University, Cleveland, OH (M.S.S.A./J.D.)
2. Graduate School of Social Work and Social Research, Bryn Mawr College, Bryn Mawr, PA (a master's of law and social policy [MLSP] degree is offered and involves a full year of study);
3. School of Social Work, University of Southern California, Los Angeles, CA (a dual degree program is available [M.S.W./J.D.] and requires four academic years of instruction);
4. School of Social Work, Virginia Commonwealth University, Richmond, VA (a dual degree program is offered in law and social work [M.S.W./J.D.]; the M.S.W. is awarded by the School of Social Work and the J.D. by the T.C. Williams School of Law, University of Richmond);
5. George Warren Brown School of Social Work, Washington University, St. Louis, MO (a joint degree is offered in law and social work);
6. School of Social Work, University of Iowa, Iowa City, IO (offers a joint degree);
7. School of Social Welfare, University of California, Berkeley, CA (a special program in law and social welfare is offered, and a M.S.W./J.D. degree is awarded).

As indicated above, the joint degree (M.S.W./J.D.) programs typically require four years of instruction. Review of the CSWE publication[151] also indicates that among the many accredited graduate programs in social work, there are at least 20 that explicitly note concentration or special interest in their M.S.W. programs that include criminal and juvenile justice and/or corrections.

Nursing

Psychiatric nursing is one of the four "core" mental health disciplines and obviously has considerable involvement in various service delivery systems pertaining to forensic mental health services. As compared with the development of special forensic/legal mental health training programs in the three preceding mental health disciplines, there has not been as much activity in the field of nursing. However, this situation appears to be changing.

The School of Nursing of the Catholic University of America (Washington, DC) has for the last three years had a master's of science in nursing program with an area concentration and specialization in the field of forensic psychiatric mental health nursing. This program prepares forensic psychiatric nurse clinical specialists who, with their knowledge of relevant legal principles, major factors at the interface of medicine and law, and academic as well as clinical training with respect to special problems and needs in large service delivery systems (security hospitals, jails, prisons, and other correctional and mental health facilities), will be able to work in a variety of forensic mental health programs.

NATIONAL STANDARDS

Our discussion of training, qualifications, and standards would be incomplete if we did not make reference to the major endeavor recently completed by the American Bar Association's (ABA) Standing Committee on Association Standards for Criminal Justice. Building upon its extensive earlier work that culminated in the ABA Standards for Criminal Justice, the standing committee continued its efforts to improve the administration of criminal justice by addressing the range of complex issues that arise when the state's criminal powers and its mental health powers come together in responding to mentally ill persons who have become involved with the criminal justice system. These ABA standards are designed to improve the administration of justice and to facilitate achievement of this goal through cooperative interprofessional programs that can foster better understanding and improved professional practice in the administration of the criminal law and in the delivery of more effective legal and forensic mental health services.

A group of 79 lawyers and mental health professionals were brought together in several task forces to draft the criminal justice mental health standards. In developing these standards the interdisciplinary groups made extensive use of the guidelines and standards of the mental disability professions involved. For example, the commentaries make frequent references to the ethical guidelines of the American Psychiatric Association and the American Psychological Association and the Standards for Providers of Psychological Services[148] and Specialty Guidelines[149] of the American Psychological Association. This ABA endeavor began in February 1981, and the draft standards and extensive accompanying commentaries were widely distributed (more than 4200 copies) for review and comments.[132] In November 1983 national public hearings were held in Washington, DC, and representatives of most major mental health and mental retardation associations testified in response to the first tentative draft that had been circulated. The draft standards and commentaries subsequently were revised and were formally adopted in August 1984 by the ABA's House of Delegates.[153]

The 96 individual but related "black-letter" standards were developed for the use of lawyers, judges, and mental health and mental retardation professionals and are presented in ten parts: (1) Mental Health, Mental Retardation, and Criminal Justice: General Professional Obligations; (2) Police and Custodial Roles; (3) Pretrial Evaluations and Expert Testimony; (4) Competence to Stand Trial; (5) Competence on Other Issues; (6) Nonresponsibility for Crime; (7) Civil Commitment of Nonresponsibility Acquittees; (8) Special Dispositional Statutes; (9) Sentencing Mentally Ill and Mentally Retarded Offenders; and (10) Mentally Ill and Mentally Retarded Prisoners.

In Part 1 the standards identify three major roles played by mental disability professionals in the criminal process: a scientific and evaluative role, a consultative role, and a treatment and habilitation role. It is recognized that these roles can produce various ethical conflicts and related dilemmas for mental disability professionals, hence the standards endeavor to delineate the primary responsibility of the professionals in performing the various obligations required of their particular roles. Moreover, it is noted, the standards help establish a framework for the basic and advanced education and training of judges, lawyers, and mental disability professionals. Clearly, therefore, the standards adopted by the ABA merit careful attention and conscientious efforts at their implementation by lawyers, judges, and mental health and mental retardation professionals who work in the criminal justice and related areas.

The following are some relevant examples from the standards that pertain to training and qualifications.

Standard 7-1.3 deals with education and training, and section (d) pertains to mental health and mental retardation professionals:

> (i) Professional and graduate schools should afford the opportunity for the students of mental health and mental retardation disciplines, as a part of their formal education, to become familiar with the issues concerning the participation of mental health and mental retardation professionals in the criminal process.
> (ii) These professional and graduate schools should also provide advanced instruction for students of the mental health and mental retardation disciplines who desire to meet the minimum criteria established by Standard 7-3.10 for qualifying as court-appointed evaluators and Standard 7-3.11 for qualifying as expert witnesses testifying about a person's mental condition.[154]

The rest of section (d) urges professional and graduate schools to address important continuing education needs in the areas of concern.

Standard 7-3.10 is concerned with qualifications for court-appointed experts for the evaluation of a person's mental condition, and **Standard 7-3.11** pertains to qualifications for testifying about a person's mental condition. Thus, with respect to requirements for qualifications as expert witnesses, section (a) of **Standard 7-3.11** states:

> (a) Qualifications. Expert opinion testimony about a person's mental condition is designed to assist the trial factfinder. Because such testimony often assumes extraordinary importance in cases that involve a person's mental condition, no witness should be qualified by the court to present expert opinion testimony unless the court determines that the witness
> (i) Has sufficient professional education and sufficient clinical training and experience to establish the clinical knowledge required to formulate an expert opinion; and,
> (ii) Has either
>   (A) Aquired sufficient knowledge, through forensic training or an acceptable substitute therefor, relevant to conducting the specific type(s) of mental evaluation actually conducted in the case, and relevant to the substantive law concerning the specific matter(s) on which expert opinion is to be proffered; or
>   (B) Has had a professional therapeutic or habilitative relationship with the person whose mental condition is in question; and
> (iii) Has performed an adequate evaluation, including a personal interview with the individual whose mental condition is in question, relevant to the

legal and clinical matter(s) upon which the witness is being called to testify. (b) Related standard. This standard refers only to qualifications for expert witnesses testifying about a person's mental condition. Qualifications for expert witnesses testifying on matters of present scientific or clinical knowledge are governed by Standard 7-3.13.[155]

Standard 7-3.12 addresses the establishment of minimum professional education and clinical training requirements for evaluators and expert witnesses, and section (a) recommends that

> Every jurisdiction should establish, by statute, regulation, or court rule, minimum professional education and clinical training requirements necessary to qualify persons for the performance of such roles.[156]

This standard also notes (section b-ii) that

> Sufficient flexibility should be provided to permit the courts to utilize persons who clearly demonstrate the requisite knowledge notwithstanding their lack of the formal education and training that may be specified in the requirements. However, experience in performing evaluations or in testifying as an expert should not, by itself, constitute a sufficient demonstration of the requisite clinical knowledge.[157]

The development of standards for service providers is a matter of much importance. The past two decades have seen increasing concerns about and interest in ensuring greater accountability on the part of various professionals. We appear to be in an Age of Accountability. Thus, as Jacobs[150] points out, mental health professionals can expect their credentials and services to be scrutinized by direct users of services, third-party payers, employers, various peer-review and quality-assurance groups, state licensing boards, and others. Eventually, it appears, all professions—including those in the mental disability area—"can expect to be held to a much higher standard of open and candid communication with the public about the services they offer."[158]

Basically, of course, standards are designed to obtain a satisfactory pattern of practice. The development and implementation of such standards (for example, those developed by the American Psychological Association[148,149]) are, first and foremost, an obligation and responsibility of the professional groups. And, although the development of such standards is easier than establishing suitable mechanisms for their implementation and enforcement, the mere formulation and wide dissemination of such standards has a valuable educational, sensitizing, and informing purpose.

It is very important, however, that in prescribing minimum educational and training levels sufficient attention be given to the broader public interest—as contrasted, perhaps, with the parochial concerns of the professional group. This point pertains to the difficult issue that confronted the ABA Task Force and the alternative formulations that were initially provided in the tentative draft.[152] If the minimum educational and training levels are set too high, clients served by public sector facilities, and areas with very few of the relevant professionals, will face even greater difficulties in the recruitment and retention of such staff and consultants. Moreover, unrealistically (and perhaps even unreasonably) high standards could create an artificial shortage of the needed "expertise," thereby affecting both the availability and the costs of such services. Thus, as the ABA interdisciplinary task forces have suggested, it is essential that more effective use be made of the various other mental health professionals (clinical social workers and clinical specialists in psychiatric nursing) to address the particular service needs. Clearly, therefore, specialized education, training, and appropriate experience in the forensic mental health area should determine the proper and effective use of available professional resources for the greater public good—rather than the social status, influence, or power of particular professional groups.

REFERENCES

1. TAPP, JL: *Psychology and the law: An overture.* Annu Rev Psychol 27:359, 1976.
2. MONAHAN, J AND LOFTUS, EF: *The psychology of law.* Ann Rev Psychol 33:441, 1982.
3. GLUECK, S: *Law and Psychiatry: Cold War or Entente Cordiale?* Johns Hopkins University Press, Baltimore, 1962.
4. BRACELAND, FJ: *Introductory remarks: Psychiatry under siege.* Psychiatric Annals 3:6, 1973.
5. RAPPEPORT, JR: *Editorial: "Belegalled."* Bull Am Acad Psychiatry Law V:IV, 1977.
6. McGARRY, AL: *Law-medicine notes: The holy legal war against state-hospital psychiatry.* New Engl Med 295:381, 1976.
7. HALLECK, SL (ED): *Coping With the Legal Onslaught.* Jossey-Bass, San Francisco, 1979.
8. HOFFMAN, PB: *Living with your rights off.* Psychiatric Annals 7:82, 1977.
9. BROOKS, AD: *The impact of law on psychiatric hospitalization: Onslaught or imperative reform?* In HALLECK, SL (ED): *Coping With the Legal Onslaught.* Jossey-Bass, San Francisco, CA, 1979.
10. SHAH, SA: *Legal and mental health system interactions: Major developments and research needs.* Int J Law Psychiatry 4:219, 1981.
11. CONRAD, P AND SCHNEIDER, J: *Deviance and Medicalization: From Badness to Sickness.* CV Mosby, St Louis, 1980.
12. FOX, RW: *So Far Disordered in Mind: Insanity in California, 1870-1930.* University of California Press, Berkeley, CA, 1978.
13. FREIDSON, E: *Professional Dominance.* Atherton, New York, 1970.
14. ROTHMAN, DJ: *The Discovery of the Asylum.* Little, Brown & Co., Boston, 1971.
15. SCULL, AT: *From madness to mental illness: Medical men as moral entrepreneurs.* Archives of European Sociology 16:218, 1975.
16. FLEMING, S: *Shrinks vs. Shysters: The (latest) battle for control of the mentally ill.* Law and Human Behavior 6:355, 1982.
17. TALBOT, JA: *Deinstitutionalization: Avoiding the disasters of the past.* Hosp Community Psychiatry 30:621, 1979.
18. BAZELON, DL: *Institutionalization, deinstitutionalization and the adversary process.* Columbia Law Review 75:897, 1975.
19. HANEY, C: *Psychology and legal change: On the limits of a factual jurisprudence.* Law and Human Behavior 4:147, 1980.
20. HALLECK, SL: *Introductory remarks.* Psychiatric Annals 4:3, 1974.
21. DIX, GR: *Expert prediction testimony in capital sentencing: Evidentiary and constitutional considerations.* American Criminal Law Review 19:1, 1981.
22. MONAHAN, J (ED): *Who Is the Client? The Ethics of Psychological Intervention in the Criminal Justice System.* APA, Washington, DC, 1980.

23. MONAHAN, J: *The Clinical Prediction of Violent Behavior.* National Institute of Mental Health. DHHS Publication No. (ADM) 81-921. US Government Printing Office, Washington, DC, 1981.

24. SHAH, SA: *Dangerousness: A paradigm for exploring some issues in law and psychology.* Psychol 33:224, 1978.

25. SHAH, SA: *Dangerousness: Some definitional, conceptual, and public policy issues.* In HAYS, JR, ROBERTS, TK, SOLWAY, KS (EDS): *Violence and the Violent Individual.* SP Medical and Scientific Books, New York, 1981.

26. MORRIS, N: *Psychiatry and the dangerous criminal.* Southern California Law Review 41:514, 1968.

27. POLLACK, S: *Psychiatric consultation for the courts.* In MENDEL, W AND SOLOMON, P (EDS): *The Psychiatric Consultation.* Grune & Stratton, New York, 1968.

28. KEILITZ, I: *Mental Health Examinations in Criminal Justice Settings: Organization, Administration, and Program Evaluation.* Final Report to the National Institute of Justice. Grant No. 79 NI AX0070. National Center for State Courts, Williamsburg, VA, September 1981.

29. SCHEIDEMANDEL, PL AND KANNO, CK: *The Mentally Ill Offender: A Survey of Treatment Programs.* Joint Information Service of the American Psychiatric Association and the National Association of Mental Health. Washington, DC, 1969.

30. ECKERMAN, WC: *A Nationwide Survey of Mental Health and Correctional Institutions for Adult Mentally Disordered Offenders.* National Institute of Mental Health. DHEW Public No. (HSM) 72-9018. US Government Printing Office, Washington, DC, 1972.

31. NATIONAL INSTITUTE OF MENTAL HEALTH. *Directory of Institutions for Mentally Disordered Offenders.* DHEW Public No. (HSM) 72-9055. US Government Printing Office, Washington, DC, 1972.

32. SHELDON, RB AND NORMAN, WB: *Comprehensive survey of forensic psychiatric facilities in the United States.* Bull Am Acad Psychiatry Law VI:93, 1978.

33. STEADMAN, HJ, MONAHAN, J. HARTSTONE, E, DAVIS, SK, ROBBINS, PC: *Mentally disordered offenders: A national survey of patients and facilities.* Law and Human Behavior 6:31, 1982.

34. DAVIS, M: *Mentally Ill Offender Systems in the Western States.* Western Interstate Commission for Higher Education, Boulder, CO, July 1983.

35. KERR, CA AND ROTH, J: *Survey of Facilities and Programs for Mentally Disordered Offenders.* Advance Report. National Institute of Mental Health, Rockville, MD, March 1984.

36. BERAN, J AND TOOMEY, BG (EDS): *Mentally Ill Offenders and the Criminal Justice System: Issues in Forensic Services.* Praeger, New York, 1979.

37. ROTH, D: *Community-based mental health services for the criminal justice system: The Ohio experience.* In BERAN, J AND TOOMEY, BG (EDS): *Mentally Ill Offenders and the Criminal Justice System.* Praeger, New York, 1979.

38. LABEN, JK AND SPENCER, LD: *Decentralization of forensic services.* Community Ment Health J 12:404, 1976.

39. LABEN, JK, KASGARIAN, M, NESSA, OB, SPENCER, LD: *Reform from the inside: Mental health center evaluations of competency to stand trial.* Journal of Community Psychology 5:52, 1977.

40. FITZGERALD, JF, PESZKE, MA, GOODWIN, RC: *Competency evaluations in Connecticut.* Hosp Community Psychiatry 29:450, 1978.

41. ROESCH, R AND GOLDING, SL: *A brief, immediate screening interview to determine competency to stand trial: A feasibility study.* Criminal Justice and Behavior 5:241, 1978.

42. SCHREIBER, J: *Assessing competency to stand trial: A case study of technology diffusion in four states.* Bull Am Acad Psychiatry Law 6:439, 1978.

43. SLOBOGIN, C: *Outpatient forensic evaluations.* Advance 31:20, 1981 (published by the Virginia Department of Mental Health and Mental Retardation).

44. PETRILA, J: *Forensic psychiatry and community mental health.* Developments in Mental Health and Law 1:1, 1981 (quarterly publication of the Institute of Law, Psychiatry and Public Policy, University of Virginia, Charlottesville, VA).

45. MEGARGEE, EI: *Reflections on psychology in the criminal justice system.* In GUNN, J AND FARRINGTON, DP (EDS): *Abnormal Offenders, Delinquency, and the Criminal Justice System,* vol 1. John Wiley & Sons, New York, 1982.

46. *District of Columbia Legal Psychiatric Service: Bronze Award.* Mental Hospitals 544, Oct. 1962.

47. RAPPEPORT, JR, CONTI, NP, RUDNICK, B: *A new pretrial screening program.* Bull Am Acad Psychiatry Law 11:239, 1983.

48. RUSSELL, DH AND DEVLIN, JH: *The Massachusetts Court Clinic Program.* Juvenile Court Judges Journal 3:3, 1962.

49. *Report to the Nation on Crime and Justice. The Data.* Bureau of Justice Statistics, US Department of Justice, Washington, DC, October 1983.

50. BRODSKY, SL: *Intervention models for mental health services in jails.* In DUNN, CS AND STEADMAN, HJ (EDS): *Mental Health Services in Local Jails.* National Institute of Mental Health. DHHS Public No. (ADM) 82-1181. US Government Printing Office, Washington, DC, 1982.

51. GIBBS, JJ: *On "demons" and "gaols": A summary and review of investigations concerning the psychological problems of jail inmates.* In DUNN, CS AND STEADMAN, HJ (EDS): *Mental Health Services in Local Jails.* National Institute of Mental Health. DHHS Public No. (ADM) 82-1181. US Government Printing Office, Washington, DC, 1982.

52. BENTZ, WK AND NOEL, RW: *The incidence of psychiatric disorder among a sample of men entering prison.* Correctional and Social Psychiatry 29:22, 1983.

53. COLLINS, JJ AND SCHLENGER, WE: *The prevalence of psychiatric disorder among admissions to prisons.* Paper presented at the 35th Annual Meetings of the American Society of Criminology, Denver, CO, November 1983.

54. COMPTROLLER GENERAL OF THE UNITED STATES: *Jail inmates' mental health care neglected: State and federal attention needed.* US General Accounting Office, Washington, DC, 1980.

55. DANTO, B, OLSZEWSKI, R, SHANNON, AW: *Crisis Behind Bars: The Suicidal Inmate.* The Dale Corporation, Warren, MI, 1981.

56. AMERICAN PSYCHIATRIC ASSOCIATION: *Diagnostic and Statistical Manual of Mental Disorders,* ed 3. APA, Washington, DC, 1980.

57. MONAHAN, J AND STEADMAN, HJ: *Crime and mental illness: An epidemiological approach.* In MORRIS, N AND TONRY, M (EDS): *Crime and Justice: An Annual Review.* University of Chicago Press, Chicago, 1983.

58. MORGAN, CH: *Service delivery models: A summary of examples.* In DUNN, CS AND STEADMAN, HJ (EDS): *Mental Health Services in Local Jails.* National Institute of Mental Health. DHHS Public No. (ADM) 82-1181. US Government Printing Office, Washington, DC, 1982.

59. MCCARTY, D, STEADMAN, HJ, MORRISSEY, JP: *Issues in planning jail mental health services.* Federal Probation 56-63, December 1983.

60. MORRISSEY, JP, STEADMAN, HJ, KILBURN, HC: *Organizational issues in the delivery of jail mental health services.* In GREENLEY, J (ED): *Research in Community and Mental Health. Vol 3.* JAI Press, Greenwich, CT, 1983.

61. RAPPEPORT, JR: *Editorial.* Bull Am Acad Psychiatry Law I:i, 1974.

62. POLLACK, S: *Forensic psychiatry: A specialty.* Bull Am Acad Psychiatry Law I:1, 1974b.

63. ROBEY, A AND BOGARD, WJ: *The compleat forensic psychiatrist.* Am J Psychiatry 126:519, 1969.

64. SUAREZ, JM AND HUNT, J: *The scope of legal psychiatry.* J Forensic Sci 18:60, 1973.

65. ROBITSCHER, J: *The many faces of forensic psychiatry.* Bull Am Acad Psychiatry Law 6:209, 1978.

66. RAPPEPORT, JR: *Differences between forensic and general psychiatry.* Am J Psychiatry 139:331, 1982.

67. WORLD HEALTH ORGANIZATION, REGIONAL OFFICE FOR EUROPE. *Forensic Psychiatry. Report of a Working Group, Siena: Oct. 13-17, 1975.* World Health Organization, 1977.

68. GUNN, J: *Forensic psychiatry as a subspecialty.* Int J Law Psychiatry 5:65, 1982.

69. BARR, NI AND SUAREZ, JM: *The teaching of forensic psychiatry in law schools, medical schools, and psychiatric residences in the United States.* Am J Psychiatry 122:612, 1965.

70. LEBLANC, TR AND HENDERSON, MD: *Forensic psychiatry: A comprehensive residency program at Southern Illinois University School of Medicine.* Bull Am Acad Psychiatry Law 7:363, 1979.

71. ZUSMAN, J AND CARNAHAN, WA: *Psychiatry and the law: Changing the system through changing the training.* Am J Psychiatry 131:915, 1974.

72. DIETZ, PE: *Educating the forensic psychiatrist.* J Forensic Sci 24:880, 1979.

73. SADOFF, RL: *Comprehensive training in forensic psychiatry.* Am J Psychiatry 131:223, 1974.

74. SADOFF, RL, THRASHER, JW, GOTTLIEB, DW: *Survey of teaching programs in law and psychiatry.* Bull Am Acad Psychiatry Law 2:67, 1974.

75. ROSNER, R: *Accreditation of fellowship programs in forensic psychiatry: the development of the final report on standards.* Bull Am Acad Psychiatry Law 10:281, 1982.

76. SCHWITZGEBEL, RK: *Development and Legal Regulation of Coercive Behavior Modification Techniques with Offenders.* National Institute of Mental Health. PHS Public No. 2067. US Government Printing Office, Washington, DC, 1971.

77. SCHWITZGEBEL, RK: *Legal Aspects of the Enforced Treatment of Offenders.* National Institute of Mental Health. DHEW Public No. (ADM) 79-831. US Government Printing Office, Washington, DC, 1979.

78. MCGARRY, AL, CURRAN, WJ, LIPSITT, PD, LELOS, D, SCHWITZGEBEL, RK, ROSENBERG, AH: *Competency to Stand Trial and Mental Illness.* National Institute of Mental Health. DHEW Public. No. (HSM) 73-9105, US Government Printing Office, Washington, DC, 1973.

79. MCGARRY, AL, SCHWITZGEBEL, RK, LIPSITT, PD, LELOS, D: *Civil Commitment and Social Policy.* National Institute of Mental Health. DHHS Public. No. (ADM) 81-1011. US Government Printing Office, Washington, DC, 1981.

80. STONE, AA: *Mental Health and Law: A System in Transition.* National Institute of Mental Health. DHEW Public. No. (ADM) 75-176. US Government Printing Office, Washington, DC, 1975.

81. WEXLER, DB: *Criminal Commitments and Dangerous Mental Patients.* National Institute of Mental Health. DHEW Public No. (ADM) 76-331. US Government Printing Office, Washington, DC, 1976.

82. FREDERICK, CJ (ED): *Dangerous Behavior: A Problem in Law and Mental Health.* National Institute of Mental Health. DHEW Public. No. (ADM) 78-563. US Government Printing Office, Washington, DC, 1978.

83. DUNN, CS AND STEADMAN, HJ (EDS): *Mental Health Services in Local Jails.* National Institute of Mental Health. DHHS Public. No. (ADM) 82-1181. US Government Printing Office, Washington, DC, 1978.

84. MUNSTERBERG, H: *On the Witness Stand: Essays on Psychology and Crime.* Clark, Boardman, New York, 1908.

85. WHIPPLE, GM: *The observer as reporter: A survey of the "psychology of testimony."* Psychol Bull 6:153, 1909.

86. HUTCHINS, RM AND SLESINGER, D: *Legal psychology.* Psychol Rev 36:13, 1929.

87. McCARTY, DG: *Psychology for the lawyer.* Prentice-Hall, New York, 1929.

88. BURTT, ME: *Legal Psychology.* Prentice-Hall, Englewood Cliffs, NJ, 1931.

89. BERSOFF, DN: *Regarding psychologists testily: the legal regulation of psychological assessment.* In SCHEIRER, CJ AND HAMMONDS, BL (EDS): *The Master Lecture Series: Vol 2. Psychology and the Law.* American Psychological Association, Washington, DC, 1983.

90. DIAMOND, SS: *Order in the court: Consistency in criminal court decisions.* In SCHEIRER, CJ AND HAMMONDS, BL (EDS): *The Master Lecture Series: Vol 2. Psychology and the Law.* American Psychological Association, Washington, DC, 1983.

91. MONAHAN, J: *The prediction of violent behavior: Developments in psychology and law.* In SCHEIRER, CJ AND HAMMONDS, BL (EDS): *The Master Lecture Series: Vol 2. Psychology and the Law.* American Psychological Association, Washington, DC, 1983.

92. ROSENHAN, DL: *Psychological abnormality and law.* In SCHEIRER, CJ AND HAMMONDS, BL (EDS): *The Master Lecture Series: Vol 2. Psychology and the Law.* American Psychological Association, Washington, DC, 1983.

93. SALES, BD: *The legal regulation of psychology: Scientific and professional interactions.* In SCHEIRER, CJ AND HAMMONDS, BL (EDS): *The Master Lecture Series: Vol 2. Psychology and the Law.* American Psychological Association, Washington, DC, 1983.

94. SCHEIRER, CJ AND HAMMONDS, BL (EDS): *The Master Lecture Series: Vol 2. Psychology and the Law.* American Psychological Association, Washington, DC, 1983.

95. BRODSKY, SL (ED): *Psychologists in the Criminal Justice System.* University of Illinois Press, Urbana, IL, 1973.

96. COOKE, G (ED): *Readings in Forensic Psychology.* Charles C Thomas, Springfield, IL, 1980.

97. FERSCH, EA: *Psychology and Psychiatry in Courts and Corrections: Controversy and Change.* John Wiley & Sons, New York, 1980.

98. GRISSO, T: *Juveniles' Waiver of Rights: Legal and Psychological Competence.* Plenum, New York, 1981.

99. GUNN, J AND FARRINGTON, DP (EDS); *Abnormal Offenders, Delinquency, and the Criminal Justice System. Vol 1.* John Wiley & Sons, New York, 1982.

100. MEGARGEE, EI AND BOHN, MJ: *Classifying Criminal Offenders.* Sage, Beverly Hills, 1979.

101. MONAHAN, J (ED): *Community Mental Health and the Criminal Justice System.* Pergamon, New York, 1976.

102. ROESCH, R AND GOLDING, SL: *Competency to Stand Trial.* University of Illinois Press, Urbana, IL, 1980.

103. TOCH, H (ED): *Psychology of Crime and Criminal Justice.* Holt, Rinehart & Winston, New York, 1979.

104. HICKEY, JE AND SCHARF, PL: *Toward a Just Correctional System.* Jossey-Bass, San Francisco, 1980.

105. KOOCHER, G (ED): *Children's Rights and the Mental Health Professions.* John Wiley & Sons, New York, 1976.

106. TAPP, JL AND LEVINE, FJ: *The Jurisprudence of Youth.* American Bar Foundation, Chicago, 1971.

107. TAPP, JL AND LEVINE, FJ (EDS): *Law, Justice and the Individual in Society: Psychological and Legal Issues.* Holt, Rinehart & Winston, New York, 1977.

108. CLIFFORD, BR AND BULL, R: *The Psychology of Person Identification.* Routledge & Kegan Paul, London, 1978.

109. ELWORK, A, SALES, BD, ALFINE, J: *Making Jury Instructions Understandable.* Michie, Charlottesville, VA, 1981.

110. LOFTUS, EF: *Eyewitness Testimony.* Harvard University Press, Cambridge, MA, 1979.

111. YARMEY, AD: *The Psychology of Witness Testimony.* Free Press, New York, 1979.

112. ABT, LE AND STUART, IR (EDS): *Social Psychology and Discretionary Justice.* Van Nostrand Reinhold, New York, 1979.

113. GREENBERG, M AND RUBACK, BR: *Social Psychology and Criminal Justice.* Brooks/Cole, Monterey, CA, 1981.

114. KONECNI, VJ AND EBBESEN, EB: *The Criminal Justice System: A Social Psychological Analysis.* Freeman, San Francisco, 1982.

115. SAKS, MJ AND HASTIE, R: *Social Psychology in Court.* Van Nostrand Reinhold, New York, 1978.

116. SAKS, MJ AND BARON, CH (EDS): *The Use/Nonuse/Misuse of Applied Social Research in the Courts.* Abt Books, Cambridge, MA, 1980.

117. BERMANT, G, NEMETH, C, VIDMAR, N: *Psychology and the Law.* DC Heath, Lexington, MA, 1976.

118. BRAY, R AND KERR, N (EDS): *The Psychology of the Courtroom.* Academic Press, New York, 1982.

119. COHN, A AND UDOLF, R: *The Criminal Justice System and its Psychology.* Van Nostrand Reinhold, New York, 1979.

120. FARRINGTON, DF, HAWKINS, K, LLOYD-BOSTOCK, SM (EDS): *Psychology, Law and Legal Processes.* Macmillan, London, 1979.

121. FELDMAN, MP: *Criminal Behavior: A Psychological Analysis.* John Wiley & Sons, New York, 1977.

122. LIPSITT, PD AND SALES, BD (EDS): *New Directions in Psycholegal Research.* Van Nostrand Reinhold, New York, 1980.

123. LLOYD-BOSTOCK, SM (ED): *Psychology in Legal Contexts.* Macmillan, London, 1980.

124. MONAHAN, J (ED): *Who Is the Client? The Ethics of Psychological Intervention in the Criminal Justice System.* American Psychological Association, Washington, DC, 1980.

125. MONAHAN, J AND STEADMAN, HJ (EDS): *Mentally Disordered Offenders: Perspectives from Law and Social Science.* Plenum, New York, 1983.

126. NIETZEL, MT: *Crime and its Modification: A Social Learning Perspective.* Pergamon, New York, 1979.

127. ROBINSON, DN: *Psychology and Law.* Oxford University Press, New York, 1980.

128. SALES, BD (ED): *Perspectives in Law and Psychology: Vol 1. The Criminal Justice System.* Plenum, New York, 1977.

129. SALES, BD (ED): *Psychology in the Legal Process.* Spectrum, New York, 1977.

130. SALES, BD, POWELL, DM, VAN DUIZEND, R: *Disabled Persons and the Law: State Legislative Issues.* Plenum, New York, 1982.

131. SALES, BD (ED): *The Professional Psychologist's Handbook.* Plenum, New York, 1983.

132. SCHWITZGEBEL, RL AND SCHWITZGEBEL, RK: *Law and Psychological Practice.* John Wiley & Sons, New York, 1980.

133. THIBAUT, JW AND WALKER, L: *Procedural Justice: A Psychological Analysis.* Erlbaum, Hillsdale, NJ, 1978.

134. VAN HOOSE, WH AND KOTTLER, JA: *Ethical and Legal Issues in Counseling and Psychotherapy.* Jossey-Bass, San Francisco, 1978.

135. ZISKIN, J: *Coping with Psychiatric and Psychological Testimony,* ed 2. Law and Psychology Press, Beverly Hills, 1975.

136. NIETZEL, MT AND MOSS, CS: *The psychologist in the criminal justice system.* Professional Psychology 3:259, 1972.

137. SPEILBERGER, CD, MEGARGEE, EI, INGRAHAM, GL: *Graduate education.* In BRODSKY, SL (ED): *Psychologists in the Criminal Justice System.* University of Illinois Press, Urbana, IL, 1973.

138. FENSTER, CA, LITWACK, TR, SYMONDS, M: *The making of a forensic psychologist: Needs and goals for doctoral training.* Professional Psychology 6:457, 1975.

139. KASLOW, FW AND ABRAMS, JC: *Forensic psychology and criminal justice: An evolving subspecialty at Hahnemann Medical College.* Professional Psychology 7:445, 1976.

140. SALES, BD AND ELWORK, A: *Issues in training forensic psychologists.* In COOKE, G (ED): *Readings in Forensic Psychology.* Charles C Thomas, Springfield, IL, 1980.

141. POYTHRESS, NG: *A proposal for training in forensic psychology.* Am Psychol 34:612, 1979.

142. SALES, BD: *The context of professional psychology.* In SALES, BD (ED): *The Professional Psychologist's Handbook.* Plenum, New York, 1983.

143. LEVINE, D, WILSON, K, SALES, BD: *An exploratory assessment of APA internships with legal/forensic experiences.* Professional Psychology 11:64, 1980.

144. ROSS, MV AND SALES, BD: *Legal/forensic training in psychology internship programs.* In GUNN, J AND FARRINGTON, DP (EDS): *Abnormal Offenders, Delinquency, and the Criminal Justice System, Vol 2.* John Wiley & Sons, New York, 1984.

145. GRISSO, T, SALES, BD, BAYLESS, S: *Law-related courses and programs in graduate psychology departments.* Am Psychol 37:267, 1982.

146. ROESCH, R: *Psychology and Law: Course Syllabi and Reading Lists.* Criminology Research Center, Simon Fraser University, Burnaby, BC, Canada, 1983.

147. ROESCH, R, GRISSO, T, POYTHRESS, NG: *Training programs, courses, and workshops in psychology and the law.* In KAPLAN, MF (ED): *The Impact of Social Psychology on Procedural Justice.* Charles C Thomas, Springfield, IL.

148. AMERICAN PSYCHOLOGICAL ASSOCIATION. *Standards for Providers of Psychological Services.* American Psychological Association, Washington, DC, January 1977.

149. AMERICAN PSYCHOLOGICAL ASSOCIATION. *Specialty Guidelines for the Delivery of Services: Clinical Psychologists, Counseling Psychologists, Industrial/Organizational Psychologists, School Psychologists.* American Psychological Association, Washington, DC, June 1981. (Reprinted from the Am Psychol 36:640-681, June 1981).

150. JACOBS, DF: *The development and application of standards of practice for professional psychologists.* In SALES, BD (ED): *The Professional Psychologist's Handbook.* Plenum, New York, 1983.

151. COUNCIL ON SOCIAL WORK EDUCATION: *Summary Information on Master of Social Work Programs.* 1983. Council on Social Work Education, New York, 1983.

152. AMERICAN BAR ASSOCIATION: *First Tentative Draft: Criminal Justice Mental Health Standards.* Standing Committee on Association Standards for Criminal Justice, American Bar Association, Washington, DC, 1983.

153. AMERICAN BAR ASSOCIATION: *Proposed Criminal Justice Mental Health Standards.* Standing Committee on Association Standards for Criminal Justice, American Bar Association, Chicago, IL, 1984.

154. Op cit, note 153, p 5.

155. Op cit, note 153, pp 25-26.

156. Op cit, note 153, p 26.

157. Op cit, note 153, pp 26-27.

158. Op cit, note 150.

APPENDIX

Standards for Fellowship Programs in Forensic Psychiatry*

A REPORT BY THE JOINT COMMITTEE ON ACCREDITATION OF FELLOWSHIP PROGRAMS IN FORENSIC PSYCHIATRY

Academic Affiliation

The Fellowship Program in Forensic Psychiatry should be built upon the foundation of a residency program in psychiatry that has been accredited by the Accreditation Council for Graduate Medical Education.

Director of the Program

The Director of the Fellowship Program in Forensic Psychiatry should be an experienced forensic psychiatrist. By the year 1983, the Director must be certified by the American Board of Forensic Psychiatry. The Director should hold a faculty position at the medical school that operates the underlying residency program in general psychiatry; his or her rank in that program should be at the level of Assistant Professor or Clinical Assistant Professor at the minimum.

Faculty of the Program

It is important that Fellows have exposure to more than one perspective in forensic psychiatry, so that at least one member of the faculty (i.e., in addition to the Director) should be an experienced forensic psychiatrist. It is not necessary, although it is highly desirable, that this person be certified by the American Board of Forensic Psychiatry. It is necessary that this person is also on the

The Joint Committee on Accreditation of Fellowship Programs in Forensic Psychiatry is co-sponsored by The American Academy of Forensic Sciences (Psychiatry Section) and The American Academy of Psychiatry and the Law.

Prepared for the Committee by Richard Rosner, MD, Medical Director, Forensic Psychiatry Clinic for the New York Criminal and Supreme Courts (First Judicial Department) 100 Centre St.—Room 124, New York, NY 10013. Clinical Associate Professor, Dept. of Psychiatry, New York University School of Medicine, 550 First Ave., New York, NY 10016.

Committee Members

David Barry, MD	Seymour Pollack, MD
Elissa Benedek, MD	Joseph Palombi, MD
Harvey Bluestone, MD	Jonas Rappeport, MD
John Bradford, MD	Phillip Resnick, MD
James Cavanaugh, MD	Richard Rosner, MD (Chairman)
J. Richard Ciccone, MD	Robert Sadoff, MD
Park Dietz, MD	Selwyn Smith, MD
Mark Mills, MD	Henry Weinstein, MD
Thomas Mould, MD	Howard Zonana, MD

* From Rosner,[75] with permission.

faculty of the medical school that operates the underlying residency program in general psychiatry, but he or she need not be of professorial rank.

An attorney must be part of the faculty of the Fellowship Program in Forensic Psychiatry, although (in deference to the requirements for medical school faculty appointments) that attorney need not be a formal member of the faculty of the medical school that operates the underlying residency program in general psychiatry.

An experienced forensic psychologist should be a member of the consultants available to the Fellowship Program, although that person need not be a formal member of the faculty of the Fellowship Program. It is desirable, but not required, that the forensic psychologist be certified by the American Board of Forensic Psychology.

An experienced child and adolescent psychiatrist should be a member of the consultants available to the Fellowship Program, although he or she need not be a formal member of the faculty of the Fellowship Program. It is desirable, but not required, that the consultant be certified by the American Board of Psychiatry and Neurology in the sub-specialty of Child and Adolescent Psychiatry.

It is recommended, but not required, that a family systems therapist, preferably a psychiatrist, be available as a consultant to the Fellowship Program. It is not necessary that the therapist be a formal member of the faculty of the Fellowship Program.

Management by Objectives

The Fellowship Program should have a clear statement regarding the desired outcome of its training. A formal statement should be made of the goals, the objectives, the methods, and the mechanism for the assessment of the effectiveness of the training program. An assessment of the effectiveness of the program in meeting its own objectives, and the relevance of those objectives for the goals of the program, should be made annually. Based on that assessment, the program's goals, objectives, and methods should be reviewed annually by the Director and the program faculty, with the aim of increasing the program's effectiveness, if necessary by the modification of those goals, objectives, and methods.

Didactic Core Curriculum

The didactic core curriculum represents that body of information and skills that is to be communicated to the fellow by means of lectures, seminars, demonstrations, and formal teaching. The subjects to be included are:

Civil Forensic Psychiatry including, at minimum, conservators and guardianships, child custody determinations, parental competence, termination of parental rights, child abuse, child neglect, psychiatric disability determinations (e.g., for social security, workers compensation, private insurance coverage), testamentary capacity, psychiatric negligence and malpractice, personal injury litigation issues.

Criminal Forensic Psychiatry including, at minimum, competence to stand trial, competence to enter a plea, testimonial capacity, voluntariness of confessions, insanity defense(s), diminished capacity, sentencing considerations, release of persons who have been acquitted by reason of insanity.

Legal Regulation of Psychiatry including, at minimum, civil involuntary commitment, voluntary hospitalization, confidentiality, right to treatment, right to refuse treatment, informed consent, professional liability, ethical guidelines.

Special Issues in Forensic Psychiatry including, at minimum, the history of forensic psychiatry, assessment of dangerousness, amnesia, organic brain syndromes, neuropsychiatric assessment, forensic use of hypnosis/amytal/polygraphy, psychopathic or sociopathic or antisocial personalities, the role and responsibilities of forensic psychiatrists.

Correctional Psychiatry including, at minimum, approaches to the treatment of incarcerated persons, administrative considerations in the operation of a treatment program in a secure setting, rape and sexual problems in a secure setting, gradations of security within the correctional system, psychological aspects of inmate riots, history of correctional psychiatry, ethical issues in a secure setting.

Basic Issues in Law including, at minimum, the nature of law and its foundations in case law/common law/statutes/administrative regulations, the structure of the federal and state court systems, use of a law library, theory and practice of punishment, basic civil procedure, basic criminal procedure, jurisdiction, mens rea, responsibility, tort law, legislative processes, equal protection.

Landmark Cases including, at minimum, the cases specifically listed in the syllabus of the American Board of Forensic Psychiatry.

Supervised Clinical Experiences

The fellow should spend a minimum of 15 hours, but not more than a maximum of 25 hours, each week in supervised clinical experiences. Emphasis should be placed on meeting the educational needs of the fellow, rather than on the service needs of the constituent clinical components of the Fellowship Program.

In the course of the fellowship year, each fellow should have performed a minimum of thirty clinical case assessments in the areas of civil and criminal forensic psychiatry, at least ten of those assessments in the civil area and at least ten in the criminal area. A written case report should be required in at least twenty-five of those thirty assessments. Related to these thirty assessments, the fellow should have the responsibility/opportunity of testifying in court on at least five cases. In addition, the fellow should have an opportunity to witness at least ten in-court appearances by a forensic psychiatrist. Among the written reports that the fellow prepares in the course of the training year there should be, at the minimum, three assessments related to aiding the court in the sentencing of criminal offenders, one assessment in a domestic relations case, one civil commitment assessment, one personal injury assessment, and one civil competency assessment.

Criminal Forensic Psychiatry experiences should include male and female adolescents and adults covering a variety of ages. Incarcerated defendants and defendants on bail, i.e., persons seen both as inpatients and outpatients, should be available for assessment. Evaluations should encompass such issues as the competence of the defendant to stand trial, competence to confess, criminal responsibility, and post-conviction reports in aid of sentencing by the Court. Opportunities should be provided for consultation with lawyers, probation officers, judges. Written reports should be drafted to conform to the special requirements of forensic psychiatry and training should be provided in report writing.

Civil Forensic Psychiatry experiences should include such cases as child custody, termination of parental rights, child abuse, child neglect, spouse abuse, assessment of psychiatric impairment in cases for Social Security/Workers Compensation/private insurance coverage, civil commitment.

Legal Regulation of Psychiatry experiences should provide the fellow with a minimum of ten cases for assessment. Preferably the fellow should do the assessments himself or herself. However, if that is not possible, intensive seminar case review, averaging two hours per case for ten cases, may be substituted. The cases should include civil commitment, and it is recommended that such other cases as confidentiality, patients' rights, professional liability, and ethical issues also be included (if need be, by the use of seminar case reviews). It would be desirable for the fellow to assess patients who are refusing their medication, are contesting their involuntary hospitalization, and whose capacity to provide competent/voluntary/informed consent is at issue.

Special Issues in Forensic Psychiatry should provide the fellow with a minimum of five cases for assessment including examples of potential or present dangerousness, psychopathy, organic brain syndromes, neuropsychiatric testing, and double-agent ethical problems. While it is preferable for the fellow to examine the cases, if that is not possible, then an intensive seminar case review may be substituted, averaging two hours per case for five cases.

Correctional Psychiatry experiences, at minimum, should occupy twenty-five hours in the course of the training year. Among the clinical settings that are appropriate for the fellow to experience are state and federal prisons, municipal and federal and state detention centers, court detention areas for persons awaiting arraignment/hearing/trial, secure court clinics, secure areas for persons contesting involuntary hospitalization, secure units for persons who have been acquitted by reason of insanity.

Clinical Supervision should be in addition to the didactic program. It should be scheduled weekly and be provided by a forensic psychiatrist. Where appropriate to the case material, supplemental supervision (in addition to that provided by the forensic psychiatrist) may be provided by a forensic psychologist, child psychiatrist, or family systems therapist.

Library Resources

The following publications should be part of the core library.

Textbooks

American Psychiatric Association: Clinical Aspects of the Violent Individual. Washington, DC, American Psychiatric Association, 1974

Bromberg W: The Uses of Psychiatry in the Law: A Clinical View of Forensic Psychiatry. Westport, CT, Quorum Books, 1979

Brooks A: Law, Psychiatry and the Mental Health System. Boston: Little, Brown and Co, 1974. Also, obtain the *1980 Supplement* to the text, by the same author, same publisher, with the same title

Cleckley H: The Mask of Sanity: An Attempt to Clarify Some Issues about the So-called Psychopathic Personality. St. Louis, C.V. Mosby Co., 1976

Goldstein A: The Insanity Defense. New Haven, Yale University Press, 1967

Goldstein J, Freud A, Solnit A: Beyond the Best Interests of the Child. New York, Macmillan Publishing Co., 1973. Also obtain the companion volume,

Before the Best Interests of the Child, by the same authors and the same publisher [new edition, 1979]

Halleck S: Law in the Practice of Psychiatry: A Handbook for Clinicians. New York, Plenum Publishing Co., 1980

Keiser L: Traumatic Neurosis. Philadelphia, J.B. Lippincott Co, 1968

Leedy J: Compensation in Psychiatric Disability and Rehabilitation. Springfield, IL, Charles C. Thomas Co., 1971

Rosner R: Critical Issues in American Psychiatry and the Law. Springfield, IL, Charles C. Thomas Co., 1982

Sadoff R: Forensic Psychiatry. Springfield, IL, Charles C. Thomas Co., 1975

Schetky D and Benedek E: Child Psychiatry and the Law. New York, Brunner/Masel, 1980

Slovenko R: Psychiatry and Law. Boston, Little, Brown & Co., 1973

Stone A: Mental Health and Law: A System in Transition. New York, Jason Aronson, 1975

Ziskin J: Coping with Psychiatry and Psychological Testimony, 3rd ed. Venice, CA, Law and Psychology Press, 1982

Reference Books

Allen, Ferster, Rubin: Readings in Law and Psychiatry, rev. ed., Baltimore, Johns Hopkins University Press, 1975

American Medical Association: Guides to the Evaluation of Permanent Impairment. Chicago, American Medical Association, 1971

Curran WJ, McGarry AL, Petty CS (Eds.): Modern Legal Medicine, Psychiatry, and Forensic Science. Philadelphia, F.A. Davis Co., 1980

Curran WJ, Shapiro ED: Law, Medicine, and Forensic Sciences, 2nd ed. Boston, Little, Brown and Co., 1970

Glaser D (Ed.): Handbook of Criminology. Chicago, Rand-McNally, 1974

Holder AR: Medical Malpractice Law. New York, John Wiley & Sons, 1975

Laboratory of Community Psychiatry, Harvard Medical School: Competency to Stand Trial and Mental Illness. New York, Jason Aronson, 1974

Rada RT (Ed.): Clinical Aspects of the Rapist. New York, Grune & Stratton, 1978

Radzinowicz L, Wolfgang ME (Eds.): Crime and Justice (3 vols.). New York, Basic Books, 1971

Spitz WU, Fisher R (Eds.): Medicolegal Investigation of Death: Guidelines for the Application of Pathology to Crime Investigation. Springfield, IL, Charles C. Thomas, 1973

Wadlington W, Waltz JR, Dworkin RB: Cases and Materials on Law and Medicine. Mineola, NY, Foundation Press, 1980

Waltz JR, Inbau FE: Medical Jurisprudence. New York, The Macmillan Co., 1971

Research Monographs

1. Gunn J, Robertson G, et al: Psychiatric Aspects of Imprisonment. New York, Academic Press, 1978
2. Guze SB: Criminality and Psychiatric Disorders. New York, Oxford University Press, 1976
3. Lewis DO, Balla DA: Delinquency and Psychopathology. New York, Grune & Stratton, 1976

4. Mednick S, Christiansen KO: Biosocial Bases of Criminal Behavior. New York, Gardner Press, 1977

5. Mohr JW, Turner RE, Jerry MB: Pedophilia and Exhibitionism. Toronto, University of Toronto Press, 1964.

6. Monroe RR: Episodic Behavioral Disorders. Cambridge, Harvard University Press, 1970

7. Robins LN: Deviant Children Grown Up. Baltimore, Williams and Wilkins Co., 1966

8. Roesch R, Golding SL: Competency to Stand Trial. Urbana, IL, University of Illinois Press, 1980

9. Simon RD: The Jury and the Defense of Insanity. Boston, Little, Brown and Company, 1967

10. Steadman HJ: Beating a Rap? Defendants Found Incompetent to Stand Trial. Chicago, University of Chicago Press, 1979

11. Steadman HJ, Cocozza JJ: Careers of the Criminally Insane: Excessive Social Control of Deviance. Lexington, MA, Lexington, Books, 1974

12. Thornberry TP, Jacoby JE: The Criminally Insane: A Community Follow-up of Mentally Disordered Offenders. Chicago, University of Chicago Press, 1979

13. West DJ: Murder Followed by Suicide. Cambridge, Harvard University Press, 1967

Training in Law

Included in the core didactic curriculum in forensic psychiatry, the fellow must be provided with a minimum of twenty-five hours of formal training devoted to acquisition of legal information. Among the essential elements to be addressed are foundations and sources of law, the structure of the court systems, use of a law library, criminal procedure, civil procedure, theory and practice of punishment, responsibility, jurisdiction, due process, and mens rea.

The attorney on the faculty of the training program should have particular responsibility in the development and presentation of the legal segment of the formal educational program. Elective opportunities for legal learning are recommended as a supplement to the training provided by the attorney on the faculty. Such opportunities may be found in law school courses, consultation with Public Defenders and Prosecutors, consultation with the law departments of hospitals, governmental agencies, and guest lectures from visiting private practitioners of law.

Training in Research

The training program should provide the fellow with basic skills in research in forensic psychiatry, such that the fellow learns to obtain and critically evaluate published research findings in the sub-specialty and such that the fellow is equipped to make some contribution to the scholarly or scientific development of forensic psychiatry.

The fellowship training program must include a research requirement for completion of its course. Suitable research projects include a scholarly review or a clinical study suitable for publication in a refereed journal, participation in ongoing externally funded research at a level of effort equivalent to at least two months of full-time work, production of a video-tape or film suitable for presentation at a major national meeting, production of a practice manual in some selected area of forensic psychiatry, preparation of an annotated bibliography on some topic in the sub-specialty.

The training program must include the resources that would make such research possible. These include, at minimum, accessibility to a major medical library, accessibility to a major law library and accessibility to at least one behavioral science research (e.g., computer processing, a programmable calculator, a one-way mirror observation room, videotape equipment, endocrine assays, psychotropic drug assays, electroencephalography, computerized tomography, polygraphy, penile plethysmography, or a medical examiner's office).

Training in Teaching

The training program must provide opportunities to foster the fellow's development as a teacher of forensic psychiatry. Such opportunities should be consistent with the fellow's acquisition of the essential knowledge and skills of the sub-specialty, so that the bulk of the fellow's teaching should be scheduled after the fellow has received basic training in forensic psychiatry. It is recommended that the fellow have exposure to senior teachers in the field, who can provide effective role models.

Among the suitable teaching opportunities are: teaching basic psychiatry to lawyers, probation, and correction officers; teaching residents in general and child psychiatry; teaching forensic psychiatry to parole and police officers; teaching revelant topics to non-psychiatric physicians (e.g., professional liability, informed consent, confidentiality).

CHAPTER 2

ETHICAL PERSPECTIVES: FORMAL CODES AND STANDARDS

William J. Curran, J.D., LL.M., S.M.Hyg.

This chapter and the next deal with issues of definition and standard setting in the interdisciplinary field of law and mental health. Primary concerns are with ethical concepts and the clash of ethical values that are a part of the environment of mental health professional activity in the American legal and correctional systems.[1-6] Many of these issues are historically based and can be explained only by reference to deeply felt, historically imbedded, cultural and social circumstances found in this field.[7-11] Other issues are related to differences in professional and technical language in which effective cross-disciplinary communication may help to achieve greater understanding and cooperation in the everyday contacts of mental health professionals with lawyers, judges, probation officers, correctional officials, prison security personnel, parole officers, and parole board members.

In this chapter, concentration is placed upon formal definitions and standards, particularly as they are found in the official codes of ethical conduct adopted by the organized professional groups in psychiatry and psychology. Two types of codes are examined: (1) codes of a general nature covering the basic professional specialties and containing provisions of relevance to forensic and legal activities, and (2) more specific codes and standards dealing directly with forensic and legal applications in psychiatry and psychology.

In the next chapter, the analysis will be more generalized, with attention given to conflicts in ethical values, particularly those concerning therapeutic goals and legal and correctional demands for security and conformity of conduct to set rules of behavior in the legal context. It is realized that psychiatrists and psychologists practice their professions in a wide variety of settings of private clinical practice, research, education, training, and public areas of responsibility. The ethical issues discussed in these chapters concern practitioners particularly in roles of clinical treatment, assessment and diagnosis, counseling, and consultation. Many of these areas are recognized subspecialties in the professional fields. However, throughout these two chapters, the general terms "psychiatrist" and "psychologist" are used to describe these various roles of professionals in working with the legal and correctional fields.

DEFINITIONAL ROLES

Psychiatrists and psychologists who work with the legal and correctional systems of this country play a variety of roles, most of them related to communicating scientific, technical, and clinical information to personnel in these systems who may have only a limited understanding of the full implications of the information conveyed. At times, the legal or correctional system may seem to accept the information too readily, too uncritically. At other times, there may seem to be an obstinate refusal to accept the information at all or to allow it to affect serious decisions.

The conveying of information by the mental health professional may be a part of the role of expert witness in the court or more broadly as a consultant to attorneys, judges, probation or parole departments, and so forth (Figs. 2-1 and 2-2).[5,6,12,13] The specialty functions are usually described as either "forensic" or "legal," with the terms used interchangeably. In a proper definitional sense, the term "forensic" should be used only when the relationship is to a court or other judicial agency, because the term means "of the court" or "of the forum."[14] The "forum" reference derives from the ancient Roman municipal meeting place in the towns and cities of the Roman Empire where legal matters were considered and where political debates took place concerning matters of community

---

PROFESSIONAL ROLES

"FORENSIC" PSYCHIATRY AND PSYCHOLOGY
- Related to the courts
- Courtroom testimony
- Preparing courtroom reports
- Evaluating parties and witnesses
- Advising trial lawyers and judges

"LEGAL" PSYCHIATRY AND PSYCHOLOGY
- Above roles in courts
- Clinical treatment for courts and prison systems
- Clinical treatment and evaluation of selected patient populations of concern to legal system
- Interdisciplinary research in legal and prison systems
- Legal policy advice and formulation for legislatures, courts, prison systems, etc.

FIGURE 2-1. Professional roles in legal areas for mental health professionals are listed here.

CONSULTATION FUNCTIONS

EXPERT WITNESS:

- Formal testimony in court
- Reports prepared for use in court (ordered by judge or requested by attorneys)

GENERAL CONSULTANT:

- Evaluate parties or witnesses who are scheduled to appear in court (usually at request of attorneys)
- Advise judges on certain aspects of litigation
- Advise attorneys on jury selection, trial tactics, questioning techniques, and oral arguments

---

FIGURE 2-2. Consultation functions in court of mental health professionals are described here.

interest.[15,16] Thus, there was an overlap in function between lawcourt presentation and public speaking or debating. Most modern dictionaries still carry both definitions of "forensic" activities.

Psychiatrists and psychologists do, however, play broader roles in the legal-correctional systems than those related to court trials. They provide treatment for criminal offenders and for persons otherwise in trouble, or potentially in trouble, with the law. Also, they offer policy recommendations to these systems based upon their clinical and research work in the interdisciplinary field. These broader roles are usually grouped under the titles of "legal psychiatry" and "legal psychology." The former term was originated in France by psychiatrists interested in the legal and penal systems of the nineteenth century, particularly by Jean Esquirol (1772-1840), Guillaume Ferrus (1784-1861), and Francois Leuret (1797-1840).[8] Esquirol was the chief psychiatric consultant in the drafting of the famous French mental health code of 1838, which is still the basic foundation of French law.

The term "legal psychology" was probably first used by Hugo Munsterberg (1863-1916), professor of psychology at Harvard University, in his lectures across the country in 1908.[17] His essays on various aspects of applied psychology related to law were also published in 1908 in the book *On The Witness Stand*.[18] The book contained chapters on complex issues of memory, illusion, emotion, bias, and the power of suggestion. The author fell under severe criticism from lawyers, judges, and law professors, largely because of the extravagance of some of his claims for the superiority of psychological methods over traditional legal practices, most of which he ridiculed strongly in his lectures and writings.[19-21] The severity of the reaction to Munsterberg's work spilled over into a widespread hostility toward psychology in legal circles and probably accounted for the long period of absence of psychological research and consultation in legal areas throughout the earlier decades of this century.[9,22-25] Since at least the 1960s, however, there has been a renewed and invigorated interest in interdisciplinary work in legal psychology. (See the descriptions of the field in chapter 1.)

FORMAL CODES OF CONDUCT

Importance of Ethical Standards

Much of the discourse in general ethics texts seems to be conducted without extensive reference to formal provisions of codes of ethical conduct adopted by professional organizations. Why, then, does this chapter place so much emphasis on the formal codes?

There is a practical reason for this stress on formally adopted standards. Whenever a **professional person** is in trouble concerning aspects of professional conduct, it is the **formal code** that will be examined, that code which was in force at the time of the alleged events. A professional person is usually questioned seriously and reprimanded or censured by a professional society or a licensing or certification body only when the alleged conduct can be found to violate specific provisions of the formal codes. When dealing with licensing penalties (fines, suspension, or revocation) for ethical matters, the American courts have referred the substance of the violation to the prevailing ethical code of the professional group involved.[26,27]

Reference to the formal professional ethical codes is also highly informative as a means of following the historical development of general policies concerning particular types of conduct or of interrelationships between professionals and their patients or clients, with their colleagues in the same profession, and with other cooperating or competing groups in the society. In nearly all instances, considerable care was taken in the drafting of these codes, and they were not formally adopted without widespread dissemination and discussion within the profession. (This type of discussion was particularly widespread and elaborate in the case of American psychology in the 1940s and 1950s before the adoption of the first national ethical code of the American Psychological Association, described later in this chapter.)

At casual review, some code provisions will seem quite general and vague, and others will seem specific and narrow. Actually, most codes contain a mixture of general and narrow standards. The opening provisions are usually of a broadly worded nature, describing general obligations of fidelity and fair dealing with patients or clients. Later provisions and newly adopted guidelines reflecting recent changes in policy are usually more precise and specific in describing ethical obligations. Careful examination of the standards will reveal these differences of approach. Also, when the codes have been in effect for a period of time, the professional groups usually produce a set of further interpretive guidelines based upon experience in enforcing the code and in answering formal inquiries about the meaning and scope of particular provisions.

It should also be noted that there is often considerable overlap between specific legal obligations placed upon professional people and what are called ethical obligations. For example, there was very little mention in ethical codes concerning an obligation to obtain "informed consent" from patients for treatment or experimental procedures before these obligations were examined and spelled out in considerable detail in legal decisions and regulations.[28-31] Some ethical codes have been newly established or quite drastically revised in direct response to legal actions or efforts toward official punishment of professional persons. The most dramatic example in this area is the ethical code for medical experimentation resulting from the Nuremberg Trials after World War II.[32,33]

Recent revisions in the code of the American Medical Association (AMA) were also adopted at least in part owing to legal actions against physicians and the association concerning violations of antitrust and restraint-of-trade laws.

Academic courses and seminars in ethics for psychiatrists and psychologists and published curriculum suggestions for such courses also are found to reflect this overlap between ethical standards and legal requirements.[34-36] In one paper by two distinguished psychiatrists, the discussion of ethical issues is more a review of legal decisions and rules than of general or professional ethics.[37]

Ethical Codes in Medicine and Psychiatry

The general ethical standards for physicians, including psychiatrists, and those for psychologists were quite recently revised. In both cases, the revisions amount to entirely new codes, not merely rewording or reinterpretation of older provisions. The medical standards date from 1980; the psychological standards were revised in 1981.

As noted earlier, the ethical standards of the American Medical Association were changed at least in part because of legal action concerning antitrust and restraint-of-trade complaints. In a broad way, the criticism concerned ethical restrictions against dealing with other "nonscientific" competing groups, such as osteopaths and chiropractors, and restrictions that seemed to discourage disclosure to the public or enforcement agencies and courts of shortcomings of fellow physicians. The new code of 1980 sought to change these policies. Whereas all other AMA ethical standards had been becoming increasingly detailed over the years, this new code struck new ground not only in substance but in length. The new code contains only seven provisions, all quite brief. Significantly more attention is given to the physician's obligations to the general society; to other, nonmedical, health professionals with whom cooperation is encouraged; and to the physician's local community. References to avoiding contact with "nonscientific" healers is omitted. There is no provision against "contract medicine," or salaried service, with organizations under the control of nonphysicians, such as health maintenance organizations or clinics. There is a strong new provision, Section 2, quite specific in wording, requiring physicians **to expose** practitioners who are deficient in either ethical character or professional competence. It establishes an **affirmative duty** to disclose deficiencies in medical colleagues to peer-review groups, accreditation agencies, or licensing boards, especially when those deficiencies could endanger or have already endangered patients. Another provision, Section 4, admonishes against breach of patient confidences. These are the most important legally related standards in the new medical pronouncements. There are no specific provisions concerning forensic activities or work with legal or correctional agencies.

There are two other important ethical documents specifically related to psychiatric practice that should be noted here. In 1978, the World Psychiatric Association adopted the *Declaration of Hawaii*,[38] an important statement of modern ethical principles for psychiatrists. Considerable attention was given to a very important legal psychiatry issue: treatment of mentally ill persons under legal restraint in closed mental hospitals or prisons. The code requires psychiatrists to seek the permission of the individual patient for treatment modalities and drug use even when the patient is under restraint or court order unless the patient is incapable of expressing his or her own wishes or cannot understand or realize what is in his or her own best interest. Also, the declaration admonishes psychiatrists to release compulsory patients from confinement and restraint as soon as clinical conditions for compulsory treatment no longer exist. The provision on informed consent also requires that when a patient is incompetent or is a child, such consent be sought from someone close to the patient. There is a specific reference to forensic psychiatric relationships: It is required that when a psychiatrist is interviewing or treating a patient under court order or on behalf of prison authorities, the psychiatrist must reveal this relationship to the patient. (For a sensitive examination of the declaration, see several commentaries by a Swedish psychiatrist with an excellent background in ethics, the late Clarence Blomquist.[39-41])

The other very important document is a set of **official annotations** to the AMA ethical code concerning psychiatric practice.[42] These guidelines were first produced in 1973. They were completely revised in 1981, in accordance with the new AMA ethical code of 1980 reviewed earlier. The new annotations were prepared by the Ethics Committee of the American Psychiatric Association (APA) and were approved by the board of trustees of the association. They constitute the official ethical code of American psychiatry.

Because of the brevity of the new AMA code, the APA group obviously had some difficulty relating the many annotations to particular provisions of the new seven-section AMA code. In several instances, the annotations seem quite irrelevant to the provision to which they are tenuously attached. Whenever the AMA provision itself is entirely new and imposes new ethical obligations, as it does in regard to a duty "to expose" physicians deficient in character or competence or who engage in fraud or deception, it is notable that most of the annotations are only rather indirectly related to the key thrust of the AMA code provision. The most relevant of the annotations seems actually to disagree with the AMA principle. The annotation states:

> When a member [of the APA] has been found to have behaved unethically by the American Psychiatric Association or one of its constituent district branches, there should not be an automatic reporting to the local authorities responsible for medical licensure, but the decision to report should be decided upon the merits of the case.[42]

The AMA's requirement "to expose" unethical conduct of physicians seems not to be observed in this annotation. The duty created by the AMA is affirmative and contains no qualifications. The obvious group to whom exposure should be made is the licensing board of the state. Many state licensure boards, either by statute or administrative regulation, require professional groups such as the state medical society to report ethical violations by members.[43,44]

There are several annotations of particular relevance to forensic psychiatric activities. Most important, there is an annotation related to Section 4 of the AMA code. The annotation reads as follows:

> Ethical considerations in medical practice preclude the psychiatric evaluation of an adult charged with criminal acts prior to access to, or availability of, legal counsel. The only exception is to the rendering of care to a person for the sole purpose of medical treatment.[42]

The above annotation will be examined in the next chapter and also in chapter 22.

As an annotation to Section 4 of the AMA code, there is a requirement concerning courtroom testimony involving patient confidences. It reads:

> When the psychiatrist is ordered by the court to reveal the confidences entrusted to him/her by patients, he/she may comply or he/she may ethically hold to the right to dissent within the framework of the law. . . . In the event that the necessity for legal disclosure is demonstrated by the court, the psychiatrist may request the right to disclosure of only that information which is relevant to the legal questions at hand.[42]

This annotation is in accordance with the rules of evidence in most states. The court should not allow a questioning attorney to force answers from a psychiatrist or psychologist concerning patients they have treated on issues not relevant to the legal case involved.

There are also two important annotations regarding freedom of the psychiatrist in therapeutic practice situations. The first appears as an annotation to Section 1 of the AMA code. It states: "A psychiatrist should not be a participant in a legally authorized execution."[42] This annotation was adopted in reaction to the laws passed in several states authorizing capital punishment by lethal drug injection. The participation of physicians in any way to order, to prepare, to administer, or to supervise other personnel in administering such drugs with the purpose of killing a condemned person had been severely criticized as unethical and as a violation of medical licensure acts in an article by this author and a physician.[45] The American Medical Association and several state medical societies have also declared unethical the involvement of physicians in lethal drug injections for capital punishment purposes.

The other annotation (related to Section 6 of the AMA code) is directed at discouraging forced or involuntary psychiatric treatment for political dissenters or radicals who are not mentally ill. The annotation would also apply to involuntary psychiatric treatment for social deviance not amounting to mental illness, such as homosexuality. The provision states: "An ethical psychiatrist may refuse to provide psychiatric treatment to a person who, in the psychiatrist's opinion, cannot be diagnosed as having a mental illness amenable to psychiatric treatment."[42]

The above annotation is similar to a provision in the *Declaration of Hawaii*: "The psychiatrist must not participate in compulsory psychiatric treatment in the absence of psychiatric illness."[38] The provision in the international document was adopted in reaction to the internment of political dissenters in Soviet Russian mental hospitals with the cooperation of Russian psychiatrists. The last annotation of particular significance to forensic work relates to certification of patients for involuntary treatment. The annotation states:

> The psychiatrist may permit his/her certification to be used for the involuntary treatment of any person only following his/her personal examination of that person. To do so, he/she must find that the person, because of mental illness, cannot form a judgment as to what is in his/her own best interests and that, without such treatment, substantial impairment is likely to occur to the person or others.[42]

The provision was adopted because some psychiatrists were signing commitment papers (usually indicating that they had seen and examined the person within the past 3 to 10 days) without ever seeing the patient, relying on hearsay statements of other physicians, family members, or arresting police.

Ethical Principles for Psychologists

Psychologists in the United States have given considerable attention in the past two decades to ethical principles covering both clinical practice and research activities. The literature of the field is extensive and impressive.[34,46-50] The national professional organization, the American Psychological Association, has produced a series of useful and influential reports over recent decades.[51-56]

Golann[46] has reviewed the progress of American psychologists in developing ethical standards since the 1930s. In 1939, a special committee on ethical matters recommended the establishment of a standing committee on ethics in the American Psychological Association. Such a committee was established in 1940. Over the next decade, there were great interest in the development of a professional ethical code and widespread discussion of draft provisions. In 1948, the association solicited from the membership descriptions of ethical problems encountered in practice and an indication of what the members believed were the ethical implications of the examples. Over 1000 case reports were collected and classified into five different areas of professional work: (1) public responsibility, (2) client relationships, (3) teaching, (4) research, and (5) professional relationships. The novel approach to gaining experience for producing a professional code of ethics resulted in the publication of several papers by the association suggesting ethical standards for psychologists.[54,55] State, regional, and local associations considered the issues over a period of years. The first code of ethics of the association was adopted in 1953. The code was revised in 1959. It became apparent over the years that the most serious issues of an ethical nature occurred in clinical practice and research activities. Golann gave particular attention to the controversy over Milgram's studies[57] of conditions under which research subjects would obey commands to inflict what the subjects were led to believe were levels of pain upon other persons.[58-60] The Milgram studies were later significant to the adoption of federal regulations on human research.

The American Psychological Association adopted an entirely new code in 1981.[61] The psychologists opted for an approach different from that of the physicians. Whereas the new medical code is briefer and more general in scope, covering essentially only clinical services, the psychological code is quite long, detailed, and comprehensive. There are a total of 64 different subsections gathered under 10 principles, or standards, each introduced by an important and substantive **preamble.**

The principles are introduced with a **general preamble** which outlines the entire document. Like the medical code, the psychologists' code begins with an affirmation of respect for the dignity of the individual and protection of "fundamental human rights." The code covers not only clinical practice but research, education, psychological assessment techniques, confidentiality, issuance of public statements, advertising of services, and the care and use of animals in research. The provisions on human and animal research are particularly well prepared and sophisticated, as well may be expected in a profession with a significant portion of its members engaged in research.

In Principle 1 the code of ethics cautions psychologists to realize that they often carry a heavy social responsibility in their work and that their recommendations and professional actions "may alter the lives of others." Members are also admonished to avoid relationships which limit their objectivity or create a conflict of interest. These cautionary statements are of particular concern in forensic work. The recommendations of a forensic psychologist can effect the criminal responsibility of a defendant charged with a serious crime or influence a decision on child custody or involuntary hospitalization. Practitioners in the forensic field must take particular cautions concerning conflict of interest, because the legal area requires the taking of positions in adversary settings. Evidence of conflict of interest can be used to discredit expert witnesses in courtroom trials and before administrative and regulatory agencies.

In the section on professional responsibility, Principle 7 (g), the psychologist is admonished to report serious ethical misconduct of members to the appropriate ethical committee of the association. The new code does not contain a similar requirement to report or to expose professional incompetence or malpractice. There are also no special provisions in this otherwise highly exhaustive code concerning psychologists' dealings with patients or clients under forms of constraint in mental institutions, prisons or schools, even though large numbers of professional members of the group serve in these settings.

It should be noted, however, that in 1978 a Task Force of the American Psychological Association made important recommendations concerning the role of psychologists in the criminal justice system.[62] (See also a publication reporting fully on the work of the Task Force.[63]) The group dealt particularly with ethical issues of confidentiality. It was suggested that the psychologist should inform prison inmates and defendants under criminal charge of any limits on the confidentiality of the relationship. It was further suggested that these limitations be spelled out in advance of any testing or therapy and be done in writing. In an ideal way, the Task Force suggested that the level of confidentiality for therapeutic services in a criminal-penal setting should be the same as that which exists in an "outside" or voluntary setting. Disclosure should be required only where necessary to avert serious harm to the patient, to others, or to the community—in this case, to the prison. The Task Force cited the well-known case of *Tarasoff v. Regents of the University of California*[64] as supporting this obligation. The decision is analyzed later in this text in chapter 3.

Principle 5 of the code of ethics of the association contains a detailed provision on confidentiality. Psychologists are required to respect the confidentiality of patients and clients. They are allowed to reveal confidences only with the consent of the person or the person's legal representative, except in those "unusual circumstances in which not to do so would result in danger to the patient or client or to other persons" (Principle 5 Preamble). Where appropriate, psychologists are advised to inform their patients or clients of the **legal limits** of confidentiality. It is not entirely clear whether the code provision on revealing confidences in matters of potential danger is mandatory or discretionary on the psychologist's part. Until the *Tarasoff* decision, the similar provision in the medical ethics code was interpreted as discretionary within the professional judgment of the practitioner. Since the *Tarasoff* case, both psychologists and psychiatrists have been advised to be ready to breach confidences and to provide warnings to individuals known to be in potential danger owing to threats of violent action by patients or clients.

Ethical Codes in Forensic Areas

Neither psychiatry nor psychology has produced an ethical code dealing directly and exclusively with forensic or legal activities in the mental health field. The closest specific document is the earlier mentioned Task Force Report of the American Psychological Association relating to the role of psychologists in the criminal justice system.[62] This is not a formal ethical code, however.

Attention should be called to the American Bar Association's efforts to prepare standards for mental health aspects of criminal justice.[65] These standards were approved by the ABA in August 1984. They contain provisions regarding qualifications required to be found an "expert" in this field. (A review of these educational and training qualifications can be found in chapter 1.)

The ABA standards also adopt a strongly conservative position on the allowable limits of psychiatric and psychological testimony. The limitations are essentially expressed in terms of the professional capacity of mental health professionals to form expert judgments or opinions on these matters, but there are indications that to go beyond these expressed limitations should be found unethical as well. These limitations can be summarized as follows. The mental health expert should not be asked and should not offer an opinion

1. concerning an "ultimate question" of law, or a moral or social value properly reserved to the court or jury;
2. concerning a prediction that a particular person will or will not engage in dangerous behavior in the future (There are specific conditions, however, which would allow testimonial opinion about future mental condition or behavior of an individual when the testimony is limited to general observations on such matters as the clinical significance of past history and criminal acts, scientific studies of a relevant nature, effects of therapeutic or habilitative interventions, and factors tending to enhance or to diminish the likelihood of such dangerous behavior in future.);
3. concerning the mental condition of a person that the expert witness has not personally interviewed or examined.

The draftsmen admitted the novelty of their proposals and the fact that none of these limitations is currently supported in the federal rules of evidence. (The evidentiary and ethical aspects of these proposals will be examined in chapter 22, "The Psychiatrist as Expert Witness.")

THE CODE OF FORENSIC SCIENTISTS

The most specific code of ethics in the United States concerning forensic activity by mental health professionals is that of the American Academy of Forensic Sciences. The academy includes within its membership forensic science specialists in a broad variety of disciplines. The code was adopted in 1977.[66] The academy's code deals primarily with testimonial matters and the preparation of reports for the courts. It also provides guidance to forensic scientists concerning advertising of their services to lawyers. The code stresses the following key matters.

1. **Qualifications:** Completeness in stating one's background in terms of training, experience, and area of expertise; avoidance of overstatement of qualifications.
2. **Findings and Conclusions:** Technical and scientific accuracy and honesty in all written reports of data and in oral statements and testimony; avoidance of misleading or inaccurate claims upon which one's opinion or conclusions are based.
3. **Impartiality:** An impartial manner at all times with stress on objectivity and clear expression of one's findings and conclusions; doing nothing that would lead to the impression of partisanship or personal or financial interest in the outcome of any matter in litigation or legal controversy.

The Academy of Forensic Sciences was very careful in circumscribing the ethics of reporting technical data. These provisions should be of particular importance to psychologists reporting test results on individuals to the courts. No excuse can be made for inaccurate, fraudulent, or incomplete reporting of objective findings. The academy was particular in distinguishing opinion statements from the reporting of objective test data. Opinion statements are obviously more subjective and less open to scrutiny for clear ethical violation. However, an expressed opinion that is based on inaccurate data or on no data at all can be questioned ethically when it is shown that the scientist was aware of the lack of adequate support for the opinion and did not reveal its scientific weakness. There have been legal prosecutions against mental health professionals for perjury in an expert opinion.[67,68] Most commonly, however, the expert's opinion is subjected to strong attack on cross-examination, and all credibility for the opinion is destroyed when its foundation is found inadequate or totally baseless.

The academy was also very clear in admonishing forensic scientists to maintain objectivity and impartiality throughout their work in the legal setting despite the fact that the legal system is itself based on the adversarial model. In fact, this system of adversarial parties in the law—the framing of issues to present the controversy in the litigation—is at the core of the ethical concerns of most forensic scientists.[4,5,69-71] Most scientists would prefer that their appearances in legal matters be as impartial examiners and reporters for the court or the public, not for the parties.

The most serious breach of the impartiality rules in an ethical sense would come when the expert is a "hired gun," a person willing to provide any opinion if paid enough to do it. The out-and-out fraudulent purveyor of opinions is, sad to relate, readily available. There are also weak personalities in the professions or sciences who are not quite fraudulent purveyors but are close to it. They are notorious for being easily swayed by clever and dominant personalities who entice them to join in "the game" of the court litigation. These dominant personalities, unethical lawyers or investigators hired by lawyers to prepare a case, make a practice of getting to these slim-charactered "experts" and talking quickly and enthusiastically about what they "need" in an opinion. They will, or course, pay little or nothing unless the expert agrees to become involved, and then the fees are usually quite attractive. Many of these "hired guns" enjoy notoriety and publicity. They consciously or unconsciously warp their opinions in order to satisfy the legal advocates seeking their services in sensational litigation.

It should also be noted that it is a clear ethical violation for either psychiatrists or psychologists to be paid in a litigation only if the party for whom they appear wins the case or if their fee is increased when the party wins the litigation and receives money damages. Such conduct means that the forensic expert has a financial interest in the outcome of the litigation, thus compromising required impartiality.

CRUELTY, TORTURE, AND INHUMAN TREATMENT

All forensic scientists must avoid involvement in situations in which excessive force, cruelty, or torture is used to interrogate criminal suspects. Psychiatrists and psychologists should avoid any participation that would condone or seem to sanction such conduct by police or other investigators. The *Declaration of Toyko*,[72] an ethical statement by the World Medical Association in 1975, admonished physicians not to engage in any practices on prisoners or accused persons that could be found to be cruel or inhuman treatment. Included in such cruel or inhuman treatment are forcible treatment with drugs to obtain a confession and forcible feeding of prisoners on a hunger strike. The admonition against forcible feeding applies to competent prisoners refusing food for political or personal reasons and not to actions of mentally disturbed prisoners and committed mental patients.[73]

It is unethical for a psychologist or psychiatrist to use improperly the skills of the profession to obtain or to aid in the obtaining of a confession from an accused person. The use of deception or coercion is improper conduct. For example, it would be unethical to tell a suspect that he or she "had flunked the test" (such as a psychological assessment, or a polygraph examination) when the results were otherwise, equivocal, or meaningless, with the purpose of frightening the suspect into confessing.

In a landmark case, the United States Supreme Court severely criticized the conduct of a psychiatrist in using subtle, persuasive techniques to extract a confession from a youthful suspect.[74] The Court appended to the opinion a transcript of the psychiatrist's interview with the accused to demonstrate its impropriety and coercive nature. Among other things, the psychiatrist said:

> I want you to recollect and tell me everything. . . . It's entirely to your benefit to recollect them because, you see, you're a nervous boy. . . . Tell me, I'm here to help you. . . . I am going to put my hand on your forehead, and as I put my hand on your forehead, you are going to bring back all these thoughts that are coming into your mind. . . . If you tell us the details and come across like a good man, then we can help you. We know that morally you were just in anger. Morally, you are not to be condemned. Right?[75]

This questioning was considered improper, particularly because it was used by a person who had misled the accused into assuming he was there to help him. Also, as a mental health professional, he was said to be using skilled techniques in a corrupt manner. The form and substance of the questions above are not, however, uncommon in police interrogation where "gentle persuasion" is used in place of, or in alternating fashion with, more aggressive confrontation. This type of questioning by police has been recommended to police examiners as quite successful by leading authorities on interrogation and confession seeking.[76]

The above decision was rendered before the establishment by the Supreme Court of the so-called *Miranda warning*.[77] Under that 1966 decision, police investigators were required to provide substantial information and warning to criminal suspects before interrogation concerning their constitutional rights to remain silent and their right to legal counsel of their own choice or provided by the state if they could not afford an attorney. Recently, in *Estelle v. Smith*,[78] the Supreme Court extended this requirement to court-appointed examining forensic experts. In that case, a forensic psychiatrist had performed a court-appointed pretrial examination of the defendant and had found him competent to stand criminal trial. After conviction of first-degree murder, the state was compelled by statute to offer further evidence of the violence potential of the defendant in order to support the newly established death penalty in Texas. The state decided to call the same psychiatrist, Dr. Grigson, to testify at the postconviction hearing. His opinion on the dangerousness of the defendant was based on the same 90-minute interview he had conducted for the purpose of trial competency. Dr. Grigson testified and gave his opinion that the defendant was a severe sociopath whose condition could not be treated and was sure to worsen in future. He observed that he felt the defendant had no regard for human life and would commit similar crimes if given the opportunity. The jury condemned the defendant to death.

The Supreme Court described Dr. Grigson's testimony as having a devastating and conclusive effect on the jury. The Court extended the ruling of the *Miranda* case to an examining psychiatrist and excluded his testimony for failure to provide the warning.

It can be argued that the Supreme Court might not have required the warning merely for the competency examination alone. The majority opinion stated that when the psychiatrist went **beyond** merely reporting on the defendant's competency to stand trial and testified at the death-penalty-imposing hearing on the crucial issue of future dangerousness, his role changed and he became essentially "an agent of the State."[79] The admission of the testimony would thus violate not only the defendant's Fifth Amendment rights (self-incrimination) but also his rights under the Sixth Amendment (right to counsel). This may have seemed a strange conclusion because the defendant was represented by counsel at the time of the pretrial examination and counsel had not objected to it. Nevertheless, the Court held that counsel was not informed at that time of the potential use of the interview material by the psychiatrist for the much more damaging purpose of the postconviction hearing on the death penalty—as the Court described it, "literally a life or death matter."[80]

Another issue of participation by psychiatrists in application of the death penalty has been raised recently in Florida. Along with reinstatement of the death penalty, the state has installed a three-person psychiatric panel to advise the governor on whether a condemned person is mentally competent to be executed.[81] The American Psychiatric Association is currently considering whether to oppose this new procedure on ethical grounds. Many states and nations have traditionally prohibited the execution of mentally ill persons. The ground has usually been that mentally ill persons cannot repent their sins and obtain mercy and religious comfort before death. Under the Florida law the issue is that of mental competency to understand the nature of the punishment and the reason for it. The general prohibition against psychiatrists "participating" in legally ordered executions may be interpreted to bar psychiatrists from joining such panels.[42] The prohibition was noted earlier in this chapter in regard to executions by lethal injection.

UNETHICAL ADVERTISING AND PUBLICITY

Psychiatrists and psychologists should avoid the use of newspaper and journal advertising of their services in legal investigations and litigation when the advertising is false, misleading, or professionally undignified. Discretion should be used in stating qualifications and experience, avoiding breaching confidences or clients' privacy, and avoiding overstatement about the effectiveness of one's methods or special technology.

The psychologists' ethical code discussed earlier in this chapter contains highly useful provisions on these issues. The section on **public statements** (Principle 4) provides direct guidance on what psychologists may include in public advertisements of their services and also what should **not** be included. For example, psychologists are admonished not to include testimonials from patients regarding the quality of their psychological services or products, statements intended to create false or misleading expectations of favorable results, statements implying unusual or unique abilities, or direct solicitation of individual clients. A paid advertisement must be identified as such unless it is obvious from the context. Because advertising by professional persons is now ethically acceptable, paid advertisements are appearing more and more frequently in legal periodicals. These advertisements contain solicitations for hire by attorneys as consultants and expert witnesses. Some solicitations contain the name of the professional, and others list a corporate organization or perhaps a post office box number. These solicitations should follow the requirements of the ethical code as noted above.

Mental health professionals should avoid personal publicity concerning their views about legal matters in litigation. Forensic examiners should not reveal to the press the results of their examinations or their scientific-clinical opinions reached in conducting tests for litigation purposes before these results or opinions are given in court. Even after testimony it is usually best for such examiners to avoid elaborating on their testimony in press or other mass media interviews. A useful expression of professional standards in this area is contained in the Ethical Code of the California Association of Criminalists (technicians and scientists working in criminal justice laboratories):

> Section 5(C). In the interests of the profession, the individual criminalist should refrain from seeking publicity for himself or his accomplishments on specific cases. The preparation of papers for publication in appropriate media, however, is considered proper.
>   Section 5(D). The criminalist shall discourage the association of his name with developments, publications, or organizations in which he has played no significant part, merely as a means of gaining personal publicity or prestige.[82]

These principles are equally applicable to psychiatrists and psychologists involved in forensic work. They are not easy standards to follow, especially in

FORENSIC ETHICAL PRINCIPLES

- Technical and scientific accuracy in reporting findings and conclusions
- Impartiality and objectivity in all dealings with courts and attorneys
- Honesty and completeness in expressing professional opinions, based only upon adequate data to support the opinion
- Avoidance of overstatement of expert qualifications; completeness in reporting background, training, and experience
- Avoidance of use of deception or coercion
- Avoidance of conducting personal examinations or interviews or use of specimens or other material obtained by force or without consent of the person
- Avoidance of excessive publicity or releasing data or results improperly
- Dedication to justice

FIGURE 2-3. Shown here is a summary of forensic ethical principles of mental health professionals.

cases involving sensational, brutal crimes, or when a series of crimes has terrified a whole community.[83-85] Nevertheless, the rights of litigants and persons under investigation can be seriously compromised by premature and often inaccurate media reporting.

SUMMARY OF FORENSIC ETHICAL PRINCIPLES

Figure 2-3 presents a summary of forensic ethical principles for mental health professionals. In general, a posture of dignity and impartiality is advisable for all forensic work by psychiatrists and psychologists, emphasizing a devotion to justice and truth and a resistance to the many pressures to compromise ethical standards in favor of one party or another in litigation, or in the temptation to gain personal notoriety in the public press or television medium of the day.

REFERENCES

1. STONE, A: *Law, Psychiatry, and Morality.* American Psychiatric Press, Washington, DC, 1984.
2. KETAI, R: *Role conflicts of the prison psychiatrist.* Bull Am Acad Psychiatry Law 2:246, 1974.
3. TUNSTALL, O, GUDJONSSON, G, EYSENCK, H, HOWARD, L: *Professional issues arising from psychological evidence presented in court.* Bull Brit Psychol Soc 35:329, 1982.
4. BONNIE, RJ AND SLOBOGIN, C: *The role of mental health professionals in the criminal process: The case for informed speculation.* Virginia Law Review 66:427, 1980.
5. ANDERTEN, P, STAULCUP, V, GRISSO, T: *On being ethical in legal places.* Professional Psychologist 3:173-180, 1980.
6. MILLER, RD: *The treating psychiatrist as forensic evaluator.* J Forensic Science 29:825, 1984.

7. MOORE, RA: *Ethics in the practice of psychiatry: Origins, functions, models and enforcement.* Am J Psychiatry 135:2, 1978.

8. CURRAN, WJ: *Legal psychiatry in the nineteenth century.* Psychiatric Annals 4:8, 1974.

9. LOH, W: *Perspectives on psychology and law.* Journal Applied Social Psychology 11:4, 1981.

10. REIK, LE: *The Doe-Ray correspondence: A pioneer collaboration in the jurisprudence of mental disease.* Yale Law Journal 63:183, 1953.

11. DIX, GE: *The death penalty, "dangerousness," psychiatric testimony, and professional ethics.* American Journal of Criminal Law 5:151, 1977.

12. ROTH, L: *Treating the incarcerated offender.* Journal Social Therapy 15:4, 1969.

13. CONVIS, CL: *Testifying about testimony: Psychological evidence on perceptual and memory factors affecting the credibility of testimony.* Duquesne Law Review 21:579, 1983.

14. CURRAN, WJ: *The confusion of titles in the medicolegal field: An historical analysis and a proposal for reform.* Med Sci Law 15:270 (1975) (reprinted in Am J Law Med 1:11, 1975).

15. ACKERKNECHT, EH: *Early history of legal medicine.* Ciba Found Symp 2:1286, 1950.

16. GIBBENS, TCN: *The development of forensic psychiatry.* In KLARE, HJ (ED): *Changing Concepts of Crime and Its Treatment.* Pergamon Press, Oxford, 1966.

17. MUNSTERBERG, M: *Hugo Munsterberg, His Life and Work.* Appleton and Co, New York, 1922, p 150.

18. MUNSTERBERG, H: *On the Witness Stand: Essays on Psychology and Crime.* Clark, Boardman Publishers, New York, 1908.

19. WIGMORE, JH: *Professor Munsterberg and the psychology of testimony.* Illinois Law Review 3:399, 1909.

20. WIGMORE, JH: *The Science of Judicial Proof,* ed 3. Little, Brown & Co, Boston, 1937.

21. CAIRNS, H: *Law and the Social Sciences.* Harcourt, Brace Publishers, New York, 1935.

22. HUTCHINS, RM: *The law and the psychologists.* Yale Law Review 16:678, 1927.

23. MOSKOWITZ, MJ: *Hugo Munsterberg: A study in the history of applied psychology.* Am Psychol 32:824, 1977.

24. REISMAN, D: *Some observations on law and psychology.* University of Chicago Law Review 19:30, 1951.

25. MARSHALL, J: *Law and Psychology in Conflict.* Bobbs-Merrill, New York, 1966.

26. Forziati v. Board of Registration in Medicine, 333 Mass. 125, 1955.

27. Pepe v. Board of Regents, 295 N.Y. 209, 1968.

28. See extensive references in Canterbury v. Spence, 464 F 2d 772 (D.C. Cir. 1972).

29. HOWELL, T AND SACK, RL: *The ethics of human experimentation in psychiatry: Toward a more informed consensus.* Psychiatry 44:113, 1981.

30. BEECHER, HK: *Experimentation in man.* JAMA 169:461, 1959.

31. FREEDMAN, B: *A moral theory of informed consent.* Hastings Cent Rep 5:32, 1975.

32. ALEXANDER, L: *Medical science under dictatorship.* N Engl J Med 241:39, 1949.

33. LADIMER, IJ: *Ethical and legal aspects of medical research on human subjects.* Journal Public Law 3:467, 1955.

34. KOOCHER, GP: *Ethical and professional standards in psychology.* In SALES, BD (ED): *The Professional Psychologist's Handbook.* Plenum Press, New York, 1983.

35. BLOCH, S: *The Teaching of psychiatric ethics.* Br J Psychiatry 136:300, 1980.

36. SALLADAY, SA: *Teaching ethics in the psychiatry clerkship.* J Med Educ 56:204, 1981.

37. REDLICH, F AND MOLLICA, R: *Overview: Ethical issues in contemporary psychiatry.* Am J Psychiatry 133:125, 1976.

38. *The declaration of Hawaii.* J Med Ethics 4:71, 1978.

39. BLOMQUIST, CDD: *From the oath of Hippocrates to the declaration of Hawaii.* Ethics in Science and Medicine 4:139, 1977.

40. BLOMQUIST, CDD: *Declaration of Hawaii: A commentary.* J Med Ethics 4:72, 1978.

41. BLOMQUIST, CDD: *A new era in European medical ethics.* Hastings Cent Rep 6:2, 1976.

42. *The Principles of Medical Ethics With Annotations Especially Applicable to Psychiatry,* rev ed. American Psychiatric Association, Washington, DC, 1981.

43. VOGEL, J AND DELGADO, R: *To tell the truth: Physician's duty to disclose medical mistakes.* UCLA Law Review 28:52, 1980.

44. California Business and Professional Code, Section 2100 (California Board of Medical Quality Assurance). See also FAMA, AJ: *Reporting incompetent physicians: A comparison of requirements in three states (Florida, Massachusetts, and New York).* Law, Medicine, and Health Care 11:111, 1983.

45. CURRAN, WJ AND CASSCELLS, W: *The ethics of medical participation in capital punishment by intravenous injection.* N Engl J Med 302:226, 1980.

46. GOLANN, SE: *Ethical standards for psychology: Development and revision, 1938-1968.* Ann NY Acad Sci 169:398, 1970.

47. See a three-part article by SHAH, SA: *Privileged Communications, Confidentiality, and Privacy: Part 1, Privileged Communications.* Professional Psychology 1:56, 1969; *Part 2, Confidentiality,* idem, 1:159, 1970; *Part 3, Privacy,* idem, 1:243, 1970.

48. JACOBS, DF: *The development and application of standards of practice for professional psychologists.* In SALES, BD (ED): *Professional Psychologist's Handbook.* Plenum Press, New York, 1983.

49. RUEBHAUSEN, OM AND BRIM, OG: *Privacy and behavioral research.* Am Psychol 21:423, 1965.

50. GOLANN, SE: *Emerging areas of ethical concern.* Am Psychol 24:454, 1969.

51. *Ethical standards for psychologists.* Am Psychol 6:427, 1951.

52. *APA report: Discussion of ethics.* Am Psychol 7:425, 1952.

53. *APA Casebook on Ethical Standards of Psychologists.* American Psychological Association, Washington, DC, 1967.

54. *Ethical standards for psychologists.* Am Psychol 23:357, 1968.

55. *Ethical issues in psychological research.* Am Psychol 23:689, 1968.

56. *APA guidelines for psychologists conducting growth groups.* Am Psychol 28:933, 1973.

57. MILGRAM, S: *Behavioral study of obedience.* Journal of Abnormal and Social Psychology 67:317, 1963.

58. BAUMRIND, D: *Some thoughts on ethics in research: After reading Milgram's behavioral study of obedience.* Am Psychol 19:421, 1964.

59. KELMAN, HC: *Human use of human subjects: The problem of deception in social psychological research.* Psychol Bull 67:1, 1967.

60. MILGRAM, S: *Issues in the study of obedience: A reply to Baumrind.* Am Psychol 19:848, 1964.

61. *Ethical principles of psychologists.* Am Psychol 36:633, 1981.

62. *Report of the task force on the role of psychology in the criminal justice system.* Am Psychol 35:1100, 1978.

63. MONAHAN, J (ED): *Who Is the Client? The Ethics of Psychological Intervention in the Criminal Justice System.* APA, Washington, DC, 1980.

64. 542 P2d 553, 1974; 551 P2d 334, 1976.

65. AMERICAN BAR ASSOCIATION: *Proposed Criminal Justice Mental Health Standards.* ABA, Chicago, IL, 1984.

66. *Code of Ethics.* Newsletter 3:1, 1977. American Academy of Forensic Sciences, Chicago.

67. State v. Sullivan, 24 N.J. 18 (1957); cert. denied, 355 U.S. 840 (1957).

68. See 38 Amer L Rep 3d, 1971.

69. WALLS, HJ: *Whither forensic science?* Med Sci Law 6:183 (1966).

70. PETERSON, JL: *The team approach in forensic science.* In CURRAN, WJ, McGARRY, AL, PETTY, CS (EDS): *Modern Legal Medicine, Psychiatry and Forensic Science.* FA Davis, Philadelphia, 1980.

71. MOENSSENS, J: *"Impartial" medical experts: A new look at an old issue.* Med Trial Tech Q 25:63, 1978.

72. *Declaration of Tokyo.* World Medical Journal 22:87, 1975.

73. See also *Health Aspects of Avoidable Maltreatment of Prisoners and Detainees.* Document A/Conf. 56/9, World Health Organization, Geneva, 1975.

74. Leyra v. Denno, 347 U.S. 556, 1953.

75. Ibid, 580-585.

76. INBAU, FE AND REID, JE: *Criminal Interrogation and Confessions.* Williams & Wilkins, Baltimore, 1962.

77. Miranda v. Arizona, 384 U.S. 436, 1966.

78. 451 U.S. 454, 1981.

79. Ibid, 467.

80. Ibid, 471.

81. *Competency for execution.* Psychiatric News, Sept. 7, 1984, p 1.

82. *Code of Ethics*, California Association of Criminalists, 1974.

83. KENEFICK, DP: *The "Boston Strangler" investigation.* Am J Psychiatry 125:4, 1968.

84. WHITTINGTON-EGAM, R: *A Casebook on Jack the Ripper.* John Wiley & Sons, London, 1975.

85. JOHNSON, PH: *On Inquiry: Some Reflections on the Moors Murder Trial.* Charles Scribner's Sons, New York, 1967.

CHAPTER 3

MENTAL HEALTH AND JUSTICE: ETHICAL ISSUES OF INTERDISCIPLINARY COOPERATION*

William J. Curran, J.D., LL.M., S.M.Hyg.
Seymour Pollack, M.D.

When participating in functions relating to the courts and the penal system, mental health professionals constantly face issues of value conflict between their own disciplines and the values expressed and enforced in the administration of justice. These issues are most starkly apparent in the forensic aspects of the work, the offering of testimony, and the making of reports.[1-6] They appear also, however, in treatment settings, either in the courts or in jails and prisons.[7-10] As pointed out in earlier writings by Pollack,[11,12] these activities require that mental health professionals apply their specialized knowledge and skills to the ends of law. The rules of law must be followed in these activities. The forensic psychiatrist or psychologist cannot substitute personal values or personally determined clinical judgment inappropriately when the legal requirements call for a particular standard to be applied. For example, the current legal standards in most American states for involuntary commitment to a mental hospital are quite strict and limited in application to seriously mentally disturbed patients who, unless hospitalized and treated, present an immediate threat to themselves or to other people. An examining clinician must apply this standard in order to effect a commitment order. The clinician cannot apply a lower, less urgent standard because the clinician wants, or the patient or family requests, an involuntary hospitalization. The same requirements apply to other civil and criminal law areas where legal standards are combined with certain mental status determinations. These are what lawyers call "mixed questions" of law and fact, or law and expert scientific determinations. Examples of these mixed questions are the criminal responsibility of the mentally ill or retarded, mental capacity to stand criminal trial, and mental capacity to prepare a valid will

---

* This chapter contains material from the chapter "Psychiatry and the Administration of Justice" by the late Dr. Pollack, which appeared in Curran, WJ, McGarry, AL, and Petty, CS (eds): *Modern Legal Medicine, Psychiatry, and Forensic Science.* F.A. Davis, Philadelphia, 1980. The current chapter was prepared by Dr. Curran.

passing property after death. In past years, many—if not most—mental health professionals preparing reports for court on patients sent to mental hospitals for observation and evaluation on these questions had only a smattering of knowledge about the required legal standards. No matter what the questions asked, the clinicians would answer in regard to the existence of serious, treatable mental illness (psychosis)—in total disregard of the legal standards.[13-15] Currently, forensic training in the required rules of the mental health–legal field is required in accreditation of residency training programs in psychiatry for board certification by the American Board of Psychiatry and Neurology. Also, minimum standards of training and experience are currently being developed for the subspecialties of forensic psychiatry and psychology. (See the review of these standards described in chapter 1 of this text.)

This chapter deals with ethical problems and dilemmas that mental health professionals face in performing forensic services. Later parts of the chapter deal with ethical conflicts in other settings, particularly treatment programs in high-security facilities for criminal offenders.

FORENSIC PSYCHIATRY AND PSYCHOLOGY AS LEGAL FACT-FINDING

The subspecialties of forensic psychiatry and psychology are now well recognized in the administration of justice and in penal settings. The instrumental application of these subspecialties to court matters is highly visible to other participants in the system, including judges, lawyers, the litigating parties, and witnesses, and to the observing mass media. The tasks of the forensic expert are very broad, because the mental status of the person and that person's functioning behavioral capacity are relevant to a range of significant legally related activities. These include areas of both civil and criminal law. The range of issues is summarized in Figure 3-1.

The role of the mental health forensic expert is essentially that of a fact-finder for the court. In performing these fact-finding roles, the forensic specialist is an instrument of the law following legal requirements. As a witness, he or she is immune to suit for the consequences of the testimony. When serving as a court-appointed impartial expert to determine a convicted defendant's potential for future dangerous conduct, the U.S. Supreme Court in *Estelle v. Smith* described the activity as that of "agent of the State."[16] There are, however, decisions to the contrary in other types of court-appointed examinations.[17] When the forensic examination is conducted on behalf of a party to the litigation, we would nevertheless hold the activity to be legally oriented and instrumental, seeking proper ends and cooperation between law and mental health objectives. In these situations, the forensic mental health expert must follow legal standards applicable to the particular examinations and the ethical requirements described in the previous chapter.

REQUIREMENTS FOR FORENSIC EXAMINATIONS

The forensic examination, as noted above, must be conducted under both legal and ethical requirements. Clinical standards for assessment by forensic psychologists are described in chapter 5, "Psychological Assessment in Legal Contexts" and chapter 21, "The Psychologist as Expert Witness." Clinical standards

Criminal Defendant $\longrightarrow$	Competent to stand trial?
Criminal Defendant $\longrightarrow$	Criminally responsible, or "insane"?
Child Witness $\longrightarrow$	Mature enough to testify?
Rape Victim $\longrightarrow$	Credible, or psychotic fantasy?
Offender $\longrightarrow$	Dangerous to release?
Mental Patient $\longrightarrow$	Dangerous to community?
Parent $\longrightarrow$	Responsible enough to have custody of child?
Testator $\longrightarrow$	Competent to make a valid will?
Contracting Party $\longrightarrow$	Competent to make binding contract?

FIGURE 3-1. The range of legal issues examined by forensic psychiatrists and psychologists as fact-finders is summarized here.

for psychiatric assessments are reviewed in chapter 4, "Forensic Psychiatric Reports" and chapter 22, "The Psychiatrist as Expert Witness." For assessments in special legal categories, see particularly chapters 6, 7, 8, and 11.

The forensic examination should be limited to exploration of those aspects of the person's mental status and past history that are relevant to the questions asked by the court or the attorney retaining the examiner. Other extraneous areas should be avoided. Efforts of the persons to seek advice or comment from the examiner either on their legal problems or on possible treatment opportunities should be avoided. The only exception to the latter area would be when a part of the legal questions to be addressed include the person's suitability for a treatment program. Examples of these evaluations in recent years are those of drug- and alcohol-dependent persons who are criminal defendants. Laws in several states provide for court-ordered examinations of such persons and allow diversion from the criminal system for defendants found suitable for treatment for these conditions.[19]

The forensic examination should be voluntary and conducted with the **informed consent** of the person. As noted in chapter 2, the *Miranda*-type of warning should be provided in all instances of a pretrial examination. As indicated in that chapter, a court-ordered examination prior to appointment of counsel for the accused defendant is regarded as unethical. In any type of forensic examination, court-ordered or privately provided, the person to be examined should be told the name of the examiner, his or her background (psychologist, psychiatrist, and so forth), the circumstances of the examination and evaluation, and their relationship to the person's problem. The person should be told that the examination is for legal purposes and not for treatment. In those instances in which the examination is imposed by judicial order, the person should still be informed that he or she may decline to cooperate, subject to possible legal sanctions. For example, in some jurisdictions, if the person refuses to be examined in a court-ordered evaluation, he or she may be foreclosed from introducing into evidence any private practitioner's opinion about his or her mental condition or from raising mental condition issues at a subsequent trial.

The forensic examiner should become accustomed to the fact that the person's legal counsel will often wish to be present during any interviewing or psychological testing. Statutes in some jurisdictions provide for the presence of the person's attorney in criminal action court-ordered examinations.[20]

The person should be informed that the forensic examination is not confidential in the United States.[11,15] Under current law in Canada, the forensic examination under court order for clinical defendants is described as confidential.[21] However, the actual practice may be similar to that of American states, because most American jurisdictions now bar court-ordered forensic examiners from testifying on any statements to them by the defendant concerning commission of the crime.[22]

When the psychiatrist or psychologist is retained by a private attorney to examine a client for forensic purposes, the attorney often accompanies the person to the interview and remains throughout the evaluation. Some professionals are not comfortable with the attorney present during the entire interview and they feel that the examined person will not disclose necessary material in such circumstances. When statutes do not apply to private evaluations, the matter of attorney presence will need to be settled cooperatively between the mental health professional and the attorney. It is common for the private attorney or the client to assume that the forensic examination will be confidential and that the examiner cannot be required by a court to reveal confidences and the results of an evaluation. Under many circumstances, this will be true. However, modern legal discovery practice requires disclosure of the names of experts retained and intended for use in court actions, including criminal defenses. In personal injury cases, including medical malpractice, it may be necessary to provide a private evaluator's report to the defendant or insurance company counsel in order to obtain an adequate settlement. In a criminal action, an important federal court opinion[23] ruled that a psychiatrist privately retained by the defense to evaluate criminal responsibility but not called as a witness for the defense could be called to the witness stand and required to reveal the results of the evaluation as a witness for the prosecution. We know of no other case coming to this conclusion prior to this opinion.

CONFLICTS OF VALUES FOR WITNESSES

The most serious problems occur when the forensic specialist has difficulty accepting the ends sought by the law. The issue of capital punishment probably arouses the most intense emotional and ethical conflicts. Many professional practitioners refuse to examine a party subject to the death penalty or refuse to examine a convicted person who is subject to sentence to death. Since involvement in the trial of Sirhan Sirhan for the murder of Senator Robert Kennedy, Seymour Pollack regularly refused participation in trials in which capital punishment might result.

Some practitioners regularly refuse to examine a party who seeks to use the insanity defense in a criminal trial on the ground that they find the legal standards inconsistent with their personal value systems or with their opinions of what psychiatry can offer to the functional issue contained in the legal standard. Earlier objections were concerned mainly with the M'Naughten-type right-wrong test unmitigated by an irresistible-impulse rule. In later years, refusal to testify has been extended to include most of the known legal rules of criminal responsibility.

Any practitioner is, of course, ethically justified in refusing participation in legal cases where he or she has a fundamental ethical or moral disagreement with the standards or ends of the law. The practitioner cannot, however, accept involvement and then, without disclosing the intention, apply a personal standard in place of the law. For example, a forensic examiner cannot ethically make a knowingly false report of "insanity" because the examiner does not personally accept the morality of capital punishment or disagrees with the jurisdiction's legal standards of criminal responsibility. Forensic examiners cannot ignore the legal tests of competency to stand criminal trial and find every psychotic person incompetent. In each of these situations, the professional forensic scientist corrupts his or her role as a legally authorized fact-finder and becomes a self-appointed social decision-maker in secret defiance of the rules of society.

FORENSIC CONSULTATION AND ADVOCACY

The question is often posed whether or not a forensic psychiatrist or psychologist, or any other forensic scientist, may ethically limit consultations to one side in litigation; for example, appearing for only the local prosecutor or for only the defense counsel who retains one's services.

There seems to be no specific ethical rule against this practice. It should be observed, of course, that some forensic scientists work full-time in a police scientific laboratory available only to the local police and prosecutors for investigations.

Many forensic specialists evaluate largely for one side or another and are rarely called by lawyers opposed to that side. It does seem inadvisable, however, for independently practicing forensic specialists to answer requests for evaluations only from one side. The reputations of such professionals are usually hurt by this limited availability. The impression is created that the forensic consultant is a "hired gun" for prosecutors or defense lawyers, respectively. The problem is compounded for psychiatrists because of the subjective nature of their examinations and findings. It is often said that psychiatrists' opinions can be "bought" more securely because their fraudulent views cannot easily be exposed. As it was put by a New York City lawyer, later turned sociologist:

> The brutal fact, which every criminal lawyer learns early in his career, is that psychiatric testimony is for sale. . . . The entire glossary of psychiatry is available for purchase, not because of corruption, but simply because

of the incredible flexibility and vacuousness of its diagnostic labels and pigeonholes.[24]

This observation was made in the mid-1960s and could be considered out-of-date, owing to more recent tightening up of diagnostic classifications and acceptable methods of evaluation as required in the *Diagnostic and Statistical Manual*, ed 3 (*DSM III*). Nevertheless, the subjective nature of some psychiatric testimony makes it difficult for the honorable professional to prove that opinions are unbiased and responsible. Psychiatric witnesses should follow the requirements of *DSM III* and be ready to support opinions with objective findings. To avoid accusations of bias, forensic specialists should, where feasible, vary their legal work in terms of side represented (prosecution, plaintiff, or defense) and content areas (criminal, civil of different types, and so forth). Of course, many forensic specialists do conduct nonpartisan psychiatric evaluations as full-time or part-time professional staff in court clinics[25,26] or in municipal, county, and metropolitan area forensic service programs.[27] The temptation in these settings is to become unduly close to the police and prosecutors with whom one associates quite routinely over a period of time. One should try to keep a professional distance from these law enforcement officials in order to maintain a nonpartisan and objective attitude and role.

JUSTICE AND THE TREATMENT ROLE

When psychiatrists and psychologists provide treatment to criminal offenders, they are often in conflict concerning the selection of patients and the purposes of therapy. The selection of patients should always constitute an independent judgment by the therapist based on clinical diagnosis, need for treatment, and the therapist's estimate of the effectiveness of treatment with the particular offender-patient. Realistically, however, the court or prison has a limited population base of persons with particular psychiatric diagnoses. Prison authorities would prefer that the therapists concentrate on offenders who are "causing trouble," or "acting strange and bothering people," or who are clearly emotionally disturbed, such as those making suicide attempts by trying to hang themselves or by swallowing ground glass. Suicides in prison, or in jail cells, are understandably very embarrassing and disturbing personally for prison authorities. In this respect, the referring group is often the prison, not the prisoner. The experienced psychiatrist and psychologist learn to listen to the prison keepers but not to answer every request. Clinical forensic services are a liaison function, not an independent therapeutic practice. There must be an accommodation between what the therapists believe they can do effectively and what the prison or court authorities press upon them, often quite unrealistically, both in numbers of referrals and in expectation that the therapists can do anything with the offender's problem. (For further discussion, see chapter 19 "Correctional Psychiatry.")

The psychiatrist or psychologist in a prison setting is often said to represent the expected morality of the social world outside the prison. The therapist is expected to help the offender-patient examine his or her past life and to take personal responsibility for antisocial conduct. Actually, this role is not very different from that of the therapist "on the outside." In an important paper on ethics in psychiatry, the late Swedish psychiatrist, Clarence Blomquist, opened

FOUNDATIONS OF FORENSIC PSYCHIATRY AND PSYCHOLOGY

his review by asserting, "Psychotherapy can be said to be a sort of applied ethic. The hidden question is always: 'How ought I (to) live my life?'"[28]

Blomquist observed that all of psychotherapy deals with values. It acts on certain assumptions about what it is good to seek in life and what it is best to avoid in the search for happiness, peace of mind, security, and success. It also assumes a basic capacity in most people to assume responsibility for their conduct.

As expressed by Seymour Halleck in a recent paper, "Because psychotherapy deals with issues such as explanation, volition, reinforcement, and punishment, it is a process in which the issue of individual responsibility regularly arises."[29]

In the same paper, Halleck associated his concern for responsibility with his work in a legal setting:

> As a psychiatric criminologist who has struggled with the issue of insanity defense for almost thirty years, I have become convinced that the extent and manner to which we hold people responsible for their behavior is a critical factor not only in governing them, but also in educating them and helping them to change their behavior.[30]

It should also be realized, however, that prisons do not encourage inmates to take responsibility, inasmuch as so much of prison life is controlled and channeled toward conformity to the security system. As Halleck[31] pointed out in an earlier book on legal psychiatry, the prison system contains elements that are more apt to aggravate or to cause mental illness than the stress experienced in most environments outside the prison (Fig. 3-2). Any newly appointed prison-based therapist should be aware of these stresses, individually and in various combinations, when examining, diagnosing, and treating patients in a prison setting.

PRISON STRESS LEADING TO MENTAL ILLNESS

1. **The absence of close interpersonal relationship with family and loved ones.**
2. **Denial of normal or acceptable sexual outlets.**
3. **Enforced idleness and physical inactivity for prisoners in young adult years, usually the most vigorous in life.**
4. **Denial of participation in socially useful activities that can add a feeling of personal worth and contribution to family and social life.**
5. **Vigorous discouragement of activist tendencies such as political reform and prisoner organization.**
6. **Deprivation of a sense of autonomy and personal decision making.**
7. **Frequent imposition of solitary confinement and cell "lock up" which constitutes a form of sensory deprivation.**

FIGURE 3-2. Seymour Halleck's[32] configuration of prison-life stresses leading to mental illness are summarized here.

CONFIDENTIALITY IN LEGAL
AND CORRECTIONAL SETTINGS

Among the most difficult ethical issues for mental health professionals in the forensic field are those relating to patient confidences. The pressures of the setting are designed to make the preserving of confidences difficult. At times, the professional may wish to reveal confidences in order to gain important considerations on behalf of the best interests of a defendant or inmate. Such disclosures should be made only with permission of the patient or client.

The *Tarasoff* decision[32] of the Supreme Court of California is currently being cited as controlling for all types of situations, including legal and correctional settings, as noted in chapter 2, when disclosures of confidences are made without permission of the patient or client in the interest of patient safety or the safety of other persons. It is therefore important to review the circumstances of that case and the reaction to it in the professions. In that decision, the court imposed an affirmative duty on psychologists and psychiatrists to warn a young woman of threats against her life by a patient in therapy at the health service of the Berkeley campus of the University of California. The court cited the AMA Code of Ethics, which at that time allowed, but did not require, physicians to breach patient confidentiality when advisable for the protection of the patient or the community. The court converted the discretionary breach of confidence into an affirmative obligation to disclose the threats to the person threatened, even though the university health service had tried to get the patient committed as mentally ill. The campus police had refused to file the commitment papers and had, in their discretion, been satisfied to warn the patient (a graduate student) to stay away from the young woman. The young man promised the police he would do no harm to the woman and so they released him.

The university health service and its psychologists and psychiatrists were apparently satisfied with the campus police disposition of the matter and took no further action. The young man later killed the young woman. The parents brought a negligence action against the campus police and the health service personnel. The case against the police, the primary defendants, was dismissed on the basis of a statutory immunity in the discretionary action of not moving to commit the young man. The case was brought forward and sustained against the health service personnel. The California Supreme Court concluded that the affirmative duty to protect the third party was defined by the scope and severity of the threatened danger; in this case, death. The court found it foreseeable to the mental health professionals that if nothing were done, the young man would kill the woman.

The *Tarasoff* decision sought and found negligence liability in a quite remote source from those directly at fault. The young graduate student who killed the woman was the obvious key perpetrator, but he had no money. The California Supreme Court, being unable to find the police responsible because of the immunity statute, reached behind them and found the therapists (and the university as employer) responsible. Were not the therapists' ethical and legal duties fully discharged when they reported the matter to the police and sought the commitment of the mentally disturbed patient? The court refused to rule so. The judges concluded that the therapists should have known that there was a continuing danger to the young woman despite the police warning to the patient. Therefore, the therapists should have warned her parents. (The young woman was out of the country but was due to return to California in a few months.)

The *Tarasoff* case was generally supported by legal commentators, with some exceptions.[33-36] Stress in law review comments was usually upon the need to compensate victims of severe violence. Reaction by mental health commentators was more mixed. Those who favored the decision tended to point to the consistency of the opinion with ethical obligations, albeit discretionary in the ethical codes, to breach confidentiality when specific dangers of violent conduct to others were revealed to the professional by the patient.[37-39] Stone criticized the case as disruptive of the patient-therapist relationship, in which the need to protect confidences needs support and understanding by the courts.[40] The decision had repercussions upon therapists' malpractice insurance premiums because of the potential for increasing the vulnerability of therapists to suit by victims of violently disturbed patients.[41]

The California courts have not retreated from the decision, although later cases have tended to limit its application to identifiable persons threatened by the patient.[42,43] A psychologist was held to have a duty not only to an identified victim but to the victim's minor child.[44] Other state courts have followed the *Tarasoff* rule in cases involving threatened personal violence not only to an identifiable person[45] but to a more general public.[46,47] One case extended the rule to negligent release of a disturbed patient from a state hospital wherein the patient drove a motor vehicle recklessly, injuring the plaintiff.[48] Actually, several courts have held hospitals liable for injuries to the patient or other persons following negligent release of the patient without need to cite the *Tarasoff* rule.[49-51]

The *Tarasoff* ruling tends to provoke less opposition from therapists in legal and correctional settings than from those in private practice. The patient in legal and correctional settings is already under considerable restrictions on freedom of action. The therapist is not privately retained by the inmate or defendant but is supplied by and paid by the facility. It is clear that the mental health professional has obligations to the facility in regard to matters of safety and security. Experienced therapists in such settings will keep confidences about previous misconduct in the lives of patients, with the possible exception of a serious crime for which another innocent person was convicted or is now being held on the charges. In both outpatient and in-prison treatment, the therapist remains free ethically to disclose information concerning the patient's future plans to commit violent acts against others or to commit other serious misconduct that could develop into harm to others or to the patient or result in serious property loss. In the prison setting, the therapist is bound to tell prison authorities of disclosure of plans to commit a prison break, serious disruption, or serious violation of prison rules. In such situations, the mental health professional should inform the prisoner-patient before therapy begins and again, if possible, as the disclosures are about to be made that the therapist is bound to disclose such plans to the prison authorities. Professionals new to the prison setting, uncertain of their role between the correctional staff and the prisoners, often make the mistake of disregarding their obligations to the prison authorities on these matters in order to gain "the trust of the prisoner-patients." This posture can be quite dangerous. The therapist may become compromised and may become part of the secret conspiracy. The prisoner or prisoners then "have something on the doctor," and they may use it against the therapist to induce him or her into further helping the effort, concealing material evidence of misconduct, and helping in other illegal actions such as supplying drugs and other contraband to the inmates. (The problems of therapist relationships, of being a "double agent" in such settings, are reviewed in the next chapter.)

There is no doubt that a prison setting in particular can be very disturbing to a professional person trained in the helping and healing arts. The prison can be a brutalizing experience, not only for the offender inmates but for all the prison staff. The bitter concentration on security, the unmitigating enforcement of what will often seem dehumanizing rules, and feelings of despair of ever accomplishing therapeutic goals will make prison work discouraging and unrewarding for many professionals in psychology and psychiatry. Many will not continue the work; those who do will develop professional standards that allow their roles to be clear and unambiguous. They will remain dedicated to trying to help many deserving, sick inmates going through an experience no one in the outside community can understand or appreciate. (For further examination of these issues, see Dr. Roth's discussion in chapter 19, "Correctional Psychiatry.")

Therapist as "Double Agent"

In response to concerns over what were felt to be abuses of the role of psychiatrists in the Soviet Union, particularly their role in involuntary commitment and forced psychiatric "treatment" of political dissenters in Russia, the American Psychiatric Association and the Institute of Society, Ethics, and the Life Sciences cosponsored a conference on "The Psychiatrist as a Double Agent" at Hastings, New York. The published proceedings contain discussion by several leading psychiatrists and ethicists gathered at the conference.[52] The participants reviewed the role and the conflicting loyalties of psychiatrists in the United States in serving the state as therapists and as forensic specialists in the American courts, prisons, mental hospitals, the military, and in public schools (Fig. 3-3). The proceedings as a whole are fully worthy of reading and reflection.

It was not made evident from the discussion that conflict of loyalties was any worse in one setting than in another. In each field, therapists experienced problems in representing the best interests of patients and in maintaining

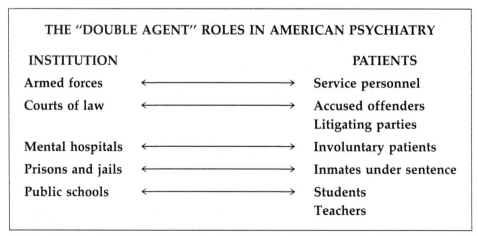

FIGURE 3-3. Conflicting loyalties discussed at the conference "In the Service of the State: The Psychiatrist as a Double Agent,"[52] are illustrated here.

FOUNDATIONS OF FORENSIC PSYCHIATRY AND PSYCHOLOGY

confidentiality from the officials of the system. In each setting, the therapist is said to prefer following "the private-practitioner model," not a coercive one. Psychiatrists do not enjoy viewing themselves as agents of social control or as administrators within the various systems.

Dr. Gerald Klerman asked, "Is it possible to separate the clinical role from the administrative one? In general, we in psychiatry have a tremendous propensity to mix these roles. We want to treat people clinically, but we also want to save the world. We do this anywhere: in schools, in prisons, in the military."[53]

When addressing problems of prison psychiatry more specifically, the participants stressed the dilemma of encouraging "adult behavior" on the part of prison inmates, thereby siding with society's interests in social control. They also discussed the demoralization of the therapist in being forced to deal with the famous question from Plato: Is it possible to be a just man in an unjust society?

Dr. Fritz Redlich, however, expressed doubt about differences between moral obligations in private psychiatric practice and in prison work. In the key area of confidentiality, for example, he asserted that a "serious risk of a crime" would have to be reported in private practice as well as in prison.[54] Dr. Alan Stone urged full disclosure to persons in courts and prisons about the fact that the psychiatrist is not free to keep confidences. He urged that such psychiatrists should wear a large "I" for "inquisitor" on their foreheads as a visible warning that they were interviewing the person for administrative purposes or legal purposes. Dr. Klerman returned to the discussion to disagree, saying that his experience was "the exact opposite."[55] Prisoners, or students at medical school, were not fooled into trusting psychiatrists. On the contrary, the psychiatrists in these settings generally found that their patients were very careful not to reveal damaging information. He observed that the same practice took place in mental hospitals where the patients knew that they couldn't tell the high-status psychiatrist what was "going on" because the therapist would surely tell the hospital administrators.

Although little in the way of consensus was revealed in the published proceedings, it was made clear that most of the participants recognized that psychiatrists in these settings have administrative or instrumental obligations to the systems in which they practice as well as ethical obligations to their patients.

In the legal settings of the courts and prisons, the primary obligations of the mental health professional must be to serve justice, to perform effectively in professional work, and to maintain respect for fundamental human rights within the American legal system.

REFERENCES

1. MILLER, RD: *The treating psychiatrist as forensic evaluator.* J Forensic Sci 29:825, 1984.

2. PERLIN, MD: *The legal status of the psychologist in court.* Mental Disability Law Reporter 4:194, 1980.

3. STONE, AA: *Law, Psychiatry, and Morality.* American Psychiatric Press, Washington, DC, 1984.

4. BEIS, EB: *Mental Health and the Law.* Aspen, Rockland, MD, 1984.

5. BLOMQUIST, CDD: *Some ethical problems in psychiatry.* Ethics in Science and Medicine 6:105, 1979.

6. LOFTUS, E AND MONAHAN, J: *Trial by data: Psychological research as legal evidence.* Am Psychol 35:270, 1980.

7. TARDIFF, K: *The Psychiatric Uses of Seclusion and Restraint.* American Psychiatric Press, Washington, DC, 1984.

8. HERMANN, D: *Assault on the insanity defense: Limitations on the effectiveness and effect of the defense of insanity.* Rutgers Law Journal 14:241, 1983.

9. ROTH, L: *Treating the incarcerated offender.* Journal of Social Therapy 15:4, 1969.

10. KETAI, R: *Role conflicts of the prison psychiatrist.* Bull Am Acad Psychiatry Law 2:246, 1974.

11. POLLACK, S: *The role of psychiatry in the rule of law.* Psychology Annals 4:8, 1974.

12. POLLACK, S: *Psychiatric consultation for the court.* In MANDEL, J AND SOLOMON, P (EDS): *Psychiatric Consultation.* Grune & Stratton, New York, 1967.

13. SZASZ, T: *Psychiatric expert testimony—its covert meaning and social functions.* Psychiatry 3:313, 1957.

14. SLOVENKO, R: *Psychiatry and Law.* Little, Brown & Co, Boston, 1973.

15. MCGARRY, AL: *Competency for trial and due process via the state hospital.* Am J Psychiatry 122:623, 1965.

16. 451 U.S. 454 at 467, 1981.

17. Anderson v. Glismann, 577 F. Supp. 1506 (D. Colo., 1984).

18. PORTER, AL, ARIF, A, CURRAN, WJ: *Legislation on Treatment of Drug and Alcohol Dependent Persons.* World Health Organization, Geneva, 1984. (This is a comparative survey of legislation in 43 countries.)

19. See, for example, Massachusetts General Laws, Ch. 111E; P.L. 89-793, Federal Narcotic Addict Rehabilitation Act.

20. See, for example, New York Criminal Process Law, Section 250.10(3).

21. Canadian Criminal Code Sections 465 and 738; For analysis, see SHARPE, G: *Discussion paper, mental disorder project.* Department of Justice, Ottawa, Canada, 1983.

22. See, for example, Massachusetts General Laws, Ch. 223, Section 12.

23. United States v. Smith, 425 F. Supp. 1038 (U.S. DC, E.D., N.Y., 1976).

24. BLUMBERG, AS: *Criminal Justice.* Quadrangle Books, Chicago, 1967, p 148.

25. ROBITSCHER, JB: *The new fact of legal psychiatry.* Am J Psychiatry 129:315, 1972.

26. HOFFMAN, J, SHOWALTER, FC, WHITEHEAD, C: *A forensic psychiatry clinic in evolution.* Journal of Psychiatry and the Law 2:423, 1974.

27. WEBSTER, CD, MENZIES, MA, BUTLER, MD, TURNER, RE: *Forensic psychiatric assessment in selected Canadian cities.* Can J Psychiatry 27:455, 1982.

28. BLOMQUIST, op cit.

29. HALLECK, S: *The concept of responsibility in psychotherapy.* Am J Psychother 36:292, 1982.

30. Ibid, 293.

31. HALLECK, S: *Psychiatry and the Dilemmas of Crime.* Harper & Row, New York, 1967.

32. Tarasoff v. Regents of the University of California, 529 P.2d 553, 1974; 551 P.2d 334, 1976.

33. *Tarasoff and the psychotherapist's duty to warn.* San Diego Law Rev 12:932, 1975.

34. *Untangling Tarasoff: Tarasoff v. Regents of the University of California.* Hastings Law Journal 29:179, 1977.

35. *Professional obligation and the duty to rescue: When must a psychiatrist protect his patient's intended victim?* Yale Law Journal 91:1430, 1982.

36. CURRAN, WJ: *Confidentiality and the prediction of dangerousness in psychiatry.* N Engl J Med 293:285, 1975.

37. Leonard, JB: *A therapist's duty to potential victims: A non-threatening view of Tarasoff.* Law and Human Behavior 1:309, 1977.

38. Roth, L and Meisel, A: *Dangerousness, confidentiality and the duty to warn.* Am J Psychiatry 13:508, 1977.

39. Shah, SA: *Dangerousness: A paradigm for exploring some issues in law and psychology.* Am Psychol 33:224, 1978.

40. Stone, A: *The Tarasoff decisions: Suing psychotherapists to safeguard society.* Harvard Law Review 90:358, 1976.

41. *Where the public peril begins: A survey of psychotherapists to determine the effects of Tarasoff.* Stanford Law Review 31:165, 1978.

42. Thompson v. County of Alameda, 27 Cal. 3d 741, 1980.

43. Mayroudis v. Superior Court, 102 Cal. App. 2d 594, 1980.

44. Hedlund v. Superior Court, 194 Cal. Rptr., 243, 1983.

45. McIntosh v. Milano, 168 N.J. Super. 466, 1979.

46. Davis v. Lhim, 124 Mich. App. 291, 1983.

47. Lipari v. Sears, Roebuck and Co., 497 F. Supp. 185 (D. Neb., 1980).

48. Petersen v. Washington, 671 P. 2d 230 (Washington, 1983).

49. Homere v. State of New York, 370 N.Y.S. 2d 246, 1975.

50. Martin v. Washington Hospital Center, 423 A. 2d 913 (Fed. D.C. App., 1980).

51. Bradley Center, Inc. v. Wessner, 161 Ga. App. 576; aff'd., 250 Ga. 199 (1982).

52. *In the service of the state: The psychiatrist as a double agent: A conference on conflicting loyalties.* Hasting Cent Rep (Special Suppl) 5:1, 1978.

53. Ibid, 5.

54. Ibid, 8.

55. Ibid, 9.

PART 2
ASSESSMENT AND TREATMENT IN FORENSIC SETTINGS

This section of our text is the longest and most ambitious. It contains the largest number of chapters, reviewing a wide spectrum of applications of professional skills in forensic psychiatry and psychology. In great measure, these chapters form the core of the practical substance of everyday professional activity. Without these skills, the forensic specialist is incompetent to provide quality service to the American system of justice.

The authors in this section had the obligation of providing an up-to-date description of the knowledge and skills needed for professional assessment and treatment in their subject areas. They also were expected to describe relevant research developments and to give attention to applicable legal standards of concern for that area. Unlike many other fields of forensic medicine and science, the mental health field contains specific legal standards imposed upon scientific assessment. Forensic specialists in psychiatry and psychology must be aware of these legal rules and must be able to apply them in clinical situations in which the legal standards are controlling.

The six chapters in this part are organized structurally in relation to the skills demanded in practice. The first two chapters are of a general nature, and the next four deal with more particular applications to special legal subjects.

The first two contributions outline the basic knowledge and skills required in forensic psychiatry and psychology. There is material of benefit to both professions in the two efforts, but differences in approach and testing procedures are stressed in order to avoid unnecessary overlapping.

Chapter 4 on forensic psychiatry by Dr. McGarry is a complete reworking of his contribution to the earlier text, owing in large part to a fundamental development in psychiatry since that writing: the publication of the third edition of the official diagnostic manual of the American Psychiatric Association, generally known as *DSM III*. In Dr. McGarry's judgment, the new manual ushers in a new era of greater precision and rigor in psychiatric diagnosis of particular significance to forensic psychiatry. He offers warnings, however, of some problems in courtroom application of the new material in *DSM III* in relation to broad implications of criminal and civil intent and the standards of criminal responsibility of the mentally disturbed. He points also to inconsistencies and confusions in the manual that can lead to difficulties in legal interpretation.

Chapter 5 on psychological assessment is comprehensive and scholarly in a manner probably not achieved in any other publication on forensic psychology. Dr. Grisso emphasizes that psychological assessments in legal settings require more than the mere application of traditional procedures developed for clinical and general research purposes. Throughout his review, he stresses the special demands placed upon the mental health examiner in forensic work. The chapter provides practical advice concerning courtroom testimony based upon specific forensic psychological tests constructed to answer complex legal issues. It is pointed out that these test results have such high relevance to the ultimate legal questions in the litigation that they may lead psychologists and courts to believe that the test results essentially answer the legal question. The author agrees with assertions by Monahan, Shah, and others that the ultimate decision should be that of a judge, not a mental health forensic specialist. This is the first chapter in the text in which "ultimate question" issues are discussed; it will not be the last.

The other four chapters in this part deal with specific areas of forensic assessment.

Chapter 6 examines one of the most controversial questions in the entire field of forensic behavioral science: the prediction of future dangerous conduct on the part of mentally ill persons and criminal offenders. Unlike most writers in this field, Dr. Gable also offers observations on treatment of dangerous persons. The extensive literature in this field on the reliability—and unreliability—of predictive efforts is thoroughly analyzed. The central problem addressed in most of the writing has been related to overprediction of dangerousness in persons who, in follow-up studies, have proved otherwise. In an updated version of his chapter from the earlier text, Dr. Gable examines recently proposed limitations on psychiatric and psychological testimony on issues of future dangerousness. These proposals are also discussed in later chapters concerned with courtroom testimony.

The remaining chapters in part 2 are completely new contributions, not built in any appreciable degree on work in the previous text. The earlier book, covering legal medicine and all the forensic sciences, concentrated attention on state-of-the-art methods as practiced by the foremost leaders in each of the specialties examined. In a single volume of 56 chapters, we could hardly do more. Only limited space could be afforded to essentially legal issues and legal reforms. The approach of this new volume is quite different. Much more attention is given throughout the book to the legal environment and to needed legal reforms. This is nowhere more evident than in these three chapters on mental competency to stand criminal trial, legal responsibility of the mentally ill, and responsibility and competency issues in the criminal field for the developmentally disabled.

Chapter 7, "Assessment of Competency to Stand Criminal Trial," offers an in-depth analysis of the forensic assessment issues involved in the field. Dr. Grisso and his colleague, Ms. Seigel, describe the legal standards for trial fitness and the procedural stages of a competency determination. Varying judicial practices are reviewed, and data are provided on the significance of competency determinations in the criminal justice and correctional systems. The special forensic assessment instruments available for trial competency evaluations are analyzed in detail. The most widely accepted are the competency screening test (CST) and the competency assessment instrument (CAI). The different uses for each are explained. In reporting results to the courts, the authors note the differing views on whether the forensic assessment should include an answer to the so-called ultimate question: the defendant's fitness to stand trial. The authors seem reluctant to answer the ultimate question, although they conclude that the matter of limitations on the forensic evaluator's testimony has not as yet been resolved.

Chapter 8 in this section concerns criminal responsibility. Even more than in the competency field, a review of issues of criminal responsibility in the middle and later 1980s must be an examination of reform movements. The climate of the law has changed dramatically since the preparation of the previous volume, owing greatly to certain highly publicized cases, particularly the trial and acquittal of John Hinckley, Jr., on insanity grounds for the attempted assassination of President Reagan. Other factors that have provided a favorable environment for these reform efforts are described in this chapter. In a thoughtful concluding portion, Dr. Shah examines policy matters not necessarily addressed in any of the reform efforts. These concern such issues as the significance of mental health diagnostic categories to the legal definition of mental illness or defect (especially in the advent of the expansive nature of *DSM III*), the scope of expert forensic testimony by psychiatrists and psychologists in this field, the dispositional questions left to the court when defendants are acquitted on insanity grounds, and the insidious effect of certain highly publicized crimes and trials upon rational discussion and analysis in this field. In this editor's opinion, these observations may well prove to be the most compelling aspect of the author's contribution to this subject.

The last chapter in this part examines issues in the criminal justice system concerning the developmentally disabled. Leading figures in university programs in psychology and law, authors Kindred and Sales review the problems in this field for persons diagnosed as having experienced mental disability from birth or early childhood, including mental retardation, autism, cerebral palsy, epilepsy, and other brain dysfunctions. The authors carry us through the various stages of an offender's contact with the law enforcement system and the courts and describe the difficulties and stresses that can be experienced by persons who are developmentally disabled. It is not a comforting view. Misunderstanding and worse can await the innocent and the guilty trying to cope with the experience. As the authors vividly point out, the person with cerebral palsy walking home at night may easily seem to be drunk; the patient having an epileptic seizure may be thought to be an illicit drug user; a mentally retarded youth's slow responses under questioning at a crime scene or in a jail cell may make him or her appear to be resistant and dissimulating. A developmentally disabled suspect under interrogation may waive his or her rights to counsel and to the privilege against self-incrimination because of a lack of awareness and understanding of the situation.

The chapter concludes with an examination of posttrial issues. It is suggested that judges and correctional systems should examine particular needs of this patient population when determining whether an offender should be placed on probation or in prison. There are several arguments against incarceration, including the potential for sexual exploitation of retarded persons and the limited resources and services for epileptic and other brain-damaged persons in closed institutions. The authors assert their position that offenders in this category are legally entitled to adequate treatment specific to their conditions while in prison facilities. They present a convincing argument that developmentally disabled offenders should not be subject to sentence to capital punishment under newly enacted reform statutes in this field.

CHAPTER 4

FORENSIC PSYCHIATRIC REPORTS: SELECTED CLINICAL TOPICS AND MODELS FOR REPORT PREPARATION

A. Louis McGarry, M.D.

The purpose of this chapter is to consider a series of applications of clinical psychiatric knowledge and skills to the needs of the American legal system. Included are discussions of memory, hypnosis, malingering, and the use and misuse for legal purposes of the diagnostic system found in the current psychiatric manual, *DSM III*.* These general discussions will be followed by an analysis of psycholegal issues in civil commitment proceedings. The chapter closes with a presentation of the principles to be applied and the elements required in preparing forensic psychiatric reports for the courts. An outline of a psychiatric report and excerpted examples of two such reports are included. These subjects have been chosen for analysis because of their importance to the pragmatic workings of the legal system.

MEMORY

Nothing in the clinical realm affecting the administration of justice is as pervasive or fundamental to credibility and probative value as memory. The testimony of every witness in a legal proceeding stands or falls on the accuracy of his or her memory. Although there is a vast literature on memory in general and there has been increased attention in recent years to the unsettling effects of hypnosis on the later testimony of hypnotized witnesses (this will be dealt with below), relatively little has been written that brings the insights and knowledge of the behavioral sciences specifically to the matter of memory in the legal system.

A massive amount of literature on perception and memory has emanated

---

* American Psychiatric Association: *Diagnostic and Statistical Manual of Mental Disorders,* ed 3. APA, Washington, DC, 1980.

from research psychologists. The extent to which the knowledge accumulated can be applied to the courtroom, however, is highly controversial.[1] On the matter of assisting juries in evaluating the credibility of eyewitness identification of perpetrators, for example, McCloskey and Egeth[2] are highly critical and see only a very limited acceptable role. Although acknowledging that this is a "stormy story," Loftus[3] defends the legitimacy of attempting to develop and to bring the findings of experimental psychology to jury consideration.

Throughout his astonishingly productive writings, Sigmund Freud was much preoccupied with memory. Indeed, this preoccupation could be described as the fundamental métier of the science and art of psychoanalysis. As early as 1906, Freud recommended in his paper *Psychoanalysis and the Ascertaining of Truth in Courts of Law*[4] that the techniques of word association then being developed, particularly by Jung, be applied, albeit cautiously and on an experimental basis, to the matter of revealing true and credible memory in legal matters. The use of projective psychological testing in legal settings may be seen as an indirect application of Freud's suggestion. (See description of forensic use of psychological testing in chapter 5.) Furthermore, Freud's central point, that we selectively and unconsciously do not remember that which is disagreeable or find it necessary to distort when we do remember that which is disagreeable, is directly applicable to legal situations. As Freud expressed it, "The view developed here, that distressing memories succumb especially easily to motivated forgetting, deserves to find application where no attention, or too little, has so far been paid to it. Thus it has still not been sufficiently strongly emphasized in assessing testimony in courts of law."[5]

Except when there has been the intervention of organic destruction of brain tissue, especially of the areas in and around the medial aspects of the temporal lobe, it appears that a significant memory once perceived and stored is never completely forgotten. For example, there is the extraordinary, well-known phenomenon of subjects who had spoken a foreign language at a very early age but had "forgotten" it, through long lack of use of that language, who then recover under hypnosis the ability to converse fluently in that language.

The process of remembering is tripartite, and each of the three subprocesses is subject to distortion. The first subprocess of memory involves perception. Courts of law are familiar with the extraordinary diversity with which an event is described by multiple observers of the event. An example of such a distortion is that of a college class being given only a brief glimpse of a chaotic scene involving violent participants, one of whom is a young black man. The class is then asked whether or not the black man had a knife in his hand. Some reply yes and some no. Whether a knife was perceived or not, aside from the fact of whether or not one was actually present, may well be affected by stereotypic racist or antiracist biases unique to the individual observer. Clearly differential perception will lead to different memories of the same event.

The second subprocess of memory is that of encoding or storage. There appears to be good evidence of a spatial locus in the brain for unique memories. For example, when discrete loci fire off abnormal electric discharges in certain temporal lobe epileptics, uniquely remembered visual scenes of the person's life may be hallucinated. Penfield[6] demonstrated that discrete memories could be triggered by the direct microelectrode stimulation of loci in the cortex of the temporal lobe of the brain of conscious patients. It is also true, at least empirically, that like or linked memories are either stored physically adjacent to each other or are otherwise connected and may "spill over" to one another in recall. Recalling a trip to Geneva, I misremembered the name of an unpleasantly expensive restaurant with demeaning service for those with rusty French as "The Diplomat." Actually the restaurant was named "The Senator." "The Diplomat" was in fact the name of a pleasant hotel where I stayed on the same visit.

The memory storage that we tend best to recall is mediated by pictorial as opposed to verbal referents.[7] With verbally encoded or stored memory, recall is consistently better with semantic cues in the form of subject categories as compared with structural cues in the form of the beginning letters of individual words.[8,9] But even in a student's attempt to recall a verbal passage in a textbook for purposes of delivery at examination time, its spatial locus on a page may be envisioned—thus the so-called photographic memory—and the student is thereby resorting to pictorial memory. The precision of police artist portraits drawn from eyewitness memory is another case in point supporting the superiority of pictorial memory. Recourse to spatial pictorial referents is well established in the courtroom as an effective means of recalling the scene and events of a crime.

The third subprocess of memory is retrieval. The example above of the misremembered name of a Geneva restaurant will do double duty as an example here. Contiguous in time and semantically similar, the name of the pleasant hotel, "The Diplomat," was inaccurately retrieved in place of the name of the unpleasant restaurant, "The Senator." Psychotherapists, for whom the precise language and manner of expression of their patients is of great significance, are familiar with the difficulties of exact retrieval of the spoken word or phrase. However, they often will astonish their patients with what appear to be feats of memory. Obviously the uniquely focused attention of the practiced and skillful therapist applies here. But relatively little can be precisely recalled even by the most conscientious and dedicated professional in postinterview recall. In examinations for psycholegal purposes, I have found audiotaping to be almost indispensible to precise recall for legal purposes. This practice also serves to unfetter the clinician so that verbal and affective communication, uninterrupted by note taking, leads to optimal data collection. Videotaping is, of course, even better because it sensitively records facial and bodily affectivity as well.

The conceptualization of memory discussed here is given some scientific support by disease states of the brain. In the Klüver-Bucy syndrome[10] the temporal lobes of Rhesus monkeys were discretely removed (a very rare event in human pathology, in which pathological states are almost invariably more diffuse.) The monkeys gave evidence that they perceived visual stimuli in the sense that the optic nerve "saw" the stimuli. The process of storing the memory of these new visual stimuli, however, was stopped by the destruction of the temporal lobes (a state described as visual agnosia) and other senses (touch, mouthing) had to be relied upon in the process of storage of a retrievable memory. Recent or new or "anterograde" memory in the Klüver-Bucy pathology is therefore severely compromised. In Korsakoff's psychosis, or Alcohol Amnestic Disorder (due to thiamine deficiency), such a state of severe recent memory loss is observed. In the Korsakoff pathology the afflicted person may confabulate or tell conflicting inaccurate stories in rapid succession. In doing so he or she is necessarily drawing upon older stored memories in order to communicate even the inaccurate material he or she reports. Thus although recent or anterograde memory is defective, some remote or retrograde stored memory is available, presumably from somewhere in the brain other than in the temporal lobes.[11]

With respect to memory in the psychological realm, trained clinicians do not or should not need a review of the meanings of the terms repression, denial, and suppression, but it has been my observation that in legal settings these psychological terms of art are often used imprecisely and give rise to confusion. This is especially true among lay consumers of our work, because the terms have lay connotations with moralistic overtones. The matter is rendered more complex by the fact that distorted or defective memory is often a mixture of these phenomena and may even be further complicated by an admixture of conscious lying. American courts have generally rejected amnesia as a basis for a finding of incompetency to stand trial or of lack of responsibility for a criminal act largely because the condition is thought to be too easily feigned.[12] An exception to this generalization is amnesia arising from severe head injury.[13] On those few occasions when I have been persuaded of the validity of an amnesia of psychogenic origin, as in a fugue or dissociative state, it has been noteworthy to me that the amnesia was not total. Scraps and flashes of the otherwise amnestic period were remembered.* In contrast, the claimed amnesia of the malingerer as well as many valid amnesias of genuine physical origin tend to be total.

For the sake of accuracy, then, it should be clear that the physically sound mind, at least in the unconscious, appears to remember everything of significance that has been stored. The liar consciously remembers but dissembles. In the use of denial as a defense, memory is preconscious. Thus it is available for recall, but it is not operative in decision making or behavior and may represent severe pathology when it is grossly discordant with reality. In repression, although sometimes recoverable through chemical, hypnotic, or psychoanalytic techniques, the forgetting is unconscious. In suppression, the memory is consciously and deliberately put out of one's mind; "I will not think about that now."

Textbooks usually have the virtue of containing clear, authoritative, general statements about the state of the art or science; what is known, at least, and optimally, what the limitations of that knowledge are. But they suffer from the impediment of being necessarily general and are at risk of being simplistic. The subject of memory should not be left without noting the complex and deleterious effects of various toxic and drug impingements on memory nor the effects of brain injury or disease. These have not been dealt with adequately here. Neither have I dealt with the phenomenon of deja vu in which events or places or persons appear to have an uncanny familiarity, not because they are in fact known or remembered but because they are reminiscent of psychodynamically familiar and displaced themes and events. I have not covered a great deal else, such as the biochemical bases of memory, which become increasingly esoteric for a chapter of this nature, designed to be of utilitarian application to the legal process.

---

* In the matter of memory, those of us who publish in texts such as this one cannot usually accurately remember where much of our knowledge or insights are acquired. Our gifted teachers and colleagues are unconsciously honored by the appropriation of their ideas. In this instance I do remember that this clinical insight originated with Dr. Alan A. Stone and was shared with me.

HYPNOSIS

The application of hypnosis in the courts has been fraught with confusion and even mischief. Unfortunately, the technique too readily lends itself to unreliable distortions, and in the wrong hands, even quackery.

Authorities in the field, notably Martin Orne,[14] have attempted to provide stringent safeguards for the acceptable introduction of hypnosis-derived data into legal proceedings, meeting the traditional *Frye* test[15] of judicial standards for admissible scientific evidence. In my opinion these suggested safeguards have not been successful and probably do not deserve to be. The problem of the reliability of recovered memory by means of hypnosis (and inferentially narcoanalysis as well) has been given recent attention in the appellate courts.[16,17] The psychiatrist Bernard Diamond has recently published a law review paper[18] in which he unequivocally states, "testimony by previously hypnotized witnesses should never be admitted into evidence." There is a clear trend that this view is being adopted in case law, although prehypnotic recall is not necessarily rejected.[16,17,19] Diamond's persuasive argument against the legal evidentiary use of the memory of the hypnotized subject rests on several clinical observations, especially those described by the authority Hilgard. This point of view is not surprising, considering the high suggestibility of the hypnotizable subject. Compounding the unreliability of memory that has been distorted by the process of hypnosis is the tendency of post-hypnotic memory to become "concretized."[20] Thus the infusion of the distortions of related fantasies by the subject and the suggested distortions by the hypnotizer are, subsequently, firmly and clearly recalled as part of the remembered events. The hypnotized witness with such firmly held inaccuracies in memory is very vulnerable to cross-examination and is deservedly diminished in credibility. Diamond, however, does not reject the use of hypnosis for investigative uncovering of half-remembered information which may be brought into clearer focus and may prove to be at least partially accurate and useful. He gives as an example the Chowchilla kidnapping of a number of children several years ago. At the investigative phase, a hypnotized person was able to recall a fragment of a license plate of a vehicle, which led to the apprehension of the criminals. Such investigative use of hypnosis may compromise or sacrifice the hypnotized subject for later testimonial purposes, however.

MALINGERING

Nowhere in clinical psychiatry are the skills and knowledge of the clinician more challenged, especially in legal settings, than in the diagnosis of malingering.[21-23] The nature of the phenomenon is highly idiosyncratic, and accordingly I have relied heavily on my own experience in the following discussion. It is well to remember that a trained clinician knows a great deal more about psychiatric and medical pathology (and normality) than does the clever but untrained malingerer. Malingerers often gain their knowledge by viewing motion-picture dramas or from television, even when they have been so sophisticated as to consult psychiatric textbooks. Thus the malingerer who described to me the Schneiderian criteria for the diagnosis of schizophrenia involving thought insertion and thought broadcasting also expressed, in paranoid fashion, the seeming delusion that his life was bedeviled by a mysterious force identified as Bora-Din. The malingerer later acknowledged that he had derived this name from a late-night oft-repeated television advertisement selling a record of classical melodies in which one of the Polovtsian Dances by Alexsandr Borodin was the theme featured and so identified. The only instance in my clinical experience of a supposed psychosis involving the possession of a man with a female-sounding falsetto voice was highly reminiscent of the performance of the psychotic killer in Hitchcock's classic movie *Psycho*. The same man was possessed of competing devils, one of which, identified as "Lila" (substitute Lola), spoke in falsetto, but there was another rather stentorian, authoritarian, male devil voice as well. In my opinion, the resemblance to the play and movie *Damn Yankees* was not accidental.

The theatrical (literally and otherwise) nature of the malingerer's presentation is illustrative of the generalization that malingerers tend to be grossly overdetermined in their conception of what constitutes mental illness. The clinical data are histrionic, variegated, and inconsistent and require multiple diagnostic labels in contradistinction to the principle of diagnostic parsimony in good medical practice. Of course, the phenomenology of the schizophrenic can be dramatic, and that of the histrionic personality even more so, but the malingerer may be discernible nonetheless.

Secondary gain is always present in the true malingerer, and its existence should raise one's suspicions. The major differential point between the malingerer and a factitious disorder is precisely the presence of secondary gain. The malingerer has difficulty in sustaining the feigned symptoms over prolonged periods, especially when the syndrome he or she presents is so varied and histrionic. Often when out of sight and hearing of mental health professionals, there is a falling away of malingered behavior. One should therefore inquire about the suspected malingerer's behavior as observed by correctional officers, attendants, other nonprofessionals, and certainly nurses. Nonprofessionals are not accorded expert status in the courtroom and cannot render a diagnosis, but they can as lay witnesses describe manifest behavior, such as the fact that seemingly dazed and prolonged delays in responses to the questions of the professional examiner in the examination room have never been observed back on the ward where the malingerer is an active poker player. Such fact testimony is acceptable in court.

Psychological testing can contribute a great deal to the making of the diagnosis of malingering. For example, an impressive pattern may emerge of incorrect answers to easy items on the Wechsler Adult Intelligence Scale beside correct answers to more difficult items. It takes a great deal of expertise to "look sick" consistently and persuasively on the Rorschach and figure drawings. Also, the "fake good," "fake bad" lie score and other validity scales of the Minnesota Multi-Phasic Personality Inventory can be quite revealing.

There are many other differential criteria which the experienced mental health professional can bring to the diagnosis of malingering. For example, the anhedonia of schizophrenia make the existence of a sense of humor most unlikely in the true schizophrenic. Even the silly behavior of the disorganized schizophrenic, formerly diagnosed as hebephrenic, has a grim, desperate, anhedonic quality. Manics, however, can appear to be genuinely funny. It cannot be disputed, despite all of the above, that malingering can go undetected and undiagnosed even by the best of clinicians. When one does make the diagnosis there is an understandable tendency to ignore or to dismiss too lightly the possibility of coexisting psychopathology. As Macdonald[22] emphasizes, malingering may mask or even serve as a defense against another significant psychiatric illness.

DSM III

The publication of the third edition of the official *Diagnostic and Statistical Manual of Mental Disorders (DSM III)* by the American Psychiatric Association in 1980 has ushered in an era of much greater precision and rigor in the making of psychiatric diagnoses.[24] Indeed, it is a level of diagnostic rigor exceeding that of most of the other medical specialties. The legal profession in general and trial lawyers in particular are very much aware of these new diagnostic standards. According to the publisher, two mailings of promotional material for *DSM III* were sent to the 24,000 trial-lawyer members of the American Bar Association, with return orders for the book of an "impressive" 17.6 percent or about 4600 copies.[25] The estimate is that far greater numbers of lawyers have bought the book than is reflected in this traceable return of orders. It can be assumed by any mental health professional who is called into the courtroom that this official diagnostic manual is virtually a standard part of the armamentarium of attorneys with regular involvement in the mental-health–legal field.

The data required by *DSM III* in order to reach a diagnosis often involve the utilization of extensive and reliable historical material. In a psycholegal issue such as the assessment of competency to stand trial, particularly when performed in large numbers by heavily burdened psychiatrists in public service, the acquisition of sufficient data to make a defensible diagnosis can be very difficult. The mental health professional is then most vulnerable in the courtroom if his or her opinions or diagnoses are challenged. Criminal defendants and other examinees involved in litigation are quite often unreliable in providing accurate histories. This tendency compounds the difficulties of the evaluation and makes the gathering of reliable historical data, independent of the examinee, of even greater importance than in the pre-*DSM III* era.

The attorney may also be familiar with the *Psychiatric Glossary*,[26] published as a companion piece to *DSM III*, and, even more dismaying, with the massively comprehensive and authoritative three-volume *Comprehensive Textbook of Psychiatry*, edited by Kaplan, Freedman, and Sadock[27] and published in the same year as *DSM III*. With such an armamentarium the courtroom challenge to the opinion offered by mental health experts can become formidable. Under such scrutiny and with such challenges to their knowledge and skills, forensic mental health professionals need to be well prepared in order to meet these challenges. It would be highly valuable in the training of clinicians for them to experience the rigor of courtroom attack and defense of their clinical problems.

Problems have already arisen in the applications of *DSM III* to the courtroom, especially in criminal matters. There is a disclaimer in the introduction to the manual, which reads as follows:

> The use of this manual for nonclinical purposes, such as the determination of legal responsibility . . . must be critically examined in each instance within the appropriate institutional context.[28]

A particular source of confusion and potential misapplication of the diagnostic manual relates to the critical issues of criminal and civil intent and criminal responsibility. There are a number of instances in the manual in which volitional elements are required in a variety of diagnostic entities that are confusing and inconsistent. Thus, in the following description of pathological gambling we read, "The essential features of pathological gambling are a chronic and progressive **failure to resist** impulses to gamble." This is in contradistinction to the language of the definition of the entity, which requires that the individual be **"unable to resist"** impulses to gamble. In the same section of the manual, in dealing with the impulse disorders, the diagnoses of pyromania and kleptomania require only the "failure to resist" these actions in order to justify these conclusions. Furthermore, in the large subclass of the paraphilias and sexual perversions, it is provided, "The essential feature of disorders in this class is that unusual or bizarre imagery or acts are **necessary** for sexual excitement. Such imagery or acts **tend** to be **insistently** or **involuntarily** repetitive." In contrast to this equivocation, in alcohol abuse there is an **"inability to cut down or stop,"** whereas dependence on alcohol, barbiturates, opiods, cocaine, and so forth requires only a **"need for"** these substances (emphases have been added throughout this paragraph).

Despite the caveat in the introduction to the *DSM III*, the "unable to resist" language in the definition of pathological gambling has already provided an inappropriate basis for courtroom findings of not guilty by reason of insanity in several jurisdictions.[29]

The volitional diagnostic nuances in *DSM III*, which were designed for treatment and prognostic purposes, have great potential for misapplication in criminal matters apart from the insanity defense, because they can affect sentences, plea bargaining, and many instances of the assessment and adjudication of intent in the legal system, both criminal and civil. They may be inappropriately applied in the legal system for purposes of punishment or even excessive detention.

The borderline personality, in contradistinction to its largely discredited predecessors, pseudoneurotic schizophrenia and pseudopsychopathic schizophrenia, has been given a legitimate place in the new psychiatric nosology. With its transient psychotic states, it has considerable potential for misapplication and mischief in its application to the legal system. This is particularly true for the difficult exercise in our society of litigating morality and culpability. There seems little reason to doubt that in the future, borderline affective states will be given a legal as well as a psychiatric legitimacy.[30] Similar difficulties exist for forensic application in such diagnoses as the dissociative states or organic confusional states, which are also borderline conditions. I do not think that we should be apologetic or defensive about this development. We are dealing, after all, with the marvelous complexity of the human mind, which does not lend itself to a simplistic moral calculus.

With respect to the other Axes of the five included in a full *DSM III* diagnosis, the application of Axis V (Level of Adaptive Functioning) has obvious application in personal injury or workmen's compensation matters. The psychosocial stressors (Axis IV) associated with a psychiatric disorder may be of great significance in criminal matters. For example, New York (and at least eight other jurisdictions) provides that criminal acts committed under the duress of "extreme emotional disturbance" that has been provoked or causally precipitated by severe psychosocial stressors may lead to conviction of crimes of much less seriousness than those originally charged, with a concomitant lesser sentence consistent with the concept of diminished responsibility (see also chapter 8).[31-33]

Despite the difficulties, confusions, and potential legal misapplication of *DSM III* adumbrated in this section as applied to courtroom settings, the development of the new manual has probably been very healthy for the mental health disciplines in general. In the forensic psychiatry field it should contribute to more soundly based and more useful contributions by our discipline to the system of justice in America.

CIVIL COMMITMENT

It is not within the purpose and scope of this chapter to deal with the very complex matter of the competing social values involved in the involuntary civil commitment of the mentally disabled. It has been dealt with, if inconclusively, by the US Supreme Court,[34] other authors,[35,36] and me[37] extensively elsewhere. Given the complexities of human behavior and the shifting mores of a free society, the issue may never be dealt with definitively, at least not by legislative or judicial mandate. Nevertheless, a cardinal principle of the clinical involvement of psychiatrists and psychologists in civil commitment proceedings is that the legal standards or criteria justifying commitment be understood and adhered to by the involved clinician. This section will summarize the present state of the matter.

Until relatively recently the legal questions the clinician has had to deal with were (and still are in many jurisdictions) broad, vague, and lacking in operational clarity. We have been required, somewhat simplistically, to address whether there is a "need for treatment" and/or whether the person for whom commitment is sought is "dangerous to self or others." In the early 1970s, however, in Massachusetts,[38] California[39] and Arizona,[40] more precise statutory definitions of behavior that qualifies as dangerous, along with due process considerations modeled on criminal standards and procedures, emerged. This was also seen in case law.[41]

These new statutes provide more precise phenomenological standards for those behaviors associated with mental illness which justify commitment. These changes represent a departure from the old statutes in at least two respects. First, the harmful behavior that justifies commitment has to be based on manifest evidence of acts or words demonstrated in past behavior. Thus the clinician is required to give to the judge behavioral descriptions that are substantially more justiciable than the vagaries of diagnosis alone.

Massachusetts's statutory standard, which was substantially adopted by at least ten other states in the 1970s,[42] defines the "likelihood of serious harm" required for commitment as follows:

> likelihood of serious harm means 1) a substantial risk of physical harm to the person himself, as manifested by evidence of threats of, or attempts at, suicide or serious bodily harm; 2) a substantial risk of physical harm to other persons as manifested by evidence of homicidal or other violent behavior or evidence that others are placed in reasonable fear of violent behavior and serious physical harm to them; or 3) a very substantial risk of physical impairment or injury to the person himself as manifested by

evidence that such person's judgment is so affected that he is unable to protect himself in the community and that reasonable provision for his protection is not available in the community [Mass. Gen. Laws, ch. 123, sec. 1, 1971].[38]

The second important operational consideration in the adjudication of commitment under these new statutes is that the prior manifest behavior justifying commitment does not exclusively require the expert to testify but can be properly brought before the court by nonexpert witnesses. In addition, the California commitment statutes require proof of **continued** proscribed physically harmful behavior during specified subsequent time periods in order to justify the continued involuntary retention and treatment of the committed person.[39]

Apart from the matter of harmful behavior, the role of the psychiatric expert (less frequently that of a member of another mental health discipline) remains undiminished with regard to defining and describing mental illness per se. Here, too, the statutes are generally silent, inconsistent, or vague with regard to what constitutes mental illness for purposes of commitment. In Massachusetts the definition of mental illness for purposes of involuntary commitment is provided in the regulations of the Massachusetts State Department of Mental Health. A more behavioral or phenomenological standard rather than a nosological label is provided here as well. Department regulations define mental illness as

a substantial disorder of thought, mood, perception, orientation or memory which grossly impairs judgment, behavior, capacity to recognize reality or ability to meet the ordinary demands of life.[43]

In California the manifest harmful behavior requirement for civil commitment has been studied,[44,45] and the general principle pointed out by Stone[46] appears to have prevailed. Stone has observed that as civil commitment of the mentally ill has been made more rigorous (or their release into the community more easily achieved), the agents of social control in our society—the police and the criminal courts—have used the alternative of the criminal justice system to remove from the community the obstreperous, the bizarre, and the irritating (as well as the dangerous) who are mentally disabled, usually under the rubric of the issue of competency to stand trial. Unlike California, in Massachusetts a concurrent tightening of the laws, especially of procedure, relating to competency to stand trial not only precluded an increase in commitments in the category but substantially reduced them.[47]

The clinician in the area of civil commitment should be aware of the legal standard applicable in his or her jurisdiction, however much help or confusion these standards may provide in such proceedings. This is a role especially difficult when the clinician seeks also to engage in a treatment relationship with the patient against whom the clinician is forced to appear in an adversary legal role.

FORENSIC PSYCHIATRIC EXAMINATIONS AND REPORTS

The involvement of mental health clinicians in legal proceedings usually begins and ends with the submission of a report either to one of the adversaries or, perhaps most frequently, to the court in the early stages of the proceedings.

Such reports are of great importance and can substantially affect the outcome of legal actions.[48] The remainder of this chapter will be devoted to considerations relating to forensic psychiatric examinations and reports, the elements regarded as necessary in an adequate report, and an annotated outline of such a report. The chapter closes with two excerpted sample reports.

Examiner as Adversary Agent or Impartial Expert

Of great importance in the preparation of forensic reports is the question of which party the examiner represents and what use is made of the report. Subtle and not-so-subtle issues emerge in this context. If the examiner is hired by an adversary, then the adversary will obviously have his or her own purposes in mind and will want the examiner to support these purposes. The adversary or the adversary's attorney may wish the report to be modified and certain findings stressed. If the examiner can agree to modify—for example, to clarify or to relate the findings to specific legal issues—this may be acceptable. But there is a point beyond which so much violence can be done to the original findings and associated opinion that it becomes unethical to accept the suggested changes. The adversary who has hired the expert may choose not to use the report if it does not adequately serve his or her purposes, and this is that person's right. Those examiners who are excessively accommodating to those who hire them do not go unnoticed in the medical and legal professions, and their credibility obviously suffers, as it should. These issues are further discussed in several other chapters of this book concerning professional ethics (chapters 2 and 3) and courtroom presentation of evidence (chapter 22).

In my experience, a more desirable model for forensic evaluation is the appointment of an examiner acceptable to both sides in an adversary proceeding. Appropriate stipulations as to the payment of the fee and to the effect that both sides will receive the report and that both may use or not use it as they choose can also be worked out. This avoids the particular ethical issues raised above.

In the public service area in which the examiner is paid by governmental sources, an impartial expert model is more generally the case. The forensic examiner in such cases is the agent of the judge or the court and need not deal with the problem of accommodation to the purposes of either adversary. This model can be criticized in view of the general truth that no one is completely impartial. In my experience, psychiatrists are usually defense-minded in criminal proceedings. Nevertheless, the competent, ethical, mental health professional should not have difficulty with either an adversarial or a nonadversarial model. What matters is that the quality of the examination be high and that it be based upon adequate, accurate data soundly related to the legal questions posed.

Clearer Questions and More Relevant Answers

In my experience the single greatest source of confusion and dissatisfaction in the involvement of mental health professionals in the legal process is that they are asked to give answers to questions that are not articulated. It should be a basic principle that any forensic report to a court begin with a statement of the question or questions that have been posed by the court or by counsel and in the absence of clear questions to postulate them if they cannot be readily clarified.

Of course, the manifest questions in these encounters often serve latent purposes in forensic evaluations which may be conscious or unconscious. This must be understood in the realistic context of courts which are flooded with litigation and must seek the rapid and efficient disposition of cases. This reality is exemplified in the fact that plea-bargaining and negotiation between parties settle the great majority of criminal and civil actions. It is not surprising, therefore, that the courts have been willing to abrogate their authority to psychiatrist-mediated alternatives, notably in the area of competency to stand trial. Thus, when a court orders a pretrial mental examination of a defendant, it presumably is posing, although infrequently articulating, the common-law questions of whether the defendant understands the nature of the proceedings against him or her and whether the defendant can rationally assist counsel in his or her defense. If the court accepts the answer that "the defendant is schizophrenic" as dispositive of these legal questions, we witness the worst in both the psychiatric and judicial fields in the exercise of their respective responsibilities. A resulting mental hospital commitment of the defendant may or may not be clinically appropriate. Most important, however, the court docket then is cleared of the case, owing to the defendant's hospitalization.

The Mental-Status Examination

Whatever the legal context, the basis of an adequate psychiatric response to the questions asked or implied by the court or other tribunal should be an adequate mental-status assessment of the examined person. Those areas of psychiatric abnormality or disability uncovered in the mental-status examination can and should be applied to the particular legal question or questions asked of the clinician that are relevant to the legal inquiry. Lay persons, including lawyers, judges, and jurors, can understand the parameters of the standard mental-status examination. This is particularly true if the clinician documents the mental-status examination with direct quotations from the examinee's responses and with descriptive data of appearance and behavior which then are logically connected with the clinician's conclusions. The clinician need not sacrifice the relative precision of professional concepts or terminology in communicating to the courts. Such terminology, with added effort, can be translated into terms of common human experience which render them comprehensible.

Probative Value

The concept of probative value in the law is an important one for the clinician to understand. In the hierarchy of clinical probabilities and in ascending order of likelihood, physicians generally begin with a differential diagnosis, then a diagnostic impression, and finally an established diagnosis. It must be stressed that only the latter is of probative value in the criminal courts, although civil, including family court, settings may be less rigorous. When relying on expert opinion, however, the legal process generally suspends evidentiary rigor in the development of the opinion. This permits the expert, by virtue of his or her unique experience and competence, to sift the wheat from the chaff, even in hearsay data, in arriving at an opinion. Such status and authority conferred on the clinician in a court of law should not be assumed lightly. Thus when the expert witness is asked, as he or she must first be asked, whether or not he or she has an opinion, the answer should be no, **unless** that opinion is within reasonable clinical or medical certainty. In the field of psychiatry, the required support for certain types of forensic opinions has become more stringent in recent years, both in statutory law[38] and in court decisions.[41] This has become increasingly true, as noted earlier, since 1980, when the official *Diagnostic and Statistical Manual*, ed 3, of the American Psychiatric Association was published.

The matters of who qualifies as an "expert" and on what issues an expert opinion is acceptable are dynamic and evolving processes.[49] A trial court, for example, rejected as unreliable psychiatric and psychological opinions on the prediction of dangerous behavior,[50] although the US Supreme Court has since refused to rule that all such testimony is inadmissable on Constitutional grounds.[51] Expert opinion that was rejected concerning the unreliability of eyewitness identification was affirmed on appeal as a proper exercise of judicial discretion.[52,53] (See further discussion on this in chapter 22, "The Psychiatrist as Expert Witness.")

General Elements of a Report

This section is devoted to a delineation of the elements that should be covered in the preparation of such reports, with an emphasis on the clinical aspects. Briefly, what is required is as follows:

1. a clear understanding on the part of the examiner of the specific legal questions being asked;
2. an understanding of the circumstances relating to the legal action, including the party for whom the examiner acts when conducting the evaluation;
3. the collection and review of relevant legal, medical, and related documents, particularly if there have been prior hospitalizations—such documents include nurses' notes and physicians' notes and previous psychiatric and psychological reports;
4. an adequate personal and clinical history;
5. the conducting of an adequate mental-status examination with particular attention to those areas of functioning abilities or disabilities that have relevance to the legal questions asked;
6. a description of the degree to which psychic disability, if any, can be related to the legal questions asked, together with the degree of certainty with which the examiner offers an opinion.

Forensic examinations may be very narrow in their scope (for example, competency to stand trial) or relatively broad (for example, the complexity of a child custody trial). Nevertheless, in my opinion, the elements outlined above remain relevant and useful. Of particular importance is the last element, relating to the degree of certainty with which an opinion is offered. Competent experts will offer opinions with that degree of certainty which their data will support. This can range from "no opinion," "more likely than not," and "probably" to "within reasonable medical certainty."

A corollary to the above is that there must be adequate time for the clinician to develop the data required to form an opinion. It is recognized that clinicians involved in forensic examinations may indeed be overburdened, particularly those in public service settings. It is this fact that has been responsible for much of the justified criticism of the involvement of the mental health disciplines in legal settings. Even an attempt (Fig. 4-1) to provide an efficient instrument for the assessment of competency to stand trial, which rarely took more than one hour, has been criticized as too complex and time-consuming.

Recommended Report Outline

The annotated outline of the recommended elements of a forensic psychiatric report presented here is intended only to provide a model and not to be rigidly applied. Differing facts and circumstances require flexibility. The outline is followed by excerpts from two such reports; the first deals with competency to stand trial and the second concerns criminal responsibility.

Adequate preparation for the actual examination is essential. Depending on the richness of the material available in advance of the interview, all inconsistencies, critical themes, quotes, and specific content to be sought relevant to the questions posed in the referral should be outlined and systematically pursued in the examination. I am not suggesting rigidity in the interview protocol. Interview technique must permit flexibility and as much spontaneity and rapport as possible. It is often useful to begin the interview with relatively neutral questions or areas, seeking to correct nonprovocative historical inconsistencies in the referral material in an effort to develop effective rapport and a collaborative posture.

PSYCHIATRIC EVALUATION

Re:
Date of Examination:
Date of Report:
By:
Identifying Data:
> The examinee's legal circumstances; the examiner's principal qualifications—a curriculum vitae may be appended to the report.

Purpose of the Examination:
> The circumstances of who engaged the examiner, when, and why; the relevant legal standard or standards, statutory or otherwise, should be quoted. What are the legal questions?

Preparation:
> All activities, documents, and ancillary interviews with other persons are noted, including times and dates; included should be reference to any case law or other authorities relied on.

Relevant Past History:
> Examinee's family, employment, education, medical, and psychiatric history; uniquely traumatic life events. Appropriate and relevant quotations from documents and interviews should be included. Psychosocial stressors are particularly important with relation to the legal event or events being inquired into.

	Degree of Incapacity					
	Total	Severe	Moderate	Mild	None	Unratable
1. Appraisal of available legal defenses	1	2	3	4	5	6
2. Unmanageable behavior	1	2	3	4	5	6
3. Quality of relating to attorney	1	2	3	4	5	6
4. Planning of legal strategy, including guilty plea to lesser charges where pertinent	1	2	3	4	5	6
5. Appraisal of role of:						
a. defense counsel	1	2	3	4	5	6
b. prosecuting attorney	1	2	3	4	5	6
c. judge	1	2	3	4	5	6
d. jury	1	2	3	4	5	6
e. defendant	1	2	3	4	5	6
f. witnesses	1	2	3	4	5	6
6. Understanding of court procedure	1	2	3	4	5	6
7. Appreciation of charges	1	2	3	4	5	6
8. Appreciation of range and nature of possible penalties	1	2	3	4	5	6
9. Appraisal of likely outcome	1	2	3	4	5	6
10. Capacity to disclose to attorney available pertinent facts surrounding the offense including the defendant's movements, timing, mental state, actions at the time of the offense.	1	2	3	4	5	6
11. Capacity to realistically challenge prosecution witnesses	1	2	3	4	5	6
12. Capacity to testify relevantly	1	2	3	4	5	6
13. Self-defeating versus self-serving motivation (legal sense)	1	2	3	4	5	6

Examinee _____ Examiner _____

Date _____

FIGURE 4-1. Shown here is the Competency-To-Stand-Trial Assessment Instrument.

The Examinee's Description of His or Her Movements, State of Mind, and the Circumstances During and Surrounding the Events in Question:
Quotations are essential here when possible.

MENTAL STATUS

Circumstances:
Where did the examination take place, when, and for how long? Who was present? Was it private and comfortable, or otherwise? Audiotaped or videotaped? What medications is the examinee taking, especially psychotropic?

General Appearance:
Examinee's dress, grooming, physical characteristics, voice, tics, posture, mannerisms, behavior, and quality of relating to the examiner. (Was the person polite, hostile, guarded, open, attentive, evasive?)

Reliability:
Does the examinee appear to be truthful? Are there inconsistencies or indications of evasion, distortion, or lying?

Affect:
Examinee's psychomotor status, appropriateness to circumstances and thought content, range, and prevailing mood.

Perception:
Hallucinations, illusions.

Speech and Intelligence:
Examinee's command of the language, syntactical errors, vocabulary, pitch of voice, modulation, fluidity, responsivity, pace.

Thought Processes:
Examinee's level of abstraction, associations, neologisms.

Thought Content:
Perseverations, dominant themes volunteered or pursued on the examinee's initiative.

Orientation and Memory:
Claimed amnesias should be carefully described (global versus fragmented); recent and remote memory.

Insight and Judgment:
These should be specifically related to the referral questions.

Diagnostic Formulation:
The bases for the diagnosis with specific references to *DSM III* criteria where possible and with adequate delineation of differential diagnostic considerations.

Diagnosis:
The five *DSM III* Axes related both to the time of the events at issue and the time of the examination.

Opinion:
A marshalling of the historical and clinical findings having specific reference to the referral questions, together with the level of medical or psychological certainty of the opinion offered. Specific reference to the legal standards and language should be made.

CLINICAL EXAMPLES

The excerpted material presented here is in the public domain in that it has been submitted in public legal proceedings. Alterations have been made to protect the privacy of the individuals examined. What has not been sacrificed in the excerpts are accurate clinical and dynamic details, which are essential to a valid rendering of the cases.

In both of the clinical excerpts below, the examiner was retained by the prosecution in examining accused murderers.* In the interests of both conserving space and protecting the privacy of the examinees, only key portions of the examinations are published here. The first of these reports, which concerned competency to stand trial, required 15 double-spaced typed pages for the full report. The second report, dealing with criminal responsibility, required 29 pages.

Competency to Stand Trial

In the first case, the defendant had spent a number of years in public mental institutions after repeated findings of incompetency to stand trial. The common-law questions that the court and the examining clinician must address in competency-to-stand-trial examinations are whether the defendant understands the nature of the proceedings against him or her and whether he or she can rationally assist counsel in his or her defense. An important caveat here is that there is a presumption of mental competency, and the burden of proof rests with whoever seeks to demonstrate that by reason of mental illness or retardation the defendant is incompetent. (For greater detail on legal criteria see chapter 7.)

PSYCHIATRIC EVALUATION†

General Appearance:
Mr. L. is about 5'5" tall and weighs 150 pounds. He was dressed in loose-fitting blue pajamas and was wearing slippers. His hair is black, straight, and medium length but starting to show significant gray streaks. He looked somewhat older than his 46 years. He was clean shaven. His complexion is somewhat grayish and on the darker side but not abnormally so. The overall impression initially was that of a rather stolid, dull, underassertive man. Several times during the interview he announced that he was "stupid." Throughout the interview Mr. L. literally chain-smoked long brown wrapped cigarettes. At the outset of the interview the examiner introduced himself and identified the purpose of the examination and stated that he was examining him on behalf of the District Attorney of Mayfair County. Mr. L. gave the appearance of having some difficulty understanding who and

---

* In any forensic examination it is, of course, ethically required of the examiner to inform the examinee of who he or she is, who he or she represents, the purpose of the examination, risks to the examinee, and foreseeable uses that could be made of the examination data.

† The Competency Assessment Instrument (Fig. 4-1) was not used in this examination because the defendant proved to be a malingerer whose responses were not reliable. This is atypical.

what the district attorney was but ultimately made the statement that he was "against me."

Almost immediately after sitting down, Mr. L. commenced extreme rocking of his upper body from side to side on his chair. The arch of this rocking at the level of his head was approximately 2 feet in width. However, after about 15 minutes this rocking subsided. The interviewer then made a note that the rocking had subsided and Mr. L. was observed to lean forward in his chair and on sitting back once again he repeated the rocking motion from side to side in an exaggerated fashion for perhaps another 3 or 4 minutes. On the second subsiding of the rocking, he began rhythmically and vigorously to kick the leg of the table for several minutes. After the kicking stopped it was not resumed throughout the interview. Quite late in the interview, a young aide was in the room briefly, quickly following up on Mr. L. after he had requested and received medication when feeling upset. At this point Mr. L. once again briefly rocked in the presence of the aide and this examiner. When the aide entered the room Mr. L. stated to the examiner, "I can't feel my heart, I get that funny feeling all over my body." At this point the examiner asked to feel the patient's pulse and he agreed. His pulse at that time was regular, strong, and slow. Mr. L.'s behavior was quite consistent with what had been described on a number of occasions in the recent clinical record at this center as "panic attacks."

As this examiner began to collect his materials and clearly indicated that the interview was about to terminate, Mr. L. spontaneously stated, "See what happens. I get this funny feeling in my body, like I'm going to die and I see my mother and she tells me to follow her . . . and she has her hand and I think that if I grab her hand I think I would die." The examiner continued at this point to gather his materials and within a matter of a minute or so, Mr. L. returned to a more bantering, playful exchange with the examiner, suggesting that he put his hat on, and laughed quietly as the taping and interview concluded.

Opinion:

This opinion is offered within reasonable medical certainty. Consistent with the diagnosis of Histrionic Personality Disorder in my opinion Mr. L.'s simulation of mental illness during this examination (and at other times) was exaggerated and theatrical. The rocking behavior described in some detail above is inconsistent with any rocking that this examiner has ever seen in a mental patient. Commonly, retarded or very seriously disturbed children rock, but their trunk does not rock to the extreme that Mr. L. displayed nor is it side to side, as he displayed, but, rather, forward and back. Similarly, the vigorous rhythmic kicking of the table was only briefly displayed but also exaggerated. The behavior and content of the "panic attack" so described in the hospital records which Mr. L. displayed to this examiner was equally unconvincing. At a time of genuine panic which involves severe anxiety, the pulse rate is almost invariably significantly increased. In Mr. L. it was not. In a number of other ways, for example, the inconsistency in the facade of dull and slow mentation on the one hand but quick and challenging responses on the other when it could be inferred that his immediate self-interest was aroused (e.g., a discussion of his heavy medication regimen) provides further support for the diagnosis of malingering. Mr. L. has had some 6 years to observe the manifest psychotic behavior of many other hospitalized mental patients. Given his very demonstrative and in my opinion resourceful personality, he may well display extreme dramatic and histrionic behavior in court or elsewhere if the criminal proceedings go forward.

Throughout the interview the standard questions relating to an individual's competency to stand trial were put to Mr. L. These included whether he understood the charges against him, whether he understood the role of the various principals in a criminal proceeding, and so on. He persistently failed to respond accurately to these questions. In one area, however, with considerable discussion, he was able to understand and repeat to this examiner the concept of plea bargaining. Generally his failure to respond accurately to the questions related to his competency to stand trial in the opinion of this examiner is not credible.

In my opinion Mr. L. understands the charges against him, the nature of the criminal proceedings against him, and is aware of the possible penalties in the criminal proceedings against him. If he chooses he can rationally and adequately assist his counsel in his defense.

Criminal Responsibility

The second excerpted report involves an assessment of criminal responsibility, which is dealt with more extensively in chapter 8. The focus here is on clinical evaluation. Forensic reports and testimony have frequently been criticized when they have dealt with this issue. There has been a preoccupation with the language of the various legal tests[53] designed to guide and to instruct the trier of fact in determining criminal responsibility.

There are a number of difficulties here, arising, in part, because clinical evaluations on the issue are ex post facto, often weeks and even years after the alleged criminal act. First, there must be retrospectively credible corroboration in order that a valid and defensible opinion can be reached. Second, it is necessary to establish a causal relationship between any mental illness at the time of the crime and the crime itself. The third consideration which, in my view, is the most confounding of all, is that the determination of criminal responsibility is in large measure a question of morality and social policy and not of science.

Despite the difficulties, I do not join with those who would eschew any role for the psychiatrist or psychologist in determining criminal responsibility. (See also chapters 3 and 8 for discussion of the role of the mental health professional in assessing criminal responsibility.) It is possible in retrospect to establish the existence of severe mental illness at the time of a criminal act with adequate, credible, and corroborative data.

The illustrative case involved a 16-year-old male Vietnamese refugee named H. who had been in America for 14 months and was living with a foster family. At 4:00 AM one morning he killed his 18-year-old male sleeping room-mate, Tran, also a Vietnamese refugee, using a baseball bat. H. then proceeded elsewhere in the house to fracture the skulls of his foster mother, the sister of the young man he had killed, and two of the foster mother's children, including a 3-year-old. He then returned to his bedroom and attempted to kill himself by grasping the exposed prongs of an electrical plug, resulting in the loss of two fingers from the extensive burns he suffered. He was charged with murder and four counts of attempted murder.

New York statutory law, which applied here, provides for exculpation "if at the time of such conduct as a result of mental disease or defect, he lacks substantial capacity to know or appreciate: (a) the nature and consequences of such conduct; or (b) that such conduct is wrong."[55] It therefore did not provide for volitional exculpation. If this case had been governed by the American Law Institute criterion, provided that H. was "unable to conform his behavior to the requirements of the law," the examiner would have offered an opinion supporting the exculpation of H. in the homicide of Tran (but not the attempted murders, as the reader will see). New York law did not permit such an exculpatory opinion.

PSYCHIATRIC EVALUATION

Diagnostic Formulation

H. is an immature, appealing youngster. Despite his age of 16 years, the diagnostic considerations which come to mind here are those relating to child psychiatry. The central dynamics are those of a dependent child, taken prematurely from his mother and family, and his failure to grow and adapt from that dependent, immature state in an alien land. Certainly, he is a young person who has struggled for a year and one half with a lack of hope, a despair. The depression of quite significant dimensions could probably most accurately be described here as an anaclitic depression which derives from the forlornness and emptiness of a child taken from the attachment to the mother before being capable of surviving independently. Such a depression is at a presexual or pregenital developmental level. I would understand his violent behavior as primarily of a suicidal nature in which he took up arms against a sea of troubles and in opposing them tried to end them. However, it cannot be ignored that at an unconscious level, at least, those persons who were injured by his explosively violent behavior were the physical embodiments of his currently painful existence and became the immediate objects of his attempt to strike down that existence. The explosive behavior described has some of the characteristics of a syndrome which has been described in the psychiatric literature under the name "amok." This syndrome, although now rare, used to be common in Southeast Asia, especially in the Malayan Peninsula parallel to Vietnam. Westermeyer[56] described the behavior as follows: "A person suddenly and unexpectedly begins an indiscriminate assault on those about him."

Lehrmann[57] writes as follows: "The savage homicidal attack is generally preceded by a period of preoccupation, brooding and mild depression. After the attack, the person feels exhausted, has complete amnesia for it and often commits suicide." Frequently, as well, the person is killed by others in order to terminate the attack or as punishment.

In his published discussion of Westermeyer's paper, Cheng[58] described amok as follows: "Running amok may be seen as a peculiar type of suicide where the individual puts himself in a situation where he is killed by his 'fellows.'" This formulation would appear clearly to apply to H.'s motivation in at least part of his assaultive behavior. What does not fit is the absence of the exhaustion and amnesia described by Westermeyer. Neither does H.'s behavior stand up as entirely indiscriminate in terms of his victims. It must be noted, however, that follow-up study of such behavior is obviously limited by the fact that many or most of those who run amok do not survive.

Diagnosis:

Axis I: 312.35 Isolated Explosive Disorder.
            309.00 Adjustment Disorder with Depressed Mood.
Axis II: V71.09 No Diagnosis.
Axis III: Sexual Immaturity.

Axis IV: Psychosocial Stressors.
            Refugee; Death of Parent.
            Severity: 6—Extreme.
Axis V: Highest Level of Adaptive Functioning in Past Year: 5-poor.

Opinion:

In the chain of violent behavior exhibited by H. which led to the indictments, it is necessary to separate the homicidal behavior toward Tran from the later behavior. In my opinion, the homicidal behavior toward Tran was impulsive and not consciously premeditated.

> I felt like to hit. I felt like to hit everything. Anything or everything. I threw the chairs and then I see Tran and I just hit him. . . . If Tran is not here, so I think I will kill myself with the baseball bat or the electric wire.

It cannot be ignored, however, that Tran had been the source of taunting, demeaning, and apparently abusive behavior toward H., and one can understand H.'s behavior as a striking out at an unconscious level against a wrongdoer associated with H.'s painful existence. Given this inconsistency between the apparent lack of conscious wrongful intent and the postulated presence of unconscious hostility, I am forced to conclude that I cannot, within the standards of the statute, arrive at an opinion with regard to the homicide of Tran within reasonable medical certainty.

The subsequent behavior, however, in which four others were gravely assaulted by H., in my opinion, represented wrongdoing on H.'s part which he, himself, perceived at a conscious level. Although suicide was his ultimate purpose, this awareness of wrongfulness is clearly implicit in his expectation that his behavior toward the four others assaulted would lead, in turn, to his being punitively assaulted.

> The most thing is to kill myself. I think it's like if I hit the people, so the people can hit me so I can die.

This awareness of wrongful behavior on his part is further confirmed by his statement shortly afterward to the police that he would expect to be imprisoned for 35 to 40 years for his behavior.

In my opinion, therefore, although H. may be regarded as mentally ill at the time of these alleged offenses, with the qualifications described above, he had the substantial capacity to know and to appreciate both the nature and the consequences of his conduct and that such conduct was wrong with respect to the four counts of attempted murder in the second degree. This opinion is offered within reasonable medical certainty.

Epilogue

An outline of the model for the elements and dimensions of a complete, perhaps idealized, forensic examination and report has been presented here for heuristic purposes. As I've indicated several times, as a practical matter, such a standard and the following in detail of this model are not routinely possible in heavily burdened public agencies. The two clinical examinations and reports excerpted in this chapter required 16 hours and 21 hours, respectively, exclusive of testimony. Examinations, especially those of the complexity of a criminal responsibility evaluation, often require scores of hours. No public agency on a routine basis can support such a commitment of time and money, and therefore compromises are necessary. For example, the extensive rendering of observations in the mental-status examinations which describe both normal and abnormal findings may be shortened. When no significant abnormal mental-status findings are made, the statement "no significant abnormalities of thinking, affect, memory, orientation, or perception were found" may be made. When there are abnormalities, however, these should be fully described.

Short of optimal time, extensive legal discovery mechanisms, and considerable fiscal support, the question then arises as to what minimal standards of time and data accessibility are acceptable. In public agencies the provision of preliminary investigatory material from affiliated probation departments or other supportive staff can do much to preserve the time of the examining clinician. The examining clinician may then reserve time for the essential examination itself and the formulation of the report. In my public sector experience, approximately 2 hours of record review, conferencing, and report drafting are required for each hour of actual examination. The reports average six to eight double-spaced pages per examined person, although examinations of limited scope such as competency to stand trial may be fewer. These concrete time and report length standards are offered as having empirically sufficed for the needs of the courts for such purposes as dispositional recommendations in the juvenile and the adult criminal courts, custody determinations, neglect, child abuse and placement, and for competency-to-stand-trial examinations. These standards have proved to be adequate even when the opinions arrived at have had to be defended in the courtroom. In my own experience a caseload of more than 10 examinations per week has proved to be very difficult, and quality will usually suffer if this number is exceeded.

As the diagnostic forensic process described in this chapter yields to greater numbers of referrals and as less time and data are available for the examiner to attempt to reach an opinion, the service rendered increasingly takes on the character of a screening triage. This screening process is respectable enough for use in a hospital emergency room with its exigencies and limitations where only the grossest and most compelling pathology will be discernible. But it is not good enough for use in a forensic psychiatric evaluative setting. The work has too great an impact on the freedom and quality of the lives of the people we serve.

REFERENCES

1. LOFTUS, EF AND MONAHAN, J: *Trial by data: Psychological research as legal evidence.* Am Psychol 35: 270-283, 1980.

2. McCLOSKEY, M AND EGETH, HE: *Eyewitness identification: What can a psychologist tell a jury?* Am Psychol 38:550-563, 1983.

3. LOFTUS, EF: *Silence is not golden.* Am Psychol 38:564-572, 1983.

4. FREUD, S: *Psychoanalysis in courts of law.* In FREUD, S: *The Collected Papers,* vol 2. Hogarth Press and The Institute of Psychoanalysis, London, 1956.

5. FREUD, S: *The forgetting of impressions and intentions.* In FREUD, S: *The Complete Psychological Works,* vol 6. Hogarth Press, London, 1957, p 47.

6. PENFIELD, W: *The Excitable Cortex of Conscious Man.* Charles C Thomas, Springfield, IL, 1958, pp 23-24 and 25-27.

7. PARK, DC, PUGLISI, J, SOVACOAL, BA: *Memory for pictures, words and spatial location in older adults: Evidence for pictoral superiority.* J Gerontol 38:582-588, 1983.

8. RANKIN, JL AND HINNICKS, JW: *Age, presentation and the effectiveness of structural recall cues.* J Gerontol 38:593-596, 1983.

9. BURKE, DM AND LIGHT, LI: *Memory and aging: The role of retrieval processes.* Psychol Bull 90:513-546, 1981.

10. KLÜVER, H AND BUCY, PC: *An analysis of certain effects of bilateral temporal lobectomy in the Rhesus monkey with special reference to psychic blindness.* J Psychol 5:33, 1938.

11. JOYNT, RJ, *Human memory.* In TONER, DB (ED): *The Nervous System, Vol 2. The Clinical Neurosciences.* Raven Press, New York, 1975.

12. *Amnesia: A case study in the limits of particular justice.* Yale Law J 71:109-120, 1961.

13. Wilson v. United States, 391 F.2d 460 (D.C. Cir. 1968).

14. ORNE, MT: *The use and misuse of hypnosis in court.* Int J Clin Exp Hypn 27:328-339, 1979.

15. Frye v. United States, 293 F.1013 (D.C. Cir. 1923).

16. People v. Shirlen, 64 P2d 775 (California, 1982).

17. Slip Opinion, People v. Hughes, No. 232 State of NY Court of Appeals, July 5, 1983 (26 pages).

18. DIAMOND, B: *Inherent problems in the use of pretrial hypnosis on a prospective witness.* Cal L Rev 68:313, 1980.

19. People v. Boudin, Ind. No. 81-285 (Supreme Court of New York Opinion filed 3/11/83).

20. ORNE, op cit.

21. WEISS, JMA: *Malingering and associated syndromes.* In ARIETI, S AND CAPLAN, G (EDS): *American Handbook of Psychiatry,* Vol 3. Basic Books, New York, 1974, pp 270-287.

22. MACDONALD, JM: *Psychiatry and the Criminal,* ed 3. Charles C Thomas, Springfield, IL, 1976, pp 267-279.

23. RESNICK, PJ: *The detection of malingered illness.* Behav Sci Law, 2:21-38, 1984.

24. AMERICAN PSYCHIATRIC ASSOCIATION: *Diagnostic and Statistical Manual of Mental Disorders,* ed 3. APA, Washington, DC, 1980.

25. MCMILLEN, RE (General Manager, American Psychiatric Press): Personal communication, April 26, 1983.

26. *A Psychiatric Glossary,* ed 5. American Psychiatric Association, Washington, DC, 1980.

27. KAPLAN, HF, FREEDMAN, AH, SADOCK, BJ (EDS): *A Comprehensive Textbook of Psychiatry.* Williams & Wilkins, Baltimore, 1980.

28. Op cit (24) at p 12.

29. MCGARRY, AL: *Pathological gambling: A new insanity defense.* Journal of the American Academy of Psychiatry and the Law 11:301-308, 1984.

30. AKISKOL, HS: *Subaffective disorders: Dysthymic, cyclothymic and bipolar II disorders in the "borderline" realm.* Psychiatr Clin North Am 4:25-46, 1981.

31. New York Penal Law, Section 125.25, Subdivision 1, paragraph (a).

32. New York Civil Procedure Law, Article 250, Section 250.10.

33. People v. Cassassa, 49 NY2d 668, 1980.

34. Addington v. Texas, 441 U.S. 418 (1979).

35. MORSE, SJ: *A preference for liberty: The case against involuntary commitment of the mentally disordered.* California Law Review 70:54-106, 1982.

36. POSTEL, RI: *Civil commitment: A functional analysis.* Brooklyn Law Review 38:1-94, 1971.

37. MCGARRY, AL AND CHODOFF, P: *The ethics of involuntary hospitalization.* In BLOCH, S AND CHODOFF, P: *Psychiatric Ethics.* Oxford University Press, New York, 1981, pp 203-219.

38. Mass. General Laws, Chapter 123, Section 1 (effective Nov. 1, 1971).

39. California Welfare and Institution Code, Sections 5000-5001 (West 1972) (effective July 1, 1969).

40. Arizona General Laws, Chapter 5, Section 36-501.

41. Lessard v. Schmidt, 349 F. Supp. 1078 E.D. Wis. (1972); *Overt dangerous behavior as a constitutional requirement for involuntary civil commitment of the mentally ill.* University of Chicago Law Review 44:562-593, 1977.

42. MCGARRY, AL, SCHWITZGEBEL, RK, LIPSITT, PD, LELOS, D: *Civil commitment and social policy: An evaluation of the Massachusetts mental health reform act of 1970.* Crime and Delinquency Reports, DHHS Publication No. (ADM) 81-1011, 1981.

43. Massachusetts Department of Mental Health Regulations, Title 4, Ch 2, Sec 200.01, effective Nov. 1, 1971.

44. URMER, AH: *A study of California's new mental health law.* ENKI Research Institute, Chatsworth, CA, 1972.

45. URMER, AH: *The burden of the mentally disordered offender on law enforcement.* ENKI Research Institute, Chatsworth, CA, 1973.

46. STONE, AA: *Mental health and law: A system in transition.* Crime and Delinquency Series, DHEW, 1975.

47. McGARRY, AL, CURRAN, WJ, LIPSITT, PD, LELOS, D, SCHWITZGEBEL, RK, ROSENBERG, AH: *Competency to stand trial and mental illness.* National Institute of Mental Health, DHEW, Public No. (HSM) 73-9105, US Government Printing Office, Washington, DC, 1973.

48. BALCANOFF, EJ AND McGARRY, AL: *Amicus curiae: The role of the psychiatrist in pretrial examinations.* Am J Psychiatry 126:342-347, 1969.

49. Dyas v. United States, App. D.C., 376 A.2d827, 831 (1977).

50. *In the Matter of William Wilson* (S.C. Family Division, D.C.) M.H.1124-82, 1982.

51. Barefoot v. Estelle, 103 S. Ct.3383 (1983).

52. United States v. Amaral, 488 F.2d 1148 (9th Cir. 1973).

53. United States v. Evans, 484 F.2d 1178 (2d Cir. 1973).

54. United States v. Brawner, 471 F.2d 969, D.C. Cir. (1972).

55. New York Penal Law Section 30.05.

56. WESTERMEYER, J: *A comparison of amok and other homicide in Laos.* Am J Psychiatry 129:703-709, 1972.

57. LEHRMAN, HE: *Other psychiatric disorders.* In KAPLAN, HI, FREEDMAN, AH, SADOCK, BJ (EDS): *A Comprehensive Textbook of Psychiatry.* Williams & Wilkins, Baltimore, 1980, p 1995.

58. CHENG, LY, op cit (56) p 709.

CHAPTER 5
PSYCHOLOGICAL ASSESSMENT IN LEGAL CONTEXTS*

Thomas Grisso, Ph.D.

In recent years, psychological assessments have become important sources of information in a variety of legal contexts, including criminal courts and correctional settings, juvenile and family courts, and civil courts. Among the legal decisions that have been assisted by psychological assessments are

- **Criminal court issues:** competence to waive rights to silence and counsel, competence to stand trial, competence to plead, criminal responsibility (insanity defense), sentencing;
- **Correctional decisions:** classification and placement of offenders, unit and institutional transfer, parole predictions;
- **Mental health law decisions:** involuntary civil commitment, competence to consent or to refuse treatment, guardianship/conservatorship for the incompetent (among the elderly, developmentally disabled, or mentally ill);
- **Juvenile delinquency decisions:** preadjudication detention, transfer to adult criminal courts, postadjudication disposition;
- **Family law matters:** termination of parental rights, divorce-related child custody decisions, foster home placement;
- **Law enforcement personnel selection;**
- **Examination of discriminatory practices** in hiring and in educational placement;
- **Evaluation of disability claims.**

* Portions of this chapter contain material and concepts that were developed with the assistance of Research Grant #RO1-MH37231 (Empirical Forensic Psychological Assessment) from the National Institute of Mental Health, Center for Studies of Crime and Delinquency.

In one sense, any mental health professional or lawyer who makes observations about an individual's personality or behavioral characteristics is engaged in "psychological" assessment. In a narrower sense (the one that is used in this chapter), **we define psychological assessment as an evaluation performed by a psychologist, using methods that are in large part an outgrowth of instruments, procedures, and principles identified historically with clinical psychology and the field of tests and measurements.**

This chapter examines several of these general principles and methods of clinical psychological assessment. The emphasis is upon psychology's potential to provide an empirical foundation to assist legal decision making. In addition, a central point of this chapter is that psychological assessments in legal contexts usually require more than the mere application of traditional psychological tools and methods, most of which were developed to address clinical and nonlegal questions. Clinical psychology's traditional assessment objectives (for example, diagnosis, personality description, treatment recommendation) often will be **relevant** to legal questions. Rarely, though, are they **sufficient** to fulfill the expert's function in assisting legal decision makers to consider questions of law. Legal questions place special demands upon the mental health examiner, requiring significant additions and modifications in the psychological assessment process and in the selection of assessment methods.

There are two important reasons traditional psychological assessment is not synonymous with assessment in legal contexts.

First, the law's definition of incompetence to stand trial or of parental fitness, for example, do not presume that any particular diagnosis (mental retardation, psychosis, and so forth) is dispositive of the legal question. Diagnoses are relevant, but the law asks more. Morse[1] has observed that most mental health laws call for three kinds of evidence concerning the individual in question: (1) a mental disorder; (2) some specific behavioral or functional ability (or lack of ability) directly relevant to the legal question; and (3) a causal connection between (1) and (2). Frequently the specific functional abilities (element 2) with which the law is concerned would neither be of interest nor be assessed in relation to treatment planning. For example, assessments for competency to stand trial must determine, in part, a person's understanding of basic trial procedures, something that almost never would be evaluated in routine assessments of clinical patients. Thus psychological assessment in legal contexts must employ methods and must address questions that usually are beyond the objectives of assessments in clinical contexts.

Second, legal decisions often will have a more restrictive and controlling impact upon the lives of persons about whom legal decisions are made. Implications for public policy and community welfare, too, may be more far-reaching than for most clinical decisions about clients in routine mental health work. Arguably, then, the assessor has an even greater burden in legal contexts than in routine clinical contexts to demonstrate the validity of the methods and findings that lead to professional conclusions.

Let us first review some general **principles** of psychological assessment, noting their special applications to assessments in legal contexts. Second, we will describe traditional and specialized psychological **tests and other instruments** that are employed as a quantitative base for psychological assessments to address legal questions. Third, we will review certain **practical issues** of psychological assessments in legal contexts that require special consideration.

PRINCIPLES

Psychological Assessment as a Concept

Maloney and Ward[2] have defined psychological assessment as "a process of solving problems . . . in which psychological tests are often used as one of the methods of collecting relevant data." This definition emphasizes a perspective of psychological examinations that often is not understood by colleagues in other professions and therefore is worthy of explanation.

The "process" to which Maloney and Ward refer includes five stages:

1. **Problem definition,** in which the question to be answered or the concern of the referring person is formulated clearly;
2. **Preparation,** in which the problem definition and available background information on the examinee lead to a plan for collecting additional information in direct assessment of the examinee;
3. **Data collection,** usually involving direct observation of the individual or group using the plan developed in the preparation stage;
4. **Interpretation,** in which available data are combined with test norms, theories, or models to arrive at opinions about the original question;
5. **Communication,** in which the assessment's results are rendered in a form usable by the individual, group, or qualified third party.

Psychologists, then, perceive the objective of their assessments to be the solving of problems or the answering of goal-directed questions, not the mere collection of information or assignment of diagnostic labels. Thus their assessment process is guided from the first stage to the last by the question or problem to be addressed in a particular case.

As a consequence, the data collection stage of psychological assessments has no invariable content. Just as physicians will employ somewhat different examination techniques when faced with different presenting symptoms and circumstances, so will psychological assessments vary in relation to different legal questions. Of course, certain tests that can provide data relevant to a broad range of human problems will appear with great frequency across psychological evaluations. Yet one should not anticipate a "standard test battery" to appear in every psychological report, because each assessment is designed to meet the specific objectives in the case in question.

Maloney and Ward's definition attempts to correct a common misconception of psychological evaluations as synonymous with "testing." Cronbach[3] defined a test as "a systematic procedure for observing a person's behavior and describing it with the aid of a numerical scale or category system." Thus psychologists employ a test merely as a tool for collecting and categorizing information relevant to the problem-solving objective of an assessment. If the solving of a particular problem does not require or is not likely to be promoted by existing psychological tests, then the assessment might include no tests at all. As we will see later, psychologists have developed several methods of data collection other than standardized tests, and in some cases these will serve the interests of the problem-solving objective better. Neither tests nor test scores, then, are synonymous with psychological assessment.

Psychological tests, nevertheless, distinguish psychological assessments from evaluations by most other mental health professionals. This fact underscores the psychologist's investment in the value of measurement and quantification. Tests and other methods that quantify human behavior and emotion are employed by psychologists in order to improve the quality of observations for use in the process of solving problems. The purpose and value of this quantified approach to assessment are misunderstood frequently. Let us examine some of the reasons for psychologists' traditional emphasis on tests and other quantified methods of observation in the assessment process.

Purpose and Value of Quantification

There is a story of the country gentleman who stopped by a crossroads grocery to purchase some sugar. Having scooped the sugar from a bin into a small paper bag, he took it to the storekeeper for purchase. The storekeeper hefted the bag in his hand and said, "Sixty-five cents." The country gentleman complained loudly that this was a most shoddy and imprecise manner for determining the quantity and value of his purchase. He vowed never to return to the store and left without purchasing the sugar. Within a few days, the gentleman heard from other customers that the storekeeper had taken the lecture seriously: He was now using pounds and ounces to determine the value of merchandise. Heartened, the gentleman returned to the store and repeated his earlier attempted purchase, handing the paper bag to the storekeeper. "Eight ounces," the storekeeper said, as he hefted the bag in his hand. "That'll be sixty-five cents."

There is, of course, limited value inherent in the mere assigning of numbers to observations, be they the weights of paper bags, degrees of intelligence, or the extent of a patient's motivations or emotions. We can assume that when the storekeeper announces that the next customer's bag weighs 4 ounces, he perceives it to be lighter than the first gentleman's bag. Yet two important values of measurement are missing in his procedure.

First, we do not know whether his estimates would be consistent from one day to the next, or whether his estimates would agree with those of his assistant who manages the store on weekends. Test developers refer to these questions of consistency and dependability as matters of **reliability.** Second, we do not know whether the storekeeper's "8 ounces" conforms to a standard US half pound. This is a matter of **validity;** that is, the degree to which a procedure actually measures what it claims to measure.

RELIABILITY

Whether administering a test or observing the frequency of some specific behavior of an examinee, the psychologist is attempting to collect data that are consistent and dependable. Observations of the examinee should be as similar as possible to those that would have been made by another examiner at the same time and place. The desired reliability of scores often depends upon the degree to which the data collection procedure has been carefully **standardized.** A procedure is standardized when one has demonstrated that it can be implemented, and scores can be assigned, in very much the same manner from one case to another by any trained examiner. This depends on how clearly the test or data collection procedure has been constructed and described by its developer in a manual and how carefully the examiner adheres to the standard procedure.

Most test developers will have published normative information, or "norms," for their test. **Test norms** are descriptions of the mean ("average") and range of scores made by some relevant, usually large, sample of people for whom the test is intended. If the examiner then administers the test to an individual and uses the standardized procedure and scoring, it may be possible to compare the individual's performance with the norms. This provides an estimate of the individual's standing relative to the normative group.

This approach to reliability in assessments has at least two important values, especially for legal contexts.

First, it mitigates subjective, discretionary error and bias, which must be recognized as influencing any process of professional observation and description. The reduction of error and bias by the professional at the stage of data collection is of special importance in legal contexts, in which the implications of decisions for human lives are no less grave—and sometimes more so—than in general clinical practice.

Second, examiner observations that are standardized, reliable, and quantified promote meaningful comparisons of various types in the course of a legally relevant assessment. One such purpose is that of locating the reasons for differences of opinion between two expert witnesses. If two experts have employed the same data collection methods in the same standardized fashion, one may examine whether the discrepancies between their opinions might derive from differences in the performance of the examinee at the two different assessment times or whether, instead, the two opinions are the result of different interpretations of essentially the same information. Another value is apparent when we are comparing a given examinee's behavior at two different times; for example, before and after having received treatment for incompetency to stand trial. We may be more confident about the extent of the observed gains, or lack of them, when we know that the pretreatment and posttreatment observations were performed in the same, standardized fashion and expressed in reliable, quantitative form. Finally, by comparing an examinee's score on a reliable test with the scores of a relevant normative group, judge and jury often are given a clear, accurate, and understandable point of reference with which to form their own opinions and impressions of an examinee.

VALIDITY

When previous research suggests that we can assign certain meanings or interpretations to the performance of examinees on a test, then the test is said to possess **validity** for that purpose. A method cannot be valid unless it is reliable (dependable, consistent). However, a method may measure reliably yet produce scores that do not have the meaning intended by the test developer or the examiner. For example, a test intended to measure prisoners' impulse control might produce highly consistent scores for a given prisoner again and again; yet it may or may not be useful in predicting impulsive expressions of emotion or motivation outside the testing situation. **Whether or not the test measures what it is purported to measure is the central question of validity.**

Psychologists speak of several types of validity for a data collection method, each of which might be relevant to the application of assessment results to various legal questions. (For a more detailed yet nontechnical description of the types of validity described below, see Kerlinger.[4])

Content validity refers to the logical congruence between the content of the test and some external criterion to which the score is to be related. For example, does the verbal content of a test of a parent's childrearing attitudes reflect the parenting qualities that the law and experts in child development regard as important for children's welfare? Not all tests must possess high content validity in order to be useful in assessments for clinical or legal purposes. If they do not, however, as a general rule there is an even greater burden upon them to meet the following two standards for validity.

Criterion validity refers to the degree to which the test has been demonstrated to concur with either of two types of events external to the test: (1) its ability to predict a particular behavior of the examinee at a point in time removed from the assessment session; or (2) its ability to produce scores that concur with another measure (obtained in the same time period) that claims to assess the same ability or trait. The first of these is especially important when, for example, the mental health professional is asked for an opinion concerning an individual's likelihood of engaging in destructive behavior in the future, or of making a satisfactory adjustment to community life after a period of involuntary civil commitment to a mental hospital. Few measures are able to predict future behavior with a very high degree of certainty. Yet many tests have sufficient criterion validity to reduce error in clinical judgments, when the data are combined with the professional's experience and with other specific information about the examinee.

Construct validity refers to a test's "track record" in past research for producing results that are consistent with theoretical expectations. For example, imagine that a psychologist had developed a test for children's abilities to perform accurately in providing eyewitness testimony in the courtroom. The meaning of the test would be enhanced if children at different ages produced different scores in a manner expected on the basis of some theory of cognitive development in children. Often this type of validity will be too complex to convey in the course of expert testimony. Nevertheless, such relationships between data collection methods and psychological theories will play an important role in the reasoning and interpretation processes of the psychologist.

Quantified and standardized observations, then, can have special value for psychological assessments in legal contexts. To be of value, however, they must be employed carefully in an assessment plan or design. The logic for designing psychological assessments requires special attention, because it is here that the examiner protects against arriving at unwarranted conclusions based on test scores alone.

Logic of Assessment Design

The psychologist has literally thousands of tests and other data collection methods from which to choose when designing an assessment. One venerable reviewer of psychological tests and measures has commented that "at least half of the tests currently on the market should never have been published,"[5] primarily because their reliability or validity have never been determined. These obvious failings considerably reduce the domain of measures from which the psychologist may draw effectively. Beyond questions of reliability and validity, the following are a few of the more important considerations when methods are being selected for a psychological assessment, especially in legal contexts.

RELEVANCE

Data collection methods are chosen in part for their relevance to the question or problem that gave rise to the assessment. Generally it will be preferable to use methods that assess as specifically as possible the traits or abilities related to a given question. For example, imagine that a psychologist has been asked to evaluate a defendant's ability to assist counsel in a defense. Some measure of the defendant's interpersonal skills and perceptions probably would be more relevant to the question than would be a test purporting to measure a wide range of general personality traits. In turn, a valid measure of "ability to relate to one's attorney" (were such a measure to exist) would be even more relevant than the measure of interpersonal skills. Inclusion of the more specific measures need not exclude the more general ones; but the objective of relevance gives priority to the more specific measures when they are available.

When the legal question is, in effect, a clinical one (for example, the individual's diagnosis, a description of personality, a recommendation for treatment), the psychologist will have no difficulty selecting from clinical psychology's armament of assessment methods those which will address the question directly. Some legal questions, however, require an opinion about abilities and capacities for which few or no specific measures have been devised. In these instances, the psychologist must select from among clinical assessment methods those which assess traits or abilities that appear to come closest in meaning to the abilities with which the law is concerned.

MULTIMETHOD-MULTITRAIT PRECAUTIONS

Psychologists recognize that there is error inherent in any single method of observation. Furthermore, the usual meaning of one ability test score might require reconsideration for some individuals because of the presence of some other ability or trait. For these reasons, psychologists frequently require that their interpretations of assessment results be grounded in more than one data source and that enough information has been obtained to rule out optional interpretations. Together these safeguards constitute what is referred to as a **multimethod-multitrait** approach to an assessment.[6]

The importance of the multimethod component in this approach is exemplified in the case of a psychologist's examination of an elderly woman for whom a court had to decide whether a guardian should be appointed to manage her financial affairs. Her son claimed that she continuously overspent her bank account because her "senile condition" caused her not to remember from one moment to the next her use of her credit cards or the amounts of financial transactions. The psychologist's subsequent assessment of her memory indicated that, indeed, the woman could not recall numbers or financial transactions within a few minutes after their occurrence. The psychologist chose to assess her memory ability with more than one specific test for that purpose. Furthermore, the psychologist inquired of her (and others) regarding her actual financial transactions in the past, and several impromptu checks on her short-term and long-term memory were made in the course of a more broad-ranging interview. Consistency in observations across these very different methods (several tests, past behavioral reports, interview behavior) lent far greater confidence to the psychologist's conclusions about the woman's memory than would the evidence from any one of the methods alone. **This multimethod precaution is basic and essential for psychological assessments.**

That, however, was not the sum of the psychologist's findings. Wanting to assess for the extent of the woman's disabilities, the psychologist examined not only her memory but also several other areas of functioning. Although the woman's memory was poor, it was discovered that she was quite adaptive and clearly capable of monitoring and controlling her own behavior at any given moment. Just as she could remember at the correct times that she owned a credit card, so could she learn and remember to write down in a notebook at the beginning of a shopping trip a starting amount, and then to record and to subtract any expenditures immediately upon their transaction. This second "trait" or ability significantly altered the competency testimony that the psychologist would have provided to the court on the basis of the memory assessment alone. The multitrait component in this assessment, then, guarded against attaching unwarranted significance to any one trait or type of disability.

PERSON-SPECIFIC INFORMATION

Thus far we have emphasized the selection of tests in the psychologist's design of an assessment. It is important to note, however, that most psychological assessments will be designed to obtain a variety of additional data in nonstandardized and nonmetric ways. These data generally will include demographic information; accounts of the individual's social, medical, and behavioral history; and the individual's own perceptions of his or her present and future situation. As we will describe later, much of this information is obtained through interview procedures and the discovery and review of archival records.

These types of data are especially important in psychological assessments for several reasons.

First, as a general rule, a person's past behavior, as well as one's expectations about one's own future behavior, can be of considerable assistance in understanding and predicting the person's behavior.[7]

Second, psychologists sometimes have available to them the base rates for certain behaviors or disorders; that is, statistical information about the actual frequency of an event or a disorder for groups defined by certain demographic characteristics or behavioral histories. To provide a simple example, the frequency of a second criminal act by first-time offenders is considerably less than the frequency of a fourth crime by third-time offenders. An examiner who evaluates offenders for parole, then, is cautioned by these base rates to require considerably more convincing data concerning an offender's future prospects in the case of a third-time offender than for a first-timer. Similarly, certain psychiatric disorders are more or less frequent among the young or the old, men or women, or in relation to other demographic categories. A knowledge of these base rates is helpful in forming hypotheses to explore in assessments, and in avoiding overprediction of certain behaviors that have a relatively low base rate for a given population.

Finally, Shapiro[8] has pointed out that base rates and normative test data are merely the starting points for clinical opinion. Information of these types serves as an "anchor" for the psychologist in forming initial, norm-based hypotheses about the individual. These hypotheses are then refined by the addition of information that is relatively specific to a particular individual and for which no norms or base rates exist. Thus obtaining highly individualized information about the person often is as important as obtaining quantified, normative data in standardized ways.

Situational Determinants of Behavior

One of the most important conceptual advances for psychological assessment in recent years has been the recognition that situational and environmental variables play important roles in determining clients' behaviors. Psychology's knowledge of person-situation interactions has a strong theoretical and research base.[9-12] Much of this research indicates that a person's past and future behaviors are often explained and predicted better by a knowledge of particular environmental circumstances, combined with personal predispositions, than by a knowledge of personal traits alone. Thus the assessment of physical and social environments with which an individual has interacted (or will be interacting) has become an increasingly frequent addition to psychological assessments.[13-16] This perspective in psychological assessment has two special justifications in legal contexts.

THE SITUATIONAL CONTEXT OF LEGAL QUESTIONS

Look back to the list of legal questions for assessments, with which this chapter began. Had we the time to analyze the laws that control these legal decisions, we would find that almost all of them are questions about an individual's probable functioning in some specific environmental or social context. For example, the question of a defendant's competence to stand trial is defined legally as an inquiry into the defendant's ability to understand the nature of pending trial proceedings, to appreciate the possible consequences, and to assist counsel in one's defense. The definition clearly points to an assessment of the **individual's** abilities and capacities; yet it asks about these capacities **in relation to a particular environment**—the defendant's trial—and the demands that it might make upon the defendant.

Trials, as with any other class of environment, vary in the demands that they place upon people. Some trials are long and emotionally draining, and others are brief. Some defenses require that attorneys have the benefit of a defendant's clear memory for past events, but the circumstances of other cases and trials may not make these demands. A psychologist's opinion regarding a defendant's competency to stand trial, then, is better informed when some of the specific circumstances of the pending trial are known. To the extent that the psychologist can obtain information about that future environment, that information can direct the assessment of the defendant more fruitfully and can be combined with knowledge of the defendant's personal characteristics to improve predictions and conclusions.

Similar analyses could be made for most questions that psychologists are asked to address in legal contexts. Usually the law is interested in the "match" or "mismatch" between a person's abilities and the demands of some environmental circumstances, or in the past or future product of the person-situation interaction. The inclusion of environmental assessment in legally relevant assessments, then, is both logical and necessary.

THE SITUATIONAL CONTEXT OF ASSESSMENTS IN LEGAL SETTINGS

An examinee's behavior during an assessment may be influenced by his or her perceptions of the purpose of the assessment. An examinee who is being evaluated for legal purposes frequently has a great deal to gain or to lose as a consequence of the assessment, inasmuch as the results are intended to provide information to a decision-making body with considerable power. It is not surprising, then, that some examinees will approach the assessment with a motive to attain whatever they perceive to be a desirable outcome.

Therefore, the situational context of assessments in legal settings requires special attention in the design and interpretation of psychological assessments. Every assessment must address the possibility of malingering, attempts to make "good impressions," or whatever other conscious and unconscious products of examinee motivation might be stimulated by the situational context of the assessment. Most tests and other quantified methods of observation are not immune to the influences noted above. The psychologist must attend to consistencies and inconsistencies in the examinee's performance, across various data sources, in order to guard against misinterpretation based on situational responses of examinees in legal contexts.[17]

TOOLS FOR PSYCHOLOGICAL ASSESSMENTS IN LEGAL CONTEXTS

In this section, we describe briefly a variety of tests, techniques, and structured methods employed in psychological assessments. Emphasis is placed on their uses and limitations when applied to legal questions. References cited for each method have been chosen especially to direct the less-informed yet interested reader to basic and more detailed sources of information.

Aids to Problem Analysis

The value of a psychological assessment to address a legal question can be greatly enhanced if the evaluator begins with a clear analysis of the problem itself: a definition of the relevant legal standard and an outline or schema of the behaviors, psychological functions, and mental states that are conceptualized as related to the legal standard. This outline can serve two purposes. First, it can guide the evaluator in designing the assessment, selecting the methods to be used, and implementing a strategic collection of data. Second, if the data then are interpreted to address each of the relevant components in the original analysis, the schema provides the logic that relates the examiner's data to the original legal question.

Several researchers have analyzed and interpreted various legal standards in order to provide examiners with schemas that can be used in the above way. Exemplary of such schemas is the product of McGarry and coworkers,[18] at the Laboratory of Community Psychiatry, who developed a list of 13 critical abilities and functions logically related to legal definitions of competency to stand trial. Other legal questions for which analytic outlines and schemas have been devised include competence to waive rights to silence and counsel,[19] criminal responsibility,[20-21] child custody determinations,[22,23] and prediction of dangerousness.[24]

Demographic and Archival Data

Demographic and properly documented background information about the examinee are important to obtain for most psychological assessments. Especially relevant are criminal justice and mental health records that can describe the history of the examinee's contacts with and treatment within these systems. Demographic and historical data are essential for the proper interpretation of many tests that the psychologist might employ in the assessment of the examinee's current functioning.

One must exercise considerable caution, however, in the use of archival records, especially with examinees who have accumulated a lengthy official file through extensive contacts with the criminal justice and mental health systems. The accuracy of recorded descriptions of events and narrative descriptions of the examinee's past motives and mental states is highly dependent upon the competence and care with which they were prepared by past observers (police, court employees, mental health professionals). These qualities vary considerably among persons within any profession. The validity of archival descriptions, then, should not be assumed automatically merely on the basis of their presence in an official file.

Behavioral Observation Methods

Psychologists have developed sophisticated technology for the systematic observation and recording of people's behaviors in naturalistic environments. When these methods are employed, they will take the psychologist out of the evaluation room into the social settings in which the examinee lives, works, and interacts with others. There the psychologist may seek to record the frequencies of various "target" behaviors of key importance to the assessment question, as well as the antecedents and consequences of the behavior in the natural, social context. These observations can mitigate against possible misinterpretations of data collected only in the context of the examination room, and frequently they can provide more direct answers about specific behaviors than are possible with inferences based on test scores alone. The range of behavioral assessment methods is quite broad,[25,26] many of which are adaptable to populations and settings that are of special concern in assessments related to legal questions.

Base Rate Information

A base rate is the statistical frequency of some disorder or behavior (within a specified time period) for a given group which is defined by some easily identified characteristics (for example, demographic descriptors). Knowledge of the base rate of a particular behavior for a specified group, and knowledge that an examinee possesses the defining characteristics of that group, can provide an estimate of the likelihood that the examinee will engage in that behavior.

Monahan[27] has noted that "knowledge of the appropriate base rate is the most important single piece of information necessary to make an accurate prediction." In fact, when the base rate for a behavior is very high, one may need to know little else about the examinee beyond appropriate group membership in order to make the necessary prediction. Many behaviors of concern in legal contexts, however, are relatively low base rate events (for example, suicide, violent assault), even among groups in which the behavior occurs with much greater frequency than in the general population. The primary value of base rate information in the latter situation is to caution the examiner against "overprediction" of the behavior, an error that many mental health evaluators may commit in their concern to protect the individual or society from the consequences of the predicted behavior.

Unfortunately, base rate information is not available for many important behaviors and groups relevant to legal questions. When it is available, however, its use is highly recommended as an aid to prediction.

Interview Guides

An open-ended, relatively unstructured interview is part of almost every psychological assessment, primarily because it provides an opportunity to observe the examinee's handling of a direct interpersonal encounter without test stimuli imposed between the examiner and examinee. In addition, the information obtained often will be rich in cues concerning certain unique characteristics of the examinee that might not be revealed with more structured assessment tools.

Several specialized interview guides have been developed to assist mental health professionals in making more reliable diagnoses of examinees' mental disorders and disabilities. The Diagnostic Interview Schedule,[28] for example, is a relatively recent yet already widely recognized interview tool. It guides the examiner in a highly structured and objective way toward diagnoses as defined in the *Diagnostic and Statistical Manual*[29] (*DSM III*, the uniform diagnostic system for the mental health professions).

Specialized interview guides also have been constructed to assist evaluators in collecting information related to specific legal questions. McGarry and coworkers,[30] for example, developed the Competency Assessment Instrument as an interview and rating guide to be used in evaluations for competency to stand trial. Slobogin, Melton, and Showalter[31] describe an interview system related to questions of criminal responsibility, and others exist for a wider range of legal questions.[32] The primary value of these methods is the enhancement of reliability, comparison of data across examiners, and improved content validity of assessments. Their use does not necessarily imply greater predictive validity, although research evidence to support that claim may well accumulate in time.

Intelligence Tests

Intelligence tests are standardized measures that are intended to provide an index of general intellectual ability. The tests of intelligence found most commonly in psychological assessments are the Wechsler Adult Intelligence Scale—Revised[33] and the Wechsler Intelligence Scale for Children—Revised.[34] Others that sometimes are used in cases involving special motivational or developmental disabilities include the Peabody Picture Vocabulary Test[35] and the Stanford-Binet test.[36]

The Wechsler tests consist of eleven subscales, each of which is intended to assess different important aspects of intellectual functioning. A person's performance on these subtests can provide an indication of strengths and weaknesses in various functions (for example, short-term memory, ability to think abstractly). Scores are used to describe strengths and weaknesses relative to one's own overall performance and relative to peers (normative samples of the general, national population of persons of one's own age). A composite of the scores from all the subtests are used to provide a summary score (the "IQ score"), which also can be compared with norms in order to find the person's standing in relation to peers.

The Wechsler tests of intelligence have been shown to yield highly reliable scores.[37] Scores on any test, however, can be influenced by extreme motivational and situational circumstances in certain cases. Thus extreme anxiety, psychopathological symptoms, or inordinate lack of motivation to use one's abilities can impair intellectual functioning and produce intelligence test scores that do not accurately reflect the individual's usual or potential level of ability. These possibilities must be taken into account by the evaluator when the results of the intelligence test are interpreted and used to address the original assessment question. Similarly, interpretive caution must be employed when evaluating children whose experiences, background, or language are not in the cultural mainstream (as might be the case for certain children with rural, ethnic, urban subcultural, or bilingual backgrounds). Comparison of their scores with national norms may simply reflect differences in background or their position of disadvantage in the taking of the test, rather than their intellectual capacity to learn and to adapt to the cultural mainstream with appropriate instruction and experience. This general issue has been at the heart of recent court decisions concerning the use of intelligence tests in the placement of children in educational programs.[38-40]

Intelligence test results are relevant when addressing a wide range of legal questions, because intellectual functioning has been recognized by courts as an important component to consider when addressing legal definitions of competency or capacity. Almost never, though, have courts recognized IQ scores or intellectual functioning alone as dispositive of any question of legal competence (for example, competence to stand trial[41,42]).

This perspective on intelligence test results is in general agreement with psychological research and practice. Most psychologists view intelligence test scores as useful for describing general intellectual functioning, but most also recognize that the IQ score alone is imperfect for predicting a person's ability in most specific situations or tasks outside the testing room.[43]

Neuropsychological Assessment

Many psychological and motor abilities may be impaired by neural tissue abnormalities; that is, brain or other nervous system damage, disease, or congenital conditions. The objective of neuropsychological assessment is to describe functional deficits resulting from nervous system dysfunction, to assist in their diagnosis, and to track the course of improvement or deterioration in functioning owing to these disorders. Even when neurological conditions have been diagnosed and located through medical technology, neuropsychological assessment frequently is necessary to provide a comprehensive and reliable picture of the behavioral and psychological consequences of the disorder.

Depending upon their type, extent, and location, neurological dysfunctions can affect any of the full range of psychological functions, including formal abilities such as memory and attention, emotional and motivational conditions, and perceptual and motor functions. Neuropsychological test batteries, such as the Halstead-Reitan[44] and the Luria-Nebraska[45] tests, have been developed to evaluate this wide range of functions and to provide schemas for the diagnostic use of the test results. One may encounter the use of these test batteries to address many types of legal questions, but especially in cases of disability claims by persons who have suffered brain damage and consequent loss of certain psychological or motor functions.

Neuropsychological assessments are time-consuming and complex. Unlike other methods described in this chapter, neuropsychological test batteries usually would not be performed by the general clinical psychologist but, instead, would be administered and interpreted by a psychologist who is specialized by training and experience in brain-behavior interactions and in neuropsychological evaluation.

Briefer, less-refined methods for detecting certain forms of neurological impairment are used by many psychologists as routine screening devices in order to assess whether more extensive neurological and neuropsychological evaluation may be needed. Among these methods is the Bender Visual Motor Gestalt Test,[46] which requires the examinee to copy standard geometric designs. Objective methods for scoring this test[47] may be useful in detecting certain types of nervous system disorders (those which affect particular perceptual-motor functions) but not other types.[48] That is, critical signs on the Bender test will usually indicate the need for more definitive assessment; the absence of those signs, however, does not necessarily indicate the absence of neurological disorder, inasmuch as many of these disorders would not directly affect perceptual-motor functioning.

Personality Inventories

Psychologists have developed a large number of paper-and-pencil, true-false, or multiple-choice measures of personality traits. Many of these are referred to as "inventories," indicating that a single test contains several scales, each corresponding to a different trait or diagnostic category. The inventory will have been constructed and developed so that an examinee's responses will provide scores on each trait scale. These scores then are used to characterize the behavioral, motivational, or personality predispositions of the examinee. The validity of these inferences depends on the degree to which research with that test has shown that normative groups of high or low scorers on these scales have, indeed, shown other evidence of the behavior or trait in question.

For example, the Minnesota Multiphasic Personality Inventory (MMPI)[49] consists of 566 true-false items contributing to 13 scales, each scale suggestive of certain diagnostic categories of psychopathology or personality. One use of the MMPI in psychological assessments is to compare the examinee's profile or pattern of scale scores with typical profiles that have been manifested by normative groups formed on the basis of a commonly shared psychiatric diagnosis. (For an example of normative MMPI profiles, see Marks, Seeman, and Haller.[50]) Thus a person with an MMPI profile most like that of a schizophrenic normative group may be further examined to determine whether other data also support evidence for that diagnosis. Although the MMPI frequently is used to assist in psychiatric diagnosis, other personality inventories, such as the Jackson Personality Inventory,[51] are intended primarily as measures of general personality traits rather than of symptoms of psychopathology.

Personality inventories can play several roles of special significance in legal contexts.

First, when the question is one of psychiatric diagnosis or personality description, these inventories may provide relatively objective data with which to validate, to refine, or to question the evaluator's inferences derived from interview or projective methods (described below), which are more susceptible to error when used alone.

Second, several personality inventories have scales designed to assist in detecting faking of symptoms, conscious suppression of symptoms, or an examinee's desire to make a socially acceptable impression. These scales do not provide foolproof protection. Nevertheless, they provide an important additional check for the evaluator who, in legal contexts, must be aware that examinees may possess many test-taking motivations less commonly encountered in clinical settings.

Third, researchers have developed a number of specialized scales and norms for the use of personality inventories in specific legal contexts. For example, Megargee and Bohn[52] have developed a system for using the MMPI to classify and to describe types of criminal offenders, and the Socialization Scale of the California Personality Inventory[53] has been found to be of special assistance in differentiating delinquent from nondelinquent youths.

The examples provided here have been inventories that claim to measure several traits or characteristics within a single instrument. Many other instruments have been designed to measure a single trait or psychiatric disorder. There are a very large number of personality inventories and single-trait measures, some of which have well-established validity for various purposes and others for which no substantial evidence of validity exists. Thus one can make no general statement about the validity of personality measures; each must be considered individually for its appropriateness and utility in relation to specific legal questions.

Projective Methods

Projective instruments, such as the Rorschach[54,55] and the Thematic Apperception Test,[56,57] are not tests in the usual psychometric sense of that term; their use usually does not involve discrete items, scores, or scales. Nevertheless, their administration is relatively standardized, and responses for many instruments can be reliably categorized.

The Rorschach, for example, is a set of 10 inkblot designs on cards which are shown to each examinee in the same sequence and with the same set of open-ended questions and inquiry. Examinees differ markedly in their reports of what the relatively amorphous forms seem to be. These responses are believed to reveal examinees' individual ways of attending to and interpreting the world around them. Various aspects of their responses—what they see or their use of the various qualities of the inkblot to justify their perception—can be reliably categorized and counted. Various systems for categorizing responses have been developed over the years. The most recent one by Exner,[58] however, appears to be gaining increased acceptance because of its author's accompanying research to improve the validity of interpretations based on this categorization system.

The Thematic Apperception Test, the second most commonly used projective method, is a set of pictures of people in a number of relatively ambiguous social situations. The examinee is asked to construct a story for each picture, and the themes of the stories are interpreted to reveal perceptions and beliefs characterizing the personality of the examinee.

The status of projective techniques in psychological assessment has been a source of considerable debate among psychologists for decades.[59] On the one hand has been the argument that projective methods have not (and perhaps cannot) be validated in the manner of most psychological tests and, therefore, that they are inappropriate as data sources for professional inferences and predictions. On the other hand are those who claim that the methods are valuable sources of subtle signs of psychopathology and are of great utility in the hands of the trained expert.

One will note that both arguments could be made about mental status or psychiatric interviews as well. Yet the interview as a source of data for inferences about psychopathology and personality is almost always seen as an appropriate and important part of every assessment, despite the fact that it is considerably less standardized, and its demonstrated reliability for diagnosis less researched, than for projective methods. By this reasoning, projective methods would seem to make no less legitimate contributions to assessments than do interview procedures, as long as an inference or conclusion is not based solely on the data derived from those methods alone. Unfortunately, some psychological examiners portray projective methods to be more definitive than is warranted, a practice which can draw well-deserved challenge on cross-examination in courtroom testimony.

Specialized Forensic Measures

Many of the methods described above are traditional clinical measures that can be applied to assessments in legal contexts. In recent years, however, test developers and researchers have constructed a number of assessment instruments designed specifically to address legal questions. These can be described as being of two types.

First, a very large number of measures related to crime and delinquency have been reviewed recently by Brodsky and Smitherman.[60] Noting that the quality of these measures is quite variable, Brodsky and Smitherman have carefully analyzed the limitations and values of each of them. Their work provides an excellent resource for evaluators and for lawyers who might need information on the tests when they are used by psychologists in legal cases.

The measures that Brodsky and Smitherman have reviewed are of several types that may be relevant in forensic assessments. For example, they list a large number of instruments that have been developed for purposes of classifying offenders, making placement or rehabilitation recommendations, and predicting recidivism or parole success. They also review many measures for evaluating delinquent and criminal attitudes and lifestyles. Described are many instruments that evaluate the attitudes and capacities of persons who work with offenders: law enforcement officers, correctional officers, and parole officers.

The second type of instruments with special relevance to forensic questions is any instrument that addresses specific legal definitions of certain competencies and capacities. A comprehensive review of this domain of forensic instruments has been completed by Grisso.[61] Many of these instruments have been developed, beginning with an analysis of the legal standard applied by courts when making determinations of a person's competencies or capacities. Then, after translating the standard into specific functions or abilities, developers have constructed test items defining these functions. Other instruments in this group were not developed specifically to address legal definitions of competencies, yet their content has seemed sufficiently legally relevant to some clinicians that they have been used for that purpose.

Instruments of this type sometimes are employed to address questions in three areas of criminal law. Concerning defendants' **competency to stand trial,** Lipsitt, Lelos, and McGarry[62] constructed the Competency Screening Test, consisting of items that evaluate the examinee's knowledge and perceptions of courtroom activities, trial roles, and client–attorney relations (which are the defining components of the legal standard for competency to stand trial). The same authors,[63] as well as Golding and Roesch,[64] have developed structured interview procedures for the same purpose, both of which yield quantified ratings of the defendant on several dimensions relevant to pretrial competency.

Several instruments have been developed to address suspects' understanding of rights to remain silent and to obtain legal counsel in the context of police interrogations, a matter bearing upon **competency to waive rights** and thus the validity of confessions. Grisso,[65] for example, developed several measures of juveniles' and adults' abilities in this area of functioning. Interpretation of these tests is assisted by normative data from large samples of adults and children. Gudjonsson[66] has developed an instrument for assessing a person's suggestibility and reliability of reporting, in the context of police questioning about one's involvement in a crime.

Instrumentation in the area of **criminal responsibility and legal insanity** has focused on structured interview outlines and decision trees, primarily without quantification. Rogers[67] and Slobogin, Melton, and Showalter[68] have developed examples of these instruments.

Several areas of civil law have received similar attention by clinicians who have sought test data with which to address questions of legal competency. For example, Anderten-Loeb[69] constructed an instrument to measure capacities of the elderly to care for themselves and their property, related to questions of **legal guardianship for the elderly.** The instrument assesses very specific abilities (for example, doing bankbook debits and credits, knowing the telephone all-purpose emergency number) that were endorsed by law and mental health professionals as relevant to legal questions of elderly persons' needs for a guardian. Other measures, such as the Older Americans' Resources and Services Instrument (OARS)[70] and the Geriatric Functional Rating Scale,[71] may be used for such purposes.

Clinicians who are asked to address legal questions of **parental fitness and child custody** have used quite a number of instruments to assist in judgments about parents' childrearing abilities or attitudes. Among these are the Mother–Child Relationship Evaluation,[72] the Parental Attitude Research Instrument,[73] the Parent Attitude Survey,[74] and the Michigan Screening Profile of Parenting.[75] Specialized measures such as those by Milner[76] may be useful in examining parents' attitudes and behaviors related to child abuse.

The special value of measures specifically developed to address legal definitions of competencies lies in the fact that their content is grounded in an analysis of what the law wants to know in relation to specific competency. Thus the results may be more directly related to the legal question in expert testimony. For example, an IQ score might allow an educated guess concerning whether or not a particular juvenile understood the police warning that he or she had the right to consult an attorney. The specialized measures mentioned earlier, however, examine in several objective ways the juvenile's understanding of the warning statement itself, thus providing much more direct evidence regarding the question at hand.

Measures of this type, however, are not without their limitations and hazards. For example, there is the danger that their high content relevance will cause users to accord more validity to their results than might actually have been demonstrated in research. There are several things that the clinician can keep in mind in order to avoid placing more weight upon these test results than is warranted.

First, as with any other test, these measures render scores that require support from additional sources of clinical data before testimony related to the legal question is justified. Their high degree of content relevance does not exclude them from the requirements of the multimethod assessment approach which we discussed earlier.

Second, one must understand that low scores on virtually any of these measures may be made not only because of interference by psychopathological phenomena but also for a variety of other reasons. For example, commentators have speculated (but as yet have not documented) that some defendants may obtain low scores on the Competency Screening Test if they have ideological disagreements with our system of justice,[77] or if past trial experiences have left them feeling helpless and powerless in legal settings.[78] Furthermore, those taking the tests occasionally may attempt to score poorly for some anticipated gain. Low scores, then, may be consistent with incapacity to understand the trial process, yet they may not always be interpreted as such without other assessment data which can assist in ruling out other possible interpretations.

Finally, the high content relevance of these instruments should not tempt the examiner to treat their scores as quantitative representations of the **legal** definition of incompetency itself. Most questions of legal competency require that the court weigh many aspects of a case. These include not only the capacities of the individual in question but also the future environmental circumstances facing the individual. In contrast, these measures generally provide only one type of information: characteristics of the person under the conditions that prevailed at the time of the evaluation. These forensic assessment instruments, then, may be especially useful to the court by providing reliable, relevant information about the person. Other types of data from other sources, however, will be needed to address the wider range of information that may be encompassed by legal definitions of competencies.

Environmental Measures

The importance of considering environmental and situational influences on behavior for purpose of description and prediction in individual cases was stressed earlier in this chapter. Consistently, the examination of interpersonal environments has come to be a frequent, if not standard, practice in psychological assessments of individuals. Depending on the exact nature of the legal question, interpersonal units relevant for individual assessments might include a family, a hospital ward, a correctional setting, a classroom, or a work environment.

Psychologists have developed a number of ways to describe and to evaluate these sorts of interpersonal environments. One method is that of measuring **psychosocial climate.** This term refers to interpersonal qualities of a setting, such as cohesion, support, conflict, or order and structure. Moos[79] has proposed that settings of the types noted above will differ with regard to these characteristics, just as persons differ on personality traits, and that the dominant psychosocial climate of a group or setting has a significant influence upon the behavior of persons who enter it. Consequently, Moos and his colleagues have engaged in an extensive research program to develop and to validate measures for assessing the dominant aspects of psychosocial climate in a variety of settings. Measures such as the Family Environment Scale,[80] the Correctional Institution Environment Scale,[81] and the Ward Atmosphere Scale[82] require each member of an environmental setting to indicate on objective test items which of a variety of activities and person interactions are typical or atypical in that person's setting. The setting's climate is determined by the sum of the members' perceptions, calculated as scores on each of 9 or 10 psychosocial climate dimensions.

The process of predicting how an individual would interact and behave if placed in that setting is at present largely intuitive. For example, one might reason that a delinquent youth assessed as very immature, dependent, and naive would not be a good match for a juvenile rehabilitation unit characterized as very low on climate dimensions of support and structure and very high on autonomy. Observations of this type may be relevant for a variety of legal questions involving the institutional and community placement of juveniles, adult offenders, the developmentally disabled, and mental patients.

It is well to note that psychologists, other mental health professionals, and lawyers who are in need of information on the development or validity of any general psychological test may consult the *Buros Mental Measurement Yearbook,*[83] which is periodically updated. The new volume by Brodsky and Smitherman,[84] noted earlier, currently is the only omnibus source for descriptions of instruments related specifically to issues in crime and delinquency.

PRACTICAL CONSIDERATIONS IN LEGAL CONTEXTS

This chapter began by examining some conceptual principles for psychological assessments in legal contexts. Then it reviewed empirical tools and other instruments that assist in the psychologist's data collection and interpretations. An assessment in a legal context, though, is more than a conceptual and empirical process for problem solving. It is also a service provided within a social context and intended for use by decision makers, many of whom are legal rather than mental health professionals. Any mental health professional engaging in assessment for legal purposes must be aware—from the initial preassessment phase through the presentation in the courtroom—of a variety of practical concerns raised by the systemic and social aspects of the legal context.

Do I understand what the lawyer wants, and does the lawyer understand what I can and cannot do? How will I manage objectivity in the context of an adversarial system of justice? What is my relationship to the examinee? What special safeguards must I use in the collection and interpretation of my data, given the legal circumstances? How can I best explain my results in the courtroom?

These are practical questions that face any mental health professional, not only the psychologist, who plans and implements an assessment in a legal context. Quite a number of resources are available to psychiatrists and psychologists who seek information regarding these practical questions. (For example, see references 72 to 77.) This section, then, does not review all these issues. Instead, it provides a few observations concerning practical considerations that are relatively specific to psychological assessments. Thus the comments focus primarily on special considerations raised by the use of psychological test results and other quantitative data, because these are the major features of psychologists' assessments which distinguish them from the assessments of most other mental health professionals.

Preassessment Considerations

Certain aspects of planning and preparation for the psychological assessment require special attention in the first contacts between the psychologist and the lawyer (or agency) at whose request the assessment will be done.

The lawyer may be most helpful in defining the legal question for the psychologist. This can improve the psychologist's ability to design an assessment that will address as specifically as possible the critical components that will be relevant to the legal decision maker (judge, jury, or parole board). Definition of the legal question may require more than an explanation of statute or major case precedent. For example, local jurisdictions and even individual judges may have their own consistent patterns of logic that guide their decisions in discretionary areas of law. Lawyers who have worked in a particular jurisdiction for some time may be familiar with these patterns.

In turn, many lawyers will not be familiar with the nature of psychological test data or the technical and logical processes with which psychologists employ data to arrive at conclusions. The psychologist, then, may assist the lawyer by describing, at this preparation stage, what it is that he or she plans to do and how the data produced by the planned methods are related conceptually to the various components of the legal question.

The lawyer often can be of assistance to the psychologist in obtaining initial background information, archival data, and the results of past psychological reports on the examinee. Criminal justice, medical, and psychiatric records frequently can be obtained most readily by the lawyer's authority as counsel to the examinee or, if necessary, by a motion to subpoena records. In either case, the lawyer will require the assistance of the psychologist to determine specifically what types of records may be available and how they are to be described in order to ensure that requests produce the desired information.

Assessment of the Examinee

The use of psychological tests raises certain issues in assessment sessions in legal contexts over and above the special considerations that would apply in assessment by other mental health professionals.

For most psychological tests, the norms with which the psychologist will compare the examinee's performance will not have been collected under psychological conditions similar to those in which the present assessment is being conducted. Very few tests have been normed on persons who have just spent their first two days in a crowded city jail, have just been issued prison clothes in exchange for their own, or are waiting judgment concerning whether they will be allowed to raise their own child. The psychologist must take special care to be aware of the effects of such situations when observing the examinee's behavior during the assessment session, when administering various tests, and when using normative data to interpret them.

Standardization and reliability of tests require that they be administered and scored in a manner that closely approximates descriptions in the test manuals. When test data are to contribute to an assessment for legal purposes, there should be a very high level of accountability regarding both administration and scoring. Scoring is documented in the psychologist's records and therefore is open to inspection by parties in legal situations. Similarly, psychologists and lawyers should consider whether administration of the assessment methods also should be documented (for example, by audiotape or videotape) in order to be able to provide a complete record of the standardized conditions under which data contributing to the psychologist's conclusions were obtained. The practice may be especially important for interview procedures, in which it may be difficult to reconstruct the event during a later trial. The same argument, though, can be made for the importance of verifying the quality of more standardized assessment procedures.

Interpretation

Of the many precautions that one could describe for the interpretation of assessment data for legal purposes, one of the most important is the practice of requiring that one's inferences and conclusions be based on more than a single test score or other single sign. The practice involves a process of formulation of hypotheses based at first on single scores or observations, then searching one's other sources of data for information that would support, refute, contradict, or simply render inconclusive one's original hypothesis. This is standard for competent practice in psychological assessments within any context, because it provides some protection against error that might be inherent in each data source when employed alone. It has special significance, though, for assessments in legal contexts. For example, inconsistencies between data obtained in the examination sessions and information about an examinee's behavior in other settings are sometimes the only indicators that one's test data reflect motivated attempts by the examinee to "look good" or to "look bad."[85]

It is at this interpretive stage that the psychologist must take special care to develop the logic regarding the relation of test scores and their clinical meanings to the important elements of the legal question. For example, a finding that the examinee has a very low IQ, interpreted as a severe deficiency in general intelligence and classifying the examinee as mentally retarded, does not suffice to address the issue of competency to stand trial. One must also show how the retardation influences functioning, and how that functioning deficit relates to that which is required in order to grasp the nature of a trial and to assist one's attorney. This, of course, will be difficult to establish if the need to show these connections was not considered **prior** to the data collection, when methods for the assessment were chosen in relation to an overall plan.

Testimony

Courtroom descriptions of tests, their content, norms, reliability, validity, test scores, and their meanings can be tedious and confusing, or they can be enlightening and instructive. Thus they can frustrate or assist the court in using psychological information with which to consider the ultimate legal question. Which of these two possibilities prevails is often dependent upon the degree of discussion, planning, or even rehearsal of testimony by the lawyer and the psychologist prior to the courtroom appearance. If the lawyer cannot understand the psychologist's description of the psychological tests and their results, it is not likely that the judge or jury will find them informative.

Lawyers have been provided with strategies for challenging the results of psychological tests on cross-examination;[86] psychologists, and the lawyers who call them to testify, should be aware of these strategies. Other resources are available to help psychologists parry the thrusts of aggressive cross-examiners;[87-94] attorneys who will oppose psychological expert witnesses should be aware of these.

Earlier we described certain psychological tests that have been developed specifically to address critical components of legal competencies. The high content relevance of these tests for the ultimate legal questions addressed by courts might lead psychologists to believe that the results of the test in effect answer the legal question. Indeed, some courts themselves might accept the results in a similar, uncritical way. It is important, therefore, to remember that ultimate decisions about questions of law usually require more than facts. The matter of a defendant's competency to stand trial, for example, is more than the sum of the defendant's abilities and capacities, no matter how precisely and validly they are measured. Someone still must decide whether that particular level of ability is sufficient to satisfy the **law's** intent and **society's** standards for justice. This is the type of ultimate decision which, as Monahan[95] has warned, should be "balanced on the scales of justice by people who wear black robes rather than people who wear white coats."

FUTURE DEVELOPMENTS

During the next five years we may see the development of a formal specialization called "forensic psychological assessment." It may follow the pattern of neuropsychological assessment's recent history, adapting traditional clinical instruments for new purposes and developing new methods in response to the demands of new questions in the specialty area.

Support for this prediction is found in the growing number of forensic assessment instruments described earlier in this review. Several others currently are in preparation. Training in forensic psychological assessment exists or is beginning in several universities. Whereas at this writing there are no textbooks or handbooks devoted entirely to the topic of forensic psychological assessment, several are in preparation or in press.

The prospect for developing a specialized field of forensic assessment is exciting, but it also calls for caution. Psychologists performing assessments do not need merely more new methods. They need new methods of high quality, carefully developed and researched, so that they meet scientific standards as well as the challenge of legal scrutiny. Their success requires collaboration between test developers and lawyers in order to ensure the relevance of new instruments to the law. It has even been proposed[97] that in some areas of law, it may be possible to develop systematic methods for engaging interdisciplinary teams of mental health professionals and lawyers in the assessment process itself. With careful attention to both scientific rigor and legal relevance, forensic psychological assessments may become more frequent, valuable contributors to legal decision-making processes.

REFERENCES

1. Morse, S: *Crazy behavior, morals and science: An analysis of mental health law.* Southern California Law Review 51:527, 1978.

2. Maloney, M and Ward, M: *Psychological Assessment: A Conceptual Approach.* Oxford University Press, New York, 1976.

3. Cronbach, L: *Essentials of Psychological Testing.* Harper & Row, New York, 1970.

4. Kerlinger, F: *Foundations of Behavioral Research.* Holt, Rinehart & Winston, New York, 1973.

5. Buros, O (ed): *The Eighth Mental Measurements Yearbook.* Gryphon, Highland Park, NJ, 1978.

6. American Psychological Association: *Standards for Educational and Psychological Tests.* American Psychological Association, Washington, DC, 1974.

7. Monahan, J: *The Clinical Prediction of Violent Behavior.* Department of Health and Human Services, DHHS Publication No. (ADM) 81-921, Washington, DC, 1981.

8. Shapiro, A: *The evaluation of clinical prediction: A method and initial application.* N Engl J Med 296:1509, 1977.

9. Bandura, A: *The self system in reciprocal determinism.* Am Psychol 33:344, 1978.

10. Bem, D and Allen, A: *On predicting some of the people some of the time: The search for cross-situational consistencies in behavior.* Psychol Rev 81:506, 1974.

11. Bowers, K: *Situationism in psychology: An analysis and a critique.* Psychol Rev 80:307, 1973.

12. Mishel, W: *The interaction of person and situation.* In Magnusson, D and Endler, N (eds): *Personality at the Crossroads: Current Issues in Interactional Psychology.* Erlbaum, Hillsdale, NJ, 1977.

13. Monahan, sup.

14. Moos, R: *Evaluating Treatment Environments: A Social-Ecological Approach.* John Wiley & Sons, New York, 1974.

15. MOOS, R AND FUHR, R: *The clinical use of social-ecological concepts.* Am J Orthopsychiatry 52:111, 1982.

16. MOOS, R AND INSEL, P (EDS): *Issues in Social Ecology.* National Press Books, New York, 1974.

17. HALLECK, S: *Law in the Practice of Psychiatry.* Plenum, New York, 1980.

18. MCGARRY, AL, CURRAN, WJ, LIPSITT, PD, LELOS, D, SCHWITZGEBEL, RK, ROSENBERG, AH: *Competency to Stand Trial and Mental Illness.* Department of Health, Education and Welfare, DHEW Publication No. (ADM) 77-103, Washington, DC, 1973.

19. GRISSO, T: *Juveniles' Waiver of Rights: Legal and Psychological Competence.* Plenum, New York, 1981.

20. ROGERS, R: *Rogers Criminal Responsibility Assessment Scales.* Psychological Assessment Resources, Odessa, FL, 1984.

21. SLOBOGIN, C, MELTON, G, SHOWALTER, C: *The feasibility of a brief evaluation of mental state at the time of the offense.* Law and Human Behavior 8:305, 1984.

22. WOODY, R: *Psychologists in child custody.* In SALES, BD (ED): *Psychology in the Legal Process.* Spectrum, New York, 1977.

23. WEITHORN, L: *The Psychologist and Child Custody Determinations.* University of Nebraska Press, Lincoln, NE (in preparation).

24. MONAHAN, sup.

25. KENDALL, PC AND NORTON-FORD, JD: *Clinical Psychology: Scientific and Professional Dimensions.* John Wiley & Sons, New York, 1982.

26. HAYNES, S: *Principles of Behavioral Assessment.* Gardner Press, New York, 1978.

27. MONAHAN, sup 34.

28. ROBINS, L, HELZER, J, CROUGHAN, J, RATCLIFF, K: *National Institute of Mental Health Diagnostic Interview Schedule.* Arch Gen Psychiatry 38:381, 1981.

29. AMERICAN PSYCHIATRIC ASSOCIATION: *Diagnostic and Statistical Manual of Mental Disorders,* ed 3. APA, Washington, DC, 1980.

30. MCGARRY ET AL: sup.

31. SLOBOGIN, MELTON, SHOWALTER, sup.

32. LAWRENCE, S: *Manual for the Lawrence Psychological-Forensic Examination.* Lawrence, San Bernardino, CA, 1981.

33. WESCHLER, D: *Wechsler Adult Intelligence Scale—Revised Manual.* Psychological Corporation, New York, 1982.

35. DUNN, L: *Expanded Manual for the Peabody Picture Vocabulary Test.* American Guidance Service, Minneapolis, 1965.

36. TERMAN, L AND MERRILL, M: *Stanford-Binet Intelligence Scale.* Houghton-Mifflin, Boston, 1973.

37. MATARAZZO, J: *Wechsler's Measurement and Appraisal of Adult Intelligence.* Williams & Wilkins, Baltimore, 1972.

38. Larry P. v. Riles, 343 F.Supp. 1306 (N.D. Cal. 1972) (order granting preliminary injunction), affirmed, 502 F.2d 963 (9th Cir. 1974); 495 F.Supp. 926 (N.D. Cal. 1979) (decision on merits), appeal docketed, No. 80-4027 (9th Cir., Jan. 17, 1980).

39. PASE v. Hannon, 506 F.Supp. 831 (N.D. Ill., 1980).

40. BERSOFF, D: *Larry P. and PASE: Judicial report cards on the validity of individual intelligence tests.* In MELTON, G (ED): *Legal Reforms Affecting Child and Youth Services.* Haworth Press, New York, 1982, p 101.

41. STONE, A: *Mental Health and Law: A System in Transition.* Department of Health, Education and Welfare, Washington, DC, 1975.

42. ROESCH, R AND GOLDING, S: *Competency to Stand Trial.* University of Illinois Press, Champaign, IL, 1980.

43. McClelland, D: *Testing for competence rather than for intelligence.* Am Psychol 28:1, 1973.

44. Reitan, R and Davison, LA (eds): *Clinical Neuropsychology: Current Status and Applications.* John Wiley & Sons, New York, 1974.

45. Christensen, A: *Luria's Neuropsychological Investigation.* Spectrum, New York, 1975.

46. Bender, L: *A visual motor Gestalt test and its clinical use.* American Orthopsychiatric Association, Research Monographs, No. 3, 1938.

47. Pascal, G and Suttell, B: *The Bender-Gestalt Test: Quantification and Validity for Adults.* Grune & Stratton, New York, 1951.

48. Maloney and Ward, sup, p 269.

49. Hathaway, S and McKinley, J: *The Minnesota Multiphasic Personality Inventory Manual.* Psychological Corporation, New York, 1967.

50. Marks, P, Seeman, W, Haller, D: *The Actuarial Use of the MMPI with Adolescents and Adults.* Williams & Wilkins, Baltimore, 1974.

51. Jackson, D: *Jackson Personality Inventory Manual.* Research Psychologists Press, Port Huron, MI, 1976.

52. Megargee, E and Bohn, M: *Classifying Criminal Offenders: A New System Based on the MMPI.* Sage, Beverly Hills, 1979.

53. Gough, H: *Manual for the California Psychological Inventory.* Consulting Psychologists Press, Palo Alto, CA, 1960.

54. Rorschach, H: *Psychodiagnostics: A Diagnostic Test Based on Perception.* Hans-Huber, Berne, 1942.

55. See Maloney and Ward, sup, pp 345-381, for brief review of Rorschach.

56. Murray, H: *Manual for the Thematic Apperception Test.* Harvard University Press, Cambridge, MA, 1943.

57. Murstein, B: *Theory and Research in Projective Techniques, Emphasizing the TAT.* John Wiley & Sons, New York, 1963.

58. Exner, J: *The Rorschach: A Comprehensive System.* John Wiley & Sons, New York, 1974.

59. Goldfried, M, Stricker, G, Weiner, I: *Rorschach Handbook of Clinical and Research Applications.* Prentice-Hall, New York, 1971.

60. Brodsky, S and Smitherman, H: *Handbook for Scales for Research in Crime and Delinquency.* Plenum, New York, 1983.

61. Grisso, T: *Evaluating Competencies: Forensic Assessments and Instruments.* Plenum, New York (in press).

62. Lipsitt, P, Lelos, D, McGarry, AL: *Competency to stand trial: A screening instrument.* Am J Psychiatry 128:105, 1971.

63. McGarry et al: sup.

64. Golding, S, Roesch, R, Schreiber, J: *Assessment and conceptualization of competency to stand trial: Preliminary data on the Interdisciplinary Fitness Interview.* Law and Human Behavior 8:321, 1984.

65. Grisso, sup.

66. Gudjonsson, GH: *A new scale of interrogative suggestibility.* Personality and Individual Differences 5:303, 1984.

67. Rogers, sup.

68. Slobogin, Melton, Showalter, sup.

69. Anderten-Loeb, P: Validation of the Community Competency Scale. Unpublished doctoral dissertation, St Louis University, 1983.

70. Center for Study of Aging and Human Development: *Multidimensional Functional Assessment: The OARS Methodology.* Duke University, 1978.

71. GRAUER, H AND BIRNBOM, F: *A geriatric functional rating scale to determine the need for institutional care.* J Am Geriatr Soc 23:472, 1975.

72. ROTH, R: *The Mother–Child Relationship Evaluation.* Western Psychological Corporation, Los Angeles, CA, 1980.

73. SCHAEFER, E AND BELL, R: *Development of a parental attitude research instrument.* Child Dev 29:339, 1958.

74. HEREFORD, C: *Changing Parental Attitudes.* University of Texas Press, Austin, TX, 1963.

75. HELFER, R, HOFFMEISTER, J, SCHNEIDER, C: *A Manual for Use of the Michigan Screening Profile of Parenting.* Test Analysis and Development Corporation, Boulder, CO, 1978.

76. MILNER, J: *The Child Abuse Potential Inventory.* Psytec Corporation, Webster, NC, 1980.

77. BRAKEL, S: *Presumption, bias, and incompetency in the criminal process.* Wisconsin Law Review 1105, 1974.

78. ROESCH AND GOLDING, sup.

79. MOOS, sup.

80. MOOS, R: *Family Environment Scale Preliminary Manual.* Social Ecology Laboratory, Department of Psychiatry, Stanford University, Palo Alto, CA, 1973.

81. MOOS, R: *The assessment of the social climates of correctional institutions.* Journal of Research in Crime and Delinquency 5:174, 1968.

82. MOOS, R: *Ward Atmosphere Scale Manual.* Consulting Psychologists Press, Palo Alto, CA, 1974.

83. BUROS, sup.

84. BRODSKY AND SMITHERMAN, sup.

85. ANDERTEN, P, STAULCUP, V, GRISSO, T: *On being ethical in legal places.* Professional Psychology 11:764, 1980.

86. BRODSKY, S, AND ROBEY, A: *On becoming an expert witness: Issues of orientation and effectiveness.* Professional Psychology 3:173, 1972.

87. HALLECK, sup.

88. LOFTUS, E AND MONAHAN, J: *Trial by data: Psychological research as legal evidence.* Am Psychol 35:270, 1980.

89. MORSE, S: *Law and mental health professionals: The limits of expertise.* Professional Psychology 9:389, 1978.

90. POYTHRESS, N: *Mental health expert testimony: Current problems.* Journal of Psychiatry and the Law 5:201, 1977.

91. HALLECK, sup.

92. ZISKIN, J: *Coping With Psychiatric and Psychological Testimony.* Law and Psychology Press, Beverly Hills, CA, 1975.

93. BRODSKY AND ROBEY, sup.

94. POYTHRESS, N: *Coping on the witness stand: Learned responses to "learned treatises."* Professional Psychology 11:139, 1980.

95. MONAHAN, J: *Commitment after acquittal by reason of insanity: Dangerousness and the role of mental health professionals.* Division of Psychology and Law Newsletter 3:14, 1983.

96. ROESCH AND GOLDING, sup.

CHAPTER 6

PREDICTION OF DANGEROUSNESS AND IMPLICATIONS FOR TREATMENT*

R. Kirkland Gable, Ph.D., J.D.

The following discussion briefly examines some of the major issues and current trends in the prediction and treatment of mentally ill persons considered dangerous. The discussion does not include a consideration of persons who are dangerous only to themselves, such as suicidal or gravely disabled persons. The focus is upon mentally ill persons who present a substantial risk of physical harm to others. The concluding suggestions for improving predictive accuracy and treatment efficacy are frankly speculative and are offered to stimulate further clinical investigation and research.

Persons attempting to predict behavior and to treat dangerous patients currently find themselves in a difficult social and legal situation. On one hand, there is legislative and judicial pressure upon treatment personnel to find the "least restrictive alternative" for handling the dangerous mental patient consonant with the patient's or public's safety.[1,2] On the other hand, treatment personnel may be legally responsible if they prematurely release a dangerous person or fail to notify potential victims of the patient's dangerousness.[3] This situation is further complicated by the varying legal definitions of dangerousness found in different states and the clinical difficulty of predicting future behavior likely to be considered dangerous.

PREDICTIVE ACCURACY

Perhaps one of the best-known studies of the prediction of dangerousness is that of the "Baxstrom patients" made by Steadman and his associates.[4,5] As a result of a legal decision by the United States Supreme Court, 967 patients who were involuntarily committed to Dannemora and Matteawan state hospitals as dangerous persons were released to 18 civil facilities in their respective com-

* This chapter was supported in part by Grant No. R01 MH25955 from the Center for Studies of Crime and Delinquency of the National Institute of Mental Health.

munities in New York State.[6] Four years later, only 2.7 percent of these patients were returned to the hospitals to which they had originally been committed. A more intensive follow-up study of a subsample of these patients found that 17 percent had been arrested and 7 percent of those arrested were convicted. Not all of the convictions resulted in confinement. In summary, the vast majority of these supposedly dangerous patients were not in fact dangerous when released into the community within the 4 years of the follow-up study.[7]

Other studies of patients released by court or administrative order, contrary to psychiatric diagnoses of dangerousness, have generally produced similar results. For example, in Illinois, Rubin[8] has studied "the Menard 18." Because of an "administrative error," 17 of these 18 patients spent a total of 425 years in confinement after they legally should have been placed in less restrictive treatment or community settings. Rubin's follow-up study also indicated that these illegally confined men were probably not very dangerous, even at the time of their initial commitment. (One of "the Menard 18" has been so administratively misplaced that he cannot be located.)

In 1967, a new statute in Massachusetts required the judicial review of involuntarily committed mental patients at the Massachusetts Correctional Institution at Bridgewater. The patients there at that time were reviewed in light of the Baxstrom decision which required new, legal safeguards prior to commitment. Out of a sample of 234 patients transferred to other civil hospitals, a 33-month follow-up study found that 93 (39.7 percent) were released or escaped into the community. After an average of 13 months in the community, 15 of the patients (16.1 percent) appeared in court. There was only one conviction for a felony. All the other charges were misdemeanors, usually drunkenness.[9] It could be reasonably concluded that at least one third of the men being detained in Bridgewater were not dangerous. A higher rate of release into the community might have revealed an even higher percentage of nondangerous patients.

The professional literature almost uniformly affirms low predictive accuracy with regard to the dangerousness of mental patients. One study, however, by Kozol, Boucher, and Garofalo[10] claims that dangerousness can be "reliably diagnosed and effectively treated." The senior author, a psychiatrist, and his associates examined 592 convicted male sex offenders who had been sent to the Bridgewater Institution for diagnosis as potentially sexually dangerous persons. On the basis of initial diagnostic studies, the authors concluded that 304 of these persons were not dangerous, and 257 were diagnosed as dangerous. The remaining 31 patients were returned to prison for legal reasons and were not included in the reported diagnostic studies. After receiving treatment for an average period of 43 months, 82 patients were released. Of these, five subsequently committed serious assaultive crimes, thereby producing a recidivism rate of 6.1 percent, according to the authors.

This appears to be an excellent record of diagnosis and treatment. Fortunately, the authors also provide data on 49 patients, diagnosed and treated by them as dangerous, whom the court released from Bridgewater contrary to the medical staff's recommendation. Of these patients, 34.7 percent subsequently committed serious assaultive crimes. Conversely, 65.3 percent did not commit such crimes after approximately 5 years in the community. Thus, nearly two thirds of those patients released contrary to predictions of dangerousness by Kozol's group were not subsequently dangerous.[11] This represents a serious overprediction of dangerousness.

There has been even further criticism of the Kozol study. A reanalysis of the data in this study by Evenson and Altman[12] found an expected base rate of recidivism of 11 percent for the total group of 435 released patients. (There were 304 patients released as not dangerous at the initial diagnosis; 82 were released as not dangerous after treatment; and 49 were released by the court contrary to a diagnosis of dangerousness.) It would have been possible to obtain 89 percent accuracy with this group of patients merely by predicting that all the patients were not dangerous. Most of the project staff's predictive accuracy came from correctly identifying the large number of patients who were not dangerous. If one statistically compensates for correct prediction occurring merely by chance, one finds that the staff's predictive accuracy was about 27 percent.

A study by Carney[13] at the Patuxent Institution of Maryland also seems to support the ability of psychiatrists to predict dangerousness or the absence of it. However, the medically released group had community placements while on parole and the court-released group did not. Moreover, the data utilized in the study are incomplete.

Ennis and Litwack[14] have sharply questioned the legal qualification of psychiatrists to testify as experts on the issue of dangerousness. They comment:

An exception to the ordinary rules of evidence has been created to permit experts to testify in court as to their opinions, conclusions, and judgment. With the exception of psychiatrists, witnesses are required to prove their expertise before courts will permit them to testify as experts. If that same proof were required of psychiatrists, they could not qualify as expert witnesses. Support for this proposition may be provided by analogy to the judicial treatment of polygraph results.

There is no question that psychiatric judgments are far less reliable and valid than polygraph judgments. Although the evidence is still accumulating, a conservative estimate is that an experienced polygraph examiner can correctly detect truth or deception about 80 to 90 percent of the time.

Significantly, one study had indicated "that an examiner is more inclined to report a guilty subject innocent than he is to report an innocent subject guilty." The converse is true of psychiatrists; if doubt exists, it almost always is resolved to the patient's disadvantage; predictions of dangerousness afford the prime example.

Despite this proven reliability and validity of polygraph tests, only a handful of state and federal trial courts have received polygraph reports in evidence, and then usually for only limited purposes. Moreover, no appellate court has approved the admission of polygraph reports over the objection of a party.

Whatever may be said for the reliability and validity of psychiatric judgments in general, there is literally no evidence that psychiatrists reliably and accurately can predict dangerous behavior. To the contrary, such predictions are wrong more often than they are right. It is inconceivable that a judgment could be considered an "expert" judgment when it is less accurate than the flip of a coin.

Accordingly, psychiatrists should not be permitted to testify as expert witnesses until they can prove through empirical studies that their judgments are reliable and valid.

In an experimental study by Sweetland,[15] college students and psychiatrists agreed extensively on the degree of "dangerousness" and "nondangerousness" as indicated by various personality characteristics. This suggests the possibility that psychiatric judgment is not based upon any special knowledge or expertise beyond that of educated laymen. There are also several studies indicating that the diagnostic classifications made by psychologists are not more reliable or valid than those made by laymen.[16]

More recently, Steadman and Cocozza[17] have studied the predictive accuracy of psychiatrists evaluating the dangerousness of 257 felony defendants found incompetent to stand trial. The study groups had an average (mean) age of 31 and were predominantly nonwhite; approximately two thirds came from the New York City area, and the alleged offenses involved violent acts more often against persons than against property or drugs. Data collected over a 3-year follow-up period indicated that the group of defendants diagnosed as dangerous was not statistically more dangerous than the group of defendants diagnosed as nondangerous. The researchers concluded, "The level of accuracy by the psychiatrists was no greater than that obtainable by chance. These findings suggest that psychiatric testimony to the court in regard to applying the dangerousness standard currently should not be considered expert."

Stone[18] has commented, "The law, influenced by the reforms I have described, asks the psychiatrist to prognosticate dangerous behavior. That is absurd because it is a rare event, and the capacity for such prognostication is absent. What the mental health profession can prognosticate is the mental state and the likely course of the illness of the patient." Legal attacks upon the assumption of psychiatric expertise in the prediction of dangerousness will probably increase in the near future unless better predictive accuracy can be scientifically demonstrated.

APPROACHES TOWARD INCREASING PREDICTIVE ACCURACY

Immediate Steps

Long-term prediction of behavior is more difficult than short-term prediction. Accurate prediction is more likely for one day in the future than for one year in the future or for an indefinite period of time. Therefore, clinicians might consider shortening, or at least specifying, the time frame of their predictions. This may require the more frequent examination of patients because the time frame is shortened.

If the psychological and social conditions surrounding a patient change, prediction becomes more difficult. Therefore, prediction might be made with reference to particularly critical conditions for each patient (for example, continued employment, a stable marriage, or abstinence from alcohol). As circumstances change, the clinician should be notified and the patient reassessed. Courts do not always require an evaluation of dangerousness projected indefinitely into the future. In fact, the trend is to require more time-limited predictions. For example, the predicted dangerous act necessitating confinement must, in some states, be expected to occur within the "reasonably foreseeable future."[19] It is reasonable to require no greater prediction into the future for the release of patients.

The definition of dangerousness should be clarified prior to prediction. Does the dangerousness include harm to self? Does it include financial harm to others? Does it include public drunkenness? Does it include verbal threats or abuse? Does it include preparation or plans that might lead to violence, such as the purchase of a firearm? Without prior agreement about what behavior constitutes a dangerous act, it is likely that there will be considerable disagreement, and predictive accuracy will be poor. Increasingly, civil commitment statutes are requiring evidence of specific acts, attempts, or threats of physical harm prior to commitment. An Arizona statute defines "danger to others" as "behavior which constitutes a danger of inflicting substantial bodily harm upon another person based upon a history of having inflicted or having attempted to inflict substantial bodily harm upon another person within 12 months preceding the hearing on court ordered treatment."[20]

Another strategy for improving predictive accuracy involves the use of two or more professionals rating or assessing the patient independently, then comparing the results.[21] In this way, factors overlooked or overrated by one person may be detected by the other. It is important that the initial assessment by the two persons be conducted independently, rather than having the initial assessment passed on to the second person for confirmation. When there is poor agreement (low interrater reliability) between two persons making an assessment, it is fairly certain that at least one of them is incorrect. Low interrater reliability usually establishes the upper limit of valid (truthful) assessment. Thus, if one physician detects mammary cancer by clinical examination and another physician using the same procedure does not, one of them is in error and the validity of the result is in question. Sometimes independent assessment and comparison using different procedures or approaches is necessary to obtain sufficient validity.*

Clinical experience alone may not be sufficient to guarantee validity or even agreement among the "experts." As a part of a study of the competency of patients to stand trial, the agreement (interrater reliability) among eight psychiatrists with an average (mean) of 287 competency examinations was examined. These expert psychiatrists were generally mental hospital superintendents or chief psychiatrists. They had no greater agreement among themselves on patient's competency (R of 0.67) than psychiatrists with no previous experience in competency examination (R of 0.68).[23] In general, even among experts, agreement about assessment criteria, discussion of areas of disagreement, and the feedback of results over a series of patients can be expected to increase substantially both assessment reliability and potential validity.

Consideration of Social-Environmental Factors

There are many theories about the etiology of dangerous behavior. A part of the reason for so many theories is that the concept of "dangerousness" subsumes many different behaviors ranging from the carefully planned execution

---

* For example, in a study involving the screening and follow-up of 20,211 women for mammary cancer,[22] almost two out of five of the prevalent cancers in the initial screening would have been missed by clinical examination. Conversely, mammography alone would have missed more than two out of five cancers subsequently detected. Both clinical estimation and mammography were necessary.

of a political enemy to rage reactions inadvertently harming innocent bystanders.* Presumed causes may range from social discontent to neurologic disorders such as temporal lobe seizures.[24,25] Traditionally, legal and psychiatric conceptualizations of dangerousness have focused upon the individual as the source of these behaviors. More recently, a view has been emerging that focuses upon the interaction of a person with his or her physical and social environment in the production of behavior considered dangerous. In this view, there must be a behavior, a social context for that behavior, and an observer who labels the behavior as dangerous.[26]

The conceptualization of dangerous behavior as a product of person-environment interactions can have important legal and clinical consequences. For example, consider the proverbial "little old lady" who accidently leaves the gas jets turned on in her apartment after using her stove. She may not kill only herself but also a few of her neighbors and is, therefore, committable under many states' statutes as a dangerous person. But does the "dangerousness" lie within her, within her environment, or both? The dangerousness in this case is correctable not only by committing this woman to an institution for treatment but also by replacing her gas stove with an electric one.

Some people may be dangerous only in particular situations (for example, in barrooms), under particular conditions (for example, when intoxicated), and in a particular interpersonal context (for example, threats to self-esteem). Too often, clinicians may infer enduring personality traits from behaviors that are, in fact, responses to specific environmental conditions. A child may hit another child primarily when he is struck first or is insulted. This aggressive behavior may persist if it is reinforced by praise for being "tough" or by the other child's surrender of territory. The importance of antecedent and consequent environmental events has been observed and demonstrated frequently in experimental studies with children.[27] From a community viewpoint, O'Neal and McDonald[28] have extensively reviewed various environmental factors that might be related to increased aggression. Among these factors are noise, heat, territoriality, crowding, anonymity, diffusion of responsibility, and audience approval. In a survey of studies of animal aggression, Moyer[29] has suggested several general categories of aggression that are responsive to the environmental context. A few of these categories are fear-induced aggression, sex-related aggression, and instrumental (rewarded) aggression. The specification of the environmental factors associated with aggression would seem to be a more promising approach to predicting physically harmful acts than a general and diffuse concept of dangerousness. As will be discussed later, the consideration of environmental factors may significantly influence treatment and release decisions.

Base Rate Information in Case-Specific Decisions

Mental health personnel rather consistently overpredict dangerousness,[30] which leads to extensive confinement of patients who are allegedly dangerous but who are, in fact, not so. The reason for this overprediction is probably, in part,

---

* The issue has sometimes been raised as to whether a "hired killer" may be involuntarily committed under civil statutes because, although he is dangerous, he may not also be mentally ill. Use of habitual offender statutes may be a more appropriate approach.

the strong negative reaction of the public to errors associated with the release of dangerous persons, whereas there is relatively little concern about unnecessary confinement.[31,32] Those persons clinically predicted to be dangerous but who are in fact not dangerous represent false-positive errors in prediction. In contrast, those persons clinically predicted to be not dangerous but who are in fact dangerous represent false-negative errors in prediction. It is likely that both false-positive and false-negative errors might be reduced by incorporating statistical prediction techniques into clinical decision making.[33]

For over two decades, research has been conducted comparing clinical prediction techniques with statistical prediction techniques.[34] A review of 45 studies by Sawyer,[35] comparing statistical and clinical evaluations, revealed that statistical methods were at least equal to, and generally superior to, clinical methods. It would seem desirable, therefore, to use statistical methods at least in combination with clinical methods. Shah[33] has described one possible method of combining clinical and statistical methods:

> A fundamental rule of statistical prediction is that expected accuracy must control the relative weights assigned to the specific evidence being used for predictions (e.g., various clinical indices and "signs") and to the prior information (viz., the base rates). As the expected accuracy of the [clinical] predictions decreases (viz., in situations where the base rates are very low and the available evidence not very reliable), the prediction should become regressive and should shift closer to the base rates or the prior probabilities. For example, if only 10 percent of a particular group are expected to engage in future violent behavior on the basis of prior probability (base rates), and if the specific evidence concerning predictions is of poor reliability (e.g., clinical assessments and certain psychological test indices), then the predictions should remain close to the base rates. The greater the move away from the base rates under the above conditions, the greater will be the probability of error.
>
> Experiments conducted by Kahneman and Tversky[36] demonstrated, nevertheless, that individuals engaged in a predictive task very commonly disregard information concerning prior probability when some specific current information is provided. There is a tendency instead to resort to the representativeness heuristic, even to the extent that involves gross departures from the prior probabilities.

It appears that specific case history information often strongly influences clinical prediction, whereas relevant statistical information does not have great influence. In fact, valuable statistical information may be ignored when completely worthless case history information is given to persons making predictions. Carroll[37] found that brief case history descriptions were subjectively compelling enough to negate the use of important statistical information.

Parole Board Prediction System

One potentially useful approach involving both clinical and statistical information is the two-dimensional system used by the United States Board of Parole.[38] In actual practice, the parole board member rates the prospective parolee on the severity of the prior offense and the parole prognosis (risk of recidivism). The severity is rated from low severity (for example, minor theft) to highest severity (for example, willful homicide). Parole prognosis is determined by considering 11 factors generally found to be related to recidivism, such as age, prior incarcerations, and employment. These 11 factors are scored to produce a parole prognosis ranging from a very high probability of success to a very low probability of success. After rating the prospective parolee on offense severity and parole prognosis, the parole board member examines a statistical table that suggests a range of time to be served before release (for example, 20 to 24 months). This table is based upon the statistical analysis of the parole success and failure of similar parolees. If the parole board member wants to make a recommendation outside the suggested range, he or she must justify the decision by providing information that makes this particular case unique. The decision maker is therefore not obligated to follow a statistical formula, but an additional burden of proof is placed upon him or her if he or she wishes to exceed the statistically generated guidelines for discretion.[39] Under these conditions, decisions appear to be more uniform and in line with statistical prediction. But there still remains much room for subjective evaluation and input which may be of critical importance in certain cases.

It is not likely that such a system will soon be used in predicting dangerousness in the civil commitment area, because there is an inadequate data base and because of the reluctance of mental health personnel to subject their decisions to empirical and administrative review. The individual clinician can, however, begin to decrease reliance upon clinical case material when such reliance results in the exclusion of factors generally shown to be related to subsequent dangerous acts. In summarizing several studies, Burnham[40] has concluded that "the maximum number of data items along different dimensions which can be processed profitably at the same time, without any formal decomposition and restructuring of the decision process, is about eight. Above that number, confusion does set in resulting from a decline in decision quality. . . . We must be aware that information overload is real, likely, important, and damaging."

The above example of parole decision making required only the simultaneous consideration of two data items. Among the eight or fewer items to be considered would be those items statistically shown to be related to subsequent dangerousness for the particular population being evaluated. At least this information, even if not used, would not be as damaging to the decision-making process as irrelevant case history material. Perhaps with training and exposure to statistical data, clinicians could begin to feel more comfortable about integrating clinical and statistical information.

TREATMENT IMPLICATIONS

Although some individual patients may be greatly helped by traditional psychotherapeutic methods, the overall effectiveness of these methods is subject to serious question. There are many studies reporting negative results.[41-45] Generally it appears that the more carefully studies are designed to control for factors such as improvement without treatment (spontaneous remission), placebo effects, self-report bias, and attrition rates, the more likely they are to find negative treatment outcome. Traditional treatment methods are not necessarily to be abandoned but may be augmented by some newer forms of treatment or behavioral intervention. Although there is a great need for more research on treatment methods, relatively little research is presently being done on this important problem. The present situation with regard to public policy is somewhat like building tuberculosis sanitariums rather than treating or preventing tuberculosis. The following discussion briefly presents a few speculations about new directions for psychotherapeutic intervention.*

Desensitization Techniques

One possible approach involves the desensitization of patients to stimuli that usually elicit anger or aggressive responses. In one study,[48] research subjects who became angry while driving and also exhibited behaviors such as swearing, tailgating, or driving at excessive speeds were gradually exposed to descriptions of driving situations that made them angry. Prior to and during this exposure, the subjects engaged in deep muscle relaxation. (Most people find it difficult to be deeply relaxed and impulsively angry at the same time.) Following this treatment, the subjects reported less anger in response to driving scenes. These reports tended to be confirmed by galvanic skin response measures but not by the heart rate measures. Further study of this treatment approach is needed. To the extent that stress or fear precedes the feeling of anger, as in situations of threat, a desensitization procedure might be a reasonable approach. Systematic desensitization has rather consistently been shown to be clinically useful in reducing fear responses.[49,50]

A related approach is called "stress inoculation."[51] It assumes that anger and aggression may be produced, at least in part, by a person's perception, thoughts, and self-statements in a situation. This approach attempts to strengthen self-control primarily through cognitive means, although some relaxation procedures may also be used.[52] The person may be taught to make statements to himself or herself such as "Stay calm," "Stay cool, this will soon be over." The person may also be taught to observe himself or herself in the situation to provide emotional distance and thus reduce the impact of the situation. The person might also attempt to think about other matters or to recall a previously practiced relaxing scene.[53] Rehearsing and role playing these procedures with a therapist may be useful or even essential.[54-56]

A different approach has been used with extremely aggressive, chronic schizophrenic patients. These patients had to be restrained because their aggression presented a danger to themselves and others. Several of these patients frequently attempted to smash windows or other glass. During counterconditioning sessions, the patients received electric shocks while visualizing breaking glass. Follow-up studies indicated marked reduction of their glass-breaking behavior.[57]

More recently, covert sensitization has sometimes been used in the place of electric shock or other aversive stimuli. In covert sensitization, the patient imagines an aversive stimulus or situation, such as becoming nauseated and vomiting, immediately after imagining the performance of the prohibited behavior.[58] This method has been used with a patient having sadistic fantasies[59]

---

* An extensive survey of contemporary treatment methods using learning theory approaches can be found in *Analysis of Delinquency and Aggression* by Ribes-Inesta and Bandura,[46] and in chapter 5 of *Aggression in Man and Animals* by Johnson.[47]

and with exhibitionists.[60] This last study involved 10 exhibitionists and included the use of valeric acid, which the subjects inhaled while imagining a nausea-inducing scene. Later the subjects were given small bottles of valeric acid from which they were to inhale in those circumstances which would ordinarily have elicited exhibitionist behavior. The subjects returned for "booster" treatment at 3, 6, and 12 months. The results indicated a very substantial reduction of exhibitionist behavior and fantasies during the 12 months.

This last study illustrates an increasing concern about the limitations of treatment confined entirely to hospital, clinic, or office settings. Patients may have difficulty in generalizing experiences in an office to their daily life situations. Furthermore, the therapist may not be able to observe directly the behavior to be changed or even to get a clear description of it. In the treatment of phobias, therapists have sometimes accompanied patients on elevators, across streets, or on airplanes while using relaxation procedures. These in vivo treatment procedures have been particularly effective with many patients.[50] A midrange procedure is to bring into the treatment session objects that elicit the problem behavior or to film or to videotape scenes in the natural setting in which the behavior occurs. These scenes may then be played during the treatment session. Of course, it is difficult to duplicate exactly the natural world of the patient in a hospital or clinic because the patient will usually be aware that he or she is in an alternative setting. In some cases, there may be no adequate substitute for real-world experiences.

Conditional Release

On a limited scale, and under close supervision and in conditions that are likely to protect both the patient and public, it might be desirable to release certain patients from a hospital. A conditional release procedure might be used. For example, in *People v. Thingvold*,[61] a patient asserted that he was no longer a sexually dangerous person and should be released from the hospital. Four psychiatrists were uncertain. The court permitted conditional release of the patient, citing an Illinois statute that read in part:

> If the court finds that the patient appears no longer to be sexually dangerous but that it is impossible to determine with certainty under conditions of institutional care that such person has fully recovered, the court shall enter an order permitting such person to go at large subject to such conditions and such supervision by the Director as in the opinion of the court will adequately protect the public. In the event the person violates any of the conditions of such order, the court shall revoke such conditional release and recommit the person under the terms of the original commitment.

The court requested a lower court to consider the placement of the patient in a halfway house under whatever provisions the trial court would consider appropriate to protect the public.

Conditional releases for short periods of time with close supervision would seem preferable to the long-term confinement of patients on the basis of uncertain probabilities of future dangerous conduct. Treatment such as in vivo desensitization could then be conducted in these settings.

Because adequate predictive accuracy about future dangerousness is difficult to obtain, it might be desirable in some situations to release the patient conditionally under very precise conditions to observe his or her behavior in natural settings. These releases might be considered a part of controlled clinical studies or tests of the effects of various environments upon the patient. The patient might, for example, be interviewed and tested immediately prior to and following the conditional release. If the patient was visited in his or her natural environment, the patient might be tested there as well.

Released patients have sometimes been requested to mail a postcard to the therapist every day. The postcard may contain a schedule of the previous day's activities and the medication taken. Unusual patterns of activity, sleep, medication, or even the failure to send in a card may provide useful information about the patient. Verification of some of the information reported can be made by phone calls or visits.

Alcohol in Treatment Program

The use of alcohol in natural settings might be an important factor related to aggression in some patients, but it is seldom tested in institutions. Alcohol has also been found to increase the intensity of electric shock that subjects are willing to administer to others.[62,63] In a different experiment conducted in an informal group setting, male volunteers from the general public showed statistically significant increases in aggressive behavior after drinking.[64]

Studies have frequently reported the involvement of alcohol with aggressive crimes. In a study of persons arrested during or shortly following the commission of a felony, it was found that 47 out of 60 persons committing physical assaults had blood alcohol levels greater than 0.10 percent at the time of their arrest.[65] In a study of 588 homicides over a 5-year period in Philadelphia, alcohol was found to be present in either the offender or the victim in 64 percent of the cases.[66] A study of 77 committed rapists in California indicated that 43 percent were drinking alcohol heavily, and 6 percent were drinking moderately or lightly, at the time the offense was committed.[67]

There are several theories that might account for the relationship between alcohol consumption and aggression in certain patients. One theory postulates that aggression is inhibited by feelings of anxiety, fear, or guilt. If alcohol reduces these emotions, aggression may be disinhibited or released. Another, but not incompatible, theory is related to state-dependent learning (sometimes called dissociated learning). State-dependent learning refers to a phenomenon in which information learned under a drug condition is not transferred or remembered in a nondrug state. For example, normal persons who learn material such as nonsense syllables following the ingestion of alcohol may subsequently experience greater recall of the learned material after ingesting alcohol than without it.[68,69] In a study involving marijuana, Stillman and coworkers[70] concluded, "As predicted by a state-dependent model, subjects reproduced material best when they were in the same drug state as they had been when they first encountered the material to be recalled. In particular, marijuana-marijuana reproduction surpassed marijuana-placebo or placebo-marijuana reproduction; that is, material first encountered in a drug state was better reproduced when the subject was again in the drug state than when he was sober." State-dependent effects have also been suggested for amphetamine and amobarbital.[71] The extent to which learning is affected by state dependency is a matter of speculation, with a low estimate of about 15 percent of the learned material influenced by the alcohol.[72] That 15 percent may be socially significant or important in daily life situations. Demonstrations of state-dependent learning with socially significant material related to aggression need to be conducted.

If it is assumed that the state-dependent learning phenomenon applies to the learning and display of aggressive behavior, it is possible to hypothesize why alcohol may be related to aggression in some individuals but not in others. For certain individuals, alcohol may facilitate the recall of previously successful aggressive behaviors emitted while intoxicated, such as fights in a barroom. The recall of these behaviors and the events surrounding them may alter both the perception of the present environment and the anticipated consequences of aggression. The altered perception, combined with the anxiety-reduction effects of alcohol, may encourage learned patterns of aggression.

If certain behaviors learned during one internal state (for example, sobriety) do not generalize well to other internal states (for example, alcohol intoxication), then we could expect little therapeutic benefit from treating a sober person in a clinic setting for those aggressive behaviors which usually occur when that person is intoxicated in a different setting. Therapeutic failure would be likely, and that is what is generally found. If the consumption of alcohol cannot be readily reduced or controlled, it might be useful to consider the possibility of treating aggression under state-dependent conditions. Shealy and Shen[73] treated a patient, in a hospital setting, who presented himself to the hospital for treatment of homicidal impulses which were manifested when he was extremely intoxicated with alcohol. The treatment involved two aspects. One aspect was a cognitive technique aimed at the patient's ideas concerning his masculinity. The second aspect used a behavior-rehearsal technique that included alcohol. Following intoxication, the patient was taught to walk away from taunts from two of his brothers. This was a situation that had previously evoked aggression.

In a study of "state-dependent therapy" currently being conducted by the author, the feasibility of treating patients while they are moderately intoxicated for behaviors occurring during intoxication is being explored. In one case involving aggressive behavior, the patient was systematically desensitized to insults while intoxicated. The initial treatment sessions were conducted in a laboratory setting. After the procedures appeared to be effective and efficient in preventing aggression in the laboratory setting, treatment was conducted in barroom settings where the aggression usually occurred, to further increase generalization and the relevance of the treatment. Preliminary results during the past several months appear very positive.

CONCLUSION

Much more research is necessary to develop effective treatment interventions with dangerous behavior. If treatment could become brief and effective with minimal side effects, the issue of the accurate prediction of dangerousness would not be as critical as it is today because false-positive errors would not result in extensive deprivations of liberty. Until that time, mental health professionals may have to tolerate considerable ambiguity and legal risk while moving toward more empirical modes of prediction and more innovative forms of treatment.

REFERENCES

1. Covington v. Harris, 410 F.2d 617, 1969.
2. Delaware Code Ann, tit. 16 §5125, 3, Supp. 1974.
3. Tarasoff v. Regents of University of California, 551 P2d 334, 1976. For a discussion of policy issues related to legal decision making affecting clinicians, see SHAH, SA: *Dangerousness: A paradigm for exploring some issues in law and psychology.* Am Psychol 33:224-238, 1978.
4. STEADMAN, HJ AND HALFON, A: *The Baxstrom patients: Background and outcomes.* Am J Psychiatry 3:376-385, 1971.
5. STEADMAN, HJ AND KEVELES, G: *The community adjustment and criminal activity of the Baxstrom patients: 1966-1970.* Am J Psychiatry 129:304-310, 1972.
6. Baxstrom v. Herald, 383 U.S. 107, 1966.
7. STEADMAN, HJ: *Implications from the Baxstrom experience.* Paper presented at the American Academy of Psychiatry and the Law Convention, Atlanta, March 16, 1973 (Mental Health Research Unit, New York State Department of Mental Hygiene, Albany, New York). See also, THORNBERRY, TP: *Community follow-up and dangerous mental patients.* In FREDERICK, CJ: (ED): *Dangerous Behavior: A Problem in Law and Mental Health.* Center for Studies of Crime and Delinquency, NIMH, Washington, DC, 1978, pp 111-122. These studies as well as those cited subsequently suggest a substantial overprediction of dangerousness. This is not meant to imply that there are no categories of mentally ill patients who are not dangerous or assaultive, for example, inpatient, latency age males. See PFEFFER, CR, PLUTCHIK, R, MIZRUCHI, MS: *Predictors of assaultiveness in latency age children.* Am J Psychiatry 140:31-35, 1983. Another population presenting risk may be male, paranoid schizophrenic patients under the age of 45 years. See ROFMAN, ES, ASKINAZI, C, FANT, E: *The prediction of dangerous behavior in emergency civil commitment.* Am J Psychiatry 137:1061-1064, 1980.
8. RUBIN, B: *Prediction of dangerousness in mentally ill criminals.* Arch Gen Psychiatry 27:397-407, 1972.
9. McGARRY, AL AND PARKER, LL: *Massachusetts' operation Baxstrom: A follow-up.* Massachusetts Journal of Mental Health 4:27-41, 1974.
10. KOZOL, HL, BOUCHER, RJ, GAROFALO, RF: *The diagnosis and treatment of dangerousness.* Crime and Delinquency 18:371-392, 1972.
11. MONAHAN, J: *Dangerous offenders: A critique of Kozol et al.* Crime and Delinquency 19:418-420, 1973.
12. EVENSON, RC AND ALTMAN, H: *A re-evaluation of "the diagnosis and treatment of dangerousness."* Unpublished paper, Missouri Institute of Psychiatry, University of Missouri School of Medicine, St Louis, 1975.
13. CARNEY, FL: *The indeterminate sentence at Patuxent.* Crime and Delinquency 20:135-143, 1974.
14. ENNIS, BJ AND LITWACK, TR: *Psychiatry and the presumption of expertise: Flipping coins in the courtroom.* California Law Review 62:693-752, 1974.
15. SWEETLAND, JP: *"Illusory correlation" and the estimation of "dangerous" behavior.* Ph.D. dissertation, Department of Psychology, Indiana University, 1972. (Cited in SHAH, SA: *Dangerousness: A paradigm for exploring some issues in law and psychology.* Paper presented at the American Psychological Association Convention, September 5, 1976.)
16. ZISKIN, J: *Coping with Psychiatric and Psychological Testimony.* Law and Psychology Press, Beverly Hills, 1970, pp 147-158.
17. STEADMAN, HJ AND COCOZZA, JJ: *A natural experiment in the psychiatric prediction of dangerousness.* Unpublished paper, Mental Health Research Unit, New York State Department of Mental Hygiene, Albany, New York, 1976, p 11.

18. STONE, AA: *Mental Health and Law: A System in Transition.* Center for Studies of Crime and Delinquency, NIMH, Washington, DC, 1975. p 67. Rather than excluding expert testimony completely, GE Dix suggests that testimony be limited to expressing the opinion that the patient poses a greater risk than the average person of engaging in future assaultive or otherwise criminal conduct. See DIX, GE: *Clinical evaluation of the "dangerousness" of "normal" criminal defendants.* Virginia Law Review 66:523-581, 1980.

19. Rosenfield v. Overholser, 262 F.2d 34, 1958.

20. Arizona, Rev. Stat. Ann. ch 36-501, 3, 1974.

21. TVERSKY, A AND KAHNEMAN, D: *Judgment under uncertainty: Heuristics and biases.* Science 185:1124-1131, 1974.

22. STRAN,' P, VENET, L, SHAPIRO, S: *Man screening in mammary cancer.* Cancer Res 23:875-878, 1969.

23. McGARRY, AL, ET AL: *Competency to Stand Trial and Mental Illness.* Center for Studies of Crime and Delinquency, NIMH, Washington, DC, 1973, reprinted 1974.

24. CLEMENTE, DC AND CHASE, MH: *Neurological substrates of aggressive behavior.* Annu Rev Physiol 35:329-356, 1973.

25. BACH Y RITA, G AND VENO, A: *Habitual violence: A profile of 62 men.* Am J Psychiatry 131:1015-1017, 1974.

26. SHAH, SA: *Dangerousness: Some definitional, conceptual, and public policy issues.* In SALES, BD (ED): *Perspectives in Law and Psychology, Vol 1.* Plenum, New York, 1977, pp 91-119.

27. PATTERSON, GR AND COBB, JA: *Stimulus control for classes of noxious behaviors.* In KNUTSON, JF (ED): *The Control of Aggression.* Aldine, Chicago, 1973, pp 145-199.

28. O'NEAL, EC AND McDONALD, PJ: *The environmental psychology of aggression.* In GEEN, RG AND O'NEAL, EC (EDS): *Perspectives on Aggression.* Academic Press, New York, 1976, pp 169-192.

29. MOYER, KE: *The physiological inhibition of hostile behavior.* In KNUTSON, JF: *The Control of Aggression.* Aldine, Chicago, 1973, pp 9-38.

30. WENK, EA, ROBINSON, JO, SMITH, GW: *Can violence be predicted?* Crime and Delinquency 18:393-402, 1972.

31. SHAH, SA: *Some interactions of law and mental health in the handling of social deviance.* Catholic University Law Review 23:674-719, 1974.

32. SHAH, SA: *Dangerousness and civil commitment of the mentally ill: Some public policy considerations.* Am J Psychiatry 132:501-505, 1975.

33. SHAH, SA: *Dangerousness: A paradigm for exploring some issues in law and psychology.* Am Psychologist 33:224-238, 1978.
    J. Monahan has suggested 14 questions that might be useful in predicting violent behavior:
    1. Is it a prediction of violent behavior that is being requested?
    2. Am I professionally competent to offer an estimate of the probability of future violence?
    3. Are any issues of personal or professional ethics involved in this case?
    4. Given my answers to the above questions, is this case an appropriate one in which to offer a prediction?
    5. What events precipitated the question of the person's potential for violence being raised, and in what context did these events take place?
    6. What are the person's relevant demographic characteristics?
    7. What is the person's history of violent behavior?
    8. What is the base rate of violent behavior among individuals of this person's background?
    9. What are the sources of stress in the person's current environment?
    10. What cognitive and effective factors indicate that the person may be predisposed to cope with stress in a violent manner?

11. What cognitive and effective factors indicate that the person may be predisposed to cope with stress in a nonviolent manner?
12. How similar are the contexts in which the person has used violent coping mechanisms in the past to the contexts in which the person likely will function in the future?
13. In particular, who are the likely victims of the person's violent behavior, and how available are they?
14. What means does the person possess to commit violence?

See MONAHAN, J: *The Clinical Prediction of Violent Behavior.* Center for Studies of Crime and Delinquency, NIMH, Washington, DC, 1981, p 115.

34. MEEHL, PE: *Clinical Versus Statistical Prediction.* University of Minnesota Press, Minneapolis, 1954.
35. SAWYER, J: *Measurement and prediction, clinical and statistical.* Psychol Bull 66:178-200, 1966.
36. KAHNEMAN, D AND TVERSKY, A: *On the psychology of prediction.* Psychol Rev 80:237-251, 1973.
37. CARROLL, JS: *Prediction of recidivism: Conflicts between clinical strategies and base-rate information.* Unpublished paper, Carnegie-Mellon University, Pittsburgh, 1977. Base rates and diagnostic information might be usefully combined to get an estimate of the likelihood of dangerous behavior using the Bayes theorem. See TVERSKY, A AND KAHNEMAN, D: *Causal schemata in judgment under uncertainty.* In FISHBEIN, M (ED): *Progress in Social Psychology.* L. Erlbaum Assoc., Hillsdale, NJ, 1980. See NISBETT, R AND ROSS, L: *Human Inference: Strategies and Shortcomings in Social Judgment.* Prentice-Hall, Englewood Cliffs, NJ, 1980.
38. GOTTFREDSON, DM, HOFFMAN, PB, SIEGLER, MH, WILKINS, LT: *Making paroling policy explicit.* Crime and Delinquency 21:33-44, 1975.
39. GENEGO, WJ, GOLDBERGER, PD, JACKSON, VC: *Parole release decision making and the sentencing process.* Yale Law Journal 84:810-902, 1975.
40. BURNHAM, RW: *Modern decision theory and corrections.* In GOTTFREDSON, DM (ED): *Decision Making in the Criminal Justice System: Reviews and Essays.* Center for Studies of Crime and Delinquency, NIMH, Washington, DC, 1975, pp 92-123.
41. MILLER, RB AND KENNY, E: *Adolescent delinquency and the myth of hospital treatment.* Crime and Delinquency 12:38-48, 1966.
42. MORRIS, HH, ESCOLL, PJ, WEXLER, R: *Aggressive behavior disorders of childhood: A follow-up study.* Am J Psychiatry 112:991-997, 1956.
43. SCHORER, CE, LOWINGER, P, SULLIVAN, T, HARTAUB, GH: *Improvement without treatment.* Diseases of the Nervous System 29:100-104, 1968.
44. SINGER, JE AND GROB, MC: *Patients discharged against medical advice: A follow-up study.* Massachusetts Journal of Mental Health 5:57-66, 1974.
45. WOLKON, GH, KARMEN, M, TANAKA, HT: *Evaluation of a social program for recently released psychiatric patients.* Community Ment Health J 7:312-322, 1971.
46. RIBES-INESTA, E AND BANDURA, A: *Analysis of Delinquency and Aggression.* John Wiley & Sons, New York, 1976.
47. JOHNSON, RN: *Aggression in Man and Animals.* WB Saunders, Philadelphia, 1972.
48. RIMM, DC, ET AL: *Systematic densensitization of an anger response.* Behav Res Ther 9:273-280, 1971.
49. PAUL, GL: *Outcome of systematic desensitization. II. Controlled investigation of individual treatment, technique variations, and current status.* In FRANKS, CM (ED): *Behavior Therapy: Appraisal and Status.* McGraw-Hill, New York, 1969, pp 105-159.
50. SCHWITZGEBEL, RK AND KOLB, DA: *Changing Human Behavior: Principles of Planned Intervention.* McGraw-Hill, New York, 1974, pp 14-31.
51. MEICHENBAUM, D AND CAMERON, R: *Stress inoculation: A skills training approach to anxiety management.* Unpublished manuscript, University of Waterloo, 1973.

52. Novaco, RW: *Anger Control: The Development and Evaluation of an Experimental Treatment.* DC Heath, Lexington, MA, 1975.

53. Bower, SA and Bower, GH: *Asserting Yourself: A Practical Guide for Positive Change.* Addison-Wesley, Reading, MA, 1976, pp 56-63.

54. Kanfer, FH: *Self-management methods.* In Kanfer, FH and Goldstein, AP (eds): *Helping People Change: A Textbook of Methods.* Pergamon Press, Elmsford, NY, 1975, pp 309-355.

55. Nolan, JD: *Self-control procedures in the modification of smoking behavior.* J Consult Clin Psychol 32:92-93, 1968.

56. Roberts, AH: *Self-control procedures in modification of smoking: Replication.* Psychol Rep 24:675-676, 1969.

57. Agras, WS: *Behavior therapy in the management of chronic schizophrenia.* Am J Psychiatry 124:240-243, 1967.

58. Cautela, JR: *Covert Sensitization.* Psychol Rec 20:459-468, 1967.

59. Davison, GC: *Elimination of a sadistic fantasy by a client: A controlled counterconditioning technique.* J Abnorm Psychol 73:84-90, 1968.

60. Maletzky, B: *Assisted covert sensitization in the treatment of exhibitionism.* J Consult Clin Psychol 42:34-40, 1974.

61. People v. Thingvold. 251 N. E. 2d 553, Ill. App. 1969. If a legal offense is involved, the court may as a condition of probation restrict the patient from certain places or areas that are reasonably related to future dangerous behavior. See, for example, People v. Green, 451 N.Y.S.2d 970 (Sp. Ct. 1982).

62. Shuntick, RJ and Taylor, SP: *The effects of type and dose of alcohol on human physical aggression.* J Exp Res Personality 6:34-38, 1972.

63. Taylor, SP and Gammon, CB: *The effects of type and dose of alcohol on human physical aggression.* J Personality Social Psychol 32:169-175, 1975.

64. Boyatzis, RE: *The effect of alcohol consumption on the aggressive behavior of men.* Q J Studies Alcohol 35:959-972, 1974. See also Pihl, RO, et al: *Attribution and alcohol-mediated aggression.* J Abnorm Psychol 9:468-475, 1981.

65. Shupe, LM: *Alcohol and crime: A study of the urine alcohol concentration found in 882 persons arrested during or immediately after the commission of a felony.* Journal of Criminal Law, Criminology and Police Science 44:661, 664, 1954.

66. Wolfgang, ME and Strohm, RB: *The relationship between alcohol and criminal homicide.* Q J Studies Alcohol 17:411-425, 1956.

67. Rada, RT: *Alcoholism and forcible rape.* Am J Psychiatry 132:444-446, 1975.

68. Goodwin, DW, et al: *Alcohol and recall: State-dependent effects in man.* Science 163:1358-1360, 1969.

69. Overton, DA: *State-dependent learning produced by alcohol and its relevance to alcoholism.* In Kissin, B and Begleiter, H (eds): *The Biology of Alcoholism, Vol 2, Physiology and Behavior.* Plenum, New York, 1972, pp 193-217. See also Peterson, RC: *Retrieval failures in alcohol state-dependent learning.* Psychopharmacology 55:141-146, 1977; Cunningham, CL: *Alcohol as a cue for extinction: State dependency inhibition.* Animal Learning Behavior 7:45-52, 1979.

70. Stillman, RC, et al: *State-dependent (dissociative) effects of marihuana on human memory.* Arch Gen Psychiatry 31:81-85, 1974.

71. Bustamante, JA, et al: *State-dependent learning in humans.* Physiol Behav 5:793-796, 1970.

72. Weingartner, J and Faillace, L: *Alcohol state-dependent learning in man.* J Nerv Ment Dis 153:395-405, 1971.

73. Shealy, AE and Shen, J: *The use of state-dependent learning principles in treatment: A case report.* J Community Psychol 1:232-234, 1973. See also Reus, VI, Weingartner, H, Post, RM: *Clinical implications of state-dependent learning.* Am J Psychiatry 136:927-931, 1979.

CHAPTER 7

ASSESSMENT OF COMPETENCY TO STAND CRIMINAL TRIAL*

Thomas Grisso, Ph.D.
Sandra K. Seigel, B.A.

Our judicial heritage has carefully guarded the right of an accused person to receive a fair, impartial criminal trial. Part of this ideal holds that defendants should have every reasonable opportunity to defend themselves against criminal allegations. It has long been recognized, though, that some defendants' mental or emotional disabilities might interfere with their performance in participating adequately in their own defense. If the defendant cannot function adequately in this role, it has been reasoned, then the standard of fairness is threatened. The failure to participate effectively may alter the trial of the case and innocent persons may be found guilty who, if their cases were presented fully, might be found innocent. When it appears that a defendant's disabilities might jeopardize the fairness and thus the outcome of a trial, judicial decision makers are charged with determining the defendant's mental competency to stand trial. Mental health evaluators are often asked to assist the court in this pretrial competency determination. When they accept this task, mental health professionals are faced with difficult legal, clinical, and social issues that are different in many respects from those encountered in routine clinical evaluations.

The purpose of this chapter is to describe the legal context in which mental health evaluations for competency to stand trial are performed and to examine issues that arise in these evaluations. First, a legal definition of the standard for competency to stand trial is presented, as well as the history and legal rationale for the standard. Second, the legal process for determining competency to stand trial is described. Third, several empirical studies have found

* Portions of this chapter contain material that was reviewed with the assistance of Research Grant #RO1-MH37231 (Empirical Forensic Psychological Assessment) from the National Institute of Mental Health, Center for Studies of Crime and Delinquency.

that competency to stand trial often has been used to meet a variety of purposes other than those for which the concept was intended. These uses of the legal mechanism are reviewed in light of their implications for pretrial competency evaluations and testimony. Fourth, the process of pretrial competency evaluations is discussed, including the request for a clinician's evaluation, available assessment methods, and communication of results. Finally, several unresolved issues of pretrial competency assessments are raised for consideration by mental health professionals, researchers, and lawmakers.

DEFINITION OF THE COMPETENCY STANDARD

There is no honor in entering a battle in full armor with the intention of striking down an adversary who is without shield or sword. Similarly, early English common law recognized the unfairness of a trial in which an accused did not know the nature of the legal battle or came mentally unarmed. If the defendant could not play the proper role in testing the "strength" of the accuser, then it was as though the defendant was not present at all. A more formal statement of this logic was set forth in Hale's Pleas to the Crown in 1788 and in the Criminal Lunatics Act of 1800.[1] These early English standards cited especially a defendant's inability to communicate with counsel, to understand the nature of the trial, or to testify in one's own behalf as major considerations when determining a defendant's competency to stand trial. Each of these inabilities could affect the substance of the defense offered, and an innocent person could improperly be found guilty.

The Sixth and Fourteenth amendments to the US Constitution provide the bases for the rights of the accused to construct a defense against criminal charges. The contemporary standard for determining competency was stated in *Dusky v. United States*[2] in 1960; the defendant must have "sufficient present ability to consult with his lawyer with a reasonable degree of rational understanding" and must have "rational as well as factual understanding of proceedings against him." Most states have adopted the *Dusky* standard intact or with minor modifications in wording. Some states, though, have added to the *Dusky* standard the requirement that the defendant's deficiencies relevant to the issue of competency must be attributable to "mental disease or defect."

What qualities does a defendant need to possess in order to meet the standard for a rational and factual "understanding of proceedings" or an "ability to consult with his lawyer"? This question has been the subject of much debate in scholarly legal analyses, producing a number of lists of recommended factors for courts to consider when addressing the competency standard.[3-5] One of the most frequently cited lists of factors is drawn from *Weiter v. Settle*,[6] a 1961 Missouri case which suggested eight elements to be examined (Fig. 7-1).

An examination of *Dusky, Weiter* and other appellate court decisions makes it clear that the mental competency construct focuses primarily on the **functional abilities of the defendant as they relate directly to the demands of the trial.**[7] The primary focus is upon the degree to which the defendant knows or can do those things that are required by the defendant role. This does not mean that information about a defendant's intellectual capacities ("intelligence"), personality traits, and motivations are unimportant when addressing the pretrial competency question. They are not sufficient, however, by themselves. By analogy,

ELEMENTS OF MENTAL COMPETENCY

1. that he has mental capabilities to appreciate his presence in relation to time, place, and things;

2. that his elementary processes are such that he apprehends (i.e. seizes and grasps with what mind he has) that he is in a Court of Justice, charged with a criminal offense;

3. that there is a Judge on the Bench;

4. a Prosecutor present who will try to convict him of a criminal charge;

5. that he has a lawyer . . . who will undertake to defend him against that charge;

6. that he will be expected to tell his lawyer the circumstances, to the best of his mental ability (whether colored or not by mental aberration), the facts surrounding him at the time and place [of the alleged law violation];

7. that there is or will be a jury present to pass upon evidence adduced as to his guilt or innocence of such charges; and

8. he has memory sufficient to relate those things in his own personal manner.

FIGURE 7-1. The eight elements of a defendant's mental competency needed in order to stand criminal trial. (From *Weiter v. Settle*.[6])

the question of a person's ability to use a sword in battle is more directly addressed by observing the way a person handles a sword than by testing for general perceptual-motor capacities.

Similarly, no particular psychiatric diagnosis is dispositive of the question of competency. The presence of psychosis, mental retardation, or even amnesia is not, by itself, sufficient to support a finding of incompetency. In *United States v. Wilson*,[8] for example, the court explained that whether or not a defendant's amnesia constitutes mental incompetency depends in part on the extent of the amnesia and its relevance to the matters of concern in the trial itself. Thus the court noted that if the accused has enough evidence available to construct a defense without recall of the alleged event, amnesia may not be of great consequence for the question of competency to stand trial. Similarly, the *Dusky* standard does not simply ask about a person's mental illness; it asks whether or not the mental illness has an effect on functional abilities required to perform the defendant's role in a pending trial.

Many human abilities and disabilities are not simply present or absent; they are manifested to a greater or lesser degree. Furthermore, the question of a defendant's competency to stand trial involves no single ability but requires weighing several functional abilities. What degree of ability is "enough" to constitute pretrial competency? And which abilities (for example, in the *Weiter* list) are weighed more or less heavily? The same logic applies here as in the previous discussion. For example, Stone[9] has explained that the degree of self-protective ability that is necessary may vary across defendants, depending upon such matters as the nature of the charges and the complexity of the proceedings. There are, for example, differences in the level of competency needed (with respect to memory and recall) between a simple trial for a single act of theft and a complex trial for tax evasion or embezzlement over a period of years.

It depends, too, upon the type of battle to be waged. For example, does the defendant face hand-to-hand combat in the open field, or will matters be decided in negotiation? Shah[10] has pointed out that while much attention has been given to determining defendants' competency to participate in trials, far less attention has been given to examining their competency to cooperate with their attorneys in the plea-negotiation process and in decisions to enter a guilty plea. This discrepancy is remarkable in that the vast majority of criminal cases are handled through negotiated pleas. One might argue that less ability is required of the defendant who does not intend to do battle. Here, however, the combat analogy is misleading. The decision to plead guilty is, in effect, a waiver of Constitutional rights and is therefore a decision of great importance. Courts have noted that determinations of a defendant's competency to make this decision merits even **more** demanding criteria than those used to assess competency to stand trial.[11]

Finally, the definition of competency to stand trial in *Dusky* clearly sets it apart from the question of criminal responsibility (for example, the insanity defense). Competency proceedings address themselves only to the characteristics and functional abilities of the defendant **at the time of the evaluation and in relation to future criminal court proceedings.** In contrast, the question of criminal responsibility inquires about the defendant's mental state **at the time the offense allegedly was committed.** Pretrial competency inquires about current functioning and psychological capacities (*Dusky*'s "sufficient present ability"[12]) and criminal responsibility is a question about the past. Indeed, a defendant may be competent to stand trial but be adjudged legally insane; conversely, a defendant may be found incompetent to stand trial yet may be unable to meet the legal test for exculpatory insanity.

Let us turn now to the legal procedures that are used to determine pretrial competency.

LEGAL PROCEDURE

There are five main stages in the procedure for determining and disposing of competency cases: (1) requesting a competency determination; (2) the court-ordered competency evaluation; (3) the judicial determination and disposition; (4) treatment for mental incompetency; and (5) rehearings on competency.

Requesting the Competency Determination

The United States Supreme Court in *Pate v. Robinson*[13] held that a trial judge must address the issue of a defendant's competency if the question is raised in a way that casts "bona fide doubt" regarding competency. In most jurisdictions, the question may be raised by the defense, the prosecution, or the judge at any stage in the criminal court proceeding. The "bona fide doubt" standard is quite

ASSESSMENT AND TREATMENT IN FORENSIC SETTINGS

vague. As the court explained in *Drope v. Missouri,* "There are no fixed or immutable signs which invariably indicate the need for further inquiry to determine a defendant's fitness to proceed with trial. The question is often difficult and one in which a wide range of manifestations and subtle nuances are implicated."[14] Therefore, judges are allowed considerable discretion in their response to a request for a competency determination. This is an important threshold issue prior to the trial itself.

If the evidence is not found to create a "bona fide doubt," criminal proceedings are continued. If the evidence does raise a sufficient doubt about the defendant's abilities, the judge will allow the parties to explore the issue more fully at a hearing at which the defense and prosecution can call their own expert witnesses to present opinion evidence concerning the defendant's competency. Also, the judge may appoint one or more mental health professionals to examine the defendant and to report as nonpartisan experts to the court regarding the person's capacities relevant to pretrial competency. In some jurisdictions, however, a court may proceed directly to a competency hearing without requesting a mental health evaluation.[15]

The Court-Ordered Competency Evaluation

Competency evaluation procedures will vary in accordance with the relevant rules in various states. Most statutes specify judicial appointment of an examining psychiatrist or physician, and many offer the alternative of a psychologist as examiner. Yet variations in the selections process are numerous. The greatest attention to fairness might be represented by Arizona's procedure; it requires that both the prosecution and the defense submit to the court alternate lists of psychiatrists and/or psychologists. The judge then chooses two examiners, one from each attorney's list.[16]

In some jurisdictions, nonpartisan examiners perform brief screening procedures in order to determine whether there is a need for more extensive evaluation. Pretrial competency evaluations sometimes are conducted in detention or holding facilities or in forensic outpatient settings.[17] More commonly, though, defendants are committed to a state forensic or security mental hospital facility for an observation and evaluation period during which extensive psychiatric and psychological examinations take place. Many statutes limit the length of these commitments, often specifying 30 days.

Judicial Determination and Disposition

Judicial practice does not always provide a formal hearing on the question of a defendant's pretrial competency. Generally, however, the mental health examiner will testify in a formal hearing, at which cross-examination and opposing expert testimony may occur. Various other witnesses may also be called to testify, including the defendant. Many statutes require that the court-appointed examiner, either a psychiatrist or a psychologist, state an opinion or conclusion regarding the defendant's mental competency to stand trial, as well as provide the basis upon which the conclusion is reached. Furthermore, several states require that if this examiner believes that the defendant is incompetent, testimony and reasons must be given concerning the likelihood that psychiatric treatment can render the defendant competent in the foreseeable future.

If the defendant is found competent by the judge, criminal trial and related proceedings will continue. Courts may have a continuing legal obligation, though, to monitor the defendant's mental state throughout the trial. In *Pouncy v. United States*,[18] the court noted that "a hospital report is only a prediction that when the accused is tried, he will be able to participate adequately in the proceedings, . . . later developments may throw doubt on the prediction." If such doubts are raised, competency reevaluation by a court-appointed mental health examiner might be necessary to aid the court.

Treatment for Mental Incompetency

If the defendant is found mentally incompetent, a judicial decision about effectiveness of any suggested treatment or habilitation must be made. The issues in this decision are best understood in light of a 1972 United States Supreme Court ruling in *Jackson v. Indiana*.[19]

Prior to *Jackson*, it had been standard practice to commit all incompetent defendants to treatment facilities until they had attained competency, suspending any criminal proceedings until that time. However, among incompetent defendants were those whose disabilities were of a severity or type—for example, most cases of mental retardation or brain damage—that was very unlikely to respond to treatment. These defendants, therefore, were not likely ever to be competent enough to stand trial. Also, professionals who provided psychiatric treatment to incompetent defendants tended to perceive the treatment objective to be the remission of a diagnosed mental disorder, whereas the appropriate legal objective was more modest; that is, the development of sufficient understanding and awareness of trial procedures and the ability to cooperate with one's attorney. These abilities do not necessarily require complete remission of a psychiatric disorder. Consequently, prior to *Jackson* forensic mental hospitals often confined defendants who were in treatment for many years with little hope of hospital discharge or a return to court for trial. In fact, in one hospital the number of patients being treated for pretrial incompetency who were returned to courts for trial was exceeded by the number whose treatment was terminated by natural death.[20]

Recognizing the unfairness of indefinite commitment for essentially untreatable conditions, the court in *Jackson* ruled that incompetent defendants could not be held for long and indeterminate periods. When the mental disorder cannot be treated (or when there appears to be no progress toward regaining competency in an ongoing treatment), commitment cannot be ordered or continued, and the defendant cannot be tried. The prosecution then has the option of dropping the charges and releasing the defendant or seeking civil commitment if the relevant commitment criteria can be met, for example, if the defendant is found to be mentally ill and likely to be dangerous to self or others if left at large in the community.

If it appears that the defendant's incompetency can be treated, commitment to a state mental hospital or forensic security treatment facility is the most common disposition. Some statutes require, however, that the defendant be treated in the least restrictive setting that provides a reasonable opportunity for regaining pretrial competency. Thus outpatient treatment for pretrial incompetency does occur in some jurisdictions when indicated; that is, when the person is judged not to be dangerous in the community.

Rehearings on Competency

In order for the principle of *Jackson* to be effective, it was necessary to require that defendants being treated for mental incompetency be reevaluated periodically by the treatment facility so that courts could review treatment progress. Most states now require reevaluation and court review at least once every six months. At the review, a court must

1. rule on competency if the treating professional believes that competency has been restored; or
2. extend the commitment another six months if it appears that competency can be restored "in the foreseeable future"; or
3. terminate commitment if at any point pretrial competency does not appear to be attainable.

ISSUES IN THE PROCESSING OF PRETRIAL COMPETENCY CASES

The foregoing description has outlined the legal structure and procedures for competency determinations. A practical understanding of competency proceedings, however, requires that one consider the operations and functions of courts, lawyers, and mental health professionals at the various stages noted above. This section, then, reviews some of the important observations that have been made concerning the actual processing of pretrial competency cases.

Monahan and Steadman[21] recently published the results of a survey concerning mentally disordered offenders in state and federal mental institutions throughout the United States in 1978. They found that almost 6500 defendants—about 32 percent of all mentally disordered offender admissions in 1978—were committed as inpatients under court order for treatment for incompetency to stand trial. Based on known ratios of competency evaluations to incompetency commitments for treatment (about 3 or 4 to 1), Monahan and Steadman estimated that there must have been at least 19,000 pretrial competency evaluations in the United States that year.

Summarizing several studies, Roesch and Golding[22] found that about 30 percent of defendants who are evaluated for competency are declared incompetent by courts. This average figure can be misleading, however, when making assumptions about any specific jurisdiction, because 4 of the 10 studies reviewed by Roesch and Golding reported rates below 20 percent, and two reported rates above 50 percent. Setting aside differences in size and sociodemography of the jurisdictions involved, there are quite a number of reasons for considerable variation in frequencies of competency evaluations and rates of commitment for incompetency across jurisdictions. Several of these reasons deserve comment, because they may have an effect on the clinician's professional activities in competency evaluations.

Judicial Patterns of Interpretation

The *Dusky* case has facilitated the application of a relatively uniform legal definition of pretrial competency across almost all jurisdictions. Nevertheless, the standard itself can be interpreted in broad or narrow fashion. Over time, then, a court that is inclined to a more narrow interpretation may have a lower rate of incompetency findings than another court. A more complex dynamic is manifested by the judge who requires considerable evidence before ordering a competency evaluation. This may produce a low frequency of evaluations; yet, because the judge orders only the more "serious" cases to be evaluated, a higher percentage of those evaluated may eventually be found incompetent, thus producing a higher proportional rate of incompetency findings among those referred for evaluation. However, there may not be a very marked difference if the incompetency adjudications are compared in proportion to all defendants who stood trial.

Variations in Evaluation Mechanisms and Procedures

It is likely that rates of competency evaluations and court findings of pretrial incompetency vary across jurisdictions partly as a function of differences in the evaluation mechanisms and procedures. For example, some courts provide for competency evaluations within jails or other facilities operated by law enforcement agencies or a department of corrections, and others refer defendants to a division of mental health facilities for observation and evaluation. Some jurisdictions provide full mental health evaluations in every case in which the question of competency is raised, and others have screening procedures that are used to determine the need for more comprehensive and costly evaluations.

The possible effects of these variations in evaluation procedures are demonstrated in data collected by McGarry and coworkers[23] in Massachusetts. They documented a more than threefold increase from 1963 to 1971 in the number of competency **evaluations** but a decrease from 22.2 percent to 1.2 percent of evaluated defendants who were **found incompetent.** Both of these changes, the authors noted, apparently were due to interim revisions in evaluation and commitment procedures in that state.

Tactical Misuse of Competency Procedures

The nature and frequency of competency evaluation cases can be influenced as well by legal maneuvers and tactical uses of this issue; that is, uses which are unrelated to the intent of the law. For example, a judge's almost automatic approval of competency evaluation requests may provide relief from overloaded dockets.[24] Prosecutors may raise the pretrial competency question in order to seek extra time to prepare their case and/or in efforts to keep the defendant in confinement. Some defense attorneys may call for competency evaluations in order to obtain information with which to weigh whether an insanity plea might be supported. The legal decision to perform a competency evaluation, then, is not always motivated by concerns expressed in the legal doctrine of competency to stand trial.

Social and Treatment Goals

Pretrial competency evaluations and incompetency commitments are also used (again, inappropriately) in order to provide psychiatric treatment to disturbed defendants when other methods for obtaining treatment (for example, civil commitment) are either more difficult or unavailable. For example, there is evidence[25,26] that incompetency commitments increase when a state enacts more restrictive civil commitment laws. Furthermore, the resulting increase in incompetency commitments tends to consist of defendants facing minor criminal charges.[27] This suggests that the incompetency mechanism can be used as a means of diverting disturbed and disturbing people from jails or the community into mental hospitals; the ostensible concern for assessing competency to stand trial may serve in fact to provide temporary solutions to other social problems.[28]

Confusion and Misunderstanding of the Legal Standard

Participants in pretrial competency hearings apparently are often confused or inadequately informed regarding the competency standard or the court's proper role in competency determinations.[29] Most common is a failure to recognize that psychiatric diagnosis is not (and should not be) dispositive of the competency question. Another common confusion is the failure to distinguish between the essential criteria for pretrial incompetency and those for criminal responsibility (legal insanity). Problems in differentiating the competency and insanity questions are abetted by laws and prepackaged court order forms that promote simultaneous evaluations for both competency and criminal responsibility as a matter of routine.[30]

One consequence of this confusion has been judges' heavy reliance upon court-appointed evaluators' conclusions regarding pretrial incompetency. Roesch and Golding[31] report a survey indicating that 59 percent of judges in one state did not hold formal competency hearings but instead relied exclusively on court-appointed evaluators' reports when making competency decisions. Furthermore, the judges reported that their conclusions never (35 percent so responding) or very rarely (remaining 65 percent) contradicted the examiners' conclusions.

This apparent degree of reliance on expert evaluators' opinions is disturbing for several reasons. For one, the court-appointed experts themselves often do not understand that questions about pretrial competency should focus specifically on an examinee's abilities to perform the role of defendant in a trial, not merely on the clinical and psychiatric features of the case. Furthermore, a competency decision is intended to be a legal conclusion that encompasses more than a statement about a defendant's abilities. These abilities must be weighed against the specific functioning that will be required in the pending trial. As we will discuss later in more detail, these are matters for judicial discretion, not clinical conclusion.

In summary, mental health professionals who evaluate defendants for pretrial incompetency are faced with a complex set of definitions, motivations, and legal concerns. The best protection against confusion is a clear view of the pretrial competency assessment goal and systematic methods for achieving the goal. The next section provides some guidelines toward those objectives.

THE COMPETENCY ASSESSMENT PROCESS

The process for pretrial mental competency assessments can be described in several stages, consistent with those outlined by Grisso in chapter 5. The stages themselves are applicable to assessments performed by both psychologists and psychiatrists, although their content may vary even among evaluators within either discipline. No attempt will be made in this section to describe how competency assessments usually are performed, because reliable generalizations about the nature and quality of current assessment practices do not exist. Instead, the present section describes circumstances, demands, and objectives that the forensic evaluator faces at each stage, and some reflections on various strategies and methods for dealing with them are offered here.

Problem Definition

First, one must define the question that is asked by the court. The criteria for pretrial competency sometimes are articulated clearly in the court order, but often they are not. Moreover, court orders often appear as "boiler-plate" forms that simultaneously request an assessment of general mental health status, competency to stand trial, and mental state at the time of the crime, even when the only issue raised at that point is the question of competency to stand trial. Even greater confusion is possible when a court orders an evaluation for competency to stand trial and includes among the criteria to be evaluated the question of the defendant's ability to "know that what he did was wrong" (or some other element of the insanity defense that bears no relation to the question of competency to stand trial).

Mental health professionals who routinely perform assessments for a particular court will have discovered across time the type of information that the court believes it needs. The examiner who is less familiar with a particular court, or with competency assessments in general, should discuss the referral with the judge or attorneys in the case after receiving the examination request in order to clarify what is needed or what the examiner plans to do.

As noted in the previous section, judges and attorneys themselves often are not clear about the nature of the information they seek. The evaluator then may wish to approach the consultation with some suggested structure for the examination. Especially helpful in this regard is Morse's[32] analysis of the logical requirements of mental health laws in general, which would outline the competency question at the broadest level in the following way: (1) Is there evidence of a current mental disorder, and if so, what is the nature and extent of the disorder and its general symptomatic consequences? (2) Does the defendant manifest some specific, functional inabilities that are of special concern to the legal standard for competency to stand trial? and (3) Given evidence for both of the above elements, is there a logical causal connection between the disorder and the legally relevant inabilities? If answers to these three questions suggest that a court might find the defendant incompetent, a fourth question will arise in many jurisdictions: (4) Is there a substantial likelihood that treatment can bring the defendant to a state of legal competency to stand trial within the number of months specified by statute or case law?

Element (2) suggests the need for a clear view of which specific abilities the court might perceive as relevant when considering whether a defendant "understands the trial process" or "can assist the attorney in a defense." Quite a number of lists[33] of competency-related abilities have been developed in order to structure examination and decision making regarding the competency question. Probably the best-known of these structures is the set of 13 specific abilities and capacities outlined by McGarry and coworkers[34] in a project that was designed to clarify and to improve competency assessments. These are described below when specific assessment methods are discussed. Taken together, the key questions outlined by Morse and the categories in the McGarry instruments offer definitions of the pretrial competency question which can guide the assessment throughout the following stages.

Preparation

This stage involves collecting background information on the case and the defendant, forming initial impressions, and planning the collection of information in subsequent direct evaluation of the defendant.

Much of the background information to be obtained will be of a type similar to that which would be desired in any psychiatric or clinical psychological evaluation: demographic characteristics of the defendant, educational history, history of diagnoses and treatments, and criminal justice records. Especially relevant in the criminal justice records will be information regarding previous competency examinations and court findings for the defendant. In addition, one should seek to determine the nature and extent of the defendant's previous contacts with courts, defense attorneys, the legal system generally, and the criminal justice system specifically. Prior learning and actual experience in these contexts may be especially relevant to questions of the defendant's understanding of courtroom events and attorney-client relations.

Competency evaluation referrals often occur because the judge or defense attorney has observed behavior that suggested deficiencies in the defendant's mental capacities relevant to pretrial competency. A firsthand description of those behaviors will be especially helpful in preparation for the evaluation. The evaluator should always ask why this particular evaluation was requested and what unusual behavior was seen or described that provoked the request. Ideally, attorneys should be required to provide information about their clients' behaviors which they have observed. The forensic evaluator then can prepare to collect information that may lead to a confirming or a disconfirming explanation for the behaviors that gave rise to the evaluation request.

Various sources provide information on the general frequency (that is, the base rates) of incompetency findings, as well as demographic and diagnostic characteristics, for large samples of defendants assessed for competency to stand trial.[35] Such information may be helpful as base rate information for approaching individual competency assessments. One could not use base rate information, of course, to classify a person as competent or incompetent. Such information can assist, however, in forming initial hypotheses and impressions or in protecting against the tendency to overpredict low base rate events, such as findings of incompetency.

The degree of ability that will be required, of course, varies with the complexity or nature of the trial. The depth or type of understanding that might be required of the defendant may be considerably different, for example, for a trial on a simple misdemeanor charge versus a serious, complex felony case with several counts. Some trials may take a few minutes or an hour, but others can be expected to extend for days or weeks. The defendant may or may not be expected to testify. Certain aspects of trials may be more or less likely to serve as physical or emotional stressors for defendants.

The forensic evaluator should obtain information about the probable nature of the pending trial. He should then explore characteristics of the defendant that are relevant to the anticipated demands of **this specific trial,** not merely trials in general. It is probable that the referring judge or the defense attorney can provide the evaluator with expectations about the trial demands, if the evaluator takes the initiative to inquire. This information is essential to a useful evaluation for the trial court.

In addition to diagnostic and trial-related abilities, several psychological functions may be important to assess. For example, if the anticipated trial will be lengthy and potentially stressful, one might be especially concerned about a defendant's ability to inhibit emotional responses under stress. An opinion about a defendant's capacity in this regard might not be attained confidently by a diagnosis, mental-status examination, or an assessment of the defendant's knowledge of courtroom activities and lawyer-client relations. Assessment of certain psychological functions and capacities, therefore, might require the use of psychological tests or other techniques.

Whatever the plans that are made during the preparation stage, they should be considered tentative and alterable. In some cases, the results of a comprehensive interview will render the rest of one's assessment plan unnecessary, but in other cases the interview might raise questions suggesting a very different or more extensive assessment plan than was conceived during preparation.

Data Collection

It is very important to provide the examinee with an explicit statement of the purposes of the evaluation and the ways in which the court may use the data to determine competency. Unlike most nonforensic evaluations of adults, the competency evaluation is neither voluntary nor confidential when ordered by the court. Thus, the client needs to be informed very explicitly that communications during such assessments are not protected by the conventional bounds of confidentiality and testimonial privilege. Typically, however, an examinee's admission to the alleged offense during a pretrial competency evaluation cannot be used as evidence in the subsequent trial. Thus, in the federal system there is very specific statutory language in this regard, as well as very similar provisions in the Rules of Criminal Procedure. The relevant language in Section 4244 states:

> No statement made by the accused in the course of any examination into his sanity or mental incompetency provided by this section, whether the examination shall be with or without the consent of the accused, shall be admitted in evidence against the accused on the issue of guilt in any criminal proceeding.[36]

The proposed Criminal Justice Mental Health Standards adopted by the American Bar Association[37] endorse the practice of informing the examinee of the following:

(i) the purpose and nature of the evaluation;
(ii) the potential uses of any disclosures made during the evaluation;
(iii) the conditions under which the prosecutor will have access to information obtained and reports prepared;
(iv) the consequences of the defendant's refusal to cooperate in the evaluation.

Competency evaluators have a variety of assessment methods at their disposal. There exists a growing body of specialized forensic assessment devices such as structured interviews and psychometric instruments, many of which are described in chapter 5. Among these forensic tools are several that have been designed to assess abilities to understand trial processes and to assist in one's defense.

Among the most researched and widely disseminated of these instruments are the Competency Screening Test (CST) and the Competency Assessment Instrument (CAI).[38] These instruments were developed for use in a two-stage process for screening defendants in competency evaluations. The CST was designed to screen out clearly competent defendants from those whose competency is questionable. The CAI was intended to assist in a more in-depth examination of the latter group.

The CST consists of 22 incomplete sentence stems such as: "When I go to court the lawyer will . . . ." "The way a court trial is decided . . . ." The sentence stems are designed to tap functions, such as one's abilities to trust and to relate to one's attorney, to understand court processes, to understand possible consequences of the trial, and to be aware of peril. The sentence stems are completed by the examinee. Each response is scored 2, 1, or 0, indicating that the response suggests competency, questionable competency, or incompetency. A total CST score falling below 20 is said to suggest behavioral or cognitive deficits that may significantly impair a defendant's trial-relevant abilities.

The CAI is a structured interview device that provides for inquiry into 13 functions relevant to competent functioning in criminal proceedings. The 13 functions are (1) appraisal of available legal defenses; (2) unmanageable behavior; (3) quality of relating to attorney; (4) planning of legal strategy, including guilty plea to lesser charges where pertinent; (5) appraisal of role of defense counsel, prosecuting attorney, judge, jury, defendant, and witness; (6) understanding of court procedure; (7) appreciation of charges; (8) appreciation of range and nature of possible penalties; (9) appraisal of likely outcome; (10) capacity to disclose to attorney available pertinent facts surrounding the offense, including the defendant's movements, mental state, and actions at the time of the offense; (11) capacity to realistically challenge prosecution witnesses; (12) capacity to testify relevantly; and (13) self-defeating or self-serving motivation.

After the interview (which may take about 1 hour), the defendant is rated on each of the 13 dimensions for degree of incapacity. Ratings range from 1 (indicating total incapacity) to 5 (indicating no incapacity). A handbook supplies definitions, a structured interview protocol, and clinical examples corresponding to various ratings.

Golding and Roesch's Interdisciplinary Fitness Interview[39] also evaluates and summarizes a defendant's trial-related abilities. One of its special features, however, is provision for assessment by a team of evaluators (including mental health professionals and lawyers). The interview guide is divided into two parts—Legal Issues (specific trial abilities) and Psychopathological Symptoms/Syndromes—with several categories for inquiry (specific abilities or types of symptoms) in each part. In addition to providing ratings for each of the ability or symptom categories, evaluators indicate for each category the degree of influence that that observation had upon their final decision about pretrial competency. The final decision is stated in two ways at the end of the process: a judgment of competency or incompetency, and a rating of the examiner's confidence in the judgment.

Many traditional psychological instruments (for example, intelligence tests, projective techniques) noted in chapter 5 by Grisso are used in forensic assessment of competency, in order to assess the general intelligence and psychological and behavioral characteristics of a defendant. These measures, however, would not invariably be used in competency assessments. The results of these more general psychological and psychiatric methods are often most valuable for relating findings of incompetency to the nature of a defendant's mental deficiency or psychopathology and its likely fluctuations, addressing questions of malingering, and in weighing the likelihood that psychiatric treatment would remedy a defendant's incompetency to stand trial.

Interpretation and Reporting

Having completed the foregoing assessment task, the evaluator must interpret the data and report it to the court in an appropriate form. The evaluator examines the data in the context of the diagnostic questions and objectives that were formulated previously. Although the court order may request only the examiner's **conclusions** about the defendant, testimony and cross-examination necessitate that the evaluator formulate a clear **rationale** for any conclusions drawn from the data.

The Proposed Criminal Justice Mental Health Standards of the American Bar Association[40] endorse the following content for written evaluations:

(i) identify the specific matters referred for evaluation;
(ii) describe the procedures, tests and techniques used;
(iii) state clinical findings and opinions on each matter referred for evaluation and indicate specifically those questions, if any, that could not be answered;
(iv) identify the sources of information and present the factual basis for the clinical findings and opinions;
(v) present the reasoning which was used to reach the clinical findings and opinions.

In addition, if the defendant manifests serious deficiencies, the examiner should explain any opinion about the likelihood that the defendant's abilities could improve with treatment within a reasonable period of time.

There is disagreement among mental health professionals about whether the examiner should render an opinion on the ultimate legal issue; that is, the defendant's competency to stand trial. A report issued by the Group for Advancement of Psychiatry (GAP) cogently stated a majority opinion that the ultimate legal question should not be addressed in examiner reports.

The report should contain sufficient data to justify the conclusions reached and to indicate how they were reached. These conclusions should not set forth an opinion as to whether the defendant is legally competent. The data offered, however, will enable the Court to assume its proper responsibility and make an enlightened legal judgment as to the defendant's competency.[41]

A minority of the GAP committee, however, felt that an opinion on the ultimate legal issue should be part of the examiner's testimony. Moreover, the American Bar Association's Proposed Criminal Justice Mental Health Standards would allow examiners to render opinions on the ultimate legal question.[42] We shall examine this issue further in the final section of this chapter.

UNRESOLVED ISSUES

In recent years there have been many improvements in the general quality of competency-to-stand-trial assessments, as well as in legal procedures for determining incompetency. Competency definitions in many states have become clearer, and mental health professionals have new tools (and often an improved grasp of the competency question) with which to assist courts. Several problems and issues, however, are yet to be resolved. Concerning many of these issues, there are differences of opinion among justice personnel and mental health professionals alike regarding the desirability or feasibility of various options. This final section briefly describes a few of these issues.

Dual-Purpose Court Orders

Roesch and Golding[43] have pointed out that the purpose of mental health professionals' assessments for competency to stand trial is blurred by court orders that request simultaneously (and sometimes merge conceptually) assessments for pretrial competency and for the insanity plea. That these are two distinct and separate issues under the law has been explained earlier in this chapter. Different functional capacities and characteristics are relevant for the two issues. Diagnosis is required in both cases, but in the one case it is retrospective (at the time of the crime) and in the other it is present and prospective. To merge the two in court orders disregards these differences, Roesch and Golding argue. Furthermore, it seems wasteful of resources to perform a more lengthy evaluation for the two purposes, when the insanity defense might not even have been raised formally at the time of the competency evaluation request.

Court orders for dual-purpose competency/insanity evaluations sometimes are not the product of judicial misunderstanding but instead are supported by statutory language. Arizona's statute, for example, specifically allows both assessments concurrently, stating that "there is no reason why these two examinations cannot be combined."[44] The motivation for combining the assessments apparently is to avoid the circumstance in which a defendant, once evaluated for competency and adjudicated as competent, then decides to use the insanity plea, thereby necessitating a further delay of proceedings while an insanity evaluation is performed.

The court's convenience is only one reason dual-purpose evaluations are promoted by some statutes. One can argue also that the defendant is given speedier consideration in this manner, thus decreasing the pretrial time during which he or she is deprived of liberty or during which period critical evidence may be lost to the defense.

The arguments for and against dual-purpose evaluations might be addressed empirically by data concerning the proportion of defendants found competent who then assert an insanity plea. If this number is small, the argument that dual-purpose evaluations save time is less convincing. Relevant data, though, are not yet available.

Competency to Negotiate and to Plead

The term "competency to stand trial" is somewhat misleading, in that it suggests that the question of a defendant's pretrial competency is appropriately raised only when the defendant will contest allegations in a trial. In fact, the concept of competency applies generally to a defendant's capacity to participate in legal proceedings related to a criminal allegation at various points before trial, during the trial, before imposition of sentence, in some states at the appeals stage, and prior to execution of the sentence.[45] The vast majority of criminal cases are handled through negotiated pleas. Yet rarely are questions raised about defendants' competency to understand or to cooperate with the attorney in the negotiation process or to make decisions about entering a guilty plea. As explained earlier in this chapter, these decisions involve a waiver of Constitutional rights, which may require a more sophisticated understanding of the issues involved than that required in cases in which defendants are proceeding to a noncomplex, lower-court trial. Competency to plead or to negotiate should receive greater attention by legislators, defense lawyers, and the criminal court.

The Scope of Competency Assessments

The development of special methods for assessing abilities related to competency to stand trial has raised questions about the need for hospital confinement and 30-day commitments in order to perform such evaluations. For example, it may be that a mental health professional's interview, consisting of a mental status examination and questions such as those provided by the Competency Assessment Instrument can form clinical opinions concerning competency versus incompetency that are very similar to those resulting from the usual and more extensive psychiatric evaluation.[46] These briefer assessments usually require no hospital commitment, being performed in an hour or two on an outpatient basis.

The motivations for these suggestions include reducing financial cost, trial delays, and deprivation of freedom associated with more extended evaluation. Most important, an outpatient examination eliminates the stigma of a mental hospital commitment for the many defendants who will be found clearly competent and not mentally ill. These motives are consistent with the principle that defendants should be provided the least restrictive alternative placement for accomplishing the assessment goal.[47]

It is difficult to present the defense for "typical" competency assessments of the extensive, inpatient type (those performed in the course of 30-day observations in security hospitals), because little data about these evaluations are available in the literature.

However, some evidence is available concerning the efficacy of pretrial competency psychometric tests and interview methods[48-55] such as those described in the previous section of this chapter. Much of this research examines the degree to which these procedures, with or without other brief, supporting methods, can match the competency and incompetency decisions made for the same defendants by clinicians performing more extensive hospital evaluations during a much longer period of observation. Some brief methods appear to fare quite well against the criterion.

Is this evidence useful in deciding the efficacy of brief competency assessment methods? Many legal standards require more than a mere "yes-no" opinion about a defendant's competency. They call for an accurate diagnosis, a knowledge of the defendant's abilities and inabilities for pretrial competency, and enough information about the defendant's symptomatology, personality, and psychological functions to be able to explain specifically how the disorder accounts for the functional inabilities that have been observed. Furthermore, enough background information and cross-situational observations must be available to rule out the possibility of malingering and to describe the type of treatment (and the probability of its success) that may be needed to restore competency.

In light of these demands, comparisons of the "yes-no" conclusions of brief evaluations with those based on evaluations requiring lengthy hospitalization do not address the critical question: To what extent do either the more extensive assessments or the brief methods reliably obtain the full range of information associated with an adequate assessment for competency? Currently the answer to this question is not known within the research literature available.

Testifying about Legal Competency

Among the many questions that have been raised about expert testimony regarding mental competency to stand trial, the most controversial may be the disagreement that has surrounded the practice of addressing the "ultimate legal question."

Some statutes and many judges require that the mental health professional testify to his or her conclusion concerning whether the defendant is competent as defined by the statute. Most experts probably comply, and the American Bar Association's Proposed Criminal Justice Mental Health Standards endorse this practice.[56]

When mental health professionals testify to the defendant's competency, however, they render an opinion regarding the interpretation of law and whether or not the available evidence satisfies that which the law requires for a determination of incompetency. A number of mental health experts have voiced their discomfort about the practice of requiring or allowing mental health professionals to testify to the ultimate legal question,[57-59] and earlier in this chapter it was noted that an important report by the Group for the Advancement of Psychiatry[60] recommended against such testimony. They have argued that the statement of legal conclusions goes well beyond the expertise of mental health professionals. They contend that the expert should inform the court concerning the type, extent, and effect of the defendant's difficulties and incapacities, leaving to the court the task of weighing the facts in order to arrive at conclusions about the ultimate legal issue of competency.

To fully understand the reasoning behind this viewpoint, one must recognize that there is no clear psychological dividing line between legal competency and incompetency. The two are not defined by a fixed quantum of either symptomatic behavior or functional disability. Whether a particular amount and type of mentally related disability is enough to satisfy a legal definition of incompetency must be explained and justified in each case. Justification is necessary because the defendant's interests are not the only ones involved in questions of legal competency. There are, in addition, the interests of the state in bringing defendants to trial.

The legal process of weighing these competing interests is called procedural justice, and the desired product is substantive justice. The process inevitably requires moral judgments regarding the greatest good, and it leads to an answer to the ultimate legal question concerning whether or not the defendant will be considered competent under the law.

The argument against mental health professionals' testimony on such matters involving moral and social judgments seems strong. Nevertheless, we are far from having resolved this question of limits on forensic evaluators' testimony in competency-to-stand-trial assessments. (For further discussion and advice on the psychologist as an expert witness, see chapter 21 of this text; on testimony by psychiatrists, see chapter 22.)

CONCLUSION

Mental health professionals who perform assessments for competency to stand trial must meet three standards in order to serve best the needs of defendants and society. They must abide by **legal** definitions and procedures that apply in pretrial competency determinations. In addition, they must apply methods that represent the **technical and empirical** standards of their professions. Finally, they must exercise care with reference to **ethical** obligations established by their professions. (Several other chapters of this text deal with various aspects of these standards.)

These three standards sometimes are in conflict with each other. At times the law requests information that the professional may feel is beyond scientific or ethical parameters. At other times, the professional may have information that seems perfectly relevant to a defendant's needs but that is not legally appropriate for use in pretrial competency proceedings.

Resolution of such conflicts does not rest with opinionated pronouncements that protect one of the three standards at the expense of the others. It depends instead upon the process of many professionals—in law and in mental health—meeting the challenges of these conflicts as they arise in case after case, thereby moving gradually toward rational policies born of experience with many instances of the conflicts.

The mental health professional can do three things to contribute to this process of movement toward rational policy and practice in pretrial competency assessments.

First, the evaluator should be thoroughly familiar with the relevant law and the current state of competent professional practice in assessing defendants for pretrial competency. Preparation and self-education for this field can begin with a personal review of many of the works cited in the present chapter. No mental health professional can contribute meaningfully to the needs of defendants, the legal process, or the future of clinical practice in this area if participation occurs in ignorance of the historical and current issues mentioned in this chapter.

Second, the mental health professional should try to approach **every** pretrial competency assessment in the way that an expert guildsman approaches the handcrafting of an exquisite silver bowl or a fine piece of woodwork. Having made countless other objects of the same type in the past, the craftsman nevertheless will approach **this** one as though reputation and integrity will be judged on the basis of this instance alone. If mental health professionals perceive each pretrial competency assessment in the above manner, their practice will contribute positively to the ongoing process of refinement in the use of mental health expertise by courts in pretrial competency cases.

Third, the evaluator's experiences in pretrial competency assessments may qualify him or her to communicate concerns or to contribute insights to researchers, who may develop empirical solutions to some problems, and to legislators and judges, who are in positions to refine and to change policies concerning pretrial competency determinations.

This chapter has attempted to assist professionals at the first step: preparing for pretrial competency assessments by educating oneself to definitions, procedures, issues, and assessment methods. In a sense, the defendant who must be competent for trial and the mental health evaluator who will assess the defendant face similar circumstances. Both must enter the "battle" adequately armed, having been prepared to play a role that will safeguard the principles of fairness which the pretrial competency doctrine represents. For the mental health professional, this preparation begins with self-education concerning the legal and professional standards for assessments related to the question of competency to stand trial.

REFERENCES

1. *Amnesia: A case study in the limits of particular justice.* Yale Law Journal 71:109-136, 1961-1962.

2. Dusky v. United States 362 U.S. 402 (1960) 788.

3. AUSNESS, C: *The identification of incompetent defendants: Separating those unfit for adversary combat from those who are fit.* Kentucky Law Journal 66:666,706, 1977-1978.

4. BENNETT, D: *Competency to stand trial: A call for reform.* Journal of Criminal Law, Criminology and Police Science, 59:569-582, 1968.

5. SILTEN, P AND TULLIS, R: *Mental competency in criminal proceedings.* Hastings Law Journal 28:1053-1074, 1976-1977.

6. Wieter v. Settle, 193 F. Supp. 318 (W. D. Mo., 1961) at 321-322.

7. ROESCH, R AND GOLDING, S: *Competency to Stand Trial.* University of Illinois Press, Champaign, IL, 1980.

8. United States v. Wilson 391 F.2d 460 (D. C. Circ 1968).

9. STONE, A: *Mental Health and Law: A System in Transition.* National Institute of Mental Health, Center for Studies of Crime and Delinquency, DHEW Publications No. (ADM) 75-176, Rockville, MD, 1975.

10. SHAH, S: *Legal and mental health system interactions: Major development and research needs.* Int J Law Psychiatry, 4:219-270, 1981.

11. See Sieling v. Eyman 478 F.2d, 211 (9th Cir., 1973).

12. *Dusky v. United States*, sup.

13. Pate v. Robinson 383 U.S. 375 (1966).

14. Drope v. Missouri 95 S. Ct. 895 (1975) at 180.

15. ROESCH AND GOLDING, sup.

16. Arizona Revised Statutes Annotated (1982) Rules of Criminal Procedure, Rule 11.4 (b).

17. HOLMSTRUP, ML, FITCH, WL, KEILITZ, I: *Screening and Evaluation in Centralized Forensic Mental Health Facilities.* National Center for State Courts, Williamsburg, VA, 1981.

18. Pouncy v. United States 349 F.2d 699 (1965) at 700.

19. Jackson v. Indiana 406 U.S. 715 (1972).

20. MCGARRY, AL, CURRAN, WJ, KENEFICK, D: *Problems of public consultation in medico-legal matters: A symposium.* Am J Psychiatry 125:42-59, 1968.

21. MONAHAN, J AND STEADMAN, HJ (EDS): *Mentally Disordered Offenders: Perspectives from Law and Social Science.* Plenum, New York, 1983.

22. ROESCH AND GOLDING, sup.

23. MCGARRY, AL, CURRAN, WJ, LIPSITT, PD, LELOS, D, SCHWITZGEBEL, RK, ROSENBERG, AH: *Competency to Stand Trial and Mental Illness.* DHEW Publication No. (ADM) 77-103, Washington, DC, 1973.

24. ROESCH AND GOLDING, sup.

25. BONOVITZ, JC AND BONOVITZ, JS: *Diversion of the mentally ill into the criminal justice system: The police intervention perspective.* Am J Psychiatry 138:973-976, 1981.

26. GUDEMAN, H: *Legal sanctions and the clinician.* The Clinical Psychologist 34:15-17, 1981.

27. DICKEY, W: *Incompetency and the nondangerous mentally ill client.* Criminal Law Bulletin 16:22-36, 1980.

28. WEXLER, DB: *The structure of civil commitment: Patterns, pressures, and interactions in mental health legislation.* Law and Human Behavior 7:1-18, 1983.

29. ROESCH AND GOLDING, sup.

30. See reference 43, infra, and accompanying text.

31. ROESCH AND GOLDING, sup.

32. MORSE, S. *Crazy behavior, morals and science: An analysis of mental health law.* Southern California Law Review 51:527, 1978.

33. AUSNESS, sup; BENNETT, sup; SILTEN AND TULLIS, sup.

34. MCGARRY ET AL, sup.

35. WILLIAMS, W AND MILLER, KS: *The processing and disposition of incompetent mentally ill offenders.* Law and Human Behavior 5:245-261, 1981; ROESCH AND GOLDING, sup; MCGARRY ET AL, sup.

36. 18 U.S.C. Section 4244—Mental incompetency after arrest and before trial, p 1374. See also Rule 12.2—Notice of Defense Based Upon Mental Condition, (c) Psychiatric Examination. Appendix—Rules of Criminal Procedure, 18 U.S.C., 1976 edition, p 1428.

37. AMERICAN BAR ASSOCIATION: *Proposed Criminal Justice Mental Health Standards.* ABA, Chicago, IL, 1984.

38. MCGARRY ET AL, sup.

39. GOLDING, S, ROESCH, R, SCHREIBER, J: *Assessment and conceptualization of competency to stand trial: Preliminary data on the Interdisciplinary Fitness Interview.* Law and Human Behavior 8:321-334, 1984.

40. AMERICAN BAR ASSOCIATION, sup, p 99.

41. GROUP FOR THE ADVANCEMENT OF PSYCHIATRY: *Misuse of psychiatry in the criminal courts: Competency to stand trial.* Committee on Psychiatry and Law 8:853, 1974.

42. AMERICAN BAR ASSOCIATION, sup, p 110.

43. ROESCH AND GOLDING, sup.

44. Arizona Revised Statutes Annotated, Rule 11.2 (Comment) (1973).

45. SHAH, sup.

46. STONE, WR, JR AND BELANGER, J: *Evaluating the competency of admissions to a state maximum-security service.* Hosp Community Psychiatry 29:425-426, 1978.

47. AMERICAN BAR ASSOCIATION, sup, p 201.

48. LIPSITT, P, LELOS, D, McGARRY, AL: *Competency for trial: A screening instrument.* Am J Psychiatry 128:105-109, 1971.

49. McGARRY ET AL, sup.

50. NOTTINGHAM, EJ AND MATTSON, RE: *A validation study of the Competency Screening Test.* Law and Human Behavior 5:329-335, 1981.

51. RANDOLPH, JJ, HICKS, T, ET AL: *The Competency Screening Test: A validation study in Cook County, Illinois.* Criminal Justice and Behavior 7:495-500, 1982.

52. RANDOLPH, JJ, HICKS, T, MASON, D: *The Competency Screening Test: A replication and extension.* Criminal Justice and Behavior 8:471-481, 1981.

53. ROESCH AND GOLDING, sup.

54. SHATIN, L: *Brief form of the Competency Screening Test for mental competence to stand trial.* J Clin Psychol 35:464-467, 1979.

55. SHATIN, L AND BRODSKY, SH: *Competency for trial: The Competency Screening Test in an urban hospital forensic unit.* Mt Sinai J Med 46:131-134, 1979.

56. AMERICAN BAR ASSOCIATION, sup.

57. GUTHEIL, TG AND APPELBAUM, PS: *Clinical Handbook of Psychiatry and the Law.* McGraw-Hill, New York, 1982.

58. HALLECK, SL: *Law in the Practice of Psychiatry: A Handbook for Clinicians.* Plenum, New York, 1980.

59. STONE, sup.

60. GROUP FOR THE ADVANCEMENT OF PSYCHIATRY, sup.

CHAPTER 8
CRIMINAL RESPONSIBILITY*
Saleem A. Shah, Ph.D.

The legal issue of criminal responsibility refers to the conditions under which persons charged with crimes are to be held criminally liable or culpable for their alleged acts or omissions. Stephens[1] expressed it rather succinctly, albeit simply, a century ago when he said, "I understand by responsibility nothing more than actual liability to legal punishment." Of course, the concern here is with **criminal** liability, as distinct from various civil liabilities pertaining to private wrongs (torts) or violations of contractual obligations.

Although there is a general rule that people are to be held legally responsible for their actions, our fundamental and long-standing societal values and moral traditions allow for several exceptions in situations in which it would not be fair or just to hold persons criminally or civilly liable. In the criminal law, these exceptions are discussed under the general heading of **defenses,** which in turn have traditionally been distinguished as **justifications** and **excuses** (see, for example, any criminal law text such as Dix and Sharlot,[2] Kadish et al,[3] Low et al,[4] Vorenberg,[5] or Weinreb;[6] see also Fletcher[7]). Stated very simply, "justifications" seek to establish that, even though the prosecution has fulfilled its required burden to prove the basic facts of the offense, the act committed by the defendant was not criminal because, for example, it was taken in **defense** of self, others, or property. "Excuses" essentially concede the wrongfulness of the act but seek to establish that the defendant is not criminally responsible

* The views expressed here are the author's and not those of the agency with which he is associated. The author would like to express his thanks to Professor Richard J. Bonnie (University of Virginia Law School), Professor John M. Brumbaugh (University of Maryland Law School), and Professor David Wexler (University of Arizona Law School) for their helpful comments to a draft of this chapter.

because the act took place, for example, under conditions of **duress or compulsion, immaturity** (the defendant was under 14 years of age),* or **insanity.**

Recently, Robinson[8] has provided a systematic analysis of criminal law defenses and presents a very useful five-tiered conceptual framework for classifying and analyzing the more than 50 possible bars to criminal conviction.

The topic of the insanity defense has attracted considerable scholarly attention from lawyers, mental health professionals, philosophers, and others, and an immense literature has accumulated. Moreover, this defense continues to be the subject of considerable public and political interest and controversy—in this regard far exceeding the actual numerical importance of the issue in the criminal justice process. Thus, Norval Morris[9] has been moved to remark that "Rivers of ink, mountains of printer's lead, forests of paper have been expended on this issue, which is surely marginal to the chaotic problems of effective, rational, and humane prevention and treatment of crime." Although he notes that he has "contributed too may words to this wastage," Morris[10] has nevertheless made some further and interesting contributions to the discussion and debate on the topic. A very similar observation regarding the considerably disproportionate attention given to the insanity defense was made by Cohen[11] about 18 years ago when he pointed out:

> Indeed, few subjects concerned with the criminal law have been debated by medico-legal writers more often or with more vigor. Its inspirational qualities notwithstanding, statistically the insanity defense is only slightly more significant than the incidence of snake bites in New York City.

Although the actual incidence of insanity acquittals in New York City during the past decade or so has markedly exceeded the incidence of snake bites, the thrust of Cohen's basic point remains unchanged.

In essence, as Abraham Goldstein noted in his highly acclaimed book on the subject,[12] the trial of the defense of insanity evokes some of the deepest feelings and ideologies pertaining to the issues of responsibility, mental disorders, and the highly charged moral, political, legal, public policy, and pragmatic questions that are involved. "The trial of the defense," Goldstein points out, "is treated as if it were a contemporary morality play revolving around the issues of sickness and guilt."[13]

If there were doubts about the general accuracy of Goldstein's observation, the media, public, and political attention given to the recent trial of John W. Hinckley, Jr. (who attempted to assassinate President Reagan in March 1981) serves to illustrate the considerable publicity that surrounds the periodic notorious cases involving the insanity defense. Moreover, even though about 20 states and the United States Congress have been considering various revisions to laws pertaining to mentally disordered offenders and other criminal statutes during recent years, the Hinckley episode—especially the jury's verdict of "not guilty by reason of insanity"—appears to have been a major trigger for the

---

* By the 17th century, under common law, there was an absolute (nonrebuttable) presumption of lack of criminal capacity below the age of 7 years; between the ages of 7 and 13 there was a rebuttable presumption of criminal incapacity, and children 14 and older were presumed to be criminally liable, just like adults.[4] The defense of infancy or immaturity has largely been supplanted in function by juvenile delinquency laws.

public and political uproar and the veritable flurry of legislative activity. Of the approximately two dozen pieces of legislation introduced in Congress pertaining to mentally disordered offenders and the insanity defense, more than a half dozen were introduced in the days **immediately** following the Hinckley verdict.

Given the numerous complex and controversial issues pertaining to criminal responsibility and the defense of insanity, this chapter will address only the following major topics. First, we will briefly review the historical background of the development of the insanity defense in Anglo-American law and the fundamental societal values and moral traditions that undergird this defense. This section will also discuss the basic definition of crimes, the key notion of mens rea, and will mention the various rules or tests that have been and are currently being used for determining the criminal responsibility of defendants who raise the defense of insanity. The second major section will address a few of the perceived problems pertaining to the defense and the manner in which related policies and procedures are administered. Some of the empirical research on the general topic will be cited to indicate the extent to which certain public and political perceptions regarding the insanity defense deviate rather sharply from the actual reality. In the third major section, a few of the reforms and associated solutions that have been proposed in recent years to address the perceived problems will also be addressed. Included here will be policy statements and recommendations made recently by several of the major professional organizations such as the American Bar Association, the American Psychiatric Association, the American Medical Association, and the American Psychological Association. The last section will discuss a number of vexing policy and programmatic dilemmas pertaining to the administration of the insanity defense and the disposition and handling of persons who are acquitted (not necessarily released) for this reason.

THE BASIC PURPOSE AND THE POLICY UNDERLYING THE INSANITY DEFENSE

It was 60 years ago when Crotty noted that

> No topic in the criminal law has aroused more discussion than the question of the responsibility of the insane for crime. The discussion breaks out with renewed violence every time that this defense is raised in a criminal case. It has long been the cause of a war of great feeling between the medical and legal professions.[14]

This observation remains generally correct even today, although the erstwhile "war of great feeling between the medical and legal professions" has subsided and various understandings have been formed in reference to the "abolition brouhaha" and related reform efforts. Whatever skirmishes and controversies exist seem to pertain more to philosophical, ideological, and policy—rather than interdisciplinary—conflicts.

Given the above background, a discussion of the subject of criminal responsibility and the defense of insanity will be facilitated by a brief historical review of the development of some of the basic notions in Anglo-American law. Because the legal doctrines have evolved over a period of several centuries and are deeply rooted in the philosophical, religious, and moral traditions of

Judeo-Christian societies, such understanding seems both important and necessary for placing into proper perspective the purpose and rationale underlying the relevant policies and legal doctrines.

Historical Background and Rationale

This historical review will simply touch upon major features in the development of Anglo-American criminal law and especially the topic of criminal responsibility.

Levitt[15] points out that the roots of Anglo-American criminal law are to be found in the Roman law, the Salic law, the Irish law, the Anglo-Saxon law, the Hebrew law, and Christian theology. Prior to the Norman conquest of England in 1066 there was no common or unified law in the country. The legal systems, such as they were, were associated with the major political divisions of the country. Not only were there national courts in the major divisions, but there also existed ecclesiastic courts and private courts belonging to landowners. Under the secular legal codes of the time most forms of homicide and other personal injuries were treated as matters for compensation, under threat of the blood feud. The main principle of this early law was that any act that caused physical harm must, in the interests of peace, be paid for. This early system was summed up in the phrase "Buy off the spear or bear it." If the compensation was not paid, the injured person or his relatives might have prosecuted the feud. Defaulters were considered to be outside the law and could be pursued and killed. For several centuries the decree of outlawry remained the ultimate remedy of the state.[16-18]

During this period in England persons were held rather strictly accountable for the harm they had done (even for the harm done by their domestic animals); compensation was also required for harmful acts that were accidental, unintentional, or in self-defense. The major concern was to supplant blood feuds by inducing the victims or their relatives to accept compensation in place of revenge. Among the many Latin maxims and phrases that reflected the relevant policies and rules was *"qui inscienter peccat scienter emendet,"* meaning "he who commits evil unknowingly must pay for it knowingly."[19]

During this period of strict liability the only recourse that persons had against criminal conviction that seemed unjust was to seek the king's pardon. Such pardons were more commonly sought and obtained in cases involving children of tender years, the severely retarded (idiots), the severely mentally disordered, and in cases of clearly accidental or unintentional harms.

The growth and evolution of the legal system was gradual over the centuries. However, even with the strict liability policies and practices noted above, and as early as the sixth century, the teachings of Augustine and Pope Gregory came to England with the missionary Austin (who was later canonized as St. Augustine).[15] By the tenth century the laws of Aethelred made reference to the desirability of considering whether the injurious act had been done intentionally or voluntarily.[17] During the tenth and eleventh centuries notions derived from canon law began to focus increasingly on the intentions of the actor, not just on the act. While the secular law of the time was concerned with whether a criminal offense had been committed, the Church and its canon law were interested in the circumstances under which moral guilt or wickedness could be imputed to the actions. By the twelfth century the influence of Church law was becoming more evident and the conception of subjective blameworthiness (mens rea) as the foundation of legal guilt began to gain importance.[16-22]

Bracton, the first medieval English jurist who was also an ecclesiastic, compiled a comprehensive legal treatise entitled *On the Laws and Customs of England*.[23] Written in Latin, this work was finished about 1256 and drew heavily on earlier sources of Continental jurisprudence, especially Roman law. In this treatise Bracton dealt with a very wide range of topics and, with respect to criminal responsibility, he emphasized the importance of considering the intentions and will of the offender. Bracton's views were very much influenced by his ecclesiastic training and his knowledge of canon law; for him, children and madmen provided examples of persons who lacked the necessary qualities of will and intention that were considered essential for guilt and crime.

It should be remembered that the nature and degree of mental disorder and disability that served to excuse insane persons from criminal liability and punishment were severe and obvious disorders (what in current terminology would be called psychoses) and severe mental retardation. A few of the terms and phrases used in the relevant literature of the time (for example, "furiosus," "frenetic passione detentus," "frenetycs," and the like) refer to an almost total lack of understanding and discretion and what in more current and popular language would be translated as "raving mad."[17]

The notion that a prohibited act could not by itself involve criminal responsibility unless there was also a quality of moral blameworthiness eventually came to be enshrined in the well-known maxim *"Actus non facit reum nisi mens sit rea,"* meaning that "The act does not make a person guilty unless the intention be guilty also."[24]

Although Turner[25] notes the "grammatical clumsiness of the whole maxim" (an English judge even went so far as to describe the grammatical structure as "uncouth"[26]), he emphasizes that this ancient maxim has remained unchallenged as a declaration of principle of common law over many centuries.

Crime: Actus Reus and Mens Rea

Basically, the criminal law constitutes a description of harms that a society seeks to discourage with the threat of criminal punishment for those who commit those harms. However, before it imposes the heavy hand of criminal sanctions, as a reflection of deeply rooted societal values and related public policies the law seeks to establish the moral blameworthiness or culpability of the accused. Moreover, consistent with the values of a democratic society in which great importance is given to protecting the rights of individuals against the power of the state, the criminally prohibited acts and omissions are very carefully and precisely defined. Thus, a **crime** cannot be committed unless all required elements in the definition of the particular offense have been satisfied. These "elements" reflect the conditions under which certain acts or omissions constitute crimes.[4,27]

The preceding review of historical developments has indicated the long-standing concern in Anglo-American criminal law to consider intent and voluntariness in making the crucially important distinction between guilt and innocence. Moreover, apart from strict liability offenses which do not concern themselves with the state of mind of the actor, it is long-established doctrine in Anglo-American law that in order for there to be a criminal act there must be a forbidden or wrongful act (actus reus) and an evil, wicked, or guilty mind (mens rea). The commission of a criminally forbidden act does not, by itself, constitute a crime. There must also be mens rea, the legally required culpable state of mind. As Justice Jackson wrote about 30 years ago in *Morissette v. United States*, "Crime as a compound concept, [is] generally constituted only from concurrence of an evil-meaning mind with an evil-doing hand."[28]

ACTUS REUS

The concept of actus reus, as a legal term of art, is much more complex than the literal translation of the Latin words would suggest. Simply because an act is harmful does not make it an actus reus—unless it is a voluntary act and, in the particular instance of the case, the law has forbidden that act under pain of criminal sanctions. The principle of voluntariness reflects a legal response to the basic intuition that it would be grossly unfair to punish people for acts that were not strictly speaking "their own acts"; for example, if one pushes against and knocks down another person while being shoved from behind in a large crowd, or if one strikes another person while in the throes of a psychomotor epileptic seizure (epileptic automatism). Hence, the principle of voluntariness is applied in a very pragmatic (not metaphysical) sense in only those exceptional situations in which the defendant completely lacks control over his bodily movements.[29] Returning to the second important principle, the fact that the particular act was not prohibited by law is generally a complete defense.[25]

Most commonly, as in the crime of battery, actus reus consists of the specifically proscribed act: hitting a person. However, the term also includes the harmful results of the proscribed act when the offense is so defined (for example, the actual death of a victim in homicide offenses), as well as other special circumstances that may be included in the definition of the crime (for example, the age of the victim in statutory rape cases). The actus reus can be viewed, therefore, as designating all the elements of the criminal offense except for the mens rea.[30] In addition, the requirement of a voluntary act serves to prevent the massive costs to individual autonomy and liberty that would result were mere intentions to be subjected to criminal sanctions. Criminal liability is in very large measure predicated on observable events that clearly manifest the voluntary actions and the state of mind of the accused.[29]

MENS REA

The concept of mens rea is both murky and hydra-headed, because its precise meaning tends to change depending upon the particular context of its usage. In essence, it reflects the idea that crime requires a guilty (culpable) mind. In his excellent article on the subject some 50 years ago, Sayre[19] observed that "no problem of criminal law is of more fundamental importance or has proved more baffling through the centuries than the determination of the precise mental elements or mens rea necessary for crime." More recently, Kadish[31] observed that "the term 'mens rea' is rivalled only by the term 'jurisdiction' for the varieties of senses in which it has been used and the quantity of obfuscation it has created."

Despite the above difficulties (as also exist to some degree with the definition and meaning of concepts such as "fairness" and "justice"), and despite various developments over the centuries regarding its meanings and varying uses, the concept of mens rea has a fundamental importance that must be kept in mind when discussing the issue of criminal responsibility generally or the defense of insanity more specifically.

There are two principle categories of mens rea that need to be distinguished: (1) mens rea used in a narrow and special sense, and (2) mens rea used in a general sense to indicate blameworthiness and legal liability.

When used in its narrow or special sense, mens rea refers only to the specific mental states or elements that are required by the definition of the particular offense. For example, the offense of larceny involves the appropriation of another's property **knowing** that it is not your own and with the **intent** to deprive the owner of possession of that property permanently. Hence, "knowledge" and "intent" are the special mental elements (or the particular culpable states of mind) required for commission of the offense of larceny. Thus, if a man walks out of a restaurant with someone else's topcoat believing it to be his own and without any intent to deprive the rightful owner of that item, it would not constitute the offense of larceny. It is important to note that the inclusion of special mens rea elements in the definition of the offense is very crucial; it serves not only to indicate the specific conduct that is to be considered and handled as a crime but also to **exclude** from such definition acts or omissions that we do not wish to punish as criminal.[29]

When used in its general and earlier sense, mens rea refers to blameworthiness and legal liability. In requiring mens rea in the general sense the criminal law provides exceptions or exemptions for persons who, for example, because of seriously incapacitating mental disorder (insanity) or immaturity (a child of tender years), should not justly be held criminally responsible—even if they, for example, **knowingly** take another person's property. It is this broad notion of mens rea that pertains to the special defense of insanity. Thus, if we return to the foregoing example, even if the accused took another person's topcoat with the knowledge and intent required for larceny, if he was acting under a psychotic delusion that God commanded him to remove that particular item and turn it over to the Holy Ghost in order to save the soul of the owner from eternal damnation, questions would certainly arise whether the accused had the required general mens rea to be held criminally responsible.

Thus, although the concept of mens rea originated in the idea that some element of moral blameworthiness or culpability must accompany the prohibited act, over the centuries the concept has evolved into a rather complex notion and is now used in very technical ways to refer to the various kinds of specific mental states that are required for particular crimes.[3,19,27,32,33] American lawyers now speak more frequently of **culpability,** meaning the central notion that a particular mental state is required by statute. This change in language also reflects the increasing prominence of the American Law Institute's Model Penal Code and its decision to cut through the veritable maze of numerous common law terms and refer to four basic culpability states: "purpose," "knowledge," "recklessness," and "negligence."[34]

In sum, even though the concept of mens rea in its current legal usage more commonly refers to the specific mental elements in the definition of criminal offenses, the basic concern with a "guilty mind" (or culpable states of mind) continues to provide a fundamental underpinning for our societal views and policies regarding criminal responsibility and related issues.

Various Insanity Tests

By the sixteenth century it became regular practice in England to acquit insane defendants instead of letting them be pardoned by the king. Walker[17] notes that the earliest clear case of an insanity acquittal occurred in 1505. During this period judges gave various instructions to the jury about the nature and degree of mental impairment that must be found to have existed at the time of the alleged offense before defendants could be exculpated from criminal liability. There was, however, no single established rule or test for this purpose.

These so-called rules or tests are the verbal formulations whereby the jury is instructed and guided concerning the extant legal policy and standard that is to be applied in judging the evidence and in making the ultimate determination regarding the criminal responsibility of defendants who raise the insanity defense. Such tests are very important to facilitate proper understanding of the applicable legal standard, to guard against the possibility that the particular situation of the case or characteristics of the defendant may improperly influence the judgments, to obtain uniformity of decisions by different juries and judges, and to ensure that the triers of fact operate under the Rule of Law in order that we may attain our ideal of "equal justice under law."[35]

During the early period in English law the defense of insanity was rather narrowly and strictly construed and applied. The defendant needed to have rather clear, obvious, even gross mental impairment before exculpation was likely. Nevertheless, the difficult question still remained for cases that were not so obvious or close to the extreme: Where precisely should the line be drawn to separate those with varying degrees of mental impairment who must still be held criminally liable from those who should be excused? This crucial question has remained a source of continuing difficulty and controversy over the centuries and to the present time. More will be said about this dilemma later in this chapter.

During the later part of the seventeenth century Sir Matthew Hale[36] addressed the foregoing question. In his *Historia Placitorum Coronae*, Hale wrote:

> [I]t is very difficult to define the invisible line that divides perfect and partial insanity; but it must rest upon circumstances duly to be weighed and considered both by the judge and jury, lest on the one side there be a kind of inhumanity towards the defects of human nature, or on the other side too great an indulgence given to great crimes.[37]

Over the past five centuries a variety of instructions and more precise verbal formulations have been used to guide the judgments of juries concerning the determination of criminal responsibility. In 1582, Lambard provided the following guidance in his manual for justices of the peace:

> If a mad man, or a natural foole, or a Lunatike in the time of his lunacie, or a childe that apparently hath no knowledge of good and evill, doe kill a man, this is no felonie: for that they cannot be said to have any understanding will.[38]

Some of the language that first appeared in the writings of Bracton used the phrase "wild beast" (the expression may actually have meant something like "dumb animal"[17]) and later appeared in some instructions to juries. In the trial of Edward Arnold, who shot and wounded Lord Onslow in 1724, Judge Tracy included the following key sentences in his instructions to the jury:

> If a man be deprived of his reason, and consequently of his intention, he cannot be guilty. . . . On the other side we must be very cautious . . . it is not every kind of frantic humour, or something unaccountable in a man's actions, that points him out to be a man that is totally deprived of his understanding and memory, and doth not know what he is doing, no more than an infant, than a brute or a wild beast, such a one is never the object of punishment.[39]

A major development that apparently served to broaden the foregoing instructions regarding exculpatory insanity was Erskine's renowed and stirring defense of James Hadfield in 1800 on the charge of treason. Hadfield had fired a pistol at King George III.[40] The requirement of "total deprivation of memory and understanding," could not be taken literally, Erskine argued. Rather, it was delusion "where there is no frenzy or raving madness, (which) is the true character of insanity."[41] Hadfield was acquitted on grounds of insanity in what appears almost to have been a directed verdict.

The most famous of all insanity cases is, of course, that of Daniel M'Naghten, who shot and killed Edward Drummond (private secretary to Sir Robert Peel, prime minister of England), mistaking him for Peel. It must be remembered, however, that although the famous test carries his name, M'Naghten himself was **not** tried and acquitted by reason of insanity on the basis of that test.* In the trial of M'Naghten, Lord Tindal (the presiding judge and chief justice) included the following in his instructions to the jury:

> If he (the defendant) was not sensible at the time he committed that act, that it was a violation of the law of God or of man, undoubtedly he was not responsible for that act, or liable to any punishment whatever flowing from that act. . . . But if on balancing the evidence in your minds you think the prisoner capable of distinguishing between right and wrong, then he was a responsible agent and liable to all the penalties the law imposes.[48]

The jury's verdict of not guilty on the ground of insanity aroused considerable public uproar and was also the subject of discussion in the House of Lords. The discussion by the Lords may well have been stimulated in large measure by Queen Victoria's reaction. Having herself been the target of an assassination attempt in 1840 by Edward Oxford (who was found not guilty by reason of insanity) as well as of some other attacks,[49] the queen was obviously quite distressed by the verdict in the case of the man who had sought to assassinate her prime minister. In a letter to Sir Robert Peel a week after the *M'Naghten* verdict, the queen expressed her concerns:

---

* The different spellings of M'Naghten's name in the literature are not due to carelessness. In addition to having his name associated with the most famous of all insanity tests, Daniel also has the dubious distinction of having had his name spelled fully 12 different ways in the relevant literature—and this without benefit of any aliases.[17,42-46] The spelling used here (M'Naghten) is the most common and customary one in the legal literature. The correct spelling of the name is "McNaughtan," according to Moran.[47]

The law may be perfect, but how is it that whenever a case for its application arises, it proves to be of no avail? We have seen the trials of Oxford and MacNaghten conducted by the ablest lawyers of the day . . . and **they allow** and **advise** the jury to pronounce the verdict of **Not Guilty** on account of **Insanity**—whilst everybody is morally **convinced** that both malefactors were perfectly conscious and aware of what they did![50] [The emphasis and exclamation are, of course, the queen's.]

In any event, all 15 of the common law judges were requested to attend a hearing in the House of Lords and to respond to a list of five questions concerning the principles underlying the defense of insanity. What came to be known as the *M'Naghten* test was contained in the responses of the judges to the second and third of the questions posed. This test gave the common law what could for the first time be called an established test of insanity for criminal cases.

THE M'NAGHTEN TEST

To establish a defence on the ground of insanity it must be clearly proved that, at the time of the committing of the act the party accused was labouring under such a defect of reason, from disease of the mind, as not to know the nature and quality of the act he was doing, or, if he did know it, that he did not know he was doing what was wrong.[51]

Many questions have been raised about the overall quality and clarity of the above test which, of course, was formulated **not** in the context of the trial of an actual case but in the abstract and, as Biggs has noted, in a situation in which "the Queen and lords put a hot fire to the feet of the judges of England."[52] A reading of the transcript of M'Naghten's trial, and especially of the medical and psychiatric evidence given in the case, gives the impression that were M'Naghten to have been tried under the test that bears his name he may well have been convicted.

Before mentioning the several other major insanity tests that have been or are currently being used in the United States, the diversity of these tests requires an explanation. Because the United States Constitution does not mandate the use of a particular test, nor has the United States Supreme Court made any such holding to bind federal courts, the several states and the 11 federal circuit courts have been free to adopt the test of their choice. Although the *M'Naghten* test was for more than a century virtually the only test being used in the United States (although supplemented in some jurisdictions with the Irresistible Impulse test), when the American Law Institute (ALI) in 1962 developed a Model Penal Code, things changed. Various drafts of the Model Penal Code's proposed insanity test had been published and discussed several years prior to 1962.

THE IRRESISTIBLE IMPULSE TEST

A major criticism of the *M'Naghten* test was that it focused exclusively on "cognitive" elements (ability to "know the nature and quality of the act") but failed to consider impairments of "volition" (the ability to control one's actions). The Irresistible Impulse test—which does not have a uniform formulation, but the essential provisions of which have been enunciated in several court decisions—was designed to address this gap. In a Massachusetts murder case in 1844, Chief Justice Shaw based his instructions to the jury on *M'Naghten*, but then he went on to add that if the jury was satisfied that the accused was in a "diseased and unsound state,"

> the question will be, whether the disease existed to so high a degree, that for the time being it overwhelmed the reason, conscience, and judgments, and whether the prisoner, in committing the homicide, acted from an irresistible and uncontrollable impulse: if so, then the act was not the act of a voluntary agent, but the involuntary act of the body, without the concurrence of a mind directing it.[53]

Another early case that added the Irresistible Impulse test was *Parsons v. State*.[54]

THE NEW HAMPSHIRE TEST

In 1871, New Hampshire became the first state to reject the *M'Naghten* test. In *State v. Jones* the court held that a defendant was "not guilty by reason of insanity" if his crime "was the offspring or product of mental disease."[55]

THE DURHAM TEST

In 1954, in *Durham v. United States*, the United States Court of Appeals for the District of Columbia adopted a test modeled after the New Hampshire rule. Judge David Bazelon wrote, "An accused is not criminally responsible if his unlawful act was the product of mental disease or mental defect."[56] The court did not provide any specific legal definition for the term mental disease and mental defect, other than to indicate that "mental disease" referred to a condition that was considered capable of either improving or deteriorating, and "mental defect" referred to any mental condition not considered capable of improving or deteriorating.

Although widely hailed by the psychiatric community as a major advance in terms of its recognition of current psychiatric views and potential contributions that could be offered by mental health expert witnesses, over the following years the *Durham* test generated considerable controversy, and various problems became increasingly evident—not the least of which was the dominance of medical-psychiatric definitions and perspectives concerning the term "mental disease" that tended to control (or at least to influence unduly) the judgments of the triers of fact. Despite the considerable volume of case law generated by the circuit court to provide greater clarification as well as more precise legal definition of the term "mental disease" in *McDonald v. United States*,[57] and despite restricting mental health experts from offering opinions on the issue of "productivity,"[58] in 1972 the court abandoned the *Durham* test and adopted the ALI's Model Penal Code test in an en banc decision in *United States v. Brawner*.[59]

THE MODEL PENAL CODE TEST

The American Law Institute (ALI) devoted ten years to the drafting of its Model Penal Code and the insanity test proposed by the code. Section 4.01 (of Article 4) of this test provides:

(1) a person is not responsible for criminal conduct if at the time of such conduct as a result of mental disease or defect he lacks substantial capacity either to appreciate the criminality [wrongfulness] of his conduct or to conform his conduct to the requirements of law.

(2) As used in this Article, the terms "mental disease or mental defect" do not include an abnormality manifested only by repeated criminal or otherwise anti-social conduct.[60]

The bracketed word "wrongfulness" indicates an option in place of the word "criminality."

The ALI test combines the "cognitive" prong (capacity to appreciate the criminality or wrongfulness of the conduct) and the "volitional" prong (capacity to conform the conduct to the requirements of law).

A survey of the 62 United States jurisdictions (50 states, District of Columbia, and the 11 federal circuits) was completed by Favole[61] as of January 1980 and indicated that fully 39 jurisdictions (including all 11 federal circuits) were using the ALI test in some recognizable form (in conjunction with Irresistible Impulse in one state), and 29 were using *M'Naghten* (in four states in conjunction with Irresistible Impulse), and the remainder had unique tests.[62-63] However, several changes have taken place since Favole's survey. The following information about state laws pertaining to the insanity defense is based upon Richard Bonnie's research (related to me through personal communication) and reflects statutory revisions through the year 1983: Model Penal Code (21 states); *M'Naghten* (20); modified *M'Naghten* (appreciation of wrongfulness) (2); *M'Naghten* and some variant of Irresistible Impulse (3); *M'Naghten* and product of psychosis (1—North Dakota); "product" test (1—New Hampshire); and "mens rea" limitation (see following section) (3—Montana, Idaho, and Utah).

Very recently, in *United States v. Lyons*,[64] the United States Court of Appeals for the Fifth Circuit replaced ALI with the test proposed by the American Bar Association.[65] This test drops the "volitional" prong and states that

a person is not responsible for criminal conduct on the grounds of insanity only if at the time of that conduct, as a result of mental disease or defect, he is unable to appreciate the wrongfulness of that conduct.[66]

THE "MENS REA" LIMITATION

During the past 5 years several jurisdictions have sought to narrow and to restrict the insanity defense in various ways. One approach has been to abolish the special defense of insanity (the defense based on general mens rea or moral blameworthiness) and to limit consideration of the defendant's defense of mental impairment only to challenging the specific mens rea elements required for the particular offense. This approach has come to be referred to as the "mens rea" limitation.[67] To date, three states (Montana,[68] Idaho,[69] and Utah[70]) have adopted this approach.

Since the specific mental elements in the definitions of various crimes actually refer only to aspects of conscious awareness and occasionally to conscious intention, a rather basic—even minimal—level of functioning is typically required.[71] For example, using the illustration of the man who was acting under a psychotic delusion when he took another person's topcoat from a restaurant, under the "mens rea" limitation the issue of the defendant's mental disorder would be relevant only for determining whether the psychosis had seriously impaired (negated or vitiated) his capacity to have the specific mens rea required for commission of the offense charged. If, regardless of his psychotic condition, it could be proved that the defendant did in fact **know** that the topcoat belonged to someone else and that he took it with the **intent** of depriving the rightful owner of possession of the item permanently, then a criminal conviction could well result. Only if the defendant's mental impairment was so severe as to negate the special mental elements required for the offense charged would there be a finding of "not guilty by lack of mental state,"[72] "not guilty by reason of insanity,"[73] or some similar verdict.

Relevant language from the Utah code will serve to illustrate the wording of such formulations.

> It is a defense to a prosecution under any statute or ordinance that the defendant, as a result of mental illness, lacked the mental state required as an element of the offense charged. Mental illness shall not otherwise constitute a defense.[74]

The Basic Structure of Insanity Tests

At this point a brief analysis of the basic structure of the various insanity tests should prove useful. The structure of these legal tests, it may be observed, is essentially the same as that of various other mental health laws that require consideration of a person's mental capacities and functioning with respect to some legal issue and associated determination.[75]

Three basic findings, described below, are typically required.

1. There must be a **mental disorder.** Mental disease or defect, legally defined for the particular purpose, is the basic threshold requirement. The initial question may well be whether the defendant has been diagnosed properly as suffering from a condition that is formally or officially recognized as a "mental disorder" in the accepted nomenclature of the relevant mental health disciplines (for example, the *Diagnostic and Statistical Manual of Mental Disorders* of the American Psychiatric Association[76]). However, it must be emphasized that a diagnostic and classification system developed by the psychiatric profession for purposes of clinical practice and research obviously cannot—indeed **should** not—be viewed as providing the requisite **legal** threshold for purposes of determining criminal responsibility by the criminal justice system. What is to be considered as a "mental disease or defect" for certain public policy and legal purposes must be defined and determined by the appropriate legal system and processes. (For further discussion, see the section entitled "The Definition and Meaning of Mental Disease or Defect" later in this chapter.)

2. Various legally relevant **impairment in functioning** must be shown to have resulted from the mental disorder. With regard to the defense of insanity, these impairments pertain generally to various "cognitive" functions (for example, the ability to distinguish right from wrong, to know the nature and quality of the criminal act, to appreciate the criminality or wrongfulness of one's conduct), and/or various "volitional" functions (the ability to control one's behavior or to conform one's conduct to the requirements of law).

3. Demonstration of **a clear and direct causal connection or relationship** between the behavioral impairment resulting from the mental disorder and the criminal act. It is **not** sufficient to demonstrate that a defendant who has been charged with shoplifting, embezzlement, armed robbery, or whatever was concurrently suffering from some mental disorder. The particular criminal act must be shown to have resulted from impairments associated with the mental disorder. In other words, "but for that mental disorder and its associated impairments" the criminal act would not have taken place.

The above structure is important to keep in mind in order to understand that the key legal terms such as "mental disease or defect" relate to a **legal** purpose and determination and hence must be defined and interpreted in their appropriate legal—**not** medical, psychiatric, or psychological—context. Failure to appreciate this basic distinction leads to a variety of problems, some of which are discussed later in this chapter.

As noted earlier, insanity tests are designed to inform and to instruct the triers of fact about the relevant legal policy and standard that is to be applied in making the ultimate judgments about a defendant's criminal responsibility. The fundamental difficulty in making such determinations is intrinsic to the very nature of the task which requires the making of dichotomous distinctions with regard to characteristics (impairments resulting from mental disorders) that lie around the "invisible line" separating criminal culpability from exculpation. This difficult task is further complicated by the vexing moral, philosophical, and ideological issues involved, the basic ambiguity of the relevant legal concepts and doctrines, and the additional problems of relating various types of psychiatric and psychological evidence regarding the defendant's impairment to the specific legal issues and the associated sociomoral judgments. Hence, even though legal scholars, judges, and mental health professionals continue to argue about the precise phrasing of the insanity tests, one must surely wonder whether this obsession with the subtle nuances of particular words and their meanings actually makes very much difference to the lay persons who serve on juries. There is at least some empirical research suggesting that such variations may not make too much difference for juries.[77] Moreover, empirical research has also demonstrated that most jury instructions, including those pertaining to the test of insanity, are simply not very comprehensible to the juries that hear these trials.[78,79]

One is reminded of the observation made by Weihofen about 30 years ago while noting the importance of some easily communicable and uniformly applicable test of insanity. This noted legal scholar observed,

> No, there is no doubt that a clear and simple rule would be a Good Thing. Clarity and simplicity are always desirable, and in law, they are rare and precious jewels among the heaps of scoriaceous dross produced by the legal mind at work.[80]

Thus, with regard to the search for the ultimate test of insanity, it would be fair to say that the search for such a "rare and precious jewel" is likely to be as difficult as it will also be quite indefinite. In addition to the references cited in this chapter, some other relevant literature[81-93] might also be of interest to readers. Also, three reports of Congressional hearings offer a rich menu of comments, opinions, and recommendations regarding the insanity defense and related issues.[94-96]

Diminished Capacity

The law presumes that most individuals are sane and capable of exercising adequate control over their behavior, and hence only severe and incapacitating mental disorders will typically serve to exculpate from criminal responsibility. However, inasmuch as impairments resulting from mental disorder are not distributed in neat and discrete categories, it is obvious that among those considered to be criminally liable will be persons with quite evident but less serious degrees of mental impairment. Our basic moral intuitions suggest that such defendants should not be held equally culpable and thereby subjected to the same degree of punishment as persons without any discernible impairment. The doctrine of diminished capacity is used in several jurisdictions to address this issue.[97] This defense, which is quite separate and distinct from the insanity defense, is generally used to assert that because of mental impairment the defendant could not form the specific mental state required for the particular offense (for example, first-degree murder), but the defendant will typically be guilty of a lesser included offense (for example, manslaughter).

The historical roots of this doctrine go back to the mid-nineteenth century when Scottish courts recognized a defense of "partial insanity." As adopted later in England in 1957, the defense of diminished responsibility permits the jury to return a verdict of manslaughter (instead of murder) in cases in which the mentally ill but legally sane defendant is judged to be less culpable than "normal" defendants.[17,98-101] Clearly, the stark specter of the executioner appears to have given special meaning and importance to this defense.

As used in the United States, the doctrine of diminished capacity is rather complex and continues to be the subject of controversy and also some differing legal interpretations. Such difficulties are compounded by the fact that while some courts and commentators use the terms diminished responsibility and diminished capacity interchangeably (see the Model Penal Code Commentaries[102]), others make some important technical distinctions between them.[98-101] Arenella[100] points out that the courts have fostered considerable doctrinal confusion by using the term diminished capacity to refer to two very different principles; (1) a **"mens rea" or rule of evidence approach,** and (2) a **partial defense of diminished responsibility** that usually applies only in homicide crimes and serves to reduce first-degree murder to second-degree murder (in about 20 jurisdictions) or, in about five jurisdictions allows a further reduction to manslaughter.[103]

Under the **"mens rea" or rule of evidence** approach, evidence of mental abnormality and incapacity is admissible whenever it is relevant to prove that the defendant lacked the specific state of mind required for commission of the particular offense. This is, essentially, a rule of evidence. Unlike the special defense of insanity, which serves as a general bar to criminal liability and exculpates completely from criminal culpability, the "mens rea" approach to diminished capacity serves to negate the particular state of mind required for the offense charged and thus generally results in conviction of a lesser included offense for which the "mens rea" can be proved beyond a reasonable doubt by the prosecutor. For example, a defendant may assert that because of serious mental disorder he did not deliberate or premeditate his actions as required for first-degree murder. If this claim is successful, the requisite mental state may nevertheless be proved and conviction obtained for the lesser offense of manslaughter.

Some courts have refused to allow evidence of mental disorder unless it is being offered to establish a defense of insanity. Other jurisdictions limit such admission of mens rea only to homicide cases.[97] In contrast, the Model Penal Code endorses the presumptive admissibility of all evidence logically relevant to establish a defendant's state of mind. Article 4, Section 4.02(1) provides that "Evidence that the defendant suffered from a mental disease or defect is admissible whenever it is relevant to prove that the defendant did or did not have a state of mind which is an element of the offense."[104]

The **"diminished responsibility" approach** refers to an entirely different concept. A few American courts have broadened the inquiry into the defendant's mental condition (whether resulting from mental disease or defect, intoxication, or other trauma) to "the implicit redefinition of homicide offenses."[102] In this approach, proof of mental abnormality of a certain severity is permitted to preclude liability for first-degree murder. In essence, defendants seek to introduce their mental condition as a factor in mitigation, thereby justifying a lesser degree of culpability and severity of punishment. This approach has most actively been litigated in California. However, in 1981—following the notorious trial in San Francisco of Dan White for the murders of Mayor George Moscone and supervisor Harvey Milk, and White's successful use of the diminished capacity defense to obtain a conviction of voluntary manslaughter—California abolished this defense.[106,107] (See Winslade and Ross[105] for further details about this case.)

The defendant's mental condition is also considered by the law in other contexts with respect to the issues of provocation and mitigation. For example, the Model Penal Code provides for criminal homicide to be reduced to manslaughter (instead of murder) when a "homicide which would otherwise be murder is committed under the influence of extreme mental or emotional disturbance for which there is a reasonable explanation or excuse."[108] At least 10 states have enacted provisions that follow in large measure the Model Penal Code. For example, New York provides that it is an affirmative defense* to the crime of murder in the second degree in which "(t)he defendant acted under the influence of extreme emotional disturbance for which there was a reasonable explanation or excuse."[109]

Thus, while for reasons of public and legal policy the criminal law is quite demanding with respect to the degree of mental impairment that will serve to exculpate completely on the grounds of insanity, lesser degrees of impairment are taken into consideration in a variety of ways—starting with the legislative grading of offenses with respect to their severity and associated prescribed penalties, the diminished capacity defense, and for purposes of mitigation as

---

* Even though all statements in a complaint may be true (for example, in criminal cases both the actus reus and mens rea can be proved), an affirmative defense enables defendants to present new facts and arguments either to reduce the severity of the offense (as in the defense of "extreme emotional disturbance"), or to seek acquittal—for example, on the basis of duress, self-defense, or insanity. In essence, defendants claiming an affirmative defense assert that they have a legally recognized excuse, justification, or mitigation for their acts. In some jurisdictions defendants have the burden merely of raising the particular issue of defense, in other jurisdictions they also have the burden of persuasion (either by a preponderance of evidence or by clear and convincing evidence). The latter is presently the case in about 28 states with respect to the defense of insanity.

noted above as well as at the sentencing and dispositional stages of the criminal process. However, as we shall see later, the insanity acquittal is **not** like any other acquittal, because the law typically retains a powerful "clutch" over the acquittee through involuntary hospitalization, the duration of which confinement may well exceed the penal sentence that might have followed criminal conviction.

PERCEIVED PROBLEMS OF THE INSANITY DEFENSE

Various proposals for changes in public policies, laws, and related procedures regarding the defense of insanity are based (whether explicitly or implicitly) upon a variety of assumptions and beliefs about the perceived problems. Unfortunately, few of the proposed changes are based upon reliable and accurate information about the nature of the phenomenon of concern, the precise frequencies and rates of insanity pleas, the relative success of such pleas, the types of criminal charges and defendants that are involved, the nature of the postadjudication disposition and handling of the insanity acquittees, the duration of the involuntary hospitalization that typically follows, and the post-release relapse and recidivism rates of the acquittees. Such systematic information is very much needed in order accurately to inform and to guide needed changes in policies and practices.[110]

As in other areas, pressure for reform often tends to be triggered, or at least to be considerably heightened, by shocking and headline-grabbing incidents. At particular points in time, such incidents appear to serve as lightning rods for public and political concerns. The verdict in the Hinckley trial clearly has served this function. The Congressional hearings that were held regarding the insanity defense and related issues relevant to proposed revisions of the federal criminal code followed rather promptly on the heels of the Hinckley verdict and the resulting outpouring of public outrage.[94-96] The characterization of this verdict as "one of the greatest miscarriages of justice in our Nation's history"[111] serves nicely to illustrate the intensity of some of the reactions.

The Hinckley verdict generated considerable pressure not only on Congress but also on legislative bodies in the various states. Many legislative proposals have been made in the various jurisdictions, and several revisions have been enacted. In several instances locally notorious cases have provided both the passion and the pressure for the legislative and related changes. For example, the voluntary manslaughter verdict in the double-murder trial of Dan White in California resulted in the abolition of the diminished capacity defense and in related changes in that jurisdiction.[105] Similarly, in Alaska, the murder of four teenagers by Charles Meach not only earned him the longest prison sentence in that state's history (four consecutive life sentences for a total maximum of 396 years) but also resulted in several changes in the insanity defense and related laws.[112]

The reaction or overreaction to such shocking incidents needs to be viewed and understood against the broader background and context of the ideological, social, and political climate in the country at particular times. Bonnie[71] has drawn attention to two large forces that appear to be at work in regard to current concerns about the defense of insanity; namely, retrenchment within the discipline of psychiatry and an ideological shift in the law (which, in my view, reflects ideological shifts in the country). With respect to the first of these,

Bonnie contrasts the current self-doubt within the discipline of psychiatry with the rather bouyant and effusive optimism that characterized the profession during the 1950s and 1960s. As to the ideological shifts in the law, Bonnie notes that the interest in the "rehabilitative ideal" during the 1950s and 1960s has clearly given way to the retributivist ideology of more recent and current times. In contrast to the concerns during the 1950s and 1960s for protection of the rights of blacks, women, juveniles, and the mentally disabled,[113] the current focus is on the rights of crime victims and of the public to be protected from crime. Thus, the shocking cases might not have provided as powerful an impetus for policy changes were it not also for the larger ideological and sociopolitical forces that provide a necessary context for the public and political reactions.

With the above as introduction, this section will focus on some of the assumptions, attitudes, and beliefs pertaining to the defense of insanity and will also summarize some of the extant empirical research relevant to these issues. The various subsections are organized under headings that reflect some of the frequent concerns about the insanity defense.

Concern about the Overuse and Abuse of the Insanity Defense

A rather common perception is that not only is the insanity defense raised inappropriately quite often, but it is also too often successful. There is the further belief that such insanity acquittals enable dangerous criminals to escape criminal sanctions and to endanger the community. Inasmuch as there is no yardstick for determining what precisely should be the "appropriate" rate for use of this defense, the above beliefs essentially reflect peoples' attitudes and feelings. Unfortunately, such attitudes and perceptions appear very much to be determined by the periodic notorious and shocking cases. The irony, however, is that we lack even the basic statistical information that could provide a reliable and accurate picture of the actual nationwide use of the insanity defense, fluctuations over time, and the specific kinds of problems that seem to occur at particular points in the entire process. Hence, we must extrapolate from the limited data that are available in a few jurisdictions in order that our information and perceptions be grounded more accurately.

Steadman et al[114] conducted a national survey of facilities serving four categories of mentally disordered offenders in all 50 states, the District of Columbia, and the federal system. During 1978 there were a total of 1625 admissions to security hospitals of persons who had been found "not guilty by reason of insanity" (NGRI). This figure does not represent **all** such acquittals; undoubtedly there were some cases in which defendants may have been hospitalized as incompetent to stand trial and who, following their subsequent trial or plea negotiation and insanity acquittal, were not considered to require any further hospitalization. No information is available about the total number of insanity pleas that resulted in the 1625 plus acquittals in 1978. It is known that use of this plea varies rather markedly across jurisdictions, over periods of time, and also across the several counties within a state. For example, over a 3-year period in Wyoming there were a total of 102 insanity pleas in the 21,012 felony indictments for that period, and there was only a single insanity acquittal (success rate of 0.9 percent).[115] In Michigan there were 5920 insanity pleas over a 7-year period and 381 NGRI acquittals, for a success rate of 6.4 percent.[116]

And, during a 10-year period in Erie County, New York, the insanity plea was raised in 202 cases and resulted in 51 acquittals, for a success rate of 25 percent.[117] Steadman[118] estimates that the plea was entered in about 0.17 percent of all felony cases in New York State, or just under two insanity pleas for every 1000 felony cases. Assuming a 15 percent success rate for the plea (which may well be on the high side) and considering the 1625 admissions of NGRI cases to security hospitals in 1978, we would obtain a rough estimate of about 11,000 insanity pleas per year nationwide.

Pasewark and his associates[115,119,120] have conducted a number of studies in Wyoming to ascertain opinions and estimates about the frequency and success rate of the insanity plea among various groups such as college students, law enforcement officers, attorneys, and mental health professionals, as well as members of the state legislature. Persons were told the total number of felony indictments in the state over a 3-year period (21,012) and were then asked to estimate the number of insanity pleas entered and acquittals on this basis. All groups **greatly overestimated** both the number of pleas and the insanity acquittals. For example, the mean estimate of the state legislators for the number of insanity pleas was 4457 (median of 3052), when in fact the plea had been raised in only 102 cases; the mean estimate for the number of insanity acquittals was 1794 (median of 501), when in actuality during that 3-year period there had been only a single NGRI finding![115]

Use in Cases Involving Crimes of Violence

The general impression that the insanity defense is typically used in cases involving crimes of violence might readily be conveyed by the infamous cases that come to public attention and which receive considerable mass media coverage. Such selective media reporting also seems to facilitate rather inaccurate public perceptions and conceptions about the "criminally insane."[121] There is not much newsworthiness, it would seem, about the many cases of seriously mentally impaired persons who are found NGRI for a variety of property and other minor crimes. The report of the National Commission on the Insanity Defense[122] provides further information about the ways in which media portrayals of the mentally ill tend to perpetuate public misconceptions and stereotypes.

Again, lacking systematic nationwide empirical data on this subject, we have to turn to the limited information available from a few states and for particular periods of time. Such data have been reported from Connecticut (1970-1972),[123] Michigan (1967-1972[124] and September 1974–August 1979[125]), Missouri (1978),[126] New Jersey (1976-1977, for one county),[127] New York (1965-1978),[128] and Oregon (1978-1980).[129] The information from Michigan and New York indicates that close to half of the insanity acquittals involved murder charges (57 percent in Michigan prior to 1972 and almost 30 percent during 1974–1979; 51 percent in New York, although fully 77 percent of the female NGRI cases in New York involved murder charges). Assault offenses were also frequent among the insanity acquittees in these two urban states (20 percent in Michigan during the earlier period and 31 percent during the later period, and 13 percent in New York); rape and other sex crimes were quite infrequent (about 7 percent in Michigan and 5 percent in New York), and most of the other offenses involved less serious property crimes. In Connecticut, Missouri, New

Jersey, and Oregon, the proportion of murder charges among the NGRI cases was much lower: 28 percent, 7 percent, 26 percent, and 5 percent, respectively. Offenses such as automobile theft, bad checks, burglary, criminal mischief, disorderly conduct, illicit drugs, lewdness, menacing, sexual abuse, and trespass accounted for about 38 percent of the NGRI cases in Missouri and Oregon. On the basis of available information, a significant number of insanity pleas do involve crimes of violence—particularly, it would appear, in largely urban states. The public perception, however, tends to get markedly exaggerated because of the disproportionate publicity given to these cases.

Use in Defense of the Wealthy

This is a fairly common belief and misconception regarding the insanity defense. In fact, such bald assertions were repeatedly made in remarks by some members of Congress during the aforementioned Congressional hearings.[130] Despite the frequency of references to the "rich man's loophole," these statements are simply **not** supported by any available empirical evidence. Indeed, the evidence refutes such assertions. Once again, it appears that a few headline-grabbing cases have a truly remarkable capacity for shaping and maintaining certain attitudes and beliefs—no matter how inaccurate.

Morrow and Peterson[131] reported on 44 NGRIs who had been discharged from a Missouri security hospital unit between January 1952 and February 1962. With regard to occupational level, fully 88 percent of the acquittees were classified as unskilled or semiskilled. Cooke and Sikorski[124] found that 38 percent of the NGRI's were unemployed at the time of the offense, 53 percent were classified as unskilled, and only 8 percent were in skilled occupations. As to educational levels, about 56 percent of the insanity acquittees had **not** completed high school, 28 percent were high school graduates, and only 3.7 percent were college graduates. A recent report from Saint Elizabeths Hospital in the District of Columbia on 212 NGRI patients who had been discharged between 1974 and 1982 indicates that almost 60 percent had less than 12 years of education; the average (mean and median) was 10 years of schooling.[132]

The several studies reviewed by Pasewark[133] indicate that the median educational and occupational levels of persons entering insanity pleas were substantially lower than those for the general population. Thus, other than the relatively few notorious cases involving affluent defendants, there is simply no evidence to sustain the assertion that the insanity defense is primarily a millionaire's or rich man's defense. The available evidence indicates that the vast majority of NGRI acquittees were not rich and had to rely on mental examinations conducted in various public sector mental-health facilities (see Smith and Hall[116] Table D).

Short Periods of Confinement and High Recidivism Rates

The belief that insanity acquittees are confined for very short periods and have very high recidivism rates upon release is evidently fostered by selective media publicity given to notorious cases and is not entirely accurate. It is true, however, that the provisions for automatic, indeterminate, and prolonged postacquittal confinement in security hospitals were repeatedly challenged in the courts during the 1960s and 1970s (see *Bolton v. Harris*,[134] *State v. Clemons*,[135] *Wilson v. State*,[136] *People v. McQuillan*,[137] and *State v. Krol*[138]), and postacquittal commitment hearings, durational limits on the resulting confinement, and other Consitutional safeguards were required. These legal changes do appear to have resulted in relatively shorter periods of postacquittal confinement, compared with those of earlier periods.

Several empirical studies provide information regarding the length of post-acquittal hospitalization and also the recidivism of the NGRI acquittees following release.[123,124,128,137-143]

Steadman[128] found that the NGRIs who had been released (55 percent) had averaged 406 days of hospitalization, but the 45 percent who remained hospitalized had averaged 1701 days (or 4.5 years) of confinement. Hence, it is misleading to focus attention only on the subgroup that has been released. Moreover, the above hospitalization figures do not include the varying periods of confinement following arrest, hospitalization for evaluation, and treatment for incompetency to stand trial. Generally longer periods of confinement tend to be associated with the more serious offenses, suggesting that hospital staff are sensitive to community concerns about the nature of the offense even though the major purpose of hospitalization is to provide treatment in a secure setting for these patients. For example, the 55 released murder acquittees averaged 500 days of confinement (range of 1 to 2326 days), two rape acquittees averaged 1102 days (range of 1042 to 1162 days), eight robbery acquittees averaged 188 days of hospitalization (range of 6 to 565 days), the 28 assault acquittees averaged 398 days (range of 33 to 1033 days), and the six burglary acquittees averaged 288 days (range of 20 to 622 days).

Steadman correctly notes that it would be inappropriate to compare the arrest charges of the NGRI acquittees with the conviction charges (usually less serious because of plea negotiation) of convicted offenders. Moreover, depending upon the nature of the particular offense and the defendant's prior criminal record, many convicted offenders (about 40 percent of convicted felons) receive probationary or other sentences rather than penal incarceration. Hence, it should not be assumed that a criminal conviction necessarily leads to a prison term.

In Michigan, prior to the *McQuillan* decision* the average (mean) length of confinement of NGRI patients was 19.31 months for those who remained hospitalized, 24.19 months for patients who had been discharged, for an overall mean of 21.27 months.[124] During the post-*McQuillan* period, the average durations of confinement were shorter—a mean of 9.48 months for NGRI patients who had been discharged and 16.91 months for those still hospitalized, for an overall mean of 13.60 months.[125]

When groups of NGRI acquittees have been compared with matched convicted and incarcerated offenders, some interesting results have been obtained. Pasewark and his associates studied 46 defendants who had been adjudicated NGRI in New York State between 1965 and 1971[140] and another 50 NGRI cases in the same jurisdiction between 1971 and 1976.[141] The first study

---

* Among other holdings, the Michigan Supreme Court held that due process and equal protection required that, upon completion of the 60-day period of examination and observation following an insanity acquittal, the acquittee "must have the benefit of commitment and release provisions equal to those available to those civilly committed."[137]

revealed that, as a group, the institutional time of the acquittees did not differ significantly from that of the matched convicted felons, although the periods of confinement did differ for specific offenses. For example, the mean number of days of confinement for homicide offenses were 1296 for the NGRIs and 1191 for the felons, for robbery the means were 134 days for the NGRIs and 620 for the felons, for assault 1020 days versus 656 days, for burglary 250 versus 533 days.[140] Also, there were no marked differences regarding the postrelease arrests incurred by the NGRI subjects (24 percent) and the released felons (27 percent).

The second sample studied[141] did reveal that the NGRI subjects spent significantly less time in the hospital than the matched group of convicted felons spent in prison. For example, the mean number of days of confinement for homicide offenses was 635 for the male NGRIs and 919 for the male felons, 489 for the female NGRIs and 585 days for the female felons; for robbery offenses, 87 days for the male and 62 days for the female NGRIs versus 602 and 423 days, respectively, for the male and female felons; for assault offenses, 393 days for the NGRIs (all males) and 703 days for the felons (all males). Again, there were no significant differences between the NGRI subjects and the convicted felons with respect to their postrelease arrests (15 percent and 18 percent, respectively).

Braff et al[142] examined the detention patterns of defendants in Erie County, New York, who were successful in their use of the insanity defense and were hospitalized and those who were unsuccessful and were convicted and incarcerated. The investigators also looked at the comparative patterns of detention for felony defendants who did not use the insanity plea. There were no statistically significant differences between the successful and unsuccessful users of the insanity plea with respect to length of confinement (average of 891 days for the NGRIs versus 984 days for the convicted felons). For crimes against persons, the NGRIs had slightly longer periods of confinement, but for homicides and other felonies the unsuccessful insanity plea users had slightly longer periods of confinement. Other findings indicated that certain costs were associated with NGRI acquittals, for example, substantially more of the defendants who were **unsuccessful** with the defense (that is, were convicted) managed to avoid institutional confinement. This and other related findings led the researchers to observe that the NGRI plea may not be quite as advantageous as often believed.

This section has pointed out that many of the beliefs and perceptions about the insanity defense are inaccurate and in some instances reflect rather gross misconceptions. Such misconceptions seem to be fostered and maintained by the considerable media attention given to the periodic shocking cases, as well as by the somewhat stereotypical portrayals in the media of mental illness and of the mentally ill.[122] Not surprisingly, persons in positions of leadership seem to be just as vulnerable to the erroneous beliefs and misconceptions as the general public. In fact, the title of the report of the National Commission on the Insanity Defense ("Myths and Realities")[122] was purposely selected to reflect the finding that much of the clamor for change in the insanity defense was based on "myths and misplaced frustration." Yet, if real problems are to be addressed effectively and remedied, it seems essential that accurate and reliable information—not a "hit or myth" approach—should guide the proposed reforms.

PROPOSED SOLUTIONS

In recent years there has been increasing public and political sentiment in favor of a variety of changes in policies and procedures pertaining to the insanity defense. In addition to the larger sociopolitical forces indicating a more conservative and retributivist ideology in the law and the added pressure from periodic infamous cases, it also appears that some of the legal reforms of the 1960s and 1970s have had the effect of reducing a few of the earlier disincentives for use of the defense.[144] These disincentives pertained to various consequences of an NGRI acquittal and included such things as automatic and mandatory confinement in security hospitals and indeterminate and prolonged periods of confinement which, for the less serious offenses, could be well in excess of the likely penal incarceration following conviction. A series of federal and state court decisions during the 1960s and 1970s required provision of greater procedural and substantive due process safeguards for civilly and criminally committed patients—for example, postacquittal hearings before acquittees could involuntarily be hospitalized, durational limits on the periods of indeterminate confinement, and regular periodic reviews to determine the need for continued confinement.[145-147] It seems likely that the reduced disincentives may well have played some part in the increased use of the insanity defense.

The various proposals for reform appear to have two common purposes. First, to narrow, to restrict, and to tighten the insanity defense in order to reduce the frequency and rate of its use and inappropriate uses. A variety of substantive changes (for example, shifting to a more restrictive test of insanity) as well as procedural changes (for example, shifting the burden of persuasion to the defendant, adjusting the standard of proof, adding an additional verdict of "guilty but mentally ill") have been proposed. Second, a variety of steps have been suggested to ensure greater protection of the public by such means as facilitating postacquittal confinement of NGRI acquittees, shifting the burden of persuasion on the acquittees for seeking release, and having mandatory periods of conditional release upon discharge from the hospital. Thus, although the philosophical and ideological concerns may well differ, as do the preferred means to be employed, the various proposals seem to share the above two goals.

Although there have been numerous proposals for change, this section will focus on the recommendations and statements made by some major professional organizations. The purpose is simply to provide an illustrative—not exhaustive—list of some of the key recommendations. A much wider range of proposals is to be found in the published Congressional hearings.[94-96]

Attorney General's Task Force on Violent Crime

In April 1981, Attorney General of the United States William French Smith appointed a task force whose overall objective was to recommend ways in which the federal government could do more to combat violent crime. Inasmuch as the mandate does not deal directly with the insanity defense, only one of the 64 recommendations is relevant to our concerns. Recommendation 39 states:

> The Attorney General should support or propose legislation that would create an additional verdict in federal criminal cases of "guilty but mentally

ill" modeled after the recently passed Illinois statute and establish a federal commitment procedure for defendants found incompetent to stand trial or not guilty by reason of insanity.[148]

The second part of the recommendation addresses a major gap in current federal statutes: Except in the District of Columbia, there are no provisions in existing federal criminal statutes for the postadjudication confinement of defendants found incompetent to stand trial or not guilty by reason of insanity. The rationale for the "guilty but mentally ill" (GBMI) recommendation was that criminal defendants who suffer from mental disorders, albeit not to a degree to be excused from criminal liability, provide a difficult choice for juries who may feel compassion but have available only the choice of the "guilty" and "not guilty by reason of insanity" verdicts. The additional GBMI verdict provides a third option that, it is claimed, could reduce the number of insanity pleas and inappropriate NGRI verdicts.

The first "guilty but mentally ill" statute enacted in Michigan was in response to the strong public outcry over the release of a large group of insanity acquittees following the Michigan Supreme Court's decision in *McQuillan*.[137] For further details see Smith and Hall.[116] As of December 1983, 11 states had enacted GBMI statutes,* and similar legislation has been proposed in at least another 11 states and in Congress.[149]

As attractive as the GBMI provisions may be to many as an "in-between classification"[150] (between findings of "guilty" and NGRI), serious questions have been raised about the conceptual and theoretical bases and also the assumptions underlying such enactments.[151-155] If a major rationale is to provide mental health care and treatment for convicted and incarcerated offenders suffering from varying degrees of mental disorder, then departments of correction already have both the authority and the responsibility to do so—the necessary treatment resources that they often lack are **not** assured by these enactments. As to the purpose of reducing insanity pleas and acquittals, a few initial research findings from Michigan (the jurisdiction with the longest experience with GBMI) suggest that this may not be an assured result.[125] Slovenko has commented that the GBMI verdict "is set up as a middle ground, but in actuality it is a semantic sleight of hand, a distinction without a difference."[156]

American Bar Association Policy on the Insanity Defense

In February 1983, the American Bar Association's (ABA) House of Delegates approved several recommendations that were proposed by the ABA Standing Committee on Association Standards for Criminal Justice and the ABA Commission on the Mentally Disabled.[157] In efforts to narrow the test of insanity, recommendation 1 suggested dropping the "volitional" prong of the American Law Institute's Model Penal Code test.

> Resolved, that the American Bar Association approves, in principle, a defense of nonresponsibility for crime which focuses solely on whether a

---

* These states are listed below with the year of enactment indicated in parentheses: Michigan (1975); Indiana (1980); Illinois (1981); Alaska, Delaware, Georgia, Kentucky, and New Mexico (1982); Pennsylvania, South Dakota, and Utah (1983).

defendant, as a result of mental disease or defect, was unable to appreciate the wrongfulness of his or her conduct at the time of the offense charged.[158]

Regarding the allocation of the burden of proof in insanity cases, the ABA policy recommended that in jurisdictions using any test for insanity that focuses solely on the "cognitive" prong ("whether the defendant, as a result of mental disease or defect, was unable to know, understand or appreciate the wrongfulness of his or her conduct" at the time of the offense) the prosecution should have the burden of disproving the defendant's claim beyond a reasonable doubt. In jurisdictions using the American Law Institute's test with its "volitional" prong, "the defendant should have the burden of proving by a preponderance of the evidence his or her claim of insanity."[159] Recommendation 3 opposed the enactment of "guilty but mentally ill" (GBMI) statutes designed to supplant or to supplement the NGRI verdict.[160]

The American Bar Association's (ABA) Proposed Criminal Justice Mental Health Standards, approved in final form in August 1984,[161] also address this issue. Standard 7-6.1 pertains to the defense of mental nonresponsibility (insanity) and states:

(a) A person is not responsible for criminal conduct if, at the time of such conduct, and as a result of mental disease or defect, that person was unable to appreciate the wrongfulness of such conduct.
(b) When used as a legal term in this standard "mental disease or defect" refers to:
    (i) Impairments of mind, whether enduring or transitory; or,
    (ii) Mental retardation,
either of which substantially affected the mental or emotional processes of the defendant at the time of the alleged offense.[162]

For further discussion of this standard see the commentary in the ABA Standards volume[163] as well as the article by Bonnie.[81]

American Psychiatric Association's Statement on the Insanity Defense

In December 1982, the American Psychiatric Association (APA) approved a paper drafted by the Association's Insanity Defense Work Group.[164] This paper (later published in the APA journal[165]) addressed several major issues and questions pertaining to the insanity defense and its administration. The APA opposed efforts to abolish the special defense of insanity, noting that "retention of the insanity defense is essential to the moral integrity of the criminal law,"[166] but favored narrowing the defense. It suggested a number of other avenues that could be explored for making needed changes. The association also opposed enactment of GBMI statutes, pointing out that "the 'guilty but mentally ill' plea may cause important moral, legal, psychiatric, and pragmatic problems to receive a whitewash without fundamental progress being made."[167]

The APA indicated that it was **not** opposed to "legislatures restricting psychiatric testimony about the aforementioned ultimate legal issues [such as 'sanity,' 'insanity,' and 'responsibility'] concerning the insanity defense. We adopt this position because it is clear that psychiatrists are experts in medicine, not the law."[168] The APA statement also addressed a number of other vexing issues such as the postacquittal handling, treatment, release, and follow-up of NGRI acquittees and suggested a number of guidelines for the disposition of acquittees who had engaged in acts of violence.

Statement and Recommendations of the American Medical Association

Although the medical group specializing in matters of mental health (the American Psychiatric Association) had already developed and disseminated a carefully considered statement and recommendations, it was noteworthy that the American Medical Association (AMA) also jumped into the policy and professional debate. And although one may well wonder about the substantive expertise residing in nonpsychiatric physicians on the topics in question, there is little question about the political power of the AMA. In fact, the pointed way in which the AMA statement takes issue with the APA's position suggests some fraternal conflicts—possibly exacerbated by the public reactions to the "battle of experts" in the Hinckley trial.

The detailed report approved by the AMA Board of Trustees contains a historical background of the insanity defense and recommends four major policy positions: (1) The AMA supports, in principle, the abolition of the special defense of insanity and its replacement by the "mens rea" approach; (2) the legal standards of civil commitment should apply to commitment of criminal defendants acquitted by reason of insanity (under statutory "mens rea" provisions), with "due allowance being made for a presumption of continuing dangerousness with respect to those acquitted of offenses involving violence"; (3) the absolute or conditional release of such insanity acquittees should be based on "concurring medical certification and judicial determination that release poses no substantial public risk"; and (4) in the case of defendants who fail to satisfy the above criteria (the "mens rea" provisions) of acquittal, the fact of their mental illness should be considered as a factor in mitigation of the penal sentence.[169]

Commenting on the disagreement between the APA and the AMA, an editorial in *The Washington Post*, "Insanity: Two Medical Opinions," concluded with the observation that "lawyers and psychiatrists are the professionals most closely involved with the insanity defense, and their views should be persuasive."[170] Like many others, the editorial writer appears to have been puzzled as to the nature of the substantive expertise that informed the AMA's position on the subject.

Statement of the American Psychological Association

Having reviewed the various proposals made by the several other professional associations and groups, the American Psychological Association (APA) developed a relatively brief statement which essentially emphasized this association's view that sound empirical research should provide the needed informational base for the legal, moral, and policy decisions to be made regarding various aspects of the insanity defense.[171] More specifically, this APA (often referred to as the "big APA" because of its larger membership) did not wish to support the changes in the insanity test recommended by the ABA and the American Psychiatric Association (namely, dropping the "volitional" prong), lacking empirical research "to provide information about whether the behavioral sciences are able to render informed opinions about behavioral control and whether such opinions assist the jury." Secondly, based on the available research data and psychological analyses, this association was opposed to the enactment of the GBMI verdict to supplant or to supplement the NGRI verdict. No position was taken about whether the defendant or the prosecution should have the burden of persuasion on the question of insanity, inasmuch as this was a legal and not a psychological issue. Finally, the APA expressed particular interest in the various dispositional issues related to mentally impaired criminal defendants and felt that additional empirical research was needed to "provide a sound basis for the important policy decisions surrounding these dispositional issues."

Report of the National Commission on the Insanity Defense

The National Commission on the Insanity Defense was established as an independent commission by the National Mental Health Association and was chaired by former United States Senator Birch Bayh.[122] The commission grew out of a concern that some of the fundamental issues pertaining to societal handling of the mentally ill were being lost in the "technical, and often emotional, debate about the insanity defense."[172] Based on its studies and public hearings, the commission came to the conclusion that "much of the clamor for change in the insanity defense is based on myths and misplaced frustration in the wake of the Hinckley verdict."[173] The commission concluded that the various myths do not provide any justification for elimination of the insanity defense. Twelve unanimous recommendations were made by the commission, and they included the following:

- Retention of the insanity defense (with the test to include both the "cognitive" and "volitional" prongs), with the burden of proof on the defendant to prove that defense by a preponderance of the evidence
- Adoption of the term "not responsible by reason of insanity" instead of "not guilty by reason of insanity" to enhance public understanding and acceptance of this vital part of our system of justice
- Rejection of the alternative verdict of "guilty but mentally ill"
- The addition of a strong dispositional provision to provide additional safeguards for the community by insuring the proper custody and supervision of insanity acquittees
- A recommendation that the "media make a conscientious effort to eliminate the pejorative references to and negative characterizations of the mentally ill and to substitute descriptions and portrayals that do not perpetuate the general public's misconceptions and stereotypes"[174]

In the wake of the Hinckley verdict and other notorious cases, it remains to be seen to what extent the "rush to judgment" will be influenced by more careful considerations of the broader policy and programmatic implications and the many dilemmas inherent in trying to ensure that policies affecting the many are not unduly influenced by the rare, albeit shocking, cases.

The Insanity Defense Reform Act of 1984

Proposals for a comprehensive revision of the federal criminal code have been made and discussed in the US Congress over the past 15 or more years. Included in some of these earlier proposals was a recommendation to abolish the special defense of insanity and to adopt the "mens rea limitation" approach (for example, Senate bill S.1 during the Nixon Administration[93]). Given the complexity of the federal criminal code and the numerous and controversial proposals, no comprehensive reform was enacted until 1984.

Chapter 4 of the Comprehensive Crime Control Act of 1984[175] contains the Insanity Defense Reform Act of 1984. This enactment is the first comprehensive federal legislation governing the insanity defense and the disposition of persons suffering from a mental disease or defect who became involved with the federal criminal justice system. As noted earlier, in the past, specific insanity tests in the various federal circuits were adopted via caselaw. The most significant features of the new federal law (chapter 4) do the following: (1) significantly modify and tighten the standard for exculpatory insanity to be applied in federal courts; (2) require defendants who wish to raise the defense of insanity to assume the burden of proving this defense by a standard of clear and convincing evidence; (3) limit the scope of expert testimony on the ultimately legal issues; (4) eliminate the defense of "diminished capacity"; (5) create a special verdict of "not guilty only by reason of insanity," which triggers a federal civil commitment proceeding (prior to this only the District of Columbia jurisdiction had a statutory provision for the postacquittal commitment of insanity acquittees); and (6) provide for federal commitment for persons who become seriously mentally ill while serving a federal prison sentence.

Thus, the new federal insanity test states:

> It is an affirmative defense to a prosecution under any Federal statute that, at the time of the commission of the acts constituting the offense, the defendant, as a result of severe mental disease or defect, was unable to appreciate the nature and quality or the wrongfulness of his acts. Mental disease or defect does not otherwise constitute a defense.[176]

The limitation on the scope of expert testimony has been accomplished by amending Rule 704 of the Federal Rules of Evidence with a new subsection (b), which says:

> No expert witness testifying with respect to the mental state or condition of a defendant in a criminal case may state an opinion or inference as to whether the defendant did or did not have the mental state or condition constituting an element of the crime charged or of a defense thereto. Such ultimate issues are matters for the trier of fact alone.[177]

The above new federal enactment is the product of considerable study, discussion, debate, and analysis, and extensive hearings during which a variety of views and recommendations were expressed. The reforms clearly reflect a public policy to tighten and to delimit more carefully the special defense of insanity to come closer to what it was historically meant to be: a very narrow (even rare) exception to the general rule and policy that wrongdoers should be held criminally accountable for their acts. In sum, the above legislation accomplishes the desired public policy objectives without needing to use what, in my view, is the "most drastic alternative" of the "mens rea" limitation approach.

POLICY DILEMMAS

The preceding discussion in this chapter has made reference to the several moral, philosophical, ideological, and public policy issues inherent in the development, formulation, and administration of the insanity defense. Given the very nature of the topics involved, it is not surprising that many of these issues continue to be subjects of much controversy and debate. A number of policy dilemmas pertain to such things as the precise scope and contours of a tightened insanity defense, whether this special defense should be abolished, the particular types of mental disorders and the nature and degree of the associated impairment that should be considered for the threshold requirement of "mental disease or defect" (the new federal legislation refers specifically to "severe mental disease or defect"), the appropriate role of mental health professionals in such legal proceedings, and the postadjudication disposition and handling of persons exculpated on grounds of insanity.

It is both desirable and necessary that, within the constraints of our major societal values and Constitutional requirements, periodic revisions be made in public policies in response to changing societal needs, accurately ascertained problems, and relevant sociopolitical considerations. In what follows, only a few of the several policy dilemmas will be noted.

The Confusion and Confounding of Legal and Mental Health Concepts, Definitions, and Roles

Several of these problems have been the subject of extensive discussion in the relevant literature,[75,178-182] and hence their presentation here will be brief.

THE DEFINITION AND MEANING OF MENTAL DISEASE OR DEFECT

It has been noted that the presence of a mental disease or defect at the time of commission of the alleged criminal act is an essential **threshold** requirement for use of the insanity defense. Unless the asserted impairments in functioning can be shown to have resulted from a "mental disease or defect," the defense may not even be permitted. Therefore, an issue of crucial concern is the precise definition and meaning of the **legal** concept of "mental disease or defect" when used for this particular purpose. (See also chapter 5.)

Regrettably, there continues to be a general tendency to permit medical, psychiatric, or psychological terms and definitions to be thoroughly confounded with legal terms.[178-183] Moreover, many legislators, judges, and lawyers seem to have insufficient awareness and understanding of the conceptual complexities, value assumptions, and social judgments that are inherent in the concepts of "health" and "disease."[184-189] Nor is there sufficient realization that definitions and classifications designed for certain purposes in the mental health field do **not** have any direct relevance for the law in the making of moral and legal judgments about criminal culpability. This basic point was made more than two decades ago by the US Court of Appeals for the District of Columbia when it noted:

What psychiatrists may consider a "mental disease or defect" for clinical purposes, where their concern is treatment, may or may not be the same as mental disease or defect for the jury's purpose in determining criminal responsibility.[190]

Moreover, although a few legal scholars have viewed the medical-psychiatric concept of mental illness as having rather direct relevance and application for the law,[191] others have reflected better knowledge and understanding of the literature on medical nosology and classification systems. In an important law review article, Swartz[192] cautioned that medical definitions need to be scrutinized because of the particular value choices and matters of social philosophy embedded in them. He emphasized that when decisions between competing values will broadly affect society, these are matters of public and not just professional concern. Hence, he urged:

> Legislatures ought to be made aware that the construct of **mental disease** is a nonlegal means of classification, which must be modified for legal purposes. Modifications may be based on statutes, precedents, and, most important, on policy considerations relevant to a particular context.[193]

The above cautions and recommendations notwithstanding, the fact remains that clear legal definitions are frequently lacking in the field of mental health law. Such lack of policy guidance by legislative bodies is further compounded by the evident reluctance of many courts to formulate via caselaw the needed legal definitions and interpretations. There is, therefore, a predictable overreliance on medical, psychiatric, and mental health concepts, definitions, and related expert testimony.

For example, simply because they are listed in *DSM III*[76] does **not** mean that "disorders" such as cannabis abuse, tobacco dependence, social phobia, pathological gambling, passive-aggressive personality disorder, or even psychosexual disorders—such as inhibited sexual desire and premature ejaculation—are automatically or even necessarily encompassed within the **legal** term "mental disease or defect." The lack of needed public policy and legal guidance invites defense attorneys and their mental health experts to use novel disorders to expand what was meant to be a very narrowly conceived exception to judgments of criminal culpability. Thus, in recent years there has been increasing use of posttraumatic stress disorders,[194,195] pathological gambling,[196-200] multiple personality,[201] and premenstrual syndrome[202-204] as bases for a defense of insanity. There is also continuing controversy about whether personality disorders should be viewed as "mental disease or defect" for this legal purpose.[205,206]

In *United States v. Torniero*,[197] the opinion of a US District Court is of interest with respect to the aforementioned issues. The defendant had sought to assert his alleged "compulsive gambling disorder" as the basis for an insanity defense to the charge of transporting stolen goods in interstate commerce. In response to the government's motion to reconsider (to abolish) insanity as a defense to a criminal prosecution, the court heard testimony from 11 mental health and related witnesses. One of the witnesses, Professor Jay Katz (M.D.) of Yale Law School, expressed the view that, using *DSM III*, "you can classify all of us under one rubric or another of mental disorder."[207] Evidently Dr. Katz had not read *DSM III* very carefully and/or had failed to remember a few important points in the introduction to the manual with respect to the concept of mental disorder. Thus he provided a perfect illustration of the concern noted in the introduction to *DSM III* that "a common misconception is that a classification of mental disorders classifies individuals, when actually what are being classified are disorders that individuals have."[208] Professor Katz appears to believe that almost everyone is a fit subject for being diagnosed as suffering from one or another "mental disorder." Such a view may well regard "normality" as a type of mental disorder that simply remains to be discovered and suitably classified!

The judge in the above case did not permit Torniero to introduce expert testimony concerning his "compulsive gambling disorder." However, given the foregoing types of misconceptions and associated mental health testimony, the court noted that it

> [S]hares the widespread and growing public concern that new mental disorders appear to be fabricated in unending succession, that psychiatrists often are required to submit themselves to public grilling by skilled advocates, and the defendants increasingly seek to "explain" their alleged criminal acts as somehow compelled by pathologies of vague description and scant relevance.[209]

If, consistent with the Rule of Law, there is to be greater consistency in the application of major public and legal policies, as well as clearer signals to participants in the legal process, the foregoing legal definitions certainly require more effective legislative and judicial attention.

THE ROLE AND FUNCTIONING OF MENTAL HEALTH PROFESSIONALS

Closely related to the preceding topic is the matter of the role of mental health professionals in the legal setting, especially in regard to the insanity defense. This has also been a topic of much commentary and discussion.[75,90,113,179-183,210-215] A continuing dilemma pertains to whether mental health experts should be permitted to proffer opinions on the ultimate legal issues that are to be determined by the triers of fact (for example, whether the defendant was or was not criminally responsible at the time of the alleged criminal act).

It has been charged that the "experts" tend to arrogate to themselves, even to usurp, roles and responsibilities that properly belong to the triers of fact (jury and judge). However, it has quite accurately been pointed out that a large share of the responsibility (hence also the blame) for the state of affairs is due to legislative and judicial default.[179] After all, the legal process is governed by legal rules and procedures, the persons presiding over such proceedings are judges, and it is their responsibility to ensure that all participants (attorneys and witnesses) adhere to prescribed and enforced rules. Moreover, it must be remembered that until the very recent amendments via the Comprehensive Crime Control Act of 1984,[175] the Federal Rules of Evidence (Rule 704), and the almost identical Uniform Rules of Evidence[216] have permitted opinion testimony on the ultimate issues by expert witnesses.

In any event, inasmuch as the ultimate legal issues involve moral, public policy, and legal—**not** psychiatric or psychological—judgments, the view has been expressed for some time that the "experts" should **not** be permitted to give opinions on such matters because they are not within their expertise.[75,179] This basic point has periodically been emphasized by some appellate courts (see *Holloway v. United States*[217] and *Washington v. United States*[58]). Yet, as Monahan has observed:

> To avoid dealing with complex and problematic questions of law, judges frequently solicit conclusory opinions from mental health professionals. Oblivious to the limits of their expertise, mental health professionals sink to the occasion.[218]

Slovenko,[219] on the other hand, does not believe that this is a major problem. He points out that the law is Janus-faced; what it prohibits via one door it permits and even invites through another. As to the controversy that surrounds psychiatric testimony in criminal trials, Slovenko suggests that such "evidence is more prized for its entertainment value than for its probative worth."[220] Moreover, and using a distinctly quaint analogy, this law professor believes that "psychiatric intervention, like a diaper change, may not permanently solve any problems, but it does make life a bit more comfortable for a while."[221]

Despite the arguable desirability of providing the triers of fact some "entertainment" and also to make them "a bit more comfortable" as they deal with the mundane and even vexing day-to-day court proceedings, reforms have been urged by several professional organizations to limit expert testimony on the ultimate legal issues (for example, the American Psychiatric Association, the ABA Proposed Criminal Justice Mental Health Standards,[175]* and also in Congressional testimony[222]). Moreover, as noted earlier, the Comprehensive Crime Control Act of 1984 has heeded such recommendations and already made appropriate changes.

Reasonable Use and Regulation of the "Cleanup" Doctrine

Historically, an acquittal by reason of insanity has not been a plain acquittal for close to two centuries of Anglo-American law, and rarely does it provide a ticket to immediate freedom. Even though our societal values do not allow us to hold criminally responsible persons who were very seriously impaired in their legally relevant mental functions at the time of the criminal act, the community nevertheless needs to be protected from likely recurrences of the harmful behavior. Hence, confinement in security hospitals is the typical post-acquittal disposition. A major policy dilemma pertains to the nature and duration of such confinement. Questions of fundamental fairness are raised when those who cannot be subjected to criminal sanctions and who we claim to wish to treat with a greater degree of benevolence may nevertheless be subjected to periods of involuntary hospitalization well in **excess** of the criminal sentence that could have been imposed upon conviction.

The policies and practices that provide a powerful legal clutch over insanity acquittees have been explained in reference to the "cleanup" doctrine.[223] This

---

* *Standard 7-6.6:* "Opinion testimony, whether expert or lay, as to whether or not the defendant was criminally responsible at the time of the offense charged should not be admissible." (Note 175, page 363.)

notion assumes that "a person who commits a crime is either responsible enough to deserve punishment, or insane enough to deserve commitment." Hence, "mistakes in criminal commitment hearings are justified by their effect of 'cleaning up' the mistakes of criminal trials."[224]

As noted earlier, several federal and state courts have ruled that due process requires some durational limits on the length of postacquittal confinement (often based on the maximum penal sentence that could have been imposed had the defendant been convicted of the offense charged). If by that time the acquittee was still mentally ill and likely to be a danger to self or others, regular or special civil commitment procedures could be used for continued involuntary hospitalization. These lower court decisions (for example, *Bolton v. Harris*[134] and *State v. Krol*[138]) relied on some earlier decisions of the US Supreme Court (namely, *Baxstrom v. Herold*[225] and *Specht v. Patterson*[226]). Despite a series of such earlier decisions (*Humphrey v. Cady*[227] and *Jackson v. Indiana*[228]), in a recent 5-4 decision in *Jones v. United States*[229] the US Supreme Court held that "an insanity acquittee is not entitled to his release merely because he has been hospitalized for a period longer than he could have been incarcerated if convicted," because "the purpose of his commitment is to treat his mental illness and protect him and society from his potential dangerousness."[230] In view of the fact that Jones had been charged with attempting to steal a jacket from a department store (the misdemeanor of petit larceny), the "potential dangerousness" involved shoplifting. Thus it appears that the "cleanup" doctrine is alive and well.

It is evident, however, that even petit larceny tends to be perceived as especially "dangerous" when mentally ill persons are involved. In striking contrast to such overreactions and stigmatizing attitudes toward the mentally ill, our society displays a truly astonishing tolerance for the carnage on our highways caused by drunken drivers. The final report of the Presidential Commission on Drunk Driving points out that "at least 50 percent of all highway deaths involve the irresponsible use of alcohol. Over the past 10 years, 250,000 Americans have tragically lost their lives in alcohol-related crashes." Also, "an even more pervasive problem is the social acceptability of intoxication and drunk driving."[231]

In the face of such contrasting societal attitudes regarding the protection of the public from "dangerous" acts, the policy dilemma involves the development of reasonable durational limits on postacquittal confinement and the use of "less drastic" and "less restrictive alternatives"[232] for the continued aftercare, monitoring, and supervision of such cases under proper conditional release status. In this regard, Oregon's Psychiatric Security Review Board provides a very good model for study and appropriate adaptation in other jurisdictions.[233-236]

The Insidious Effects of Notorious Cases on Public Perceptions and Policies

It has been observed that selective media coverage of the "newsworthy" infamous cases tends to convey and to foster rather inaccurate perceptions, attitudes, and beliefs about the phenomenon. The National Commission on the Insanity Defense pointed out that myths often begin with selected facts or cases and then broaden to conclusions that are not valid. The highly publicized notorious cases both feed and perpetuate the "myth machine."[122]

There is the additional problem that the feelings generated in reaction to shocking cases tend to produce a "rush to reform." Moreover, as discussed earlier, in many instances the reforms proposed with respect to the insanity defense have often been based on exaggerated, distorted, or even entirely inaccurate beliefs and perceptions about the problems of concern. Hence, doubts arise as to whether some of the proposed "solutions" will ever manage to come into contact with—let alone correct—the "problems" they were supposed to address.

There is also reason for concern that the shocking cases tend to have a very disproportionate influence in shaping public policies and related practices. Notorious cases seem in many instances to function like the proverbial tails that tend to wag and influence policies affecting the much larger (albeit less visible) class of people. For example, stronger disincentives designed to reduce the rates of insanity pleas and acquittals and also to discourage attempted misuses (for example, by ensuring prolonged postacquittal confinement of acquittees) may well serve also to discourage very justified and proper uses of the defense. The policy challenge, therefore, is to try to ensure that the more stringent disincentives deemed necessary to deal with the few notorious cases are very carefully and narrowly formulated and specifically targeted, so that they do not work to the disadvantage of the vast majority of persons in the larger affected class. Wexler[146] has pointed out that a separate and "special" system should be fashioned for committing insanity acquittees, so that the entire civil commitment system does not get distorted by elements of what was earlier described as the "cleanup" doctrine. Moreover, further distinctions should be made with respect to acquittees who were involved in serious crimes of violence, so that the concerns about their "dangerousness" does not become generalized in loose and indiscriminate fashion to encompass acquittees who were involved in minor crimes like petit larceny.

REFERENCES

1. STEPHEN, JF: *A History of the Criminal Law of England, Vol 2*. Macmillan, 1883, p 96.
2. DIX, GE AND SHARLOT, MM: *Criminal Law: Cases and Materials, ed 2*. West Publishing, St Paul, 1979.
3. KADISH, SH, SCHULHOFER, SJ, PAULSEN, MG: *Criminal Law and Its Processes: Cases and Materials, ed 4*. Little, Brown & Co, Boston, 1983.
4. LOW, PW, JEFFRIES, JC, BONNIE, RJ: *Criminal Law: Cases and Materials*. Foundation Press, Mineola, NY, 1982.
5. VORENBERG, J: *Criminal Law and Procedure: Cases and Materials, ed 2*. West Publishing, St Paul, 1981.
6. WEINREB, LL: *Criminal Law: Cases, Comments, Questions, ed 2*. Foundation Press, Mineola, NY, 1975.
7. FLETCHER, GP: *The individualization of excusing conditions*. Southern California Law Review 47:1269, 1974.
8. ROBINSON, PH: *Criminal law defenses: A systematic analysis*. Columbia Law Review 82:199, 1982.
9. MORRIS, N: *Psychiatry and the dangerous criminal*. Southern California Law Review 41:514, 1968, p 516.
10. MORRIS, N: *Madness and the Criminal Law*. University of Chicago Press, Chicago, 1982.

11. COHEN, F: *Insanity: From abstract debate to operational reality.* Contemporary Psychology 13:386, 1968, p 386. Review of GOLDSTEIN, A: *The Insanity Defense.* Yale University Press, New Haven, CT, 1967.

12. GOLDSTEIN, A: *The Insanity Defense.* Yale University Press, New Haven, CT, 1967.

13. op cit supra, p 3.

14. CROTTY, HD: *The history of insanity as a defense to crime in English criminal law.* California Law Review 12:105, 1924.

15. LEVITT, A: *The origin of the doctrine of mens rea.* Illinois Law Review 17:117, 1922.

16. HOLDSWORTH, W: *A History of English Law, Vol 2.* Methuen, London, 1966, (first published 1903).

17. WALKER, N: *Crime and Insanity in England, Vol 1. The Historical Perspective.* Edinburgh University Press, Edinburgh, 1968.

18. DREHER, RH: *Origin, development and present status of insanity as a defense to criminal responsibility in the common law.* J History Behav Sciences 2:47, 1967.

19. SAYRE, FB: *Mens rea.* Harvard Law Review 45:974, 1932.

20. PLATT, AM AND DIAMOND, BL: *The origins and development of the "wild beast" concept of mental illness and its relation to theories of criminal responsibility.* J History Behav Sciences 1:355, 1965.

21. PLATT, AM AND DIAMOND, BL: *The origins of the "right and wrong" test of criminal responsibility and its subsequent development in the United States: An historical survey.* California Law Review 54:1227, 1966.

22. QUEN, JM: *Anglo-American criminal insanity: An historical perspective.* J History Behav Sciences 10:313, 1974.

23. THORNE, SE: *Bracton on The Laws and Customs of England. Vol 2.* Belknap Press of Harvard University Press, Cambridge, MA, 1968.

24. SHUMAKER, WA AND LONGSDORF, GF: *The Cyclopedic Law Dictionary.* Callaghan, Chicago, 1912.

25. TURNER, JWC: *Russell on Crime, Vol 1,* ed 12. Stevens and Sons, London, 1964, p 22.

26. Id., p 22, note 16.

27. HALL, J: *General Principles of Criminal Law,* ed 2. Bobbs-Merrill, Indianapolis, 1960.

28. Morissette v. United States, 342 U.S. 246, 251 (1952).

29. COHEN, MD: *Actus reus.* In KADISH, SH (ED): *Encyclopedia of Crime and Justice, Vol 1.* Free Press, New York, 1981.

30. See KADISH ET AL, op cit sup, note 3.

31. KADISH, SH: *The Decline of Innocence.* Cambridge Law Journal 26:273, 1968.

32. HOLDSWORTH, W: *A History of English Law, Vol VIII.* Methuen, London, 1966 (first published 1925).

33. EDGAR, H: *Mens rea.* In KADISH, SH (ED): *Encyclopedia of Crime and Justice, Vol 3.* Free Press, New York, 1981.

34. *Model Penal Code.* Proposed Official Draft, May 1962. American Law Institute, Philadelphia, 1962 (Section 2.20, General Requirements of Culpability, pp 25-28).

35. WEIHOFEN, H: *The Urge to Punish.* Farrar, Straus & Cudahy, New York, 1956.

36. HALE, M: *Historia Placitorum Coronae: The History of the Pleas of the Crown, Vol 1.* Robert H. Small, Philadelphia, 1847 (first published in 1736).

37. Id, p 30.

38. As quoted in WEINREB, op cit sup, note 6, p 388.

39. As quoted in WEINREB, op cit sup, note 6, pp 389-390. See notes 18 and 27.

40. Op cit sup, note 17, chapter 4. See also note 7, pp 390-391.

41. As quoted in WEINREB, note 6, p 390.

42. *The spelling of M'Naughten.* The Weekly Law Reports 1:1122, 1957.

43. *The real McNaughton.* Law Quarterly Review 74:1, 1958.

44. *The real Mhicneachdain.* Law Quarterly Reports 74:321, 1958.

45. DIAMOND, BL: *On the spelling of Daniel M'Naghten's name.* Ohio State Law Journal 25:85, 1964.

46. MORAN, R: *Knowing Right from Wrong: The Insanity Defense of Daniel McNaughtan.* Free Press, New York, 1981.

47. Op cit pp xi-xiii.

48. *Queen against Daniel M'Naughton,* 4 State Trials (NS), 847, 925 (1843).

49. Op cit sup, note 17, chapter 11. See also WEINREB, op cit sup, note 6, 384, note 2.

50. As quoted in WEINREB, op cit sup, note 6, p 384.

51. *Daniel M'Naghten's Case,* 10 Cl. & F. 200, 210-211, 8 Eng. Rep. 718, 722-723, 1843.

52. BIGGS, J: *The Guilty Mind.* Harcourt, Brace & Co, New York, 1955, p 107.

53. Commonwealth v. Rogers, 7 Metc. (Mass) 500, 502 (1844).

54. Parsons v. State, 81 Ala 577, 596-597 (1886).

55. State v. Jones, 50 N.H. 369, 398 (1971).

56. Durham v. United States, 214 F.2d 862, 874 (D.C.Cir. 1954).

57. McDonald v. United States, 312 F.2d 847 (D.C.Cir. 1962).

58. Washington v. United States, 390 F.2d 444 (D.C.Cir. 1967).

59. United States v. Brawner, 471 F.2d 969 (D.C.Cir. 1970).

60. Op cit sup, note 34, Section 4.01, p 66.

61. FAVOLE, RJ: *Mental disability in the American criminal process: A four issue survey.* In MONAHAN, J AND STEADMAN, HJ (EDS); *Mentally Disordered Offenders: Perspectives from Law and Social Science.* Plenum Press, New York, 1983, pp 257-269.

62. *Modern status of test of criminal responsibility—Federal cases (annotation).* 56 A.L.R. Fed. 326, 1982.

63. *Modern status of tests of criminal responsibility—State cases (annotation).* 9 A.L.R. 4th, 526, 1981.

64. United States v. Lyons, 731 F.2d 243 (5th Cir. 1984).

65. AMERICAN BAR ASSOCIATION: *Proposed Criminal Justice Mental Health Standards.* ABA, Chicago, IL, 1984.

66. Op cit sup, note 64, p 248.

67. Op cit sup, note 4, pp 759-767.

68. Montana Revised Codes Annotations, Sections 46-14-103 and 46-14-201(2) (adopted in 1979).

69. Idaho Code Annotations, Section 18-207 (adopted in 1982).

70. Utah Code Annotations, Section 76-2-305(1) (adopted in 1983).

71. BONNIE, RJ: *Morality, equality, and expertise: Renegotiating the relationship between psychiatry and criminal law.* Bull Am Acad Psychiatry Law 12:5, 1984.

72. Op cit sup, note 68, Section 46-14-301.

73. Op cit sup, note 70, Rules of Criminal Procedure, Section 77-35-21, Rule 21.

74. Op cit sup, note 70.

75. MORSE, SJ: *Crazy behavior, morals, and science: An analysis of mental health law.* Southern California Law Review 51:527, 1978.

76. *Diagnostic and Statistical Manual of Mental Disorders,* American Psychiatric Association, Washington, DC, 1980.

77. SIMON, RJ: *The Jury and the Defense of Insanity.* Little, Brown & Co, Boston, 1967.

78. ELWORK, A, SALES, BD, ALFINI, J: *Juridic decisions: In ignorance of the law or in light of it?* Law and Human Behavior 1:163, 1977.

79. ELWORK, A, SALES, BD, ALFINI, J: *Making Jury Instructions Understandable.* Michie, Charlottesville, VA, 1982.

80. Op cit sup, note 35, p 34.

81. Bonnie, RJ: *The moral basis of the insanity defense.* American Bar Association Journal 69:194, 1983.

82. Fingarette, H: *The Meaning of Criminal Insanity.* University of California Press, Berkeley, 1972.

83. Fingarette, H and Hasse, AF: *Mental Disabilities and Criminal Responsibility.* University of California Press, Berkeley, 1979.

84. German, J and Singer, A: *Punishing the not guilty: Hospitalization of persons acquitted by reason of insanity.* Rutgers Law Review 29:1011, 1976.

85. Goldstein, J and Katz, J: *Abolish the insanity defense—why not?* Yale Law Journal 72:853, 1963.

86. Halpern, A: *The fiction of legal insanity and the misuse of psychiatry.* J Leg Med 2:18, 1980.

87. Livermore, JM and Meehl, PE: *The virtues of M'Naghten.* Minnesota Law Review 51:789, 1967.

88. Monahan, J: *Abolish the insanity defense—not yet.* Rutgers Law Review 26:719, 1973.

89. Morris, GH: *The Insanity Defense: A Blueprint for Legislative Reform.* DC Heath, Lexington, MA, 1975.

90. Morse, SJ: *Failed explanations and criminal responsibility.* Virginia Law Review 68:971, 1982.

91. Singer, A: *Insanity acquittals in the seventies: Observations and empirical analysis in one jurisdiction.* Mental Disability Law Reporter 2:406, 1978.

92. Stone, AA: *The insanity defense on trial.* Hosp Community Psychiatry 33:636, 1982.

93. Wales, HW: *An analysis of the proposal to "abolish" the insanity defense in S.1: Squeezing a lemon.* University of Pennsylvania Law Review 124:687,1976.

94. *Limiting the Insanity Defense.* Hearings before Subcommittee on Criminal Law of the Committee on the Judiciary. United States Senate, 97th Congress, 2nd Session. June 24, 30, and July 14, 1982. Serial No.J-97-122. US Government Printing Office, Washington, DC, 1983.

95. *The Insanity Defense.* Hearings before Committee on the Judiciary, United States Senate, 97th Congress, 2nd Session. July 19 and 28, August 2 and 4, 1982. Serial No. J-97-126. US Government Printing Office, Washington, DC, 1982.

96. *Insanity Defense in Federal Courts.* Hearings before Subcommittee on Criminal Justice of the Committee on the Judiciary. House of Representatives, 97th Congress, 2nd Session. July 21, August 12, 17, and September 9, 1982. Serial No. 134. US Government Printing Office, Washington, DC, 1983.

97. *Mental or emotional condition as a diminishing responsibility for crime* (annotation, comment note). 22 A.L.R. 3rd, 1228, 1968 (Supp. 1983).

98. Dix, GE: *Psychological abnormality as a factor in grading criminal liability: Diminished capacity, diminished responsibility, and the like.* Journal of Criminal Law, Criminal and Police Science 62:313, 1971.

99. Arenella, P: *The diminished capacity and diminished responsibility defenses: Two children of a doomed marriage.* Columbia Law Review 77:827, 1977.

100. Arenella, P: *Diminished capacity.* In Kadish SH (ed): *Encyclopedia of Crime and Justice, Vol 2.* Free Press, New York, 1981, p 612.

101. Morse, SJ: *Diminished capacity: A moral and legal conundrum.* Int J Law Psychiatry 2:271, 1979.

102. *Model Penal Code and Commentaries* (Official Draft and Revised Comments), Part II, Definitions of Specific Crimes, Vol 1. American Law Institute, Philadelphia, 1980. See especially Article 210,3—Manslaughter, pp 43-73.

103. Id, p 70.

104. *Model Penal Code,* op cit sup, note 34, Section 4.02.

105. WINSLADE, WJ AND ROSS, JW: *The Insanity Plea.* Charles Scribner's Sons, New York, 1983.

106. *West's Annotated California Codes.* Penal Code, Section 28(b), which reads, "As a matter of public policy there shall be no defense of diminished capacity, diminished responsibility, or irresistible impulse in a criminal action or juvenile adjudication hearing," West (Supp.) 1984. See also Section 25(a).

107. KRAUSZ, FR: *The relevance of innocence: Proposition 8 and the diminished capacity defense.* California Law Review 71:1197, 1983.

108. Op cit sup, note 102, p 43.

109. *McKinney's Consolidated Laws of New York.* Penal Law, Section 125.25 (subd 1, para (a)). See also People v. Cassassa, 49 NY2d 668 (1980).

110. SALES, BD AND HAFEMEISTER, T: *Empiricism and legal policy on the insanity defense.* In TEPLIN, L (ED): *Mental Health and Criminal Justice.* Sage, Beverly Hills, CA, 1985.

111. Op cit sup, note 94, p 82.

112. Alaska Statutes Annotations, chapter 47, Sections 12.47.010 through 12.47.090.

113. SHAH, SA: *Legal and mental health system interactions: Major developments and research needs.* Int J Law Psychiatry 4:219, 1981.

114. STEADMAN, HJ, MONAHAN, J, HARTSTONE, E, DAVIS, SK, ROBBINS, PC: *Mentally disordered offenders: A national survey of patients and facilities.* Law and Human Behavior 6:31, 1982.

115. PASEWARK, RA AND PANTLE, ML: *Insanity plea: Legislator's view.* Am J Psychiatry 136:222, 1979.

116. SMITH, GA AND HALL, JA: *Evaluating Michigan's guilty but mentally ill verdict: An empirical study.* Journal of Law Reform 16:75, 1982.

117. STEADMAN, HJ, KEITNER, L, BRAFF, J, ARVANITES, TA: *Factors associated with a successful insanity plea.* Am J Psychiatry 140:401, 1983.

118. STEADMAN, HJ: Prepared statement, op cit sup, note 97, pp 83-87.

119. PASEWARK, RA AND CRAIG, PL: *Insanity plea: Defense attorneys' view.* Journal of Psychiatry and Law 8:413, 1980.

120. PASEWARK, RA, SEIDENZAHL, D, PANTLE, ML: *Opinions about the insanity plea.* Journal of Forensic Psychology 8:63, 1981.

121. STEADMAN, HJ AND COCOZZA, JJ: *Selective reporting and the public's misconceptions of the criminally insane.* Public Opinion Quarterly 41:523, 1978.

122. *Myths and Realities: A Report of the National Commission on the Insanity Defense.* National Association of Mental Health, Arlington, VA, 1983.

123. PHILLIPS, BL AND PASEWARK, RA: *Insanity plea in Connecticut.* Bull Am Acad Psychiatry Law 8:335, 1980.

124. COOKE, G AND SIKORSKI, C: *Factors affecting length of hospitalization in persons adjudicated not guilty by reason of insanity.* Bull Am Acad Psychiatry Law 2:251, 1974.

125. CRISS, ML AND RACINE, DR: *Impact of change in legal standard for those adjudicated not guilty by reason of insanity, 1975-1979.* Bull Am Acad Psychiatry Law 8:261, 1980.

126. PETRILA, J: *The insanity defense and other mental health dispositions in Missouri.* Int J Law Psychiatry 5:81, 1982.

127. SINGER, A: *Insanity acquittals in the seventies: Observations and analysis of one jurisdiction.* Mental Disability Law Reporter 2:406, 1978.

128. STEADMAN, HJ: *Insanity acquittals in New York State, 1965-1976.* Am J Psychiatry 137:321, 1980.

129. ROGERS, JL AND BLOOM, JD: *Characteristics of persons committed to Oregon's Psychiatric Security Review Board.* Bull Am Acad Psychiatry Law 10:155, 1982.

130. See, for example, op cit sup, note 94: "Let me also say that the insanity defense is a millionaire's defense or a rich man's defense. Unless one is a cause celebre,

there is almost no hope of a middle-income person or a poor person marshalling the type of psychiatric testimony that would be necessary to sustain such an action." (Sen. Larry Pressler, p 51.) Also see op cit sup, note 95: "The current insanity defense has also become a 'rich man's defense.'" (Sen. Orrin Hatch, pp 4, 10, and 255.) Op cit sup, note 96: "The system should not be designed with a 'rich man's loophole' that is available as a means of releasing one who can sufficiently confuse jurors with weeks of psychiatric testimony." (Rep. John T. Myers, p 10.)

131. MORROW, WR AND PETERSON, DB: *Follow-up of discharged psychiatric offenders: "Not guilty by reason of insanity" and "criminal sexual psychopaths."* Journal of Criminal Law, Criminology and Political Science 57:31, 1966.

132. BARIDON, P, SEITZ, F, ECHOLS, A: *A special report on the commitment of persons found not guilty by reason of insanity.* Division of Forensic Programs, Saint Elizabeth's Hospital, National Institute of Mental Health, Washington, DC, June 1983.

133. PASEWARK, RA: *Insanity plea: A review of the research literature.* Journal of Psychiatry and Law 9:357, 1981.

134. Bolton v. Harris, 395 F.2d 642 (D.C.Cir. 1968).

135. State v. Clemons, 515 P.2d 324 (Ariz 1973).

136. Wilson v. State, 287 N.E.2d 857 (Ind. 1982).

137. People v. McQuillan, 221 N.W.2d 569 (Mich. 1974).

138. State v. Krol, 344 A.2d 289 (N.J. 1975).

139. PASEWARK, RA, PANTLE, ML, STEADMAN, HJ: *Characteristics and disposition of persons found not guilty by reason of insanity in New York State, 1971-1976.* Am J Psychiatry 136:655, 1979.

140. PANTLE, ML, PASEWARK, RA, STEADMAN, HJ: *Comparing institutionalization periods and subsequent arrest of insanity acquittees and convicted felons.* Journal of Psychiatry and Law 8:305, 1980.

141. PASEWARK, RA, PANTLE, ML, STEADMAN, HJ: *Detention and rearrest rates of persons found not guilty by reason of insanity and convicted felons.* Am J Psychiatry 139:892, 1982.

142. BRAFF, J, ARVANITES, T, STEADMAN, HJ: *Detention patterns of successful and unsuccessful insanity defendants.* Criminology 21:439, 1983.

143. PASEWARK, RA, BIEBER, S, BOSTEN, KJ, KISER, M, STEADMAN, HJ: *Criminal recidivism among insanity acquittees.* Int J Law Psychiatry 5:365, 1982.

144. Op cit sup, note 113, pp 222-224.

145. WEXLER, BD: *Criminal Commitments and Dangerous Mental Patients: Legal Issues of Confinement, Treatment, and Release.* National Institute of Mental Health, DHEW Publ. No. (ADM)76-331, US Government Printing Office, Washington, DC, 1976.

146. WEXLER, DB: *The structure of civil commitment: Patterns, pressures, and interactions in mental health legislation.* Law and Human Behavior 7:1, 1983.

147. SLOVENKO, R: *Commentary: Disposition of the insanity acquittee.* Journal of Psychiatry and Law 11:97, 1983.

148. *Attorney General's Task Force on Violent Crime.* Final Report. US Department of Justice, US Government Printing Office, Washington, DC, August 1981, p 55.

149. INSTITUTE OF MENTAL DISABILITY AND THE LAW: *The "Guilty But Mentally Ill" Verdict: Current State of Knowledge.* Tentative Draft of Interim Report, Guilty But Mentally Ill Project. National Center for State Courts, Williamsburg, VA, April 1984.

150. People v. Jackson, 263 N.W.2d 44, at 45 (1977).

151. *Guilty but mentally ill: A historical and constitutional analysis.* Journal of Urban Law 53:471, 1976.

152. *Insanity—guilty but mentally ill—diminished capacity: An aggregate approach to madness.* John Marshall, Journal of Practice and Procedures 12:351, 1979.

153. SHERMAN, SL: *Guilty but mentally ill: A retreat from the insanity defense.* Am J Law Med 7:237, 1981.

154. *Indiana's guilty but mentally ill statute: Blueprint to beguile the jury.* Indiana Law Journal 57:639, 1982.

155. *Guilty but mentally ill verdict and due process.* Yale Law Journal 92:475, 1983.

156. SLOVENKO, R: *Commentaries on psychiatry and law: "Guilty but mentally ill."* Journal of Psychiatry and Law 10:541, 1982, p 544.

157. Op cit sup, note 65.

158. Id, p 1.

159. Id, pp 1-2.

160. Id, p 2.

161. AMERICAN BAR ASSOCIATION, STANDING COMMITTEE ON ASSOCIATION STANDARDS FOR CRIMINAL JUSTICE: *Proposed Criminal Justice Mental Health Standards.* ABA, Chicago, IL, August 1984.

162. Id, p 323.

163. Id, pp 323-339.

164. AMERICAN PSYCHIATRIC ASSOCIATION: *Statement on the Insanity Defense.* American Psychiatric Association, Washington, DC, December 1982.

165. INSANITY DEFENSE WORK GROUP: *American Psychiatric Association Statement on the Insanity Defense.* Am J Psychiatry 140:681, 1983.

166. Id, p 683.

167. Id, p 684.

168. Id, p 686.

169. AMERICAN MEDICAL ASSOCIATION: *Report to the Board of Trustees: The Insanity Defense in Criminal Trials and Limitations on Psychiatric Testimony.* American Medical Association, Chicago, IL, 1983.

170. *The Washington Post,* Friday, December 9, 1983, p A22.

171. AMERICAN PSYCHOLOGICAL ASSOCIATION: *Policy Statement on Insanity Defense Issues.* American Psychological Association, Washington, DC, January 1984.

172. Op cit sup, 122, p 5.

173. Id, p 1.

174. Id, pp 1, 3.

175. Comprehensive Crime Control Act of 1984 (Public Law 98-473).

176. Id, p 221.

177. Id, p 232.

178. SHAH, SA: *Crime and mental illness: Some problems in defining and labeling deviant behavior.* Mental Hygiene 53:21, 1969.

179. SHAH, SA: *Some interactions of law and mental health in the handling of social deviance.* Catholic University Law Review 23:674, 1974.

180. SHAH, SA: *Dangerousness: Some definitional, conceptual, and public policy issues.* In SALES, BD (ED): *Perspective in Law and Psychology, Vol 1.* Plenum, New York, 1977.

181. SHAH, SA: *Dangerousness and mental illness: Some conceptual, prediction, and policy issues.* In FREDERICK, CJ (ED): *Dangerous Behavior: A Problem in Law and Mental Health.* National Institute of Mental Health. DHEW Publ. No. (ADM)78-563. US Government Printing Office, Washington, DC, 1978.

182. DIX, GE: *Mental health professionals in the legal process: Some problems of psychiatric dominance.* Law and Psychology Review 6:1, 1981.

183. HOFFMAN, PB: *Mental health professional in the legal process: A plea for rational applications of the clinical method.* Law and Psychology Review 6:21, 1981.

184. LEWIS, A: *Health as a social concept.* Br J Sociol 4:109, 1953.

185. FABREGA, H: *The position of psychiatry in the understanding of human disease.* Arch Gen Psychiatry 32:1500, 1975.

186. PANZETTA, AF: *Toward a scientific psychiatric nosology.* Arch Gen Psychiatry 30:154, 1974.

187. REDLICH, FC: *Editorial reflections on the concepts of health and disease.* J Med Philos 1:269, 1976.

188. KLERMAN, GL: *Mental illness, the medical model, and psychiatry.* J Med Philos 2:220, 1977.

189. SLOVENKO, R: *The meaning of mental illness in criminal responsibility.* J Leg Med 5:1, 1984.

190. Op cit sup, n 57, p 851.

191. WEIHOFEN, H: *The definition of mental illness.* Ohio State Law Journal 21:1, 1960.

192. SWARTZ, LH: *"Mental disease": The groundwork for legal analysis and legislative action.* University of Pennsylvania Law Review 111:389, 1963.

193. Id, p 393.

194. GRANT, DL AND COONS, DJ: *Guilty verdict in a murder committed by a veteran with post-traumatic stress disorder.* Bull Am Acad Psychiatry Law 11:355, 1983.

195. PACKER, IK: *Post-traumatic stress disorder and the insanity defense: A critical analysis.* Journal of Psychiatry and Law 11:125, 1983.

196. United States v. Gillis, 645 F.2d 1269 (8th Cir. 1981).

197. United States v. Torniero, 570 F.Supp. 721 (1983).

198. United States v. Lewellyn, 723 F.2d 615 (8th Cir. 1983).

199. McGARRY, AL: *Pathological gambling: A new insanity defense.* Bull Am Acad Psychiatry Law 11:301, 1983.

200. RUBIN, AH: *Beating the odds: Compulsive gambling as an insanity defense—State v. Lafferty.* Connecticut Law Review 14:341, 1982.

201. FRENCH, AP AND SCHECHMEISTER, BR: *The multiple personality syndrome and criminal defense.* Bull Am Acad Psychiatry Law 11:17, 1983.

202. TAYLOR, L AND DALTON, K: *Premenstrual syndrome: A new criminal defense?* California Western Law Review 19:269, 1983.

203. MULLIGAN, N: *Premenstrual syndrome.* Harvard Women's Law Journal 6:219, 1983.

204. BOVERI, MD AND MARSHALL, BE: *Criminal law, premenstrual syndrome: A criminal defense.* Notre Dame Law Review 59:253, 1983.

205. RACHLIN, S, HALPERN, AL, PORTNOW, SL: *The volitional rule, personality disorders, and the insanity defense.* Psychiatric Annals 14:139, 1984.

206. SCHWARTZ, RA AND SCHWARTZ, IK: *Are personality disorders diseases?* Diseases of the Nervous System 11:613, 1976.

207. Op cit sup, n 191, p 733.

208. Op cit sup, n 76, p 6.

209. Op cit sup, n 191, pp 723-724.

210. DIX, GE: *Clinical evaluation of the "dangerousness" of "normal" criminal defendants.* Virginia Law Review 66:523, 1980.

211. DIX, GE: *Expert prediction testimony in capital sentencing.* American Criminal Law Review 19:1, 1981.

212. APPELBAUM, PS: *Psychiatrists' role in the death penalty.* Hosp Community Psychiatry 32:761, 1981.

213. SHAH, SA: *Dangerousness: Conceptual, prediction, and public policy issues.* In HAYS, JR, ROBERTS, TK, SOLWAY, KS (EDS): *Violence and the Violent Individual.* SP Medical & Scientific Books, New York, 1981.

214. MONAHAN, J (ED): *Who Is the Client? The Ethics of Psychological Intervention in the*

Criminal Justice System. American Psychological Association, Washington, DC, 1980.

215. TASK FORCE REPORT: *Report of the Task Force on the Role of Psychology in the Criminal Justice System.* Am Psychol 33:1099, 1978.

216. Federal Rules of Evidence for United States Courts and Magistrates. (Includes Uniform Rules of Evidence) Effective July 1, 1975, as amended to April 1, 1983. West Publishing, St Paul, 1983.

217. Holloway v. United States, 148 F.2d 665, at 667 (D.CV.Cir. 1945).

218. MONAHAN, J: *Foreword.* In ROESCH, R AND GOLDING, SL: *Competency to Stand Trial.* University of Illinois Press, Urbana, IL, 1980, p v.

219. SLOVENKO, R: *Reflections on the criticisms of psychiatric expert testimony.* Wayne Law Review 25:37, 1978.

220. Id, p 48.

221. Id, p 58.

222. See op cit sup, n 96, testimony of Sen. Arlen Specter, pp 11-12.

223. *Commitment following an insanity acquittal.* Harvard Law Review 94:605, 1981.

224. Id, p 618.

225. Baxstrom v. Herold, 383 U.S. 107 (1966).

226. Specht v. Patterson, 386 U.S. 605 (1967).

227. Humphrey v. Cady, 405 U.S. 504 (1972).

228. Jackson v. Indiana, 406 U.S. 715 (1972).

229. Jones v. United States, 103 S.Ct. 3043 (1983).

230. Id, p 3045.

231. PRESIDENTIAL COMMISSION ON DRUNK DRIVING. *Final Report.* US Government Printing Office, Washington, DC, 1983.

232. Shelton v. Tucker, 364 U.S. 479, at 488 (1960).

233. ROGERS, JL: *1981 Oregon legislation relating to the insanity defense and the Psychiatric Security Review Board.* Willamette Law Review 18:23, 1982.

234. BLOOM, JL AND BLOOM, JD: *Disposition of insanity defense cases in Oregon.* Bull Am Acad Psychiatry Law 9:93, 1981.

235. BLOOM, JD, ROGERS, JL, MANSON, SM: *After Oregon's insanity defense: A comparison of conditional release and hospitalization.* Int J Law Psychiatry 5:391, 1982.

236. ROGERS, JL, BLOOM, JD, MANSON, SM: *Oregon's Psychiatric Security Review Board: a comprehensive system for managing insanity acquittees.* In SHAH, SA: *The Law and Mental Health: Research and Policy* (in press).

CHAPTER 9

DEVELOPMENTALLY DISABLED PERSONS IN THE CRIMINAL JUSTICE SYSTEM

Michael Kindred, J.D.
Bruce D. Sales, J.D., Ph.D.

The concept of developmental disabilities is a broad one. Although it includes mental retardation, cerebral palsy, epilepsy, and autism, it is not restricted to those subcategories.[1] In fact, the developmental disabilities concept was developed in order to overcome fragmentation and compartmentalization in services among related groups with similar service needs. The stimulus to the concept's widespread adoption came from federal legislation that used it broadly to identify beneficiaries who would qualify for federal funds.

Despite the impulse to be broad and inclusive in social service legislation, the current federal legislative definition incorporates several narrowing qualifiers. These limits direct benefits to persons whose disabilities arise during youth and are severe, chronic, likely to last indefinitely, demand long-term services, and result in at least three functional limitations (for example, impairments in seeing, hearing, learning, walking, talking, or caring for self).[2]

A developmentally disabled person creates special problems for a criminal justice system because that human being may differ dramatically in his or her capabilities from the "normal" individual and because developmentally disabled persons vary greatly among themselves in the behavioral manifestations of their disorders. This problem is exacerbated by the fact that the criminal justice system is complex, consisting of many stages (for example, interrogation, arrest, trial, sentencing, incarceration, and parole)[3] and legal actors (police officers, prosecutors, judges, and wardens). Each interaction of an accused offender with an actor (suspect with police) at each stage may be affected by the fact that the person (suspect, defendant, or prisoner) is developmentally disabled.[4]

Because the problems that can arise are many, the purpose of this chapter is to survey them broadly, from first police contact through incarceration.

PRETRIAL STAGE

Arrest, Screening, and Diversion

Police officers play a complex role in American life.[5] They are the first gatekeepers, or screeners, between civilian life and the criminal justice process. Upon receipt of a complaint, a police officer must exercise discretion in deciding whether a crime has actually occurred that warrants state intervention, and whether to arrest or to take into custody an accused person.[6] When making these decisions, the officer typically will interrogate the person suspected of a crime in order to establish facts that are disputed or uncertain. Police also discharge non-law-enforcement duties[7] ranging from the provision of emergency life-saving services for the endangered to directions for the bewildered.

In discharging both law enforcement and social service functions, the fact that a suspect or person in trouble is developmentally disabled may make an important difference in how officers should respond. Thus, they must be trained to recognize the symptoms of developmental disabilities, because the behavior of these persons may appear to the untrained person to be something very different from what it is. For example, an individual with cerebral palsy walking home from a meeting late at night can easily be thought to be drunk, inasmuch as the speech and ambulation impairments sometimes symptomatic of cerebral palsy resemble drunkenness.[8] The slow response of a mentally retarded person might be confused with dissimulation. A person having an epileptic seizure might be thought to be on drugs.[9] Such a seizure might even result in serious damage to the person or property of another and yet not be criminal,[10] inasmuch as the action is often completely involuntary. (For further information about the principle of voluntariness, see chapter 8 of this text.)

It is, of course, appropriate for a police officer to investigate apparently criminal behavior, and there will be occasions when arrest of a developmentally disabled person is entirely proper. Nevertheless, the officer should make reasonable efforts to determine whether or not the developmentally disabled person's behavior is explained by noncriminal, disability-related characteristics. In that case, no further police intervention may be necessary other than to offer voluntary assistance or referral to a social service agency if the individual expresses a need for it, or if the individual is unable to do so even though he or she is clearly in need of these services. Unfortunately, research has demonstrated that police regularly fail to recognize symptoms of mental disability and are 20 percent more likely to arrest suspects exhibiting mental-disability symptoms than to arrest comparable suspects who are "normal."[11] This percentage is probably low when speaking of developmentally disabled persons because, as a group, they evince both mental and physical disabilities.

For police to carry out their social service functions properly, it is also important that they learn about the services that are available to assist developmentally disabled persons. This is certainly important when a developmentally disabled person requests assistance in securing emergency help when no criminal offense is involved. Such knowledge of available services will also be important, however, in case of minor antisocial conduct that could give rise to criminal prosecution but probably should not. For example, when a developmentally disabled person is apprehended for urinating in public, the best response may be referral to an agency that can provide instruction on socially appropriate behavior, rather than arrest for indecent exposure. Although there is debate about the extent to which police should be active decision makers in diversion programs,[12] there is little doubt that some such role will and should be played in cases of minor misconduct.[5]

Interrogation Process

Another potential problem in police interaction with developmentally disabled persons relates to interrogation. Although police place a high value upon being able to interrogate criminal suspects, a countervailing value is placed in our law on the right of an individual to refuse to provide self-incriminating information. The Fifth Amendment to the United States Constitution states, "No person shall . . . be compelled in any criminal case to be a witness against himself." This privilege against self-incrimination has long been held applicable to police interrogation[13] at both the state and federal levels.[14] Similarly, the Sixth Amendment's right to "assistance of counsel" applies during interrogation of a suspect by state officials.[15,16] Thus, when the police wish to question a person in custody who they have probable cause to believe has committed a crime, they are required to advise the person of his or her rights to remain silent, to consult counsel, and to have counsel appointed in case of indigency.[13] After being informed of these rights, a person is ordinarily free to exercise or to waive any of them.

For a waiver to be valid, however, it must be made voluntarily, knowingly, and intelligently. It is here that the problems arise. Inasmuch as many developmentally disabled persons suffer from deficits in intellectual capacity, their ability to evaluate the wisdom of waiving their right to counsel or their privilege against self-incrimination may be limited—thereby precluding an intelligent waiver of these rights. Similarly, the voluntariness of their waivers is also subject to question. Although any individual may find the atmosphere of a police station interrogation room intimidating, mentally disabled persons may feel especially vulnerable, be greatly intimidated, and be more susceptible to being led by persons in authority (such as police officers) into giving responses they feel are desired—even if such responses are falsely incriminating.[17]

The US Supreme Court has often noted the relevance of mental illness and mental retardation to the voluntariness of confessions and waivers.[13,17-21] The justices have not, however, held such a disability to constitute, per se, a constitutional invalidation of such waivers. Rather, they have held that the validity of a person's waiver, as a constitutional matter, must be determined by reviewing the totality of the circumstances in each case.[22,23]

Moreover, failure to recognize a disability can result in a questionable interrogation and a costly after-the-fact suppression of evidence hearing to determine whether the interrogation violated the rights of the disabled person. Awareness of the disability and respect for the individual's rights, however, can permit a different investigative tactic that may prevent the conviction of an innocent person, while still allowing for the preparation of a valid case.

Prosecutorial Process

The next step in the criminal justice system is the prosecutorial phase. The prosecutor's office exercises considerable discretion in determining whether to press criminal charges against a person, what level of charge to file, and whether to consider possible pretrial diversion from the criminal process.[24] Although the prosecutor must consider such factors as the accused's guilt and the seriousness of the crime, consideration is also given to other factors, such as whether the accused is intellectually or emotionally impaired.[25,26] For example, when a social service agency is prepared to provide services to the developmentally disabled person and to take some responsibility for that person, a prosecutor may feel that referral to that agency is a sufficient discharge of his or her responsibilities. The prosecutor may also have less than the usual confidence in his or her ability to secure a conviction in light of a possible finding of mental incompetence to stand trial, defenses of nonresponsibility or diminished capacity, and possible attacks on the validity of any confession. For these reasons, the discretionary aspects of the prosecutor's function are of great importance to a developmentally disabled person accused of crime, particularly when that crime is of a nongrievous nature.

In recent years a considerable body of literature has developed that is critical of the failure to regulate the manner in which prosecutorial discretion is exercised.[27-31] In cases of extreme abuse, courts have limited the exercise of that discretion,[32,33] and many prosecutors have developed guidelines to govern their staffs.

TRIAL STAGE

Following arrest and a decision to prosecute, a criminal case enters the trial stage. The object of this stage is to make a formal determination of innocence or guilt. At the trial stage there are three criminal law doctrines of particular relevance to some developmentally disabled defendants: competency to stand trial, mental nonresponsibility, and diminished capacity.

Competency to Stand Trial

It is an ancient common law doctrine that a defendant who is unable to comprehend the nature of the proceedings against him or her or to assist defense counsel cannot be subjected to trial.[34,35] (See also chapter 7 on this subject.) The doctrine is universally embraced by the states[36,37] and probably has more significance for the developmentally disabled than any other criminal law doctrine.[37] The US Supreme Court has characterized it as "fundamental to an adversary system of justice"[38] and has said that "failure to observe the procedures adequate to protect a defendant's right not to be tried or convicted while incompetent to stand trial deprives him of his due process right to a fair trial."[38] Individual states might well find it required by their own constitutions if the matter were put in issue.[39]

Although this doctrine appears to recognize the limitations of, and to provide some protection for, developmentally disabled persons, its implementation has historically often operated to the disadvantage of these persons. Although the person may be shielded from criminal prosecution, the consequence of being found incompetent to stand trial was often indeterminate or even lifelong confinement, until the US Supreme Court outlawed the practice in 1972.[40] The continued problem of the duration of confinement is discussed later in this chapter on the posttrial stage.

The negative consequences of a finding of incompetency to stand criminal trial render problematic another aspect of the doctrine. State laws have typically provided that the competency issue can be raised by the prosecutor, court, or defendant.[36,37] This has been reinforced by the US Supreme Court's requirement that trial courts inquire into competency when there are indications that the defendant may be incompetent.[41] As a consequence, a finding of incompetence to stand trial can be reached in cases in which the defendant would clearly benefit from going through the criminal trial. It should be pointed out, however, that even today, conviction and a short prison sentence or probation may be a lesser deprivation of liberty than what would result from a finding of incompetence. A defendant, or defense attorney, might have had reasonable hope of establishing the defendant's innocence or otherwise blocking successful prosecution had a trial of the criminal charge taken place. In fact, the prosecution's ability to raise the competency issue has led to concern that prosecutors might use competency determinations to secure confinement via hospitalization when they have a weak criminal case.[42] This had led most commentators who have studied this problem in recent years to argue that defendants whose competency is questioned should at least have an opportunity to establish their innocence.[37,40,43,44]

Criminal Responsibility

A second major legal doctrine that comes into play at the trial stage is the "nonresponsibility" defense, better known as the "insanity" defense. (See also chapter 8 of this text.) Because the criminal law is based upon notions of individual choice and responsibility and moral fault,[45,46] the law has long recognized a defense of "not responsible because of mental disease or defect."[47-49] The doctrine serves to separate "the mad" from "the bad" and is available to some persons who are mentally retarded.

Operationally, this defense is less intrusive than the doctrine of competency to stand trial, because in most jurisdictions it can be raised only by the defendant.[48,50,51] Therefore, it comes into play only when the defendant or defense counsel believes it to serve the defendant's interest. The defense is also less likely to short-circuit the fact-finding process than is a finding of incompetency to stand trial, because a verdict of "not responsible by reason of mental defect" must ordinarily be predicated upon a jury's finding beyond a reasonable doubt that the defendant performed the act charged.

Nevertheless, there are serious problems with the nonresponsibility defense as it relates to mentally retarded defendants who are not mentally ill. Repeated changes in the legal definition of the responsibility criteria reflect political and jurisprudential debate about the relationship between mental disability in general and criminal justice. Beyond these general concerns, developmental disabilities create special questions of criminal responsibility, because the nonresponsibility doctrines seem a bad fit for developmental disabilities problems. This is probably because the insanity defense tests were developed primarily, although not entirely, from the perspective presented by mental illness rather than that presented by mental retardation. Thus, courts trying to accommodate this doctrine to mentally retarded persons have done so with mixed results. For example, although the M'Naghten test's reference to "disease of the mind" seems to exclude mental retardation, many cases considering the matter have viewed the defense as applicable to a mentally retarded person as long as the person meets the functional test of being "unable to distinguish right from wrong." Despite this attempt at accommodation, however, a number of cases have refused to permit jury consideration of the defendant's mental deficiency as a basis for an "insanity" defense.[52-55]

These cases seem to reflect a general ambivalence about whether the nonresponsibility defense should encompass the mentally retarded. The persistence of "insanity" language is perhaps the best indication of the continued domination of the area by notions of mental illness. Also telling is the extent to which the impact of the defense on the mentally retarded has been left virtually unaddressed in the voluminous litigation, legislation, and literature on the defense. Little attention has been given to the suitability of the various test formulations to persons with mental retardation[56] or indeed to the appropriateness of criminal responsibility when mental retardation is a significant causative factor in unlawful behavior.[57-60] (See also chapter 8 regarding the basic structure of insanity tests.) It may be more appropriate to think about degrees of culpability for the diverse population that makes up the developmentally disabled. The next section addresses one approach to this problem.

Diminished Capacity

The concept of diminished capacity is succinctly stated by the American Law Institute's Model Penal Code, Section 4.02(1):

> Evidence that the defendant suffered from a mental disease or defect is admissible whenever it is relevant to prove that the defendant did or did not have a state of mind which is an element of the offense.

This simple concept, that evidence of mental retardation or mental illness should be admissible in a criminal trial to negate proof of a required mental element of a crime, seems so obvious as to be incontrovertible. Nevertheless, it is a radical departure from prior doctrine and has become one of the most hotly disputed questions in criminal law. (See also discussion in chapter 8.)

Diminished capacity as a doctrine can be understood only as an erosion of the rigidity of traditional criminal responsibility doctrine. Under traditional doctrine expert psychiatric testimony was admissible only to prove that the defendant was "insane" in the meaning of the law's test. The central corollary of this doctrine was that evidence, or at least expert evidence, of a defendant's mental illness or mental retardation was not admissible for any other purpose. It could not be used to prove that a defendant could not and did not "premeditate" a killing, even though the law punished premeditated killings more seriously than nonpremeditated killings.

The diminished capacity defense tore down this barrier. Following adoption of the Model Penal Code by the American Law Institute, the doctrine won increasing acceptance during the 1960s and 1970s.[61-63] Its apparent logic and simplicity were attractive. Recent developments, however, suggest that the apparent indisputability of this simple solution may yet fall into disfavor.[64,65] Little more than a decade after the US Court of Appeals for the District of Columbia had embraced the "diminished capacity" doctrine in the *Brawner* case,[66] the District of Columbia Court of Appeals rejected it.[67] Similarly, the

Ohio Supreme Court recently rejected evidence of diminished capacity[68] despite earlier indications that such evidence was admissible.[69,70] Most dramatically, the federal Seventh Circuit Court of Appeals held in 1978 that it would be unconstitutional to reject such evidence.[71] In 1983 it reversed itself—or at least gave its 1978 opinion an exceedingly narrow interpretation.[72]

The concept of diminished capacity seems to be a more appropriate tool to reflect the degree of criminal culpability of many mentally retarded defendants than the simple right-from-wrong test. It recognizes that for different crimes different culpable mental states are required.[63] Indeed, one study group, perhaps most attuned to the needs of the developmentally disabled, went as far as to propose that "diminished capacity" be completely substituted for the nonresponsibility defense for the mentally retarded.[37] Some commentators have proposed that this substitution be made generally.[73]

The reaction against this attractive doctrine is probably based upon a fear that it offers insufficient protection to the security interests of the public at large. Unlike the nonresponsibility defense doctrine, most states have no provision for the automatic incarceration of persons shown to lack a mental element for the crime charged. Such persons are simply "not guilty" and so will be released unless some civil confinement can be invoked independently of the criminal trial. These security concerns are central to issues that arise in the posttrial stage.

POSTTRIAL STAGE

After preliminary screening by police and prosecutorial personnel and processing through the criminal courts, other difficult issues remain. They relate to the disposition and treatment of developmentally disabled defendants.

Sentencing

In many circumstances, developmentally disabled persons will be tried and found guilty of criminal offenses. The breadth of the concept of developmental disabilities ensures this. The number of such convictions will be increased by restriction of the nonresponsibility and diminished capacity defenses discussed above. The overriding postconviction issue is whether, after conviction for a crime, the defendant's developmental disability should make a difference in determining what sentence to impose. Although it may seem self-evident that disability can make a difference, much depends on the theoretical basis of the criminal sanction, itself a matter of continuing dispute.[74] If the criminal sentence is viewed as an opportunity to rehabilitate, sentencing strategies will have to be adapted to the convict's strengths and needs; thus, facts about disability will clearly be of major significance.

Even if retribution is seen as the function of the sanction, disability may make a difference. If society is to exact a compensatory price from an offender, the sentence may depend on the degree of blameworthiness attached to the wrongdoing. One might argue that "naively" committed crime is less awful than a calculatingly committed crime. In the proper case, disability might thus attenuate the blame and lessen the appropriate sanction. But information about disability is less relevant if the criminal sentence is viewed primarily as a means to deter other members of society from criminal behavior by making an example of the one convicted. Facts of disability are also of little importance when the criminal sanction is treated as a purely objective retribution, as in "an eye for an eye." In fact, the last several years have been characterized by many as a period of shift from the rehabilitative ideal to a mix of objective retribution and general deterrence, characterized by an increase in fixed, mandatory sentences and much less judicial discretion to take into account factors such as disability.[74]

The instrumentality through which sentencing judges can receive information about a defendant's disability is the presentence report. Such reports have become a common and important feature of the sentencing process.[75] The Model Penal Code [Section 7.07(1)] would require an investigation and report before sentencing whenever the defendant is less than 22 years old, the sentence is for a felony, or an extended prison term is to be imposed. It also would give the judge discretion to order a presentence study in other cases. Whatever the correctional philosophy, presentence reports are generally important and should be ordered when the defendant may be developmentally disabled. To sentence such a person to a period of imprisonment without any information on the nature and extent of the disability is undesirable, because special medication may be required for life or health.

Nevertheless, there may be situations in which no presentence report is needed, even though the defendant is developmentally disabled. If the offense is a relatively minor one (such as a traffic offense) for which the penalty is generally a small fine or short-term probation, the cost of a thorough presentence report could exceed its utility. Also, the evaluation itself can be a real burden to a defendant, and this burden might not be justified when the offense and sanction are minor. Thus, a presentence report should be required only when the offense is relatively serious or when there is a penalty of imprisonment.

The issue of the significance that the judge should attach to a developmental disability arises at every point along the continuum of possible sentencing choices. The difficulty of the problem can be illustrated best by situations at both ends of the spectrum. A judge often has discretion to choose between an incarcerative sanction and probation or a suspended sentence. Aside from concerns about the most appropriate use of the limited prison "bed space," various considerations suggest that the prison sentence should be used with greater caution when the defendant is developmentally disabled. As noted above, there may be a sense of attenuated guilt arising from diminished comprehension or self-control. One may also have concerns about the increased possibility of sexual and other exploitation of a developmentally disabled person within the prison context. There may also be greater concern generally about the antitherapeutic nature of the prison environment, which might cause greater damage to the disabled convict than to the nondisabled convict. At the same time, one might be able to identify a specific rehabilitative community training program that is available to developmentally disabled persons and could serve as an alternative dispositional placement. In short, there may be a rationale for lessening the use of incarcerative sanctions in the case of developmentally disabled offenders.

At the opposite end of the sanction continuum is the death penalty. One must consider whether the death penalty, even when an available sanction for a particular crime, ought to be precluded when the offender is developmentally disabled. The Model Penal Code provides that a defendant's physical or mental condition may be relevant as a factor that would preclude imposition of the death penalty (Section 210.6). There is, of course, vigorous debate concerning whether the death penalty ought ever to be imposed upon anyone.[76,77] Putting this general question aside as beyond the purview of this chapter, at least it can be argued that this ultimate sanction ought never to be used in the case of a developmentally disabled offender.[78]

First, even though the disability is not sufficiently extreme to negate criminal responsibility, it may be presumed sufficiently significant to play some indirect or partial role in shaping the offender's perception and behavior and thus to preclude imposition by society of that most severe expression of moral condemnation that is implicit in the death penalty. Second, although the disability may not negate the individual's ability to receive a fair trial, disability can trigger subjective discomfort with or prejudice against a defendant or might diminish his or her ability to assist defense counsel. There is reason for increased concern about the possibility of error or prejudice creeping into the trial process. The common thread of these two arguments is that, because the death penalty is an extreme and irreversible penalty, its use ought to be limited to the most extreme and clearest cases. When the defendant is developmentally disabled, it is questionable whether the case can be fit within that narrow categorization.

The Civil Commitment Alternative

For a nondisabled defendant the criminal process has two basic possible outcomes: acquittal or a criminal sanction. For the developmentally disabled defendant, several additional options exist. As discussed earlier, the defendant may be found either incompetent to stand trial or not responsible by reason of mental defect. Disposition following these determinations is discussed in the following two sections. Problems with those dispositions, however, can be understood only if one first understands another set of restrictive alternatives: civil commitment.

Virtually every jurisdiction has a civil commitment system through which an individual can be confined in a state institution if found to be mentally ill or mentally retarded and dangerous to self or others.[36,37] This system provides an alternative incarcerative mechanism that does not depend at all upon conviction under the criminal law for an offense. Of course, much behavior indicative of "danger to others" is in fact also behavior that can be characterized as "criminal." This overlap of the two systems means that the civil commitment system is often an alternative dispositional mechanism or diversionary placement that can be used for a person suspected of "criminal" behavior. It also provides a mechanism for confining persons found incompetent to stand trial or "nonresponsible" in a criminal trial. The criminal justice system, however, has developed separate confinement tracks for those latter two categories of persons. A critical question of the last several years has been the extent to which such separate tracks can diverge from the basic civil commitment track provided by a state for the confinement of persons not convicted of a criminal offense.

Confinement of the Person Incompetent To Stand Trial

Until the 1970s persons found incompetent to stand trial were regularly committed to state mental institutions for substantial periods of time. The basis of the confinement was not a finding that the person was dangerous; rather, it was that the person was incompetent to participate in a criminal trial.[37] Because developmental disabilities are often severe and chronic, commitment "until competence is restored" was often commitment for life. Although such a permanent commitment may have protected society from the accused and untried defendant, it was a harsh result for the developmentally disabled person, whose transgression may have been minor or even nonexistent.

In 1972 the US Supreme Court examined this confinement system and held such lifetime commitments to be unconstitutional. In *Jackson v. Indiana*[40] the Court held that incompetence to stand trial does not justify such extensive confinement and that such confinement violated substantive due process of law. The Court also compared Indiana's postincompetence confinement with its civil commitment system. It held that major differences between these systems, in their criteria for commitment and their criteria and process for release, were unjustifiable and amounted to a denial of equal protection of the laws.

State courts, legislatures, and commentators have gradually begun to grapple with the implications of the *Jackson* case,[37,44] but the shape of the new system remains to be determined.

Post-Insanity Confinement

Issues similar to those for postincompetence confinement arise after a finding of "not responsible by reason of mental defect," with one very significant difference. Whereas incompetence precludes the criminal trial, a verdict of nonresponsibility generally is permitted only when the judge or jury has first found beyond a reasonable doubt that the defendant committed the act charged. Thus, it may not be surprising to find that the confinement following a determination of nonresponsibility is swift, sure, and long-lasting. The typical practice has been to require the judge to commit the defendant and to provide that the confinement shall last until the person can show that he or she is either no longer mentally ill or retarded or no longer dangerous.[36]

Since the late 1960s,[79-80] there has been debate about whether equal protection and due process notions require limitations upon this confinement. In *Jackson v. Indiana*, invalidation of the unrestricted postincompetence confinement reenforced the sense that the postnonresponsibility confinement rules might have to be limited as well. In 1983 in *Jones v. United States*,[81] the United States Supreme Court addressed this topic and approved an indefinite confinement following a determination of nonresponsibility when the confinement had already extended beyond the maximum possible prison sentence for the crime involved. The Court held that it was unnecessary to meet its own civil commitment standard of proof by clear and convincing evidence[82] to justify continued indefinite commitment.[83] Of course, the possibility exists of greater limitation under state constitutions[39] or legislation, but *Jones* certainly seems to indicate substantial federal constitutional tolerance for restrictive state postnonresponsibility systems. One must indeed wonder whether *Jones* does not even suggest a very narrow reading in the future of *Jackson v. Indiana* in its own postincompetence domain.

Right to Treatment or Habilitation

A final major legal issue requiring attention is whether a developmentally disabled prisoner has a right to treatment or habilitation within the prison system. Although the US Supreme Court has not addressed the question of whether there is a right to treatment in prison, two lines of lower court cases and some tangential US Supreme Court authority support an argument that such a right does exist. The first line of court cases deals directly with the rights of prisoners. It has been held that conviction and imprisonment for an offense do not justify denying normal medical care to the person imprisoned.[83-85] It has also been held that medical care in this context includes treatment for mental illness.[86] This obviously suggests that prison officials cannot completely ignore the therapeutic needs of developmentally disabled prisoners. Surely a person with epilepsy cannot be denied the medication needed to control seizures. How far this principle will extend remains to be seen.

The second line of cases holds that there is a right to treatment for persons civilly committed. There are numerous lower court decisions holding that there is a broad right to treatment and habilitation for persons civilly committed to institutions.[87,88] One important case[89] applied this principle to persons being held after findings of incompetence and nonresponsibility, but none has yet reached into the general prison context. Although the US Supreme Court has not recognized a broad and general right to treatment or habilitation in civil institutions, it has held that persons confined to civil institutions for the mentally retarded retain basic constitutional rights and that treatment must be provided when it is necessary for the protection of those rights.[90]

Here again, state constitutions may provide even greater protection than the US Constitution.[39] Furthermore, sound legislative and administrative policy generally will dictate the provision of services that are responsive to the special needs of developmentally disabled prisoners. When the developmental disability has somehow contributed to the criminality of the prisoner, the public interest favors treatment that will change that behavior, permit the release of the individual from prison, and make him or her a productive rather than a destructive member of society. Even when the developmental disability is not causative of the criminal behavior, the state might reasonably conclude that it should provide treatment or training during the time of incarceration in order to improve the individual's ability to cope as a productive person upon release. Indeed, simple humanity and decency may command that a person requiring medication to control seizures receive it, that a person requiring a wheelchair or crutches for mobility receive them, and that a person requiring training in a skill in order to live successfully in modern society receive such training.

CONCLUSION

The interaction between developmental disabilities and the criminal justice system raises complex issues. Much more needs to be said on each of the topics discussed in this chapter to accord full measure to that complexity. The purpose here has been to suggest the scope of the problem and to demonstrate its potential development.

The broad issue facing the criminal justice system is whether it can and indeed should accommodate the diversity of capabilities, difficulties, and needs represented by developmentally disabled persons. It seems evident that this accommodation can succeed only through full utilization of the expertise of professionals with training and experience in the developmental disabilities area. This utilization is imperative at several different levels. First, at the policy level it is clear that adequate standards of criminal responsibility and programs of rehabilitation in prisons can be built only with the assistance of such expertise. Second, at the training level, police officers and prosecutors at the intake phase and prison officials at the exit phase must be trained to recognize and to respond to the problems and needs presented by developmentally disabled persons. Third, in practical implementation of diversion programs, presentence studies, and prison habilitation, professionals with expertise in developmental disabilities are essential to the administration of a rational and humane criminal justice system. Future study will have to elaborate on both the scope of the problem and the specific roles mental health professionals can play in its amelioration.

REFERENCES

1. Developmentally Disabled Assistance and Bill of Rights Act, codified at United States Code, Sections 6001-6081. US Government Printing Office, Washington, DC, 1983.

2. WIEGERINK, R AND PELOSI, J (EDS): *Developmental Disabilities.* Paul H. Brookes, Baltimore, 1979.

3. KADISH, S AND PAULSEN, M: *Criminal Law and Its Processes,* ed 3. Little, Brown & Co, Boston, 1975.

4. FOX, S: *The criminal reform movement.* In KINDRED, M, COHEN, J, PENROD, D, SHAFFER, T (EDS): *The Mentally Retarded Citizen and the Law.* Free Press, New York, 1976.

5. GEORGE, BJ, JR: *Screening, diversion and mediation in the United States.* New York Law School Law Review 29:1-38, 1984.

6. AMERICAN BAR ASSOCIATION: *Standards Relating to the Urban Police Function.* American Bar Association, Washington, DC, 1972.

7. PRESIDENT'S COMMISSION ON LAW ENFORCEMENT AND ADMINISTRATION OF JUSTICE: *Task Force Report: The Police.* US Government Printing Office, Washington, DC, 1967.

8. CRUICKSHANK, WM (ED): *Cerebral Palsy: A Developmental Disabililty,* ed 3. Syracuse University Press, Syracuse, NY, 1976.

9. BARROW, R AND FABING, H: *Epilepsy and the Law,* ed 2. Harper & Row, New York, 1966.

10. ROBINSON, P: *Criminal Law Defenses, Vol 2.* West Publishing, St Paul, MN, 1984.

11. TEPLIN, LA: *Criminalizing mental disorder.* Am Psychol 39:794-803, 1984.

12. US NATIONAL ADVISORY COMMISSION ON CRIMINAL JUSTICE STANDARDS AND GOALS: *Report on Courts.* US Government Printing Office, Washington, DC, 1973.

13. Miranda v. Arizona, 384 U.S. 436 (1966).

14. Mapp v. Ohio, 367 U.S. 643 (1961).

15. Gideon v. Wainwright, 372 U.S. 335 (1963).

16. Argersinger v. Hamlin, 407 U.S. 25 (1972).

17. Fikes v. Alabama, 352 U.S. 191 (1957).

18. Davis v. North Carolina, 384 U.S. 737 (1966).

19. Blackburn v. Alabama, 361 U.S. 199 (1960).

20. Spano v. New York, 360 U.S. 315 (1959).

21. Powell v. Alabama, 287 U.S. 45 (1932).

22. United States v. Cassell, 452 F.2d 533 (7th Cir. 1971).

23. Brewer v. Williams, 430 U.S. 387 (1977).

24. MILLER, F: *Prosecution: The Decision to Charge a Suspect with a Crime.* Little, Brown & Co, Boston, 1969.

25. LAGOY, S, SENNA, J, SIEGEL, L: *An empirical study on information usage for prosecutorial decision making in plea negotiations.* American Criminal Law Review 13:435-471, 1976.

26. JACOBY, J, MELLON, L, SMITH, W: *Policy and Prosecution*. US Dept. of Justice, National Institute of Justice, Washington, DC, 1982.

27. DAVIS, K: *Discretionary Justice: A Preliminary Inquiry*. Louisiana State University Press, Baton Rouge, 1969.

28. GOLDSTEIN, A: *The Passive Judiciary: Prosecutorial Discretion and the Guilty Plea*. Louisiana State University Press, Baton Rouge, 1981.

29. ATKINS, B AND POGREBIN, M (EDS): *The Invisible Justice System: Discretion and the Law*, ed 2. Anderson, Cincinnati, 1982.

30. VORENBERG, J: *Narrowing the discretion of criminal justice officials*. Duke Law Journal 1976:651-697, 1976.

31. COX, S: *Prosecutorial discretion: An overview*. American Criminal Law Review 13:383-434, 1976.

32. United States v. Falk, 479 F.2d 616 (7th Cir. *en banc* 1973).

33. Dixon v. District of Columbia, 394 F.2d 966 (D.C. Cir. 1968).

34. BLACKSTONE, W: *Commentaries*. Clarendon Press, Oxford, 1765.

35. *Incompetency to stand trial*. Harvard Law Review 81:454-473, 1967.

36. BRAKEL, S AND ROCK, R: *The Mentally Disabled and the Law*. University of Chicago Press, Chicago, 1971.

37. SALES, B, POWELL, D, VAN DUIZEND, R, ET AL: *Disabled Persons and the Law*. Plenum, New York, 1982.

38. Drope v. Missouri, 420 U.S. 162 (1975) (p 172).

39. MEISEL, A: *The rights of the mentally ill under state constitutions*. Journal of Law and Contemporary Problems 45:7-40, 1982.

40. Jackson v. Indiana, 406 U.S. 715 (1972).

41. Pate v. Robinson, 383 U.S. 375 (1966).

42. FOOTE, C: *A comment on pre-trial commitment of criminal defendants*. University of Pennsylvania Law Review 108:832-846, 1960.

43. BURT, R AND MORRIS, N: *A proposal for the abolition of the incompetency plea*. University of Chicago Law Review 40:66-95, 1972.

44. AMERICAN BAR ASSOCIATION STANDING COMMITTEE ON ASSOCIATION STANDARDS FOR CRIMINAL JUSTICE: *Proposed Criminal Justice Mental Health Standards*. American Bar Association, Chicago, 1984 (adopted August 1984).

45. WILLIAMS, G: *Criminal Law: The General Part*, ed 2. Stevens, London, 1961.

46. HART, HLA: *Punishment and Responsibility*. Oxford University Press, New York, 1968.

47. GOLDSTEIN, AS: *The Insanity Defense*. Yale University Press, New Haven, CT, 1967.

48. LAFAVE, W AND SCOTT, A: *Handbook of Criminal Law*. West Publishing, St Paul, MN, 1972.

49. WEIHOFEN, H: *Mental Disorder as a Criminal Defense*. Dennis, Buffalo, NY, 1954.

50. SINGER, AC: *The imposition of the insanity defense on an unwilling defendant*. Ohio State Law Journal 41:637-673, 1980.

51. Frendak v. United States, 408 A.2d 364 (D.C. Ct. Ap. 1979).

52. Nail v. State, 328 S.W. 2d 836 (Ark. 1959).

53. Reece v. State, 94 S.E. 2d 723 (Ga. 1956).

54. Washington v. State, 85 N.W. 2d 509 (Neb. 1957).

55. State v. Huff, 102 A.2d 8 (N.J. 1954).

56. BROWN, B AND COURTLESS, T: *The mentally retarded in penal and correctional institutions*. Am J Psychiatry 124:1164-1170, 1968.

57. PERSON, J: *The accused retardate*. Columbia Human Rights Law Review 4:239-266, 1972.

58. TUPIN, J AND GOOLISHIAN, H: *Mental retardation and legal responsibility.* Depaul Law Review 18:673-682, 1969.

59. ALLEN, R: *The retarded offender: Unrecognized in court and untreated in prison.* Federal Probation 32(3):22-27, 1969.

60. BURGESS, H: *The mental defective and the law.* Intramural Law Review of New York University 23:115-134, 1967.

61. DIX, G: *Psychological abnormality as a factor in grading criminal liability: Diminished capacity, diminished responsibility, and the like.* Journal of Criminal Law, Criminology and Political Science 62:313-334, 1971.

62. *A punishment rationale for diminished capacity.* UCLA Law Review 18:561-580, 1971.

63. *Diminished capacity—recent decisions and an analytical approach.* Vanderbilt Law Review 30:213-257, 1977.

64. ARENELLA, P: *The diminished capacity and diminished responsibility defenses: Two children of a doomed marriage.* Columbia Law Review 77:827-865, 1977.

65. MORSE, S: *Diminished capacity: A moral and legal conundrum.* Int J Law Psychiatry 2:271-298, 1979.

66. United States v. Brawner, 471 F.2d 969 (D.C. Cir. 1972).

67. Bethea v. United States, 365 A.2d 64 (D.C. Ct. Ap. 1976).

68. State v. Wilcox, 70 Ohio State 2d 182, 436 N.E.2d 523 (1982).

69. State v. Nichols, 3 Ohio App. 2d 182, 209 N.E.2d 750 (1965).

70. Pigman v. State, 14 Ohio 555 (1846).

71. Hughes v. Mathews, 576 F.2d 1250 (7th Cir. 1978).

72. Muench v. Isreal, 715 F.2d 1124 (7th Cir. 1983).

73. MORRIS, N: *Madness and the Criminal Law.* University of Chicago Press, Chicago, 1982.

74. ALLEN, FA: *The Decline of the Rehabilitative Ideal: Penal Policy and Social Purpose.* Yale University Press, New Haven, CT, 1981.

75. CARTER, RM: *Presentence Report Handbook.* National Institute of Law Enforcement, US Department of Justice, Washington, DC, 1978.

76. *Symposium: The death penalty.* Criminal Law Bulletin 14:7-80, 1978.

77. VAN DEN HAAG, E AND CONRAD, JP: *The Death Penalty: A Debate.* Plenum, New York, 1983.

78. LIEBMAN, J AND SHEPHARD, M: *Guiding capital sentencing discretion beyond the "boiler plate": Mental disorder as a mitigating factor.* Georgetown Law Journal 66:757-836, 1978.

79. People v. Lally, 277 N.Y.S.2d 654 (1966).

80. Bolton v. Harris, 395 F.2d 642 (D.C. Cir. 1968).

81. Jones v. United States, 103 S.Ct. 3043 (1983).

82. Addington v. Texas, 441 U.S. 418 (1979).

83. Spicer v. Williamson, 191 N.C. 487, 132 S.E. 291 (1926).

84. Estelle v. Gamble, 429 U.S. 97 (1976).

85. KLEIN, S: *Prisoner's rights to physical and mental health care: A modern expansion of the eighth amendment's cruel and unusual punishment clause.* Fordham Urban Law Journal 7:1-33, 1979.

86. Bowring v. Godwin, 551 F.2d 44 (4th Cir. 1977).

87. Wyatt v. Stickney, 325 F. Supp. 781, 344 F. Supp. 373, 381 (M.D. Ala. 1971) aff'd sub nom Wyatt v. Aderholt, 503 F.2d 1305 (5th Cir. 1974).

88. Welsch v. Likins, 373 F. Supp. 487 (D. Minn. 1974).

89. Davis v. Watkins, 384 F. Supp. 1196 (N.D. Ohio 1974).

90. Youngberg v. Romeo, 457 U.S. 307 (1982).

PART 3

THE CHILD, THE FAMILY, AND THE COMMUNITY: LEGAL PERSPECTIVES

This part of the text does not deal with particular diagnostic categories, as will the next two parts. Rather, the focus of the three chapters here is upon family and community concerns, particularly those forensic situations involving marriage, divorce, child custody, child and spouse abuse, and criminal conduct or delinquency of children and adolescents.

Many textbooks in forensic psychiatry and psychology ignore these issues. This is due in part to the subspecialization of the field. Many forensic mental health services deal only with adults, and many serve only adult criminal courts or prisons. In recent decades, however, forensic mental health services for family courts and juvenile courts have been growing considerably.

The first chapter in this part deals broadly with issues of family violence. It is pointed out that family disturbances are by far the most common of community complaints to local police all across the United States. Dr. Rosenbaum offers estimates of the prevalence of family violence, including the prediction that some 30 percent of all marriages will experience serious violence committed on its members by others in the family unit.

Although the research literature on child abuse and neglect is voluminous, the research output—especially of empirical studies—on marital violence is sparse and of limited utility. Spousal violence is surprisingly mutual with an almost equal distribution between husbands and wives in the studies by Straus and his associates. The most serious injuries are clearly to wives, however. Therefore, the chapter's concentration is upon spousal violence as it relates to women.

Particularly compelling are the author's concerns with ethical issues in this field. They relate to problems and dilemmas of confidentiality and the prediction of violent conduct discussed in earlier chapters. All 50 states now have enacted mandatory reporting laws on child abuse and neglect. No discretion is left to therapists in complying with the reporting requirements, which apply even on a first visit of a family to a professional. The discussion focuses not only upon the effect of this lack of confidentiality and privacy in such relationships but upon the lack of effectiveness and follow-up by social agencies in coping with the cases after they are reported. The author points to large-scale underreporting of child abuse, including conscious refusal to comply with the legal requirement in the belief that the reporting could be detrimental to the child's welfare. Nevertheless, it is pointed out that professional ethical principles in medicine and psychology allow or sanction breaches of patient or client confidences when danger to a child is seriously threatened. In the case of interspousal violence, ethical principles and the *Tarasoff* decision support reporting to relevant social agencies and the police.

Chapters 11 and 12 deal with other issues concerning child welfare and community interests. Dr. McGarry's chapter reviews legal and professional aspects of child-custody disputes in divorce and separation litigation. Dr. Widom's contribution provides a wide-ranging criminological review of juvenile offenders and the juvenile justice system.

Dr. McGarry cites estimates that about 10 percent of divorces in this country involve litigation over child custody. The author reviews the legal standards for awarding child custody to one or the other parent, and he analyzes the recently enacted statutes providing for joint custody. The participation of mental health professionals in custody matters can involve three types of roles: therapeutic, mediative, and consultative. The most traditional involvement is found in providing theatment for troubled marital partners during the marriage; during the dispute period over a separation, divorce, or custody; and during the later life of one or the other of the former marital partners. Forensic psychiatrists and psychologists are most often involved in the latter two roles, those of a mediator and consultant. The professional mediator is given an opportunity to arrange a reconciliation or to work out a satisfactory arrangement for disposing of all issues, including child custody, in the separation or divorce. In consultative roles, the forensic specialist may advise the trial judge on specific custody issues—including attention to the medical, psychiatric, and psychological needs of the child or children—whatever the judge's decision on custody.

Dr. McGarry asserts that the major contribution of clinicians as forensic consultants in custody disputes lies in their exploration of the significance of mental disturbance in either or both parents, which may have a bearing on the child custody decision. These disturbances can include psychotic illness, personality disorder, or certain relevant character traits or destructive behavioral practices. The author examines research studies evaluating the impact of these factors upon the children. He notes that some children may have special vulnerabilities, but others, even in the same families, may display little or no discernible deleterious effects. In making specific recommendations and in the tone of general observations, Dr. McGarry warns against the effect upon forensic consultants of the tactics that may be employed by contesting parties in these highly volatile custody disputes. He suggests that forensic evaluators be aware of the effect of narcissistic expectations and priorities of the parents upon their handling of the custody issues. The parent who feels cheated or deprived of certain entitlements in the marriage may act out these resentments in a fight over custody, using the children as a "bargaining chip" to gain other objectives or in seeking to hurt or to embarrass the other party with accusations of unfitness for custody. The evaluator can help the parents deal with their narcissistic feelings, healthy or unhealthy, and to allow the custody issues to proceed to determination on the basis of the best interests of the child.

In chapter 12, Dr. Widom takes a broadly interdisciplinary approach to her subject, juvenile delinquency. The author is jointly appointed to the Department of Forensic Studies (particularly related to criminology and police science) and the Department of Psychology at Indiana University. Both areas of her academic interest are displayed in the chapter. The opening pages examine the major theories of delinquency causation. Research in the field has provided support for a multiplicity of etiological factors, including biological and genetic elements. Social and psychological factors are also recognized, including family disruption and disorganization, limited opportunities to achieve more conventional goals, conformity to a subculture of deviant values and behavior, academic failure, unemployment, and poverty.

The author reviews programs of deinstitutionalization and diversion from the juvenile correctional system. The programs are particularly aimed at eliminating from the criminally oriented facilities those "status offenders" who have not committed violent or antisocial actions but who are convicted only of running away from home, incorrigibility, sexual promiscuity, or truancy. These cases are estimated at nearly 40 percent of defendants before the juvenile courts of the country. Dr. Widom casts considerable doubt, however, on the assumption that this class of offenders is not involved in a wider range of delinquent conduct. She also points out that diversion to community programs does not always lead to more humane and beneficial handling of youthful offenders. This type of legal processing often results in a widening rather than a narrowing of the scope of offenders involved, because many complaints would have been dismissed under a more formal court review.

CHAPTER 10
FAMILY VIOLENCE
Alan Rosenbaum, Ph.D.

Family violence shocks us not only because of the magnitude and seriousness of the problem but also because of the contradiction it poses to the popular conceptions of what a family should be. Our conceptions of a family are fostered by the media, our religious institutions, our literary heritage, and, most importantly, by the very basic needs for love, security, and stability that humans share. Family violence has long been the undetected cancer in our society. Until 1962, when Kempe and coworkers[1] drew popular attention to child abuse by introducing the battered-child syndrome into our collective vocabularies, family violence flourished behind closed doors. It was secure from the interference of society's legal institutions, protected by laissez-faire policies—which viewed a man's home as his castle—and differential enforcement of existing assault-and-battery legislation. Over the past two decades the castle walls have been penetrated, at least to the extent that family violence has become more visible and is now the focus of social, political, legislative, and professional attention.

The statistics are truly horrifying. A person is considerably more likely to be killed by a member of his or her own family than by a stranger.[2] Domestic disturbance is by far the most common call received by police. It has been estimated that as many as 30 percent of all marriages will at some point involve the use of physical violence[2] and that, annually, as many as two million children may be abused by their parents[3] in the United States alone. Even the elderly are being victimized by their children and grandchildren. Adult abuse is the most recent addition to the family violence tree. It seems as though no family member is immune. All forms of family violence considered, it is estimated that between five and six million children, spouses, and elderly individuals are neglected, battered, and abused in the United States every year.[4] The family may very well be the most violent of our social institutions.

Historically, the use of violence against family members has been prescribed rather than proscribed. Wives and children have traditionally been considered the legal property of the husband and parents, respectively. English common law, which formed the basis for our American legal system, recognized the right of the husband to chastise his wife for misbehavior. In Massachusetts, the Stubborn Child Law of 1646 permitted the killing of a child for disobedience. Even such common phrases as the "rule of thumb" are rooted in our heritage of domestic violence. The "rule of thumb" is purported to have referred to the permissibility of beating one's wife with a rod as long as the thickness of the rod did not exceed the thickness of the husband's thumb. It is a sad commentary indeed that the Society for the Prevention of Cruelty to Animals in New York City predated its counterpart for the prevention of cruelty to children.

Although the legal status of domestic violence has changed dramatically, the family remains the only social structure, with the exception of the police and the military, for which we still describe a legitimate use of violence. Physical punishment is used by between 84 percent and 97 percent of parents,[2] and discriminating between the legitimate physical punishment of a misbehaving child and child abuse is one of the most difficult problems confronting child-protective workers, legislators, and the courts. In their nationally representative sample of 2143 husbands and wives, Straus and his colleagues[2] found violence to be so common as to necessitate creation of the construct "normal violence" to describe such acts as spanking children or slapping a spouse; acts which have traditionally "been taken for granted as necessary, useful, inevitable or instinctive" and to distinguish such acts from the more abusive and serious forms of violence. It does not speak well of our culture that phrases such as "normal violence" are acceptable parlance.

The social and legal acceptance of domestic violence, the absence of reporting laws or agencies to report to, the inadequacy of social services for victims of domestic violence, and the shame and stigma of such victimization are a few of the factors that contributed to the invisibility of family violence and to the illusion that such problems either did not exist or were insubstantial. The various mental health professions were conspicuous in their inattention to these problems, with the consequence that our knowledge of the parameters of domestic violence, the characteristics and etiology of these problems, and how to effectively treat families characterized by violence is rudimentary and inadequate. This is particularly unfortunate, given the fact that the mental health professions are commonly referral sources for the treatment of both the victims and the perpetrators of family violence.

DEMOGRAPHY, ETIOLOGY, AND THEORY

Child Maltreatment

Child abuse is defined as the nonaccidental or intentional maltreatment of a child either through the commission of a harmful act or the omission of some necessary caregiving behavior by a parent or some other caretaker.[5] Child abuse thus encompasses the more active forms of abuse, including violence, torture, and emotional mistreatment, as well as the more passive forms, normally classified as neglect. Whereas the term child abuse usually evokes images of physical violence, neglect may actually be more common and, as a few have suggested, more detrimental to the welfare of the child.[6] Neglect involves the failure to provide proper care, including nourishment, medical care, appropriate clothing, supervision, and attention to the personal hygiene of the child. Data collected by the American Humane Association[7] indicate that 58 percent of reported cases of maltreatment are for neglect only, and an additional 15 percent are for abuse and neglect. Furthermore, lethalities resulting from neglect may actually outnumber lethalities resulting from physical abuse.[6] Failure to thrive concerns the failure of a young child to grow and to develop properly and may result from neglect, physical abuse, or both. Legally and practically there is little need to distinguish among the various forms of abuse. As Fontana[8] stated, "the distinction is of little value to a child in need of help." However, from a research perspective, there is disagreement over whether abuse and neglect should be differentiated. Steele[9] stated, "The parents of infants who fail to thrive are essentially not much different from parents who abuse their offspring." But there is recent evidence to the contrary,[10,11] suggesting that neglecting parents may differ in background experiences, relationship with their own parents, and in level of pathology from abusing parents. Except where noted, this chapter will not differentiate among the various forms of abuse but, rather, will use the term child abuse to include maltreatment resulting from acts of commission as well as omission. This does not reflect a belief in the rightness of that position but a concession to the broad scope of the current chapter. It should also be noted that the definitions of abuse and neglect differ across different geographic areas[12] and across cultures,[13] further complicating the picture.

Our knowledge of the etiology of child abuse is inadequate, despite the fact that almost three hundred articles purporting to address the causative factors relating to child abuse have been published since 1967. Although it is not the purpose of this chapter to critically evaluate the research literature, a few comments are in order. Plotkin, Azar, Twentyman, and Perri[14] recently examined the existing literature pertaining to the cause of child abuse. In all, they reviewed and evaluated 270 articles. They found that only 25 percent were based on original data collected by the authors and that 75 percent were based on clinical impression. Furthermore, even those employing empirical methodologies often lacked the appropriate comparison groups and inferential statistics necessary for valid interpretation of the data. Their warning that despite the fact that "hundreds of published papers have addressed the issue of etiology, this should not foster the sense of assurance that we are approaching an understanding of the controlling variables of this phenomenon" seems well taken. However, most phenomenologists and clinicians would be quick to defend the validity of clinical impression and observation. Nevertheless, there are many inconsistencies and incongruities in the literature, and often when a widely held belief about child abuse is put to the empirical test, it fails to be substantiated. An excellent case in point concerns one of the more popular models of child abuse which posits that child abuse is related to a defect in the attachment process, resulting from a failure of bond formation.[15] Although theoretically appealing, empirical validation has not been forthcoming.[16] It is necessary to view much of the literature on etiology as suggestive rather than definitive and to bear in mind that most is based on clinical impression, which may or may not withstand empirical scrutiny.

Child abuse occurs in all cultural and ethnic groups and at all socioeconomic status (SES) levels.[17] Mothers and fathers are equally likely to be the abuser,[7] but mothers are more likely to be the perpetrators of the more serious forms of child abuse.[2,17]

It is clear from the literature that child abuse is multidetermined. There is not a typical child abuser, but there are numerous factors that are often associated with abuse. Belsky[18] presents an excellent conceptual scheme for integrating the various findings. His framework consists of four levels of analysis: (1) ontogenic development, which includes the background experiences of the parents, as well as their individual psychological structure; (2) the microsystem, the interactions within the immediate household, including the characteristics of, and interactions with, the child; (3) the exosystem, which concerns the current environmental stressors and influences; and (4) the macrosystem, the sociocultural context in which violence occurs.

The characteristic that is most consistently found in the background of abusive parents is a history of maltreatment in their own childhood.[19,20] This maltreatment may be in the form of physical abuse; however, it has been suggested that a defective relationship with the parents may be a more consistent finding.[21] Altemeier[21] reported that significantly more mothers in the abuse category did not get along with or were separated from their own mothers. The incidence of living in foster care was eight times as common among mothers of abused children. Abusive parents are often reported to have low self-esteem[22] and to abuse alcohol.[20,23] There is evidence that abusive parents are more likely to be suffering from emotional disorders, but no particular pattern of emotional disturbance has emerged.[10]

Concerning the microsystem, large families and inadequate spacing between children appear to increase the likelihood of abuse.[24,25] The most extreme example of inadequate spacing, twin births, is particularly predictive of maltreatment.[26] The most important microsystem factor may be the contributions of the child victim.

Family violence and rape are crimes for which the victim is often blamed for his or her own victimization, a phenomenon which is seldom observed in other forms of victimization. There is an undercurrent of resistance to blaming the victim,[27] yet family violence is one of the few forms of victimization in which the victim and perpetrator are involved in an intimate, often intense, relationship. There is little question that violence evolves out of this relationship, and to ignore the contributions of the victim to that interaction, merely because it might be politically unsavory, would be to ignore potentially important information, thus jeopardizing both our understanding of the phenomenon and our therapeutic effectiveness.

There has been an increasing tendency to look at the contribution of the child to the provocation of abuse. The focus has been on the characteristics of the child, "what the child is"; and on the behavior of the child, "what the child does." Various reports have suggested that abused children are often premature and have low birth weight,[29] are illegitimate or conceived premaritally,[30] have congenital defects, physical handicaps, and mental retardation.[31] Few studies have actually examined the circumstances surrounding the occurrence of abuse, but those that have generally identify the child as the provocateur.[32,33] Aggressive behavior, hostility, and general misbehavior are the most frequently cited precursors of abuse.[32,34] Although some of these child characteristics have been supported by empirical research (for example, prematurity), others have not (for example, handicaps).[29] A recent empirical study of the precursors of child abuse[29] concluded that the various circumstances surrounding the various types of maltreatment accounted for only a small percentage of the variance associated with maltreatment. Although the child's behavior may be an important part of the parent-child interactions that evolve into abuse, the parent's behavior is a major factor in determining whether the outcome is violent.

Much of the literature on family violence has been contributed by sociologists, preeminently by Murray Straus and his associates and students at the University of New Hampshire. Consequently, there has been a great deal of attention to the contributions of social stress to the production of all forms of domestic violence. These are the exosystem factors and they include job-related stress, financial difficulties and unemployment, as well as isolation and inadequate social networks. Although abuse cuts across socioeconomic groups, there is a clear relationship between economic stress and child abuse. Maltreatment is more likely to occur in families experiencing unemployment.[24,35] Declines in the work force, one of the best measures of socioeconomic stress, are significantly related to reported child abuse.[11] In addition to unemployment, there appears to be a relationship between job dissatisfaction and child maltreatment.[36] Child abuse, as well as all other forms of family violence, is more common in the lower socioeconomic strata.[37]

Socioeconomic stress is but one form of stress that has been associated with child abuse. Justice and Duncan[38] compared the life-stress inventory of 35 child-abusive families to 35 matched, nonabusive control families and found significantly more ongoing life stress in the abusive families. Utilizing a prospective approach, Egeland and coworkers[39] confirmed highly significant differences between life-event scores of mothers providing adequate care and those of mothers providing inadequate care. They concluded that environmental stress was an important factor in the etiology of child maltreatment. Another stress commonly associated with child abuse is the marital discord that frequently exists in abusive families.[18,20]

The final exosystem factor that has received considerable support concerns the social isolation of abusive families. It has been widely asserted that abusive families tend to be isolated from both family support and from the support of community organizations.[20,40,42] Kempe[43] suggested that abusive families lack a "lifeline," meaning that they do not have people to turn to, or to rely on, in times of stress. It has also been suggested that social isolation promotes abuse by depriving these families of role models of appropriate parenting behavior and also of corrective feedback.[44,45]

Finally, the influence of the macrosystem on the etiology of child abuse concerns the cultural context in which child abuse occurs. Our society is a violent one. It is one in which violence toward family members is treated differently from violence between strangers. The corporal punishment of children by parents is approved of and practiced by the majority of the population, and the right of school personnel to physically discipline misbehaving children has even been recognized by the Supreme Court. It may be significant that child abuse is rare in countries that discourage the physical punishment of children.

The interrelationships among the four levels of analysis are indeed complex. A history of maltreatment appears to be highly predictive of abusing one's own child, yet the majority of people who have been maltreated by their own parents do not abuse their children. There is a strong association between unemployment and child abuse, yet the majority of the unemployed and lower SES individuals are not abusive. Prematurity, low birth weight, birth defects, and retardation may be common among abused children, but the majority of children born with such difficulties are not maltreated. Markham[20] proposes that "child abuse occurs when the substantial stress of child rearing is super-imposed on already strained emotional and environmental resources." Perhaps a diathesis-stress model is most parsimonious. The parents' developmental history and psychological makeup (ontogenic development) predispose them to maltreat their children, given certain stresses imposed by family (microsystem) and/or society (exosystem). As Belsky[18] concludes, the response to stress takes the form of child maltreatment both because the parent has learned a violent role model as a result of childhood maltreatment (ontogenic development) and because of the values and child-rearing practices that characterize the sociocultural context (macrosystem) in which abuse occurs.

Marital Violence

Marital violence is typically defined as the nonaccidental, physical assault on one spouse by the other, with the intent to inflict pain or injury. Although most of the literature is concerned with physical violence, it is increasingly recognized that physical abuse rarely occurs in the absence of emotional or psychological abuse, whereas the latter often occurs independently of the former and may be equally—if not more—damaging to the victim. Marital violence and child abuse share many commonalities in terms of the characteristics of the perpetrators, etiological factors, and the effects on the victims; however, there are also important differences. Child abuse presents definitional problems; marital violence does not. Although there are those who might disagree, it is generally accepted that there is a legitimate use of physical punishment in raising children. There is not, however, a corresponding legitimate use of physical violence between spouses. Consequently, any use of violence between spouses can be defined as abuse, whereas in the case of children there is a much finer line between acceptable punishment and abuse. A second important distinction concerns the mutuality of spousal violence. Recent research by Straus and his associates[2] indicates that in almost half (49 percent) of the cases of spouse abuse, both the husband and wife had used violence toward each other. Perpetrator and victim are much more clearly delineated in cases of child abuse. A third distinction concerns the relative helplessness of the victim. The highest incidence of child abuse is purported to occur in children under the age of three years.[30] As such, child victims are truly helpless and at the mercy of their caretakers. Although victims of marital violence are often without adequate resources, they are somewhat better off than the child victim.

Most of the literature on marital violence contains some statement bemoaning the dearth of methodologically sound research or the lack of professional interest in this area. Gelles[46] is typical in pointing out that prior to 1970 a literature search would have yielded only two scholarly articles on wife abuse. Since 1970, a great deal has been written and published about marital violence, yet the lack of empirically validated knowledge remains a legitimate complaint.

Professional ignorance regarding the characteristics of violent couples and effective methods of dealing with marital violence is very serious, especially when one considers the magnitude of the problem. Marital violence may affect as many as 30 percent of all married couples at some time in the course of their marital relationship.[2] One estimate suggests that a woman is beaten once every 30 seconds. [47] The consequences of marital violence are equally shocking. Wife abuse often results in injuries requiring medical attention and resulting in permanent deformities, traumatic injuries, miscarriages, and possibly death. Approximately one eighth of all homicides are interspousal, and not uncommonly the abusive husband is the victim,[48] his wife driven to murder by the (not unrealistic) belief that it may be her only escape from the abuse. Abused wives frequently suffer from a host of stress-related disorders, both mental and physical. Gayford[49] reported that almost half of the abused wives in his sample had been referred for psychiatric evaluation, and 21 percent were consequently diagnosed as depressed. Almost three quarters of his sample were taking either tranquilizers or antidepressants, and more than half had attempted suicide at least once. Furthermore, families characterized by marital violence are significantly more vulnerable to child abuse, and children who witness marital violence often exhibit concurrent behavioral or emotional difficulties and frequently grow up to abuse their own spouses.[50,51]

Marital violence cuts across all socioeconomic, ethnic, and religious groups but may be especially prevalent in the lower socioeconomic strata. Although marital violence is often equated with wife abuse, it has become apparent that husbands and wives are equally likely to be violent toward each other;[2] however, there is substantial agreement that wife abuse is the more serious problem. Because the vast majority of the literature and research regarding marital violence focuses on wife abuse, for the purposes of the present chapter we will be concerned primarily with wife abuse; thus, except when it is otherwise specified, marital violence and spouse abuse will refer mainly to wife abuse.

Marital violence is particularly difficult to study, largely because the abusive husbands are frequently reluctant to participate in research or therapy. In contrast to child abuse, there are no mandatory reporting laws for spouse abuse and no agencies specifically charged with dealing with marital violence. Much of our information, of necessity, is obtained from abused wives, who may not be the best sources of information regarding their assailants, and from those husbands who are willing to participate in research or therapy and who may therefore be atypical. Additionally, many of the methodological problems discussed with regard to the child-abuse literature are equally relevant here, specifically the lack of appropriate comparison groups; the prevalence of descriptive, rather than inferential, statistics; and the failure to employ valid, standardized measures in operationalizing many of the constructs being investigated.[46,52] The "Woozle effect,"[53] which refers to the repeated citing of the results of inadequate research studies until the findings attain the status of facts and the poor quality of the research is forgotten, has unfortunately operated in this area. As a result we have numerous myths about marital violence, many of which have not been supported by empirical investigation. A case in point concerns the myth that abused wives come from violent family backgrounds, a myth supported by earlier, uncontrolled, research. The addition of comparison samples of nonabused wives from both discordant and satisfactory family backgrounds later showed the finding to be artifactual.[52] In fact, Star[54] reported that violence was actually more prevalent in the backgrounds of nonbattered women, though not significantly so.

Although Belsky[18] developed his conceptual scheme to integrate the findings regarding child abuse, his four levels of analysis appear to be equally relevant to marital violence. Ontogenic development again appears to play a most significant role in the etiology of marital violence. Coleman and associates[55] compared maritally violent men with a nonviolent sample and reported that the most significant discriminant was a history of having witnessed parental conjugal violence and being hit as a child, a finding replicated by Rosenbaum and O'Leary.[52] Abusive husbands have also been shown to have defective self-concepts,[56] to abuse alcohol,[57] to have assertiveness deficits (specifically with their wives),[52] and to have generalized aggression problems.[55]

Microsystem factors again include the contributions of the victim to the violent family system. The verbal and physical aggression of the wife toward the husband may be a significant contributing factor. It has been established that wife-toward-husband violence is as common (though perhaps not as serious) as husband-toward-wife violence. An important question for future research would be the extent to which wife-toward-husband violence is retaliatory, as opposed to initiative. Marital violence clearly emerges from a discordant marital relationship. Coleman and coworkers[55] reported frequent marital arguments to discriminate violent from nonviolent marriages, and similarly, Rosenbaum and O'Leary[52] found degree of marital discord to be the most important factor in discriminating maritally violent couples from their nonviolent counterparts. Pregnancy of the wife (especially the first pregnancy) is often associated with abuse,[58] an association that has been attributed to the prospect of sharing the affections of the wife with another, the increased financial burden anticipated, and the addition of potentially highly charged topics for argument—such as how to raise the child, what to name the child, who should care for the child, and so forth. Such potentially intense arguments become even more likely if the couple is characterized by ideological, racial, or religious differences. Interestingly, there is research supporting the prevalence of both racial[59] and religious[54] intermarriages in violent couples.

Exosystem factors in the marital violence area are similar to those reported for child abuse. Abusive husbands are more likely to be either unemployed or dissatisfied with their jobs.[60] Families characterized by marital violence are more socially isolated[61] and tend to experience more stress as measured by life change.[59] A final exosystem factor that has been empirically established concerns status inconsistency and status incompatibility,[62] both of which have been shown to be associated with an increased risk of psychological abuse, physical abuse, and life-threatening violence between spouses. Overachievement in occupation by the wife is associated with a high incidence and prevalence of spousal violence, whereas overachievement by the husband is associated with a lower incidence and prevalence of violence. Couples with educational incompatibilities, particularly if the wife's attainments are low relative to the husband's, experience a high incidence of marital violence.[62]

As with child abuse, marital violence occurs in a sociocultural context that historically and concurrently supports, legitimizes, even romaticizes its occurrence. The portrayal of violence against women is used to sell jeans, to decorate record album covers, and to get laughs in classic situation comedies such as *The Honeymooners.* The macrosystem factors also include a legal system that treats marital violence differently from violence between strangers. Marital rape exemptions in most states, for example, still permit a husband to rape his wife.[63] Statistics support the conclusion that a husband accused of wife abuse is often admonished but infrequently convicted or sentenced.[64] Police, for a variety of reasons—not the least of which is the fact that more policemen are killed while intervening in a domestic disturbance than in response to any other type of call—are reluctant to get involved, further supporting the permissibility of marital violence.

It is possible to integrate the findings that have been presented into a conceptual framework. In this scheme, wife abuse is seen as evolving out of marital discord. Many of the ontogenic, microsystem, and exosystem factors are conceptualized as contributing to the production of marital discord, thus alcohol use by the husband; financial difficulties and job dissatisfaction; ideological, racial, or religious differences; and status inconsistencies or incompatibility produce marital discord. The wife is seen as a full partner to the production of this distress; however, whether or not the discord becomes violent is seen as a function of the ontogenic development of the husband. If the husband comes from a violent family background, has low self-esteem, or has difficulty properly asserting himself with his wife, the probability of violence is increased. Other factors that may increase the probability of violence include the use of violence by the wife and the influences of the macrosystem.

LEGAL AND ETHICAL ISSUES

Child Maltreatment

Every state currently has mandatory reporting laws which require certain professionals to report known or suspected cases of child abuse and neglect to designated governmental authorities. The professions bound by the statutes vary from state to state, but most include any profession dealing with children, such as teachers, physicians, nurses, psychologists, and social workers. The states differ not only with respect to the professions that are mandated but also with respect to the agencies to whom the report is made and the penalties for failing to report. Mandatory reporting laws are based on the principle of *parens patriae*, or the right of the state to assume parental powers to protect the best interests of "defenseless" children. In addition to protecting the child, the reporting laws are designed to protect the person making the report. The law is intended to take the decision of whether to report out of the hands of the reporting professional. Most state laws protect the identity of the reporter by withholding identifying information from the family. Finally, in most states, the reporter is protected from legal liability if the report turns out to be unfounded, provided the report was made "in good faith."[65] Although the spirit of the mandatory reporting law seems laudable, the fact that reporting is mandated for even the suspicion of abuse and that each report must be thoroughly investigated by the state makes this law one of the most intrusive and questionable from a constitutional standpoint. Our society is one that values the principle of family autonomy, and protecting families from excessive control by the state has been fundamental in our legal and political processes.[20] The Supreme Court has repeatedly validated the right of an adult to privacy within the family unit and has vociferously protected that right by strictly limiting governmental interference.[66] The American Civil Liberties Union, a dedicated watchdog of our constitutional rights, referred to the mandatory reporting laws as "reminiscent of totalitarianism."[67]

Constitutional issues aside, mandatory reporting laws have been questioned on the basis of whether the best interests of the child are truly served by reporting. Most states have established child-protective agencies within their departments of social services to serve as the recipients of such reports. These agencies are often understaffed and overworked. If all cases of known or suspected child maltreatment were reported, as the law intends, these agencies could not possibly serve the population effectively. Furthermore, the remedies available to child-protective agencies are of questionable value. Removal of the child from the home, reassignment of custody, and foster care may serve to compound, rather than to ameliorate, the effects of child abuse. It is of interest that one of the more common reasons offered by physicians for failure to report is the belief that not reporting would actually be best for the child.

Despite the legal and ethical obligations imposed by the mandatory reporting laws, many physicians and mental health professionals fail to report child abuse. A recent survey conducted by the Journal of the American Medical Association found that one physician in four would refuse to report a suspected case of child abuse, even though he or she was aware that failure to report was a violation of the law.[67] A similar survey of mental health professionals concluded that a large proportion were either ignorant of or chose to ignore their legal obligation to report.[68]

Mandatory reporting laws create a conflict of ethics for many of the professionals involved. One of the foundations upon which the therapeutic relationship is built is confidentiality, and most mental health professionals consider it essential to the therapeutic process. The therapeutic contract implies that the patient can say anything, without fear that it will be used against him or her. Most practitioners fail to expound upon the possible exceptions to the doctrine of privileged communication when presenting the ground rules of therapy to the client and, therefore, consider it a breach of ethics to report knowledge or suspicions obtained under the client's mistaken belief that confidentiality will be protected. Whereas it normally is the therapist's responsibility to safeguard the confidentiality of information obtained in the context of therapy, the ethical guidelines do specify that it may be necessary to violate this principle when necessary to avoid clear and imminent danger to the client or others, or when a "specific requisite of the law takes precedence."[69]

Furthermore, the likelihood that betraying the client's confidence will ultimately result in the termination of the therapeutic relationship produces the dual negative consequences of loss of a paying customer and, perhaps more importantly, the lost opportunity to help the child and the family. This is especially relevant if the family has come in with a presenting problem of abuse and is asking for help in stopping the abuse. There do not appear to be many satisfactory ways to comply with the law without threatening (if not destroying) the therapist-client relationship. Although it is possible that a client will respect the therapist for setting limits and respecting his or her legal obligations, it seems unlikely that such understanding would coexist in a person experiencing the difficulties necessitating reporting in the first place. The consequences of informing the client at the outset of therapy as to the nature of the exceptions to the principle of privileged communication (while possibly easing the conscience of the therapist) need not be elaborated.

The consequences of failing to report vary across jurisdictions and may be quite severe. Some states provide civil consequences, some criminal consequences, and in many (for example, New York) both civil and criminal penalties may be imposed. In those states providing criminal penalties, failure to report is most commonly considered a misdemeanor. In New York State it is a Class A misdemeanor, which is punishable by up to a year in jail (NYS Penal Law #70.15). Civil penalties include the assessment of damages, monetary fines, and suspension or cancellation of professional license. The consequences of failing to report, although potentially quite severe, are infrequently invoked. Practitioners are seldom, if ever, prosecuted for failure to report. It is difficult to determine whether a practitioner had reasonable cause to suspect abuse, and furthermore, the legal obligation is to report known or suspected abuse. Therefore, the practitioner is held liable only if it can be established that he or she knew or suspected abuse (for example, from the case notes). Failure to suspect may be bad judgment, but, to date, it is not a legal or ethical violation.

There is no question that child abuse is a serious problem. The victims are harmed both physically and emotionally. The physical damage is often obvious, as are the fatalities. Child abuse is the fifth leading cause of death in children under the age of four years.[70] Less obvious are the short- and long-term emotional consequences. It has been reported that chronic abuse can impair intellectual functioning and school performance.[71] Abused children exhibit increased aggressive behavior, have difficulties interacting with peers and adults, and may have difficulties with emotional attachments and trust.[72] Adults who have been abused as children often abuse their own children and/or their spouses.[52] A study of violent inmates at San Quentin indicated that all experienced extreme violence as children.[73] Despite the reluctance of many professionals to comply with the reporting laws, the laws have coincided with a substantial increase in the volume of reported cases of abuse. There is also some evidence that the majority of reports made by professionals are authenticated. There remains the question of the value of these laws in preventing future abuse. Does the reporting of child abuse have positive consequences for the child? In one study, it was reported that abusive parents continued to abuse the child in 35 percent of the cases studied, despite the fact that a report had been made to the appropriate agency and had been followed by intervention.[74]

Marital Violence

Unlike child abuse, there are no laws requiring the reporting of marital violence. Physicians and mental health professionals, like other citizens, are permitted to report such violence to the authorities but are not protected from prosecution should the report turn out to be unfounded and the subject of the report choose to pursue legal recourse. Reports made in good faith, however, are unlikely to result in prosecution, even if they do prove to be unfounded. The question of ethics with respect to violating confidentiality in making a report to the authorities is, due to the absence of a legal mandate, not as clear-cut as with child abuse. The guiding principle again must be that confidentiality must be abrogated when there is knowledge of clear and present danger to the client or to some other person. The *Tarasoff* decision and the ethical guidelines evolving therefrom would suggest that if a therapist was working with an abusive husband (or wife) and had knowledge that the spouse was in imminent danger (or if the therapist was called by a spouse who was in the act of either beating or being beaten), it would be incumbent upon the therapist to notify the police and, if necessary, the intended victim (spouse).

Despite the absence of mandatory reporting laws, working with maritally violent populations poses some unusual ethical issues and also necessitates a knowledge of related legalities. In the course of working with abusive couples, it may become apparent that the violence cannot be controlled and that for this or some other reason the most therapeutic course would be for the couple to terminate the marriage. "With such couples, it is the therapist's ethical and moral responsibility to abdicate the role of relationship advocate and help the threatened person find protection."[75] Such help requires a knowledge of the services available for battered wives as well as a knowledge of the applicable legal procedures. The therapist should have available the telephone numbers of appropriate shelters, hotlines, social service agencies (welfare, child protective), and legal services. Most localities have legal aid societies or neighborhood legal services. Ironically, until recently if an abused wife pressed charges against her husband, he would be entitled to a public defender or court-appointed lawyer if needed, but she had to pay her lawyer, regardless of resources. Many states now provide legal counsel to either or both spouses, as needed.

Abused wives should be encouraged to document all instances of abuse with a physician. Physicians are encouraged to note the cause of injuries in the medical record when marital violence is involved and, if possible, to take color photographs, which should also be included in the medical record. Abused spouses should be advised that they might have a right to have their abuser arrested. In many states, most instances of spouse abuse are classified as misdemeanors, which means that if the police officer did not actually witness the abuse, he or she cannot make an arrest. New York City and California are two exceptions to this generality. California has made spouse abuse a specific statutory felony.

The most common protection afforded an abused spouse is the order of protection, or, in some jurisdictions, the peace bond. This is a court order that requires the husband to refrain from abusing his wife and may require him to leave the home, stay a certain distance away, cease any form of harassment, and/or to attend some form of counseling. The peace bond requires the payment of a sum of money which is held by the court and forfeited if the order is violated. Again, as with all the laws relating to family violence, the requirements of the order, the time it takes to obtain one, the penalties attached to violating it, and the agency issuing it vary from one jurisdiction to another. Some states require the initiation of divorce proceedings before an order is issued. Unfortunately, orders of protection may not be very effective in preventing abuse.[76] Penalties for violating the orders are often light and difficult to enforce.

Separation and divorce are often the most effective legal alternatives available to the abused spouse, yet even dissolution of the marriage is no guarantee of protection from abuse. All too often the abuse and harassment continue and may even intensify. Unfortunately, the judicial system frequently treats an ex-spouse more like a spouse than like a stranger, failing to provide adequate legal protection. In many states, for example, the marital rape exemption extends to ex-spouses.[63] In a rather infamous example, a woman in Central New York was convicted and sentenced to prison for murdering an ex-spouse who, she alledged, had kidnapped her and forced her to have sex with him at gunpoint—an act that would most certainly have been seen as self-defense given any other victim-perpetrator relationship.

TREATMENT

Family violence is often characteristic of couples and families presenting for a variety of marital, individual, and child problems; yet the shame, stigma, and fear of legal repercussions often prevent clients from revealing the existence of violence. Therapists are often unaware of family violence, even in families they have been treating for a long time, because they fail to specifically assess for it.

A knowledge of the risk factors can alert therapists to the need for inquiring about the possibility that abuse is occurring.

General Risk Factors

The following factors are associated with both child and wife abuse.

1. Violence in the family of origin. Clients who either witnessed parental conjugal violence or were themselves abused as children are at risk for both child and wife abuse.
2. A history of alcohol or drug abuse.
3. Low self-esteem.
4. A medical history of, or the presence of unexplained or poorly explained, injuries in the child or wife.
5. Isolation from community and/or family supports.
6. Unemployment and economic deprivation.
7. Above-average marital conflict.

Risk Factors for Child Abuse

In addition to the general factors, the presence of some combination of the following should alert the therapist to the possibilities of child abuse.

1. Child afraid of contact with adults. The child may shy away from contact or cringe when approached by the therapist.
2. Failure of the child to develop properly physically and/or intellectually.
3. Frequent unexplained absences from school.
4. Child unkempt, shabbily or inappropriately clothed, lack of appropriate hygiene.
5. Large family and/or inadequate spacing of children.
6. The existence of wife abuse.

Risk Factors for Wife Abuse

In addition to the general factors, the following should alert the therapist to the possibility that wife abuse is occurring.

1. Racial or religious intermarriage.
2. History of chronic physical illness, depression, and anxiety in the wife.
3. Status incompatibility between spouses.
4. Husband unable to assert himself properly with his wife.
5. A history of miscarriage, spontaneous abortion, or other pregnancy difficulties.

There is no formula specifying how many or what combination of risk factors predict family violence. The existence of one or more of the factors should prompt the therapist to make further inquiries. At present, there are no valid personality measures or other diagnostic instruments with assessment value for family violence. Research employing aggression and personality measures has failed to produce profiles with predictive value. Self-report inventories, such as the Conflict Tactics (CT) Scales,[77] are not generally used for clinical assessment but, rather, for quantifying family violence for research purposes. Asking appropriate questions of wives and children, when not in the presence of the husband or parents, is currently the most effective way of confirming or disconfirming the suspicions generated by the presence of the various risk factors.

Once violence is confirmed, protection of the victim becomes the ethical consideration that supersedes all others. Often protection of the victim will preclude the possibility of providing therapeutic intervention, as when the family withdraws from treatment following a therapist's report to the child protective agency or when the therapist advises the wife to call the shelter or to obtain an order of protection, thus jeopardizing marital therapy by alienating the abusive husband.

Child Maltreatment

Treatment strategies for child abuse typically involve teaching parents to handle their children more effectively. Behavioral approaches, specifically token reinforcement and contingency management, are ideally suited to teaching the parents how to control their children better without resorting to violence.[78] Approaches that reinforce positive interactions between parents and children appear to be superior to approaches that attempt to eliminate violent interactions without providing a more prosocial substitute. Reid and Taplin[79] have evaluated the effectiveness of techniques based on social learning principles in teaching and maintaining noncoercive interactions to abusive families. Their program involves the use of audiovisual and bibliographic materials on child management, modeling of appropriate parenting skills, and instruction in social learning theory. Parents are taught to observe and to monitor various aspects of their child's behavior and to use positive reinforcement and time-out procedures for appropriate and inappropriate child behavior, respectively. Such training in parenting skills can be highly effective in reducing parent-child conflict in abusive homes.[80]

It is frequently observed that abusive parents have unrealistic expectations regarding their children. The term "role reversal" has been employed to describe the fact that abusive parents often expect their children to provide emotional support and tend to be dependent on their children, whereas the reverse is true of nonabusive parents. Unrealistically high expectations which the child cannot meet contribute to the attribution of willfulness to the child's inability to comply with parental demands. It may, therefore, be helpful to employ psychoeducational techniques to teach more age-appropriate expectations to abusive parents.

Finally, physical and/or mental defects in the child are commonly associated with abuse. Several mechanisms for this association have been proposed, including attachment or bonding difficulties. Another possibility is that these defects make the child more abrasive. The colicky child, for example, exhibits behavior that would try the patience of any parent. Parents with self-esteem deficits might be predisposed to interpret the child's inconsolable crying as a result of poor parenting. The child would be behaving in ways threatening to the parental self-concept and would, therefore, be a likely target of aggression. Additionally, a retarded child, or a child with some defect affecting his/her appearance might similarly threaten the self-esteem of a parent who has a defective self-concept. The relationship between self-esteem and child abuse would suggest that dealing with parental self-esteem would be a useful therapeutic strategy.

Marital Violence

Marital violence can be treated only if both husband and wife are willing to participate in therapy. Abused wives often are unable to involve their husbands and consequently are often offered support and advocacy as individuals or in groups. Providing the woman with the strengths and skills needed to live independently of her spouse is often the goal of this therapeutic approach. However, a frequent consequence may well be the termination of the relationship.

If, however, both partners are willing to participate in therapy, more options are available. Most commonly, therapy for such couples involves either conjoint marital therapy, group therapy for the batterer, or a combination of the two. The Marital Research Program at Syracuse University typically treats couples by placing the husband into the Men's Educational Workshop, a six-week, psychoeducational group. The group focuses on teaching lessons about wife abuse, getting the men to accept responsibility for their violence, and presenting behavioral techniques for controlling violent behavior. Most of the participants (some of whom are court mandated under the provisions of the New York State Family Court Act) start out disavowing responsibility for their abusive behavior, maintaining that they lose control (often due to the influence of drugs or alcohol), or that their wives provoke the abuse. The workshop leaders (typically a dual sex team) maintain that violence is a learned behavior, that behaving violently is a choice that the men make, and that they cannot be forced (least of all by the wife, who is typically smaller and weaker) to do anything they do not want to do. Although the wives may irritate or provoke them, provocation does not equal justification. Audiovisual materials (such as the "Time-Out" series—see Wachter and Boyd[81] for an excellent description of this film series) are employed to stimulate conversation about many of these issues. Finally, the participants are taught a variety of behaviorally based techniques for dealing with their own violence, including identifying the cues that violence is imminent, taking a time-out (leaving the situation, with the understanding that the conversation will be resumed once the spouses have cooled down and can deal with the issues nonviolently), engaging in nonviolent alternative activities (for example, jogging), assertiveness training, relaxation, and a cognitive approach to replacing anger-provoking self-statements. The reader is referred to Frank and Houghton[82] and Adams and McCormick[83] for excellent descriptions of alternative group approaches for wife abusers.

Workshop programs are often only part of the treatment strategy. Often the men have alcohol- or drug-related problems which must be dealt with as well. One goal of the Men's Educational Workshop is to formulate a continuation plan for each of the participants, following completion of the workshop. Typically this plan involves placing the couple into conjoint marital therapy, but also it will include appropriate referral to alcohol- or drug-rehabilitation programs and psychiatric treatment as indicated. There is some initial evidence that such workshop programs are effective in eliminating violence immediately, but perhaps equally important is the fact that workshop graduates frequently continue in various forms of therapy postworkshop.[82]

Social learning theory and psychodynamic theories are often incompatible. Methods of counseling couples based on the psychodynamic theories emphasize the importance of catharsis—the open expression or ventilation of hostile, aggressive feelings. However, there is research evidence provided by proponents of social learning theory that indicates that greater amounts of ventilation of aggressive feelings are associated with increased physical aggression. It has been recommended that counseling couples with abusive spouses should avoid the escalation of anger and hostility and focus on a more constructive problem-solving approach.[75] The reader is referred to Margolin[75] for a more detailed description of a conjoint approach to therapy for violent couples.

Marital therapists, like most mental health professionals, have paid relatively little attention to marital violence. Therapeutic approaches, for the most part, are little more than modifications of traditional intervention strategies for nonviolent couples. Furthermore, the outcome research necessary to assess the effectiveness of such strategies remains to be done. There is a potential danger to applying traditional approaches to this population. The widespread use of assertiveness training for battered wives is a case in point. One of the myths regarding battered wives is that they are unassertive and would benefit from assertiveness training approaches;[84] however, it has also been suggested that one cause of violence is the wife's assertiveness. It is possible that the use of assertiveness training with abused wives might actually intensify, rather than reduce, the frequency and severity of the abuse.

CONCLUSION

Family violence affects large segments of the population and has serious consequences for all members of the violent household and for society in general. There is strong evidence for the intergenerational transmission of violence, suggesting that family violence is self-perpetuating. Although mental health professionals are in an ideal position to intervene in violent families, only recently have they paid serious attention to these phenomena, and consequently there are important gaps in our knowledge of them. There is a need for methodologically sound empirical research into the characteristics of the participants, the etiology of violence, and the effectiveness of current treatment strategies.

REFERENCES

1. KEMPE, CH, SILVERMAN, FN, STEELE, BR, DROEGMUELLER, N, SILVER, HK: *The battered child syndrome.* JAMA 181:17, 1962.
2. STRAUS, MA, GELLES, RJ, STEINMETZ, SK: *Behind Closed Doors.* Anchor/Doubleday, New York, 1980.
3. GELLES, RJ: *Violence toward children in the United States.* Am J Orthopsychiatry 48:580, 1978.
4. KIRKLAND, K: *Assessment and treatment of family violence.* J Fam Pract 14:713, 1982.

5. BURGESS, RL AND GARBARINO, J: *Doing what comes naturally? An evolutionary perspective on child abuse.* In FINKELHOR, D, GELLES, RJ, HOTALING, GT, STRAUS, MA (EDS): *The Dark Side of Families.* Sage, Beverly Hills, CA, 1983.

6. CANTWELL, HB: *Child neglect.* In KEMPE, CH AND HELFER, RE (EDS): *The Battered Child.* University of Chicago Press, Chicago, 1980.

7. *American Humane Association national analysis of official child neglect and abuse reporting.* AHA, Englewood Cliffs, NJ, 1978.

8. FONTANA, VJ: *Somewhere a Child is Crying: Maltreatment—Causes and Prevention.* MacMillan, New York, 1973.

9. STEELE, B: *Psychodynamic factors in child abuse.* In KEMPE, CH AND HELFER, RE (EDS): *The Battered Child.* University of Chicago Press, Chicago, 1980.

10. FRIEDRICH, WN AND WHEELER, KK: *The abusing parent revisited: A decade of psychological research.* J Nerv Ment Dis 170:577, 1982.

11. MARTIN, MJ AND WALTERS, J: *Familial correlates of selected types of child abuse and neglect.* Journal of Marriage and the Family 44:267, 1982.

12. STEINBERG, LD, CATALANO, R, DOOLEY, D: *Economic antecedents of child abuse and neglect.* Child Dev 52:975, 1981.

13. KORBIN, JE: *The cross-cultural context of child abuse and neglect.* In KEMPE, CH AND HELFER, RE (EDS): *The Battered Child.* University of Chicago Press, Chicago, 1980.

14. PLOTKIN, RD, AZAR, S, TWENTYMAN, CT, PERRI, MG: *A critical evaluation of the research methodology employed in the investigation of causative factors of child abuse and neglect.* Child Abuse and Neglect 5:449, 1981.

15. AINSWORTH, MDS: *Attachment and child abuse.* In GERBNER, G, ROSS, CJ, ZIGLER, E (EDS): *Child Abuse.* Oxford University Press, New York, 1980.

16. EGELAND, B AND VAUGHN, B: *Failure of bond formation as a cause of abuse.* Am J Orthopsychiatry 51:78, 1981.

17. BLUMBERG, ML: *Child abuse in our violent society.* NY State J Med 80:921, 1980.

18. BELSKY, J: *Child maltreatment: An ecological integration.* Am Psychol 35:320, 1980.

19. STEELE, BB AND POLLACK, CB: *A psychiatric study of parents who abuse infants and small children.* In HELFER, RE AND KEMPE, CH (EDS): *The Battered Child.* University of Chicago Press, Chicago, 1974.

20. MARKHAM, B: *Child abuse intervention: Conflicts in current practice and legal theory.* Pediatrics 65:180, 1980.

21. ALTEMEIER, WA, O'CONNOR, S, VIETZE, PM, SANDLER, HM, SHERROD, KB: *Antecedents of child abuse.* J Pediatr 100:823, 1982.

22. SPINETTA, JJ AND RIGLER, D: *The child-abusing parent: A psychological review.* Psychol Bull 77:296, 1972.

23. BLUMBERG, ML: *Psychopathology of the abusing parent.* Am J Psychotherapy 28:21, 1974.

24. LIGHT, R: *Abused and neglected children in America: A study of alternative policies.* Harvard Educational Review 43:556, 1973.

25. BALDWIN, JA AND OLIVER, JE: *Epidemiology and family characteristics of severely abused children.* British Journal of Preventive and Social Medicine 29:205, 1975.

26. GROOTHUIS, JR, ALTEMEIER, WA, ROBARGE, JP, O'CONNOR, S, SANDLER, H, VIETZE, P, LUSTIG, JV: *Increased child abuse in families with twins.* Pediatrics 70:769, 1982.

27. RYAN, W: *Blaming the Victim.* Random House, New York, 1971.

28. FRIEDRICH, WM AND BORISKIN, JA: *The role of the child in abuse: A review of the literature.* Am J Orthopsychiatry 46:580, 1976.

29. HERRENKOHL, RC, HERRENKOHL, EC, EGOLF, BP: *Circumstances surrounding the occurrence of child maltreatment.* J Consult Clin Psychol 51:424, 1983.

30. FONTANA, VJ, ET AL: *The maltreatment syndrome in children.* New Engl J Med 269:1391, 1963.

31. BERGER, AM: *The child abusing family. II. Child and child-rearing variables, environmental factors and typologies of abusing families.* American Journal of Family Therapy 8:52, 1980.

32. KADUSHIN, A AND MARTIN, J: *Child Abuse: An Interactional Event.* Columbia University Press, New York, 1981.

33. THOMSON, EM, PAGET, NW, BATES, DW, MESCH, M, PUTNAM, TI: *Child Abuse: A Community Challenge.* Henry Stewart and Children's Aid Society for the Prevention of Cruelty to Children, East Aurora, NY, 1971.

34. BURGESS, RL AND CONGER, RD: *Family interaction in abusive, neglectful and normal families.* Child Dev 49:1163, 1978.

35. GIL, D: *Violence against children.* Journal of Marriage and the Family 33:639, 1971.

36. McKINLEY, D: *Social Class and Family Life.* Free Press of Glencoe, New York, 1964.

37. FINKELHOR, D: *Risk factors in the sexual victimization of children.* Child Abuse and Neglect 4:265,1980.

38. JUSTICE, B AND DUNCAN, DF: *Life crisis as a precursor to child abuse.* Public Health Report 91:110, 1976.

39. EGELAND, B, BREITENBUCKER, M, ROSENBERG, D: *Prospective study of the significance of life stress in the etiology of child abuse.* J Consult Clin Psychol 48:195, 1980.

40. GARBARINO, J AND GILLIAM, G: *Understanding Abusive Families.* DC Heath, Lexington, MA, 1980.

41. FINKELHOR, D: *Psychological, cultural and family factors in incest and sexual abuse.* Journal of Marriage and Family Counseling 4:41, 1978.

42. SALZINGER, S, KAPLAN, S, ARTEMYEFF, L: *Mothers' personal social networks and child maltreatment.* J Abnorm Psychol 92:68, 1983.

43. KEMPE, C: *A practical approach to the protection of the abused child and rehabilitation of the abusing parent.* Pediatrics 51:804, 1973.

44. GARBARINO, J: *The human ecology of child maltreatment.* Journal of Marriage and the Family 39:721, 1977.

45. COCHRAN, M AND BRASSARD, J: *Child development and personal social networks.* Child Dev 50:601, 1979.

46. GELLES, RJ: *Applying research on family violence to clinical practice.* Journal of Marriage and the Family 44:9, 1982.

47. ROBITSCHER, J: *Battered wives and battered children.* Bull Am Acad Psychiatry Law 5:373, 1977.

48. FLEMING, JB: *Stopping Wife Abuse.* Anchor/Doubleday, Garden City, NY, 1979.

49. GAYFORD, JJ: *Wife battering: A preliminary survey of 100 cases.* Br Med J 1:195, 1975.

50. ROSENBAUM, A AND O'LEARY, KD: *Children: The unintended victims of marital violence.* Am J Orthopsychiatry 51:692, 1981.

51. ROSENBAUM, A, COHEN, BF, HERSHORN, M: *Marital violence: Short and long term effects on witnessing children.* Symposium presented at the convention of the American Psychological Association, Anaheim, CA, 1983.

52. ROSENBAUM, A AND O'LEARY, KD: *Marital violence: Characteristics of abusive couples.* J Consult Clin Psychol 49:63, 1981.

53. GELLES, RJ: *Violence in the family: A review of research in the seventies.* Journal of Marriage and the Family 42:873, 1980.

54. STAR, B: *Comparing battered and nonbattered women.* Victimology: An International Journal 3:32, 1978.

55. COLEMAN, KH, WEINMAN, ML, HSI, BP: *Factors affecting conjugal violence.* J Psychol 105:197, 1980.

56. GOLDSTEIN, DL: *Self-esteem and marital violence: A study of spouse abusive men.* Unpublished master's thesis, Syracuse University, 1982.

57. WALKER, LE: *The Battered Woman.* Harper & Row, New York, 1979.

58. STEINMETZ, SK: *The battered husband syndrome.* Victimology: An International Journal 2:499, 1977-1978.

59. WASILESKI, M, CALLAGHAN-CHAFFEE, ME, CHAFFEE, RB: *Spousal violence in military homes: An initial survey.* Milit Med 147:761, 1982.

60. APPLETON, W: *The battered woman syndrome.* Ann Emerg Med 9:84, 1980.

61. CAZENAVE, N AND STRAUS, MA: *Race, class, network embeddedness and family violence: A search for potent support systems.* Journal of Comparative Family Studies 10:281, 1979.

62. HORNUNG, CA, McCULLOUGH, BC, SUGIMOTO, I: *Status relationships in marriage: Risk factors in spouse abuse.* Journal of Marriage and the Family 43:675, 1981.

63. RUSSELL, DEH: *Rape in Marriage.* Macmillan, New York, 1982.

64. SANSON, BE: *Spouse abuse: A novel remedy for a historic problem.* Dickinson Law Review 84:147, 1979-1980.

65. MANCINI, M: *Adult abuse laws.* Am J Nurs 80:739, 1980.

66. YATES, A: *Legal issues in the psychological abuse of children.* Clin Pediatr 21:587, 1982.

67. CAIN, LP: *Child abuse: Historical precedent and legal ramifications.* Health Soc Work 80:61, 1980.

68. SWOBODA, JS, ELWORK, A, SALES, BD, LEVINE, D: *Knowledge of and compliance with privileged communication and child-abuse reporting laws.* Professional Psychology Research and Practice 9:448, 1978.

69. MARGOLIN, G: *Ethical and legal considerations in marital and family therapy.* Am Psychol 37:788, 1982.

70. CHRISTOFFEL, KK, LIU, K, STAMLER, J: *Epidemiology of fatal child abuse: International mortality data.* J Chronic Dis 34:57, 1981.

71. ELMER, E: *A follow-up study of traumatized children.* Pediatrics 59:273, 1977.

72. KINARD, EM: *Child abuse and depression: Cause or consequence?* Child Welfare 67:403, 1982.

73. MAURER, A: *Physical punishment of children.* Paper presented at the California State Psychological Association Convention, Anaheim, CA, 1976.

74. MORSE, CW, SAHLER, O, FRIEDMAN, S: *A three-year follow-up study of abused and neglected children.* Am J Dis Child 120:439, 1970.

75. MARGOLIN, G: *Conjoint marital therapy to enhance anger management and reduce spouse abuse.* American Journal of Family Therapy 7:13, 1979.

76. BERK, RA, BERK, SF, LOSEKE, DR, RAUMA, D: *Mutual combat and other family violence.* In FINKELHOR, D, GELLES, RJ, HOTALING, GT, STRAUS, MA (EDS): *The Dark Side of Families.* Sage, Beverly Hills, CA, 1983.

77. STRAUS, MA: *Measuring intrafamily conflict and violence: The Conflict Tactics (CT) scales.* Journal of Marriage and the Family 41:75, 1979.

78. GOLDSTEIN, AP AND ROSENBAUM, A: *Aggress-Less: How to Turn Anger and Aggression into Positive Action.* Prentice-Hall, Englewood Cliffs, NJ, 1982.

79. REID, JF AND TAPLIN, PS: *A social interactional approach to the treatment of abusive children.* Unpublished manuscript cited in Burgess.[80]

80. BURGESS, RL: *Child abuse: A behavioral analysis.* In LAHEY, BB AND KAZDIN, AE (EDS): *Advances in Child Clinical Psychology.* Plenum, New York City, NY, 1978.

81. WACHTER, O AND BOYD, I: *Time-Out: Description of a film series dramatizing the conflicts and consequences faced by men who batter.* In ROY, M (ED): *The Abusive Partner.* Van Nostrand Reinhold, New York, 1982.

82. FRANK, PB AND HOUGHTON, BD: *Confronting the Batterer: A Guide to Creating the*

Spouse Abuse Workshop. Volunteer Counseling Service of Rockland County, New York City, NY 1982.

83. ADAMS, DC AND MCCORMICK, AJ: *Men unlearning violence: A group approach based on the collective model.* In ROY, M (ED): *The Abusive Partner.* Van Nostrand Reinhold, New York, 1982.

84. BALL, PG AND WYMAN, E: *Battered wives and powerlessness: What can counselors do?* Victimology: An International Journal 2:545, 1977-1978.

CHAPTER 11
CHILD CUSTODY
A. Louis McGarry, M.D.

Child custody disputes, whether they involve contesting parents or other adult family members, and including governmental placement of neglected or abused children, are affected by societal change. In recent years, there have been accelerated and extraordinary changes in American society which have had direct and unsettling effects on the family. Among these are the record number of teenage parents—especially among urban minorities—the ready availability of abortion, changes in the status of women, and the extent of family violence and abuse. Excellent reviews exist of the legal evolution and mental health concepts in custody and placement proceedings.[1,2] These texts are basic and important in approaching and understanding the complex issues of child custody litigation.

The scope of this chapter is limited to legal disputes in which the parents are contesting the custody of their children in separation and divorce actions. It is estimated that by 1990 one third of American children will have experienced the divorce of their parents before they reach the age of eighteen.[3] A divorce or separation connotes at least a dysfunctional and even a destructive marriage which precedes it. The divorce or separation of the parents may therefore relieve a destructive rearing situation for the children and may create the opportunity for a healthier environment. A recent 10-year follow-up suggests that this is often the case.[4] In this study, 110 children out of 54 divorced families had resolved much of the acute distress, anger, and depression associated with the divorce and had shown a general stability with no greater rate of delinquency among the children than in the general population. In a slightly expanded study of the same population, the younger children appear to have fared the best.[5] Further support on the same point is found in the recent reporting by Thomas and Chess[6] on their longitudinal developmental studies of behavioral disorders among children who have now reached their young adult years. They found that parental conflict itself—irrespective of divorce, separation, or even death in a parent—was predictive of emotional adjustment problems in young adult-hood.

It is estimated that about 10 percent of divorces proceed to litigation on the issue of child custody.[7] These are among the most acrimonious and destructive divorces, especially for the children. Mental health professionals are frequently involved in this minority of divorce cases in which custody is contested. This chapter concerns itself with that involvement and focuses on the clinical dimensions of the role of the mental health professional in custody assessments.

HISTORY AND SOCIAL DYNAMICS

During earlier centuries in Western society, children and wives had the legal and social status of being controlled by and assumed to be the property of the father and husband. Nora, Ibsen's heroine in the famous 19th-century play *A Doll's House*, sent shock waves through the educated classes of the time by abandoning a shallow marriage in feminist protest. Had she attempted to take her children with her, she would not have succeeded in the likely legal challenge from her lawyer husband.

In the early 20th century, the "tender years" presumption came to dominate custody determinations in American courts. It was felt that quite young children should not be taken from the mother on whom they were primarily emotionally dependent. Currently, the mother still tends to receive custody in the great majority of court disputes, but the pendulum has swung back some with a moderately increased frequency of fathers being adjudicated as the custodially superior parent.

In recent years, family courts having jurisdiction over custody matters have proved to be flexible and ready for change. In 1966, in *Painter v. Bannister*[8] the Iowa Supreme Court upheld the awarding of custody to grandparents who offered a churchgoing, traditional way of life on a farm rather than give custody to a father whose unconventional lifestyle was described as "Bohemian." Relative freedom from convention is more characteristic today in custody determinations than has been the case in the past. For example, the existence of a lover in the life of one or both of the contesting parents may receive little weight in custody determinations in metropolitan areas such as New York, although such behavior may still be the grounds for the divorce itself in fault-oriented proceedings.

Among the insights contributed by Goldstein and associates[1] in their 1973 book was the concept of the superior claim of the "psychological parent" as opposed to the biological parent. By the term psychological parent they meant the parenting figure who had provided the primary developmental nurturing of the child and on whom the child was mainly dependent for support, guidance, and identification. Such a consideration is more significant in the younger, more dependent child, but it is not intended to connote exclusivity, particularly as the child grows older. The authors also pointed out the different sense of the passage of time in children as opposed to adults. Young children may find even a brief separation from their primary nurturer for a period of a few days or weeks to be an extended and painful loss. The authors urged that every effort be made to avoid or to shorten such disruptions. Unfortunately, these separations are often prolonged when they are part of a court process.

STATUTORY AND CASE LAW

Generally the "best interests" of the child or of the children is legally mandated as the governing principle in custody disputes. Statutorily, the concept of "best interests," if defined at all, is either broadly[9] or multifactorally described,[10] as it was in the first state to attempt it, Michigan, in 1970 (Fig. 11-1). This is not surprising, given the complex and idiosyncratic situations with which the court must deal in these legal disputes.

There is useful and extensive case law developed from these often appealed custody disputes. However, the multiplicity of principles and accompanying dicta laid down in the cases do not lend themselves to any simple codification. A New York court put it as well as it can be stated in a recent decision:

> In custody matters, there are no absolutes and the situation must be resolved on a case by case basis after a consideration of the totality of the circumstances with special emphasis being placed upon the best interests of the child and the stability of the home environment.[11]

The Michigan statute defines "best interests" as follows:

722.23 Best interests of the child, definition. "Best interests of the child" means the sum total of the following factors to be considered, evaluated and determined by the court:

(a) The love, affection and other emotional ties existing between the competing parties and the child.

(b) The capacity and disposition of competing parties to give the child love, affection and guidance and continuation of educating and raising of the child in its religion or creed, if any.

(c) The capacity and disposition of competing parties to provide the child with food, clothing, medical care or other remedial care recognized and permitted under the laws of this state in lieu of medical care, and other material needs.

(d) The length of time the child has lived in a stable, satisfactory environment and the desirability of maintaining continuity.

(e) The permanence, as a family unit, of the existing or proposed custodial home.

(f) The moral fitness of the competing parties.

(g) The mental and physical health of the competing parties.

(h) The home, school and community record of the child.

(i) The reasonable preference of the child, if the court deems the child to be of sufficient age to express preference.

(j) Any other factor considered by the court to be relevant to a particular child custody dispute.

FIGURE 11-1. This is the Michigan statute definition of "best interests."

Once custody has been awarded, the courts will not disrupt it except under extraordinary circumstances. These circumstances were defined in another New York case as "surrender, abandonment, persistent neglect, unfitness and unfortunate and involuntary extended disruption of custody, or other equivalent, but rare circumstances which would drastically affect the welfare of the child."[12]

It is important for mental health professionals to keep in mind that the psychological status of the parents is only one factor, albeit a very important one, in the totality of the circumstances that the court must weigh in custody determinations.

JOINT CUSTODY

In recent years, there has been a considerable interest in the desirability of joint custody of children by divorced parents, and many states have adopted statutes designed to encourage this arrangement.[13-17] Joint custody, as opposed to sole custody (given to one or the other of the parents), is usually described in terms of alternating periods of physical custody of the child with or without domiciliary change from one parent to the other.

From a psychological point of view, joint custody has as its most desirable aspect the continuation of authority in both the father and the mother as decision-sharing parents. Neither parent is downgraded or viewed as less "fit" to have custody. Such an arrangement requires adequate good faith on the part of both parents in the best interests of the child or children and the willingness not to permit marital differences to interfere with the custodial process. Benedek and Benedek[18] have defined what they regard as the major elements to be addressed in considering the wisdom of a joint custody arrangement. Generally these require "desire," "commitment," "cooperation," and a "predisposition to honor the contract" on the part of both parents as well as their continued geographic proximity—presumably to avoid school and other community disruptions for the children.

What appears obvious from these considerations is that high levels of shared maturity, civility, and goodwill are required of parents for whom joint custody is likely to work well. Therapeutic mediation may enhance the likelihood of successful joint custody.[19]

THE INVOLVEMENT OF THE MENTAL HEALTH PROFESSIONAL

Therapeutic Role

Most commonly, the involvement of mental health professionals in troubled marriages is therapeutic; that is, one or the other or all family members may now or may have been patients of the professional. This may involve individual treatment, couple therapy, marital counseling, or family therapy. If a custody dispute emanates and a parent who has been in psychotherapy enters the psychiatric status of the parents into the proceedings, the therapist may be called and required to testify. Even in those jurisdictions with a psychotherapist-patient privilege against testimony, child custody proceedings may be an exception and the psychotherapist of an involved patient or child may be required by the court to testify, even against the wishes of the former patient.

Mediative Role

Motivated by the goal of avoiding the potentially damaging partisanship, expense, and trauma of an adversary proceeding, a second mental health role involves mediation in a marriage in which the couple has decided to obtain a divorce. It is important to recognize that in 90 percent of divorces, the parties do arrive at an acceptable divorce settlement, including custody of the children.

There are now a number of organizations, such as the Family Mediation Association, that deal with all the issues of divorce, including custody. A quarterly professional journal on the subject is in its 23rd year.*

A model has emerged for the involvement of mental-health professionals as family mediators when the goal is the resolution of disputed divorce issues including custody and visitation. It should be emphasized that although the role of the mediator may be regarded as therapeutic in that such mediation is presumably less divisive and traumatic than a court battle, the primary goal is to arrive at a stipulated divorce agreement. In its most successful form an agreement is reached, signed by both parents, and then adopted as an order of the court. The mediation process is usually privileged under state law and remains confidential.[20] If no agreement can be reached, the open-court, adversary process must be used.

Consultative Role

The mental health professional may also serve as a consultant to the family courts on matters of child custody. The specialized skills of a mental health professional can be utilized effectively in such a role, and, in my opinion, the following comprise the four major rationales for their involvement. These are (1) the application of clinical skills in eliciting psychodynamic data relevant to the child custody determinations, (2) the application of specialized knowledge of psychopathological diagnosis and prognosis, (3) the application of specialized knowledge of the developmental needs of children, and (4) the provision of professional consultation relatively free from countertransference distortions. The importance of each of these skills will be expanded later in this chapter.

It should be added that when there is physical illness in either the parents or the children, the psychiatrist consultant can bring a medical perspective to the child custody determinations. If the opinions of other medical specialists are required, the psychiatrist is in a position to indicate the need to the court. The special physical treatment requirements of the child and the prognosis for physical illness in the parent can have significant bearing on custody determinations. An evaluation of the differential strengths of parents in dealing with problems of stress in coping with handicapped children may also be relevant to the custody decision itself.

---

* *Conciliation Courts Review*, Association of Family Conciliation Courts, Meyer Elkin, editor. 1217 Shadybrook Dr., Beverly Hills, CA 90210.

METHODS OF PROVIDING COURT CONSULTATION

Before expounding on the rationales for the involvement of mental health professionals in custody disputes, it is useful to consider the matter of the assessment processes and procedures that have evolved. Some clinicians prefer, in the difficult custodial assessment process, to avoid making an explicit recommendation to the court as to which parent should have custody. Nevertheless, they should be willing to articulate fully the clinically determined assets and liabilities of the contesting parents while leaving the final decision to the judge, who has the responsibility of weighing the totality of relevant factors, many of which are not clinical or psychodynamic in the usual sense. However, many mental health authorities[21,22] in this field have a firm view that the clinician should offer a final custodial recommendation. Difficulties arise when the contesting parents are almost equally healthy or unhealthy from a mental health perspective. A recommendation favoring one parent over the other is then open to serious challenge.

In the absence of significant parental psychopathology in either parent, a good case can be made that mental health consultant clinicians do not have a defensible basis for an opinion favoring either parent. If there is fault to be found here, then some of it lies with courts too eager to have positive recommendations to aid the disposition of the dispute itself. These demands for determinative recommendations are difficult to resist. This is certainly not a new problem for forensic consultants. In the criminal courts, for example, the ultimate decision on the issue of competence to stand trial is legal, but clinicians are expected, and, indeed, usually required to offer an opinion on the ultimate issue: the overall mental capacity of a defendant to stand trial. It is an honorable course of action for the clinician to decline to offer an opinion in the absence of a significant psychopathological basis for that opinion. Each clinician must choose his or her own course on this issue. Very often we can find relatively soft clinical observations to provide support for an opinion one way or another. In my experience, many of that small minority of parents who arrive at a custody dispute do in fact have significant psychopathology. If a clinician does elect to provide or yields to the pressure to offer an opinion in the absence of significant parental psychopathology, then he or she should lay bare the basis of that opinion, expose its weakness, and not falsely endow the opinion with clinical authority. Whether or not an opinion is offered in the absence of significant psychopathology, it is a service to the court to establish that there is no such pathology, especially when such has been alleged. If an opinion on custody is offered in the absence of a substantial psychopathological basis for the opinion, there is considerable risk (despite any disclaimers) that it will be accorded greater weight than it deserves.

There appears to be a substantial consensus that the mental health professional who accepts a consultative role in custody disputes should do so on an impartial basis, examining all those concerned, on both sides.[23,24] Rappeport[25] has taken the position that it is not "good medical practice" to offer an opinion on who should receive child custody based on an examination limited to one parent. He would also submit that it is unethical to offer any opinion concerning the custodial capacity or incapacity of an unexamined parent.

Consistent with this consensus, Gardner[21] has described a private sector model in which he accepts a consultation only if it is stipulated that all the parties on both sides having any material contribution to make to the assessment agree to participate. The number of participants and the process can be extensive, including not only the parents and the children but also grandparents, other concerned relatives, housekeepers, "live-in friends," potential stepparents, and other possible parental surrogates.

Our group* in Nassau County, although a public agency, operates similarly in terms of a prior stipulation under the authority of the presiding judge assuring that all the relevant persons on both sides will be examined. Such a public service program can be offered free of charge or paid for on the basis of a sliding-scale fee schedule proportional to family income. Our clinical evaluation process works in collaboration with the probation department of the courts we serve. Probation officers conduct a preliminary investigation and provide a family history. There is usually a home visit, and relevant medical and psychiatric reports, school records, and other documents are collected. Thus, at the point at which mental health clinicians become involved, considerable preliminary data have already been collected and organized; hence, expensive clinical time is more efficiently deployed.

Our practice is to assign to the case a general psychiatrist and/or a child psychiatrist, often aided by clinical psychologists or social workers. Generally, the psychiatrist sees the parents and may see one or more of the children. It is the psychiatrist who is usually called to court to defend the recommendations if testimony is required. The other disciplines may examine other pertinent parties. At the conclusion of all examinations, a conference is held by the clinicians who have been involved and, after a meeting of the minds, the psychiatrist who has examined the central figures in the matter drafts a summary of the findings and makes recommendations in a report to the court which all of the involved clinicians sign. A recommendation is usually made favoring one or the other of the contesting parties—usually, but not always, a parent. Occasionally a temporary custody recommendation is made conditional on psychotherapeutic intervention or other condition, with a follow-up evaluation requested before a definitive recommendation is made. Although it occurs rarely, there is provision for a minority report and recommendations or at least a noting of reservations or a lack of unanimity if such is the case. The report is submitted to the court, and either party may require any or all of the clinicians to testify in court to support or to challenge the opinions offered.

It is Gardner's[21] practice to share and to review his report and recommendations with the parents prior to submitting his report to the court. Such a practice provides an opportunity for correcting errors of a historical or other nature. This is likely, however, to be a painful experience for the parent who is not favored in the report.

The question can be raised as to the vulnerability to suit of a psychiatrist or other mental health clinician who serves in this court-appointed consultative role and makes a recommendation to a court on child custody. In a recent federal court case,[26] the disgruntled husband sued the psychiatrist who had recommended custody to be granted to the wife over the one child of the

---

* The Forensic Services Section, Nassau County Department of Mental Health, New York.

marriage. The suit was brought for professional malpractice, invasion of privacy, fraudulent misrepresentation, negligence and violation of Constitutional rights. The court dismissed all the claims as having no merit and also found the consultant to have immunity from suit as a common law witness. The husband based his claim for invasion of privacy on the theory that the psychiatrist was in a physician-patient relationship to him and was bound to keep confidences revealed in the examination unless released by the husband. The judge denied this theory, asserting that the consultation was on behalf of the court and not for treatment. Therefore, no physician-patient relationship existed upon which a duty of confidentiality would rest. The claim of violation of Constitutional rights was based on the Federal Civil Rights Act (42 US Code S 1983). That law requires that the violation be a matter of state action or under color of law. The judge denied this claim also on the basis that the psychiatrist consultant was not acting on behalf of or under color of federal law. He was found by the court not to be "an agent of the court" because neither the judge nor any other federal officer controlled his decision or recommendation regarding custody of the child. The court cited a similar decision in another federal court.[27] Also, the court cited two cases in which suits were brought against psychiatrists who certified patients for commitment to state mental hospitals.[28,29] In both cases, the physicians were acting under state statutes but were held not to be state actors in their clinical capacities of certification of mental illness. It should be noted that in neither of these cases was the physician a court-appointed impartial examiner. No matter what the weakness of the court's reasoning, the important point for this discussion is the fact that the federal court granted a full immunity from suit by the losing party as long as the consultant testifies in court as an expert witness or as long as the consultant's report is filed in court and reviewed by the trial court.

CLINICAL ASPECTS OF THE CONSULTATIVE ROLE

Among the rationales offered earlier in this chapter in support of the involvement of mental health clinicians in custody disputes was the interviewing skill which the clinician brings to these matters. Such a skill would appear to be especially useful when the parents have reached such a degree of polarization that communication between them is only through their attorneys. The courtroom and even the judge's chambers, with their inherent procedural and situational constraints, limit the spontaneity and rapport that a clinical setting and clinicians' skills can enhance. Gardner[21] finds family interviews and joint interviews of the parents to be of great value in discerning the psychodynamics and in gathering critical data in the assessment process. The affective displays of children regarding one or the other parent in such settings can tell a great deal that their words may not. The children's biological functions also are revealing: A toilet-trained child who regresses to soiling, or the older child who is enuretic while visiting with the parent with whom his or her relationship is more conflicted, is communicating something to which we should pay attention.

When accurately and properly interpreted, the drawings and play of children when oriented to parental or family scenes often are revealing of their relationships with each parental figure. There is also often an important contribution to be made by projective psychological testing, although I do not find such testing to be routinely necessary in all custody assessments.

PSYCHOPATHOLOGY IN THE PARENTS

The major contribution that clinicians can make is in regard to the diagnosing of significant psychopathology in the contesting parents. Sound clinical opinions can usually be offered regarding the prognosis and likely course of psychiatric illness, especially in the more severe forms, such as the psychoses. These and other illnesses, especially the personality disorders, often have predictably long-term status and are therefore of relevance in the longitudinal prediction of parental quality. In the absence of sufficient psychopathological data to arrive at a full formal diagnosis, the clinician may find no more in the way of psychopathology than the discernment of certain character traits. Often no greater psychopathology can be found than that which is attributable to transient adjustment disorders associated with the psychosocial stressors of the divorce itself.

Extreme parental character traits and destructive parental practices would certainly appear to deserve weight in custody determinations. Among these are schizoid coldness, rigidity and excessive controls, inconsistent setting of limits, instability of judgment, impulsivity, psychopathy, and pathological narcissism. Drug and alcohol abuse, physical abuse of the children and spouse or others, and sexual abuse of the children have rather obvious implications for parental quality. The impact of these negative parental traits and practices will be assessed below.

CHILD DEVELOPMENTAL ASPECTS

The mental health professional does bring specialized knowledge and insights to the developmental needs or tasks of children in custody determinations, but the ease of appropriate or valid application of this knowledge should not be exaggerated. Rather, one needs to be both careful and cautious in this regard. For example, Eriksonian concepts such as basic trust, autonomy, industry, and identity do not lend themselves to precise determinations or quantification in the child, and the assessment of parental art and skill in their promotion may be even more complex and subtle.

The paramount question is whether psychopathological states or extreme personality traits in parents or abusive parental practices are, in fact, likely to damage children and therefore are predictive of their later dysfunction. Although there are a number of discrete studies that retrospectively associate later problems with some earlier parental practices or other experiences, it is difficult to draw valid inferences from such studies because of biases of ascertainment and other limitations.

In order to have sound and valid empirical evidence relevant to the above paramount question, ideally one would wish to have some systematic prospective longitudinal studies that follow the developmental course for a wide range of children (not only those from socially disadvantaged or other special groups) over a period of several years (optimally until their young adult years), with regular periodic assessments of the children and the family situation. It is in the context of such long-term prospective studies that one could more precisely discern the nature and frequency of various social and psychopathological problems in the children and how they are affected by various parental traits and practices. Such prospective studies would also indicate the continuities and discontinuities with regard to early and later manifestations of various problems. Many of the earlier manifestations may **not** continue over a period of time. In many youngsters the problems may tend to have delayed onset, and other children may have no significant problems. However, in the absence of long-term and systematic follow-up, the above continuities and discontinuities will not be known, and incorrect inferences may well be drawn.

Although there is a considerable volume of research and related literature in the fields of child and developmental psychology, relatively few longitudinal studies have been reported in the psychiatric literature. Understandably, such studies are difficult to conduct and are also very expensive. Among the few highly regarded longitudinal studies have been those of the Gluecks[30] (acclaimed more for their pioneering aspects than for the rigor of their design), Robins[31] and, more recently, Long and Vaillant,[32] Vaillant and Milofsky.[33] In the chapters on family violence (chapter 10), juvenile delinquency (chapter 12), and child sexual abuse (chapter 14), there are reviews of the relevant literature pertaining to the sequelae of parental psychopathology for the children in those families. The vast majority of such studies were, of course, retrospective in nature. Many of the sequelae may indeed be rather serious and even devastating for the futures of many of the children, but the findings suggest potential problems rather than certain or definite outcomes. Moreover, within the very same psychopathological families some children may be much more vulnerable and thus display obvious deleterious effects, and other siblings may show relatively little or even no discernible indications of harmful effects.

There does appear to be a fairly consistent trend of empirical evidence (albeit derived primarily from retrospective studies) pointing to the increased likelihood of long-term damaging sequelae of parental dysfunctioning associated with physical abuse of the children. Such children appear to be at increased risk for later abusing their own spouses and children. Often they exhibit aggressive behavior and interpersonal deficits reflecting lack of trust.[34] Similarly, many violent criminals provide retrospective reports of having been victims of parental violence.[35]

Psychiatric illness and hospitalization of parents has been found to be associated with higher rates of delinquency and related problems in their children.[36] The parents of delinquent children are generally less supportive and more coercive than those of nondelinquent children.[37] Parents who are very aggressive, alcoholic, or have criminal records, and whose parenting behavior involves punitive and erratic discipline, are more likely to produce delinquent and violent children.[38] More equivocal—possibly owing to the limited research in that area thus far—are the long-term developmental outcomes and emotional sequelae of the sexual abuse of children. (See chapter 14.)

In contrast to some of the studies of delinquent or otherwise disturbed youngsters that point to histories of severe abuse and deprivation, there appears to be relatively little research reported in the psychiatric literature that relates to less severe parental dysfunction or rearing circumstances and destructive sequelae for their children. The prediction, for example, of Lidz and his colleagues that mothers who are "dominant, over-protective, but basically rejecting" are more likely to be "schizophrenogenic" does not appear to have stood up to critical reassessment.[39] Freud was cautious about simplistic psychodynamic applications in the legal system.[40]

Although there are not many research reports in the psychiatric literature with respect to pathological sequelae for children reared by parents with less severe psychopathology, this should not be interpreted as suggesting that there is no damage to the children. Nor, for that matter, could one readily assume that such damage is either an invariable or even a common occurrence. Furthermore, long-term predictions in any science are problematic, and they are certainly no less so in such follow-up research in which there may be a multiplicity of intervening variables.[4,5,32]

As noted earlier, one must always be alert to the ascertainment biases inherent in retrospective studies, especially studies involving highly selected groups (for example, adjudicated and incarcerated violent delinquents or criminals) who have already come to attention precisely because of their obvious and serious problems. Lacking appropriate information derived from unselected and more general study samples, one does not have an opportunity to learn about persons who had very similar developmental histories (for example, abusive and emotionally disturbed parents) but who do **not** display any serious dysfunctioning. In short, it is important to exercise much care in drawing conclusions and inferences from particular research studies. Of course, even greater caution is required in trying to generalize broadly on the limited basis of one's own clinical experience.

In essence, clinical assessments and recommendations should be guided as much as possible by a knowledge and understanding of the available empirical research evidence and not simply on one's own clinical experience and intuitions. In summary, the major curent psychiatric knowledge indicates the following: (1) severe parental psychopathology, marital conflict, and abusive parental practices are associated with a much higher incidence of significant demonstrable dysfunction in the children of such parents; (2) lesser degrees of parental psychopathology may only be inferred to result in dysfunction in the children of such parents. It must be emphasized, however, that these inferences have neither been proven nor disproven. Hence, much care and caution should be exercised regarding the predictions, conclusions, and recommendations that are offered to courts.

COUNTERTRANSFERENCE ASPECTS

The training, traditions, and values of mental health professionals profess an approach to patients that is as nonjudgmental as possible. Child custody evaluations, on the contrary, are an inherently judgmental task. Which parent is to be "awarded" custody of the children by virtue of his or her superior character and "fitness"? Nevertheless, it is assumed that dynamically trained clinicians are aware of and better equipped to guard against countertransference distortions; that is, the potential intrusion of the personal values and reactions of the evaluator into these custody evaluations.

The objectivity that clinicians strive to maintain is strained in custody matters. The problem arises in part from the fact that, in the short term of the custody dispute, desperate parents may adopt tactics that are not necessarily representative of their long-term behavior and fitness as parents. In custody matters, otherwise decent people may offer the most outrageous fabrications about their divorcing spouses. In such a context, when clinicians perceive that they have been lied to, or that attempts have been made to manipulate them, they may be tempted toward a too precipitous rush to judgment. Evaluators are at risk of feeling offended and even responding in a punitive fashion against the objectionable parent.

In the adversary process, the accepted norm is for each side to stress its own strong points in order to arrive at the closest approximation of the truth, which is usually expected to lie somewhere between. The extent to which attorneys may contribute to or encourage what may be seen as fabrication and manipulation by the contesting parents is not a very useful preoccupation for clinicians. In the adversary process, the usual legal remedy for such distortions lies in mutual confrontation of the parties and their stories and the "test of cross-examination"[41] on the witness stand. It is well to remember that clinicians are relative amateurs in cross-examination, compared with experienced trial attorneys. Although it is necessary in a clinical examination to have concern for the reliability of those examined—particularly when confronted with grossly inconsistent marital, parental, and family histories—the extent to which the clinician adopts aggressive and partisan tactics is a corruption of the clinician's role. The adversary process should remain in the hands of the appropriate professionals in court.

It is, however, a legitimate concern to the clinician when the children themselves are forced to become involved in the manipulations of their contesting parents. The parent who finds it necessary to exploit the children in custody determinations by exposing them to or tutoring them in the deficiencies of the other parent is **not**, in my opinion, acting in the "best interests of the child"—at least not in the short-term exigencies of the custody dispute. Even if the deficiencies are true, the child is not well served if unnecessary awareness of such deficiencies is forced on the child. The maligned parent remains a parent and will always be a greater or lesser part of what the child identifies as himself or herself. In the totality of relative assets and liabilities, such short-term involvement and exposure of children should not, in and of themselves, be dispositive of which parent can better serve the best interests of the child in the long term of custody. It is tempting to be sweepingly judgmental about such parental behavior.

Another issue with potential for highly judgmental reactions by the clinical evaluator arises from the fact that the psychoanalytic concept of narcissism is often a key operating factor. This factor may be explicit or implicit, conscious or even unconscious, on the part of the evaluator. I believe it is necessary to discuss the usefulness and confront the risks inherent in this concept.

The lay use of the word narcissism connotes egocentrism, and its current use by clinicians is almost always pejorative. Freud, however, used the term not only in a narrow technical sense but also in a very broad sense, encompassing, for example, the need for self-preservation.[42] In this broad and non-judgmental sense he intended a spectrum of entitlements, ranging from healthy to unhealthy narcissism. At the healthy end of the spectrum, for example, we all have expectations that decency and fairness on our part will be similarly honored by others and that hard work merits just rewards. The sacrifices of genuinely altruistic parenting from which the parent may expect to derive a measure of appropriate self-esteem belongs at this healthy end of the spectrum. At the unhealthy end of the spectrum, one may see an excessively selfish and even bizarre sense of entitlement, which is imposed as a demand on others with little or no regard for the needs or rights of the others. An obvious pathological example is the sexual exploitation of a child.

In custody determinations, clinicians are concerned about the relative narcissistic expectations of the parents in Freud's broad use of the term. What are the parents' individual priorities? How healthy or unhealthy are these needs, and where and how do the developmental needs of the children fit within the narcissistic interests and priorities of each of the parents? Insofar as clinicians can utilize the concept to include healthy—even altruistic—narcissistic dimensions in their evaluations, as well as the unhealthy and problematic aspects, this conceptual framework is useful and constructive. Insofar as clinicians are oriented only toward pathologically narcissistic features, there is a risk of being excessively judgmental. It is nevertheless true that when it is the children in a custody dispute whose needs are in fact subordinated to the dysfunctional or even destructive needs of a parent, such a consideration deserves balanced and appropriate weight in the custody determination.

In custody disputes, it is very often the case that one or both of the parents have been and/or feel seriously injured in terms of what he or she has felt entitled to, reasonably or unreasonably, from the marriage and the marital partner. It is this perceived and felt injury—a narcissistic injury, if you will—which often fuels the striking intensity of most of these disputes and the protracted litigation that may continue around such issues as visitation. Custody and visitation litigation may have more to do dynamically with themes of narcissistic injury than primary concern about the care and custody of the children. Litigation, particularly repetitive and prolonged litigation, may be secondary to or a displaced arena for the continuation of the marital conflict itself, despite the parental separation. Among the common themes of narcissistic injury are those arising from sexual unfaithfulness and the emergence of a more actively feminist posture in a wife whose husband cannot adapt to the shift. The distribution of the family estate may involve a custody dispute as a "bargaining chip" in the process. The familiarity and expertise of psychodynamically trained clinicians with such themes and with their countertransference risks should add to the objectivity and value of their evaluations.

CHILDREN'S CHOICE

The choice of the children in custody disputes ordinarily deserves considerable weight. However, this, too, is a complex matter. The natural hedonism of children, especially the younger ones, may dominate; they may choose based on short-term, shallow, pleasure-oriented considerations. The parent who is the most generous or who is in the financial position to be the most generous with gifts or who is the less severe disciplinarian may be chosen. In older children, the choice may be dictated by considerations of not wishing to change domiciles, friends, or schools; hence, they may not choose wisely in their own long-term best interests. Emotionally disturbed children may make choices for psychopathological reasons; for example, out of an unhealthy symbiotic relationship with one of the parents.

The matter of eliciting a choice from the children involved must be sensitively handled. Although they should be given the opportunity to express a preference, and most importantly, their reasons for doing so should be ascertained, they should not be forced to do so. Children often do not wish to choose, preferring that their parents, even their warring parents, remain together. They should be allowed to remain outside the decision-making arena. The process is painful enough without forcing the children to make a choice they don't wish to make and don't feel capable of making at that time.

REFERENCES

1. GOLDSTEIN, J, FREUD, S, SOLNIT, AJ: *Beyond the Best Interests of the Child*. Macmillan, New York, 1973 (rev ed, 1979).

2. GOLDSTEIN, J, FREUD, S, SOLNIT, AJ: *Before the Best Interests of the Child*. Macmillan, New York, 1979.

3. GLICK, PC: *Children of divorced parents in demographic perspective*. Journal of Social Issues 35:170-182, 1979.

4. WALLERSTEIN, JS: *Children of divorce: A preliminary report of a follow-up*. Unpublished material from a paper given at the Annual Meeting of the American Academy of Psychiatry and the Law, Portland, OR, October 1983.

5. WALLERSTEIN, JS: Unpublished material from a paper given at the annual meeting of the American Orthopsychiatric Association, April 1984, as reported in the New York Times p C 1, April 10, 1984.

6. THOMAS, A AND CHESS, S: *Genesis and evolution of behavioral disorders: From infancy to adult life*. Am J Psychiatry 141:1-9, 1984.

7. FOSTER, HH AND FREED, DJ: *Joint custody: Legislative reform*. Trial 16:22-27, 1980.

8. Painter v. Bannister, 258 Iowa 390, 140 N.W. 2d 152, 1966.

9. Uniform Marriage and Divorce Act (1970), Part IV—Custody. In the GAP Report, New Trends in Child Custody Determinations, Appendix A, Harcourt Brace Jovanovich, New York, 1980, pp 151-152.

10. Mich. Comp. Laws Ann. Section 722.23 (Supp 1971).

11. Yeo v. Cornaire, 485 N.Y.S. 2d, 743, 1983.

12. Bennet v. Jeffreys, 387 N.Y.S. 2d 821, 1976.

13. STEINMAN, S: *Joint custody: What we know, what we have yet to learn, and the judicial and legislative implications*. University of California at Davis Law Review 16:739, 1983.

14. KELLY, JB: *Further observations on joint custody*. University of California at Davis Law Review 16:762, 1983.

15. SHULMAN, J AND PITT, V: *Some second thoughts on joint child custody: Analysis of legislation and its implications for women and children*. Golden Gate University Law Review 12:538, 1982.

16. MILLS, BG AND BELZER, SP: *Joint custody as a parenting alternative*. Pepperdine Law Review 9:853, 1982.

17. *Joint custody: The best interests of the child*. Tulsa Law Journal 18:159, 1982.

18. BENEDEK, EP AND BENEDEK, RS: *Joint custody: Solution or illusion*. Am J Psychiatry 136:1540-1544, 1979.

19. SUAREZ, JM, WESTON, NL, HARFSTEIN, MB: *Mental health interventions in divorce proceedings*. Am J Orthopsychiatry 48:283, 1978.

20. See, for example, New York Family Court Act. McKinney's Consolidated Laws of New York, Annotated, Book 29A, Section 915, 1983.

21. GARDNER, RA: *Family evaluation in child custody litigation*. Creative Therapeutics. Cresskill, NY, 1982, pp 213-214.

22. DERDYN, AP: *A consideration of legal issues in child custody contests*. Arch Gen Psychiatry 33:165-171, 1976.

23. Report, Group for the Advancement of Psychiatry, New Trends in Child Custody Determinations. Harcourt Brace Jovanovich, New York, 1980, pp 127-130.

24. HOFLING, CK (ED): *Law and Ethics in the Practice of Psychiatry*. Brunner/Mazel, New York, 1981, p 202.

25. RAPPEPORT, JR: *Ethics and forensic psychiatry*. In BLOCK, S AND CHODOFF, P (EDS): *Psychiatric Ethics*. Oxford University Press, Oxford and New York, 1981, pp 280-281.

26. Anderson v. Glismann, 577 F. Supp. 1506, D. Colo., 1984.

27. Watkins v. Roche, 529 F. Supp. 327, S.D. Ga., 1981.

28. Hall v. Quillen, 631 F. 2d 1154, 4th Cir., 1980.

29. Landry v. Odom, 559 F. Supp. 514, E.D. La., 1983.

30. GLUECK, S AND GLUECK, E: *Delinquents and Nondelinquents in Perspective.* Harvard University Press, Cambridge, MA, 1968.

31. ROBINS, LN: *Deviant Children Grown Up: A Sociological and Psychiatric Study of Sociopathic Personality.* Williams & Wilkins, Baltimore, 1966.

32. LONG, JVF AND VAILLANT, GE: *Natural history of male psychological health, XI: Escape from the underclass.* Am J Psychiatry 141:341-346, 1984.

33. VAILLANT, GE AND MILOFSKY, E: *Natural history of male psychological health, IX: Empirical evidence for Erikson's model of the life cycle.* Am J Psychiatry 137:1348-1359, 1980.

34. ROSENBAUM, A AND O'LEARY, KD: *Marital violence: Characteristics of abusive couples.* J Consult Clin Psychol 49:63, 1981.

35. MAURER, A: Unpublished material. A paper presented at the convention of the California State Psychological Association, Anaheim, CA, 1976.

36. LEWIS, DO, BALLA, DA, SCHANK, SS, SNELL, L: *Delinquency, parental pathology, and parental criminality.* J Am Acad Child Psychiatry 15:665, 1976.

37. HETHERINGTON, EM AND MARTIN, B: *Family interaction.* In QUAY, HC AND WERRY, JS (EDS): *Psychopathological Disorders of Childhood.* John Wiley & Sons, New York, 1979.

38. McCORD, J, McCORD, W, HOWARD, A: *Family interaction as antecedent to the direction of male aggressiveness.* Journal of Abnormal and Social Psychology 66:239, 1963.

39. PARKE, G: *Re-searching the schizophrenogenic mother.* J Nerv Ment Dis 170:452-462, 1982.

40. GOLDSTEIN, RL: *Sigmund Freud: Forensic psychiatrist.* Bull Am Acad Psychiatry Law 11:273-277, 1983.

41. United States v. DeSisto, 329 F.2d 929, 2d Cir. 1964, at p 934.

42. FREUD, S: *On narcissism: An introduction.* In FREUD, S: *The Complete Psychological Works, Vol 14.* Hogarth Press, London, 1957, pp 73-102.

CHAPTER 12
JUVENILE DELINQUENCY
Cathy Spatz Widom, Ph.D.

Juvenile delinquency has become a particularly troubling social problem. Readers of daily newspapers are regularly exposed to stories of crime and violence associated with individual youths and juvenile gangs. Juvenile delinquency refers to a variety of law-violating behaviors by youths. In most states, juvenile status ends with the 16th birthday.

On the national level, one in five persons arrested for violent crimes (murder, forcible rape, robbery, and aggravated assault) and 43.5 percent of those arrested for property crimes are under 18 years of age.[1] It has been estimated that one in every nine children in the United States will be referred to a juvenile court for an act of delinquency before his or her 18th birthday. Of all men born in Philadelphia in 1945, over one third have had recorded contacts with the police between their 7th and their 18th birthdays.[2] It should be noted, however, that only a small portion of the offenders account for a very large portion of the total offenses committed during that time.

In addition to the large number of youths who acquire an official record, it is important to distinguish between delinquent behavior and official delinquency. Official delinquency is an official response to delinquent behavior. The great majority of youth engage in some form of delinquent behavior at some point in their development. Thus, court and police records of offenses are of limited usefulness as an index of actual delinquent behavior.[3]

Official records underestimate the volume of delinquency because not all acts are officially recorded. For example, in one self-report study of delinquency in a national sample of youths ages 13 to 16 years, Williams and Gold[4] found that 88 percent of the sample had done something that could have resulted in trouble with the law, but only 22 percent had ever had any contact with police, and only 2 percent had contact with the courts for their behavior. The magnitude of the discrepancy between officially recorded delinquency and self-reported delinquency is the focus of continuing debate among criminologists; however, both kinds of information are relevant to understanding the phenomena.

Because of the very broad scope and range of this topic and the truly voluminous nature of the relevant literature, I have chosen to limit my discussion in view of space restrictions. However, references have been provided to assist the reader who wishes more details on particular subtopics or issues.

This chapter begins with a review of the major theories of the causes of delinquency, emphasizing the failure of unidimensional, single-factor approaches. The second part focuses on the correlates of delinquency through a review of empirical research. Part three describes recent attempts to categorize delinquents, including the American Psychiatric Association's *Diagnostic and Statistical Manual of Mental Disorders*, edition 3 *(DSM III)* criteria for conduct disorder. The final sections deal with issues of diversion, treatment, recidivism, and proposals for early intervention projects.

DELINQUENCY CAUSATION

Since the early work of Lombroso and the Gluecks, researchers have searched for **biological** or **constitutional** factors in the etiology of delinquent behavior. Recently, evidence from a variety of studies suggests that biological factors play a role. For example, individual differences in responsiveness to pain[5] and the need for stimulation and sensation-seeking have been related to delinquent and criminal behavior,[6] and differences in autonomic nervous system responsivity have been linked to psychopathy.[7]

Lewis[8] examined the incidence of medical problems in juveniles who had been referred for neuropsychiatric assessment, finding that behavioral difficulties were associated with physical trauma, such as head and facial injuries or perinatal difficulties. Based on these findings, she suggested that injuries involving the central nervous system contribute to the development of aggressive and delinquent behavior. Penner[9] also found a high incidence of vision, speech, and hearing problems associated with antisocial behavior.

Here, as elsewhere in this chapter, it is important to bear in mind the nature and possible limitations of study samples, research methodologies, or designs which could influence the generalizability of the findings. It is quite clear that serious neurological injuries may produce major behavioral deficiencies in youths from adequate to excellent environmental circumstances. However, minor neurological injuries may simply reflect the negative impact of rather adverse environmental conditions on cognitive and psychological development. Similarly, group differences in neurological problems may reflect social class differences in the quality of medical care, rather than factors fundamental to delinquency. Because these problems would be likely to occur before the onset of antisocial behavior, they would lead to difficulties in school, at home, and among peers, thus contributing to the development of delinquent behaviors.

Causal involvement of **genetic factors** in delinquency and criminal behavior has also been demonstrated,[10,11] although the mechanism for the intergenerational transmission of such behavioral tendencies is not understood. Some studies show higher concordance rates for criminality among monozygotic (identical) twins as compared with dizygotic (fraternal) twins.[12] However, in Norway Dalgaard and Kringlen[13] compared fraternal and identical twins who had been exposed to similar environments and found low concordance for criminality among indentical twins. Adoption studies reveal that boys are more likely to follow in the footsteps of their **biological** fathers than to follow in those of their adoptive fathers in exhibiting delinquent and criminal behavior.[14] However, adoption studies have been criticized because children are often placed in homes similar to those of their biological parents. In addition, differences in the age of placement, number of foster home placements, and other factors may influence the likelihood of future antisocial behavior problems.[15]

For a long time, **psychodynamic** theories have emphasized the importance of psychological problems encountered during the "formative years" and their influence on growth and development. Delinquent behavior was thought to be symptomatic of deep emotional conflicts and unconscious motivations[16] and a form of neurotic behavior, frequently associated with a compulsive need for punishment and hostility directed outward.[17] In these theories, delinquency is attributed to weak ego and superego controls, resulting from the failure to develop strong identification with a parental figure.

In contrast, **social learning** theorists[18] assume that delinquent behaviors are acquired through direct and observational learning experiences, poor examples, or lack of reinforcement of prosocial behaviors. They point to the tangible rewards associated with delinquent behavior (particularly when attractive alternatives are not available) and nontangible rewards such as approval by and social status among peers or attention from a parent. Once a youth has engaged in delinquent behavior, both the promise of future rewards and the threat of future punishment exist. But, inasmuch as the probability of getting caught (arrested) is fairly low and the youth may "get away with" delinquent behavior (an experience that serves to reinforce the behavior), the criminality or delinquency is likely to persist.

To **social control** theorists, delinquent behavior is a function of the strength of the individual's bond to conventional goals, values, persons, and institutions. In Hirschi's[19] model, an adolescent with a strong commitment and bond to society is not likely to become delinquent. As the bond is weakened by neglectful or rejecting parents, poor school performance, and deviant peers, the chances of delinquent behavior increase. Social control theory has been criticized as having some circularity, because delinquency is, by definition, behavior that is counter to conventional societal norms. Furthermore, although some social control theorists address issues of motivation, the primary emphasis is on the mechanisms that prevent or deter delinquency.

Other theories focus on the conflict between our society's emphasis on success and the limited opportunities for achievement in educational, social, and/or financial spheres experienced by youths from socially disadvantaged backgrounds. This **limited opportunity theory**[20,21] postulates that youths initially want to conform to conventional goals and standards of acceptable behavior. However, after experiencing frustrated economic and status aspirations, and finding that access is limited, they search for alternative means of obtaining sources of satisfaction. Thus, being denied access through legitimate means, the delinquent finds illegal channels to obtain desired resources.

Another sociological perspective views delinquency as the product of "successful socialization" into a **subculture** whose values are at odds with the dominant culture.[22] For example, urban slums and ghettos often provide environments where opportunities for crime are numerous, yet barriers against crime or delinquency are weak.[23] In these subcultures, role models provide firsthand knowledge of the behaviors and rewards, seldom the penalities. Not all children, however, exposed to the subcultural or delinquent environments become delinquent. The results of Elliott and Voss's[3] longitudinal study suggest that delinquent friends may result from, rather than cause, delinquent behavior.

Several of these explanations emphasize strong bonds and emotional attachments necessary to produce a socialized individual. The approaches differ, however, in their emphasis on early childhood factors. Psychodynamic theorists attach particular importance to early childhood experiences and maternal relationships, whereas social learning and sociological perspectives view behavior as a function of continuous experiences throughout one's lifetime. In the less deterministic models, delinquency arises from what is happening in the present; that is, reinforcement of current behaviors.

These theories have been based on the assumption that youths who commit delinquent acts differ in measurable ways from those who do not. Involvement in delinquent behavior is explained by environmental and institutional forces or factors residing within the individual. However, some argue that there is no difference between delinquents and nondelinquents, except that one group has been caught and processed by the system. Thus, officially labeling a youth as delinquent causes others to respond to that youth differently, with the consequence of promoting and encouraging further delinquency. As a causal explanation of delinquency, this theory is limited. Labeling may explain why a person continues to behave in a delinquent manner, but it does not explain initial delinquent behavior. Furthermore, labeling effects appear to be most pronounced among white, middle-class youths with no prior records;[24] moreover, the idea that labeling fosters a delinquent identity is being challenged on empirical grounds.[25]

Each of these theories can point to some supporting evidence; however, none by itself provides an adequate explanation of delinquent behavior. There is no single causal factor. Biological predispositions, family disruption and disorganization, personality characteristics, deviant subcultures, academic failure, unemployment, or poverty do not individually explain the delinquency. Rather, delinquent behavior is the result of many variables associated with the individual and her or his environment which interact in an ongoing and reciprocal manner.[26]

CORRELATES OF DELINQUENCY

Investigators have examined the relationship of numerous factors to delinquency. Here we selectively review some of the correlates of delinquency, focusing on sex, cognitive and intellectual factors, and a variety of environmental variables.

Sex

It has been said that sex is the most important correlate of official crime statistics. While there is general agreement that boys are more involved in delinquent behavior than girls, there has been disagreement about the magnitude of the differences, the pattern, seriousness, changes over time, and so forth. In official arrest statistics, boy:girl ratios have varied considerably, from 3:1 up to 8:1, depending on the study reviewed. According to the Uniform Crime Reports, for youths under 18 the arrest ratio for boys to girls in 1981 was 3.9:1.[27] Because of the problems and inadequacies of official statistics, however, self-report surveys have been used to assess incidence, patterns, and correlates of delinquent behavior. For self-reported delinquency, boy:girl ratios have been much lower.[3,28,29]

Official and self-report studies disagree on the nature of sex differences in delinquency. Official statistics indicate greater differences in delinquency involvement between boys and girls, with boys primarily involved in property and violent crimes and girls more involved in traditionally female crimes (for example, prostitution, running away from home, and so forth). In contrast, self-report studies indicate smaller sex differences in patterns of delinquent involvement.[28,30-32]

In a recent analysis of sex differences in self-reported delinquency, using data from the National Youth Survey (a national probability sample of 1725 adolescents ages 11 to 17), Canter[33] found small but consistent sex differences in all subcategories of crime examined, with the exception of illegal service crimes, hard drug use, home delinquency, felony theft, and minor theft. Boy:girl ratios varied from 7:1 for robbery to no difference (1:1) for hard drug use. Canter also found large sex differences in the proportion of high-frequency offenders (that is, boys were more likely to report a large number of delinquent behaviors).

Elliott[24] examined the stability of sex differences across time by comparing 1977 National Youth Survey data with Gold and Reimer's[34] data from 1967 to 1972. Limiting her analysis to 13- to 16-year-olds and across eight similar items, Canter[33] compared the three samples (1967, 1972, 1977) and found stable sex differences across the 10-year period. Although there were dramatic increases in marijuana use, truancy, and alcohol across time, these increases were similar for boys and girls. According to Canter, "while females have closed the gap with males somewhat on alcohol use and have demonstrated sizable increases in their participation in drinking and other delinquent behaviors, their involvement in delinquent behavior relative to males has remained lower."

Despite increased interest and publications on this topic, researchers are only just beginning to appreciate the ways in which sex or gender affects our understanding of crime and delinquency. In a recent examination of the relationship between sex roles and adult criminality, Widom[35] illustrates how assumptions and societal expectations about appropriate sex-role behavior influence choice of causal theories and models, diagnosis and labeling, research designs, and society's responses to behavior.

Cognitive and Intellectual Factors

A number of studies have found an inverse relationship between **intelligence quotient (IQ)** and delinquency. Some interpret this relationship as an example of the problems faced by children from educationally deprived backgrounds. However, the findings from two Danish longitudinal studies suggest that the relationship is not spurious. Moffitt and associates[36] found a negative relationship between IQ and delinquency, controlling for socioeconomic status (SES). They note that "low IQ children may be likely to engage in delinquent behavior because their poor verbal abilities limit their opportunities to obtain rewards in the school environment."

Hyperactivity or "Attention Deficit Disorder* with hyperactivity" *(DSM III)*[37] has been linked to delinquency. Children with this disorder display "signs of developmentally inappropriate inattention, impulsivity, and hyperactivity." Support for an association between hyperactivity and later antisocial behavior comes from a number of sources: (1) Longitudinal studies have indicated a relationship between hyperactivity and later antisocial behavior;[38] (2) retrospective studies have indicated that parents of delinquents, who may themselves be impulsive and violent, often have histories of hyperkinetic syndrome as children;[39,40] and (3) hyperactivity has been related to alcoholism, psychopathy, and other neurological disorders in adulthood.[41,42]

Numerous studies have documented a link between juvenile delinquency and specific **learning disabilities** (see Lane[43]). Most are based on children from predominantly lower-class backgrounds, so that the relationship between learning disabilities and children arrested for delinquency is confounded with social class. For example, a recent study by Broder and coworkers[44] challenges the hypothesis that learning-disabled children necessarily engage in more delinquent behavior. Although there was a higher incidence of learning disability problems in adjudicated delinquents, the authors found that self-reported delinquency had a low but **negative** relationship to learning disability. Although not necessarily involved in more delinquent activity, learning-disabled youths had a greater chance of being found delinquent in juvenile court. On the other hand, in a recent study addressing many of these concerns, Wolff and associates[45] found that delinquents differed markedly from both lower- and upper-middle-class controls on language measures but not on nonlinguistic neuropsychological measures. Group differences were not removed by adjusting for nonverbal intelligence. The authors concluded that the delinquents were "selectively impaired in language functions and that the language deficits were a characteristic of the delinquent index group, rather than a nonspecific correlate of social-environmental factors."

Delinquents have also been characterized by egocentrism, inability to demonstrate empathy, and lack of foresight about the consequences of their actions, thereby suggesting a certain similarity to what Piaget referred to as "preoperational children." **Preoperational,** in Piagetian usage, refers to the transitional period between the development of sensorimotor skills and adaptations typically associated with infancy and the first signs of the development of the capacity for conceptual and symbolic thinking. Empirically, it has been noted that delinquents perform at a lower stage of ego development than nondelinquents.[46,47]

Environmental Factors

Delinquency is **not** primarily a lower-class problem. Findings from self-report studies of delinquency question a bias toward the lower class. Only in **arrest** rates is the apparent skewness maintained.[48,49]

---

* Attention Deficit Disorder may encompass different subtypes with respect to etiology, because children with this syndrome exhibit differences in physical, neurological, and biochemical indicators. Some types of Attention Deficit Disorder may promote antisocial behavior, whereas others might not.

Historically, the **family** has probably received more attention than any other factor associated with delinquency. It has been suggested that as family size increases, the likelihood of delinquency in children also increases.[50] Psychiatric disturbance in parents[8] as well as hospitalization and/or treatment for mental illness[51] has been linked to delinquency in children. Interactions between delinquent adolescents and their parents have consistently been found to be less supportive and more coercive than those between nondelinquents and their parents.[52]

Farrington[53] found that harsh parental attitude and discipline was the best predictor of later criminal violence, better than rated aggressive behavior in school. These results are similar to those of McCord and coworkers,[54] who also found that violent delinquents, as children, tended to have parents who were rejecting and punitive, who supervised them poorly, disciplined erratically, and who themselves were aggressive, alcoholic, or convicted. In a recent review of 71 delinquency prediction studies from the United States and abroad, Loeber and Dishion[55] found that the principal predictors of delinquency were parents' family management and techniques (supervision and discipline); the child's conduct problems (stealing, lying, and truancy); parental criminality; and the child's poor academic performance (poor educational achievement).

The effect of **broken homes** on delinquency has received considerable attention and continues to be of concern. In a longitudinal study of British youths, Wadsworth[56] found that delinquency was strongly associated with early disruption of a parent-child relationship through death or marital separation. But in a study of middle-class delinquency, Hennessey and associates[57] found that family structure had only a small effect on self-reported delinquency. Findings from other research also indicate that the impact of family structure varies with other factors such as sex, race, type of offense, and community attitudes toward broken homes.[26,58-60]

Recently, **child abuse** has been implicated as a factor in later delinquent behavior (see also chapter 10). In addition to the failure to provide adequate supervision and socialization for their children, abusive parents might also serve as models for aggression and impulsivity, thereby fostering the development of these behaviors in their offspring. If the child is afraid to retaliate against abusive parents, then he or she might retaliate against others in the form of antisocial and aggressive behavior. Some reports have noted a relationship between parental child abuse and later delinquency (for example, Alfaro[61]). However, because of serious limitations in samples studied and research designs, there are a number of confounds which make any relationship reported very tentative at best.

Delinquent behavior has been related more clearly and consistently to success or failure in **school** experiences. High academic achievement has consistently been associated with lower rates of delinquent behavior.[62] This relationship has also been found in self-report studies[17,28] and appears to hold across races and socioeconomic levels.[63]

Nutritional deficits have also been implicated in the development of delinquency. For example, it has been hypothesized that iron deficiency may cause perceptual alteration, which in turn might lead to learning and behavioral problems.[64] Diet, food additives, insufficient nutrients, and food allergies have also been linked to delinquent behaviors.[65] Despite these suggested links, the relationship between nutritional factors and delinquency remains controversial.

Population, growth, change, and mobility associated with industrialization have been linked to higher delinquency rates, owing to the breakdown of traditional forms of control, such as family, school, religion, and community. Changing patterns of community composition (racial and ethnic patterns) have been related to changing levels of delinquent behavior.[66] Rates of crime and delinquency as well as offense patterns have been reported to differ for rural and urban settings.[67]

TYPES OF DELINQUENTS

Over the years there has been increasing recognition that delinquency is not a unitary phenomenon and that delinquents are not a homogeneous group of antisocial young people. Although no single theory can account for all types, there are certain similarities in characteristics and behaviors of groups of delinquents.

By creating more manageable and homogeneous subgroups, classification schemes and typologies may facilitate further understanding of delinquency. Typologies can and do serve a variety of purposes and may differ in theoretical perspective, methodologies used to develop them, and subject samples. Because of obvious space limitations, only a few examples of typologies are presented. Those discussed here have implications for the development of different kinds of treatment and intervention programs.

Warren's[68] I-level classification system is based on the **interpersonal maturity** level of the person. The theory, originally stated by Sullivan, Grant, and Grant,[69] assumes that individuals pass through a series of developmental stages, which increase in complexity over time, culminating in the interpersonal competence of the adult. Although nine categories are identified within the typology, the most frequently occurring types are referred to as conflicted/anxious, conflicted/acting-out, power-oriented, passive conformist, and cultural conformist.[70] Warren's classification has been used on a large scale in an attempt to match treatments to types of clients. For example, the I-level system has been used to classify numerous correctional populations (for example, the California Youth Authority classifies each youth sent to its reception center according to I-level).

In a series of factor-analytic studies based on some earlier work by Jenkins,[71] Quay and Parsons[72] used behavior ratings and personality measures from a variety of samples (normal, disturbed, and delinquent children of varying ages) and consistently identified and demonstrated the existence of four to five factors. Four of the basic dimensions were (1) **inadequate-immature,** which included behaviors such as preoccupation, being easily flustered and confused, laziness, short attention span, and excessive daydreaming; (2) **unsocialized-psychopathic,** associated with lack of socialization and concern for others manifested in impulsiveness; assaultiveness; and a rebellious, antiauthority, amoral, attitude; (3) **neurotic-disturbed,** characterized by social withdrawal, guilt, anxiety, and depression; and (4) **socialized-subcultural,** involving the acceptance of social norms of a delinquent subgroup, rather than neurotic conflicts or lack of socialization. Quay's factorial system is being applied to predicting correctional treatment outcomes in a study at the National Training School of Boys.

In the third and most recent edition of the American Psychiatric Association's *Diagnostic and Statistical Manual of Mental Disorders (DSM III),*[37] there is no category labeled "juvenile delinquent." The *DSM III* refers to the diagnosis of

conduct disorder, the essential feature of which is "a repetitive and persistent pattern of conduct in which either the basic rights of others or major age-appropriate societal norms or rules are violated." The conduct thus categorized is "more serious than the ordinary mischief and pranks of childhood adolescence." An individual is further classified as either aggressive or nonaggressive and socialized or undersocialized, resulting in four specific subtypes: (1) undersocialized, aggressive; (2) undersocialized, nonaggressive; (3) socialized, aggressive; and (4) socialized, nonaggressive.

Two recent studies suggest the usefulness of *DSM III* criteria in predicting differential social outcomes. Henn, Bardwell, and Jenkins[73] examined criminal activities of male juvenile delinquents who had been classified according to *DSM III* criteria (using behavior, personality, psychological test results, and family background characteristics). During the 10 years following discharge from the Iowa State Training School for Boys, undersocialized aggressive boys were involved in more crimes of violence than were the boys of the other groups. The socialized delinquents had significantly less chance of being convicted on an adult charge and of going to prison as an adult than undersocialized delinquents. Similarly, Kashani, Horwitz, and Daniel[74] in their study of delinquent boys at the Missouri State Training School found classification according to the *DSM III* criteria useful in regard to prognosis and management.

Although samples, classification procedures, and dependent variables differed across these studies, there is remarkable similarity in some of the basic types or dimensions that have been isolated. Typologies of adult male offenders,[75] female juvenile delinquents,[76] and adult female offenders[77] also reveal characteristics strikingly in common with the types of delinquents described above.

DIVERSION, TREATMENT, AND RECIDIVISM

Youths become delinquent in a variety of ways and by committing a variety of offenses, and their motivations, needs, personalities, and backgrounds vary considerably. Deciding how to handle juvenile delinquents thus presents a number of problems. At one end of the spectrum, juveniles may be sent to state institutions (such as training schools) designed to isolate the "dangerous delinquent" from society. Residential care facilities and outpatient treatment programs are less restrictive, and probation represents minimal formal supervision. Informal kinds of adjustments made by the police or juvenile court intake staff are the least restrictive and most diversionary form of treatment.

The United States has a "two-tiered" system of justice, one for juveniles and one for adults. The juvenile justice system was originally created to protect juveniles from the harshness of the adult system. However, over the last decade, it has been argued that youths should also be diverted from the juvenile justice system itself as much as possible.

Diversion

Since the 1960s, many courts have adopted the "least restrictive alternative" principle, partially out of concern for the "overprocessing" of young offenders. Interest in **diversion** arose from recognition of the potential negative effects of stigmatization through involvement in the formal juvenile justice system, increased awareness of the limits of rehabilitation via correctional institutions and of the inefficiency of traditional strategies for treatment and prevention of delinquency, and genuine concern for the effective and humane treatment of delinquent youth.

One source estimated that **status offenders** (juveniles convicted only of running away from home, truancy, sexual promiscuity, or incorrigibility rather than of criminal law violations) represented nearly 40 percent of the cases referred to juvenile court.[78] The Federal Juvenile Justice and Delinquency Prevention Act of 1974 was designed to encourage the removal of status offenders from detention and correctional facilities through various diversion and deinstitutionalization programs. However, these efforts have been criticized because at least one basic assumption about status offenders is highly questionable. Findings from recent research indicate that most delinquents commit a range of offenses; the "pure" status offender is relatively rare.[81-83] Thus, more complexity is involved in diverting status offenders from the formal juvenile justice system than was originally realized. Despite attempts to deinstitutionalize the juvenile justice system,[79] there were 45,251 juveniles in public custody facilities and 28,707 in private facilities in 1979. An additional 7175 youths (ages 17 years and younger) were prisoners in state and federal adult correctional facilities.[80]

Rutherford and McDermott[84] have outlined three types of diversion programs. **Legal diversion** operates from within the system and attempts to minimize penetration of individuals into the formal system. **Paralegal diversion** occurs in agencies outside, but still connected to, the formal system (for example, youth service bureaus). The third type of diversion is **nonlegal** and takes place entirely outside the juvenile justice system; participation is voluntary.

Different kinds of evidence for the effectiveness of diversion programs have been presented. Theoretically, diversion allows the system to be more efficient by decreasing the number of cases handled in court. This should permit the remaining cases to receive more effective and prompt treatment, enabling courts to concentrate their resources on the more serious or difficult cases. Indeed, diversion programs have been found to reduce court caseloads and to decrease expenses.[85]

In 1972, Massachusetts closed its juvenile training schools and reformatories and placed over 1000 youths in new, small, nonsecure community-based residential or nonresidential programs. Less than 5 percent of the youths—those considered dangerous enough to require secure facilities—were detained traditionally. According to one report,[86] communities varied as to their success in absorbing the youths, but the Massachusetts experiment with deinstitutionalization did not lead to any major increases in juvenile crime. On the other hand, deinstitutionalization programs have proved to be inconsequential in reducing recidivism rates.[85,87]

California's Community Treatment Program,[88] incorporating Warren's I-level classification system, has been among the most thoroughly evaluated diversion programs. Participants were 13 to 19 years of age and were first randomly assigned to the program (before incarceration) or were first institutionalized prior to being paroled. Each parole agent had a caseload of no more than 12 youths, and the development of individualized treatment programs for each youth was encouraged. The results suggested that certain "neurotic" types functioned as well or better under conditions of intensive parole supervision without initial incarceration, whereas others (for example, power-oriented youth) did better with a short period of incarceration or residential treatment before release to the community-based programs.[70]

Lerman[89] criticized dependence on parole violations and suggested that there was a broader, system-wide, impact of the treatment program. Although delinquent behaviors for both groups were probably similar, according to Lerman, the rate of being noticed was different. The delinquent behavior of the experimental group received more official notice, yet it was less often labeled as a parole violation.

Although diversion programs were originally designed to provide more humane treatment of juveniles and to reduce the number of juveniles in contact with the criminal justice system, the effect of these programs may not be so salutary. Community-based treatments may not be more beneficial or humane than juvenile court processing. Young offenders often get caught between community agencies vying for clients and funds.[90] Rather than diverting children who would have been brought into the legal system, diversion programs are bringing in children who would previously have been excluded. Many cases that previously would have been dropped after initial contact with the police are now being diverted into new programs. Hence, diversion appears to represent a supplement to rather than a substitute for court disciplinary proceedings. Moreover, there is broader discretion in handling some of the less serious cases, and diversionary programs may inadvertently produce harsher treatment of those who are not diverted.[91] Finally, Bullington and coworkers[92] suggest that formal diversion is incompatible with due process ideals.

Treatment Programs

A review of the history of the treatment of delinquents reveals few positive results, so that any discussion of effective programs could be quite brief. This review is illustrative and selective and makes no attempt to be comprehensive. Rather, the goal is to summarize the major approaches, particularly those with significant evaluation components.

For example, although individual examples of success can be cited, **professional counseling** has consistently been found not to be effective with delinquents. Thus, the success of conventional psychotherapy methods with delinquents is basically much less than with children having other psychological and behavioral disorders.[93,94]

In probably the most famous longitudinal research on delinquency prevention and treatment, the Cambridge-Somerville Youth Study, juvenile delinquents and a group of matched controls were given guidance and counseling, with treatment lasting from 5 to 8 years. In an early follow-up, the recidivism rate for youths given counseling was about the same as for those who had not received counseling.[95] A further 30-year follow-up indicated that the counseling interventions failed to prevent later crime. Indeed, the results were somewhat better for the untreated youths! Participation in the treatment program was associated with various negative outcomes; for example, a higher incidence of alcoholism, mental illness, stress-related diseases, and early death.[96]

When treatments have been routinely applied to all types of offenders, overall outcomes have been generally negative. However, one product of the work on delinquent typologies has been the effort in some projects to design differential treatments and interventions on the basis of characteristics shared by similar types of delinquents. When client, treatment program, therapist, and location are considered, there are more examples of success. For example, the "conflicted" or neurotic offender, who exhibits evidence of considerable neurotic symptoms (for example, guilt or anxiety over the offense), usually does better in and benefits more from individual counseling and psychotherapeutic experiences.[97-99]

Among the **behavioral approaches** used, delinquents have been exposed to such procedures as reinforcement by peers, token economies, and contingency contracting. Interpretations of the effectiveness of these procedures have varied. Initial reports of behaviorally oriented treatments were quite optimistic, demonstrating that the behavior of delinquent adolescents could indeed be modified.[100] For example, a number of studies evaluating the effects of contingent consequences on discrete behaviors have shown reductions in aggressive behavior and speech and increases in prosocial behavior.[101] However, the long-term benefits of these treatment programs have not been maintained, particularly once the youths have been returned to their natural environments.[100,102-104]

Sarason[105] reported positive results with children at the Cascadia Juvenile Reception–Diagnostic Center in Washington. Follow-up studies conducted 4 and 5 years later showed lower recidivism rates among the boys in modeling and discussion groups than among those in the control group. Another successful program was a behaviorally oriented family-therapy program developed by Alexander and Parsons.[106] Teenagers assigned to this treatment program (involving efforts to improve communication among family members and to negotiate contingency contracts) were less likely to become reinvolved in the juvenile justice system than teenagers in psychodynamic group therapy, client-centered family counseling, or a no-treatment group.

Another behavioral intervention program for the treatment of juveniles within a group-home setting is the Achievement Place Project.[107] Based on behavioral principles, the treatment approach was developed on the premise that deviant behavior might be reduced or eliminated by "providing youths with relationships with adults who have high reinforcing value, who provide differential consequences for youth behavior, and who teach requisite social, academic, and self-care skills for successful community living."[107] Since 1967, the Achievement Place group home model in Lawrence, Kansas (originally developed and evaluated as a community-based program), has served as the prototype for the Teaching-Family programs.[108] The program incorporates skill teaching, self-government, motivation, relationship development, and youth advocacy within the context of a structured family setting and under the guidance of a married couple (the teaching parents). As of January 1981, there were six regional training sites and approximately 170 Teaching-Family group homes operating throughout the country. Although Kirigin and associates[108] are careful to point out the limitations associated with the design, sample size, and outcome measures used in their evaluation studies of their group homes, they concluded that the Teaching-Family programs provided a set of conditions that reduced delinquent behavior during treatment to a greater degree than the comparison programs and did so in a manner that produced more positive ratings by the youth participants. In contrast to the during-treatment differences favoring the Teaching-Family programs, there were no posttreatment differences in the rates of criminal offenses or in the percentage of youths institutionalized or involved in further offenses.

Although treatment programs have not yet been shown to have an appreciable impact on failure rates, this finding should not be misinterpreted as providing a basis for a return to harsher methods of treatment. There is no evidence that more humanitarian approaches necessarily lead to greater failure rates.

Recidivism

Although there is little conclusive evidence as to what constitutes effective treatment for juvenile offenders, the evaluative criterion used most frequently is the rate of recidivism: the number of offenders involved in further criminal activities, as determined through arrests or convictions. This dependence on recidivism rates has received much criticism. Specifically, recidivism rates are seriously confounded with the discretionary actions of juvenile justice system personnel.

For example, recontact with the criminal justice system represents one measure of potential failure. Although it is common to measure the success of correctional treatment programs by determining whether youths released from custody have refrained from known violations of the law, Lerman[89] has argued that this criterion of known violations is misleading. He points out that youths released from an institution who are not "renoticed" might be considered successes. Similarly, youths who have been involved in offensive behavior but who have not been reinstitutionalized could be counted as successes. This would be a questionable practice.

There are a number of administrative decisions and actions (from arrest to conviction to revocation of parole) that affect recidivism rates. Persons on probation or parole can be returned to an institution not because of rearrest or reconviction but because they have violated certain conditions of their probation or parole. Such "technical" violations, it should be noted, do not appear to be very frequent bases for revocation of probation or parole. Nevertheless, recidivism depends not only on the behavior of the individual but also on policies, practices, and associated responses of criminal justice system officials. Recidivism rates may also be too crude to assess accurately the benefits of a particular correctional program.

What other factors affect whether a juvenile will persist in antisocial behavior into adulthood? One of the clearest is age of onset of delinquency. Wolfgang[109,110] found a strong relationship between juvenile and adult arrests and reported that the probability of rearrest reaches a peak of about 80 percent for youths with six or more arrests. Hamparian and coworkers[111] found a strong inverse relationship between age of first arrest and average number of arrests. In their study, the average number of arrests decreased from 7.27 for those whose first arrest was at age 10 years or younger to 4.10 for those whose first arrest was at age 13 years. West and Farrington[112] also found a close relationship between juvenile and adult delinquency. More than 75 percent of those with four or more juvenile convictions also had four or more adult convictions, and the youths first convicted at the earliest ages (10 to 12 years of age) were likely to be the most persistent offenders.

DELINQUENCY PREVENTION: CAUSE FOR FUTURE OPTIMISM?

The fact that the juvenile court system has not been able to demonstrate success has encouraged some to develop different proposals involving fundamental changes in approach. Intervention projects with youths have typically been secondary prevention efforts, that is, diverting youths who have already had official contact with the legal system toward some form of psychotherapeutically oriented treatment program. However, intervention programs have been plagued with weak methodologies, poor evaluations, and lack of comprehensive, well-grounded, multidimensional theories guiding the projects.

For a number of reasons, early intervention projects have been proposed. Extremely antisocial delinquents do not appear to outgrow the problem;[113,114] rather, retrospective[115] and prospective longitudinal[116] studies indicate considerable continuity of antisocial behavior in juveniles, adolescents, and adults.

In a series of outcome-evaluation studies of parent-training programs for preadolescent children, Patterson and his colleagues at the Oregon Social Learning Center have demonstrated significant decreases in deviant child behavior.[117] More recently, Loeber,[55] Patterson, and colleagues have been developing a predictive model involving "proto-delinquent behaviors" that can be incorporated into prevention programs; this model systematically applies a multiple-stage assessment and screening procedure to a successively reduced sample of youngsters who are determined to be at risk for serious delinquent behavior.[55]

Another intervention effort by Shure and Spivack[118] is focused on approximately 600 children who entered kindergarten in a predominantly black, lower-class, urban center in 1968. Utilizing a competency building model, and assuming that there are individual differences in the ability to solve typical interpersonal problems with peers and adults and that these differences can be reliably distinguished among children, Shure and Spivack designed an interpersonal cognitive problem-solving intervention with young children aimed at reducing and preventing impulsive and inhibited behavior. Because these behavior patterns typically elicit negative responses from parents and teachers, these adult responses in turn are likely to trigger hostile reactions and increased likelihood of engaging in further antisocial behavior in the children. According to Shure and Spivack,

> Helping inner-city black four- and five-years-olds learn to think through and solve interpersonal problems reduced aberrant impulsive and uninhibited behaviors, maintained those improvements over time, and prevented behavior problems from occurring in already adjusted children.[118]

Despite the potential for success in these intervention projects, there is still an urgent need to identify critical variables and relevant risk factors in delinquency, to develop accurate screening instruments with minimal levels of false-positives, and to implement and to evaluate interventions.

CONCLUSION

Delinquency is a complex social and legal phenomenon. There is no single homogeneous entity that can be labeled delinquency nor is there a clear dichotomy between delinquents and nondelinquents. Current approaches to delinquency and its treatment are influenced by past and present social norms and values, which in turn influence public policy. As with attempts to address other social problems, such as the "war on poverty," policies regarding delinquency are influenced by public opinions and ideologies.

In the 1960s there was concern for the overprocessing of young offenders. The 1970s produced attempts to deinstitutionalize delinquents through community-based treatment programs. Given the experiences of the last 20 years, what can we expect and hope for in the 1980s?

Delinquency is not caused by any single factor. Rather, behavioral and social scientists are adopting multivariate and multistage systems approaches. The results of past studies are being re-examined in the context of these more complex multidimensional models. Loeber and Dishion,[55] for example, discuss consistencies in studies of the predictors of delinquency, noting that the earliest predictors identified were factors related to adverse family functioning. Problem behaviors, such as troublesomeness and daring behavior on the part of the youth, appeared later in the developmental process. However, these predictors occur prior to the manifestation of antisocial or delinquent behavior and before the onset of significant school problems in particular.

One of the most consistent findings that has emerged in recent years is the importance of school experiences. School problems may be critical in the early stages of delinquency and may serve as a crucial marker for the child. However, at the same time it is important to avoid the trap of self-fulfilling prophecies and the potential stigmatizing effects of being labeled "predelinquent."

Results from some of the early intervention projects, such as the work of Shure and Spivack[118] and of Patterson and his colleagues[117] suggest that it may be possible to reverse the outcome of early school difficulties. These studies also underscore the complexity of the problem.

From a research perspective, these findings and reanalyses are exciting developments in understanding delinquency. However, further research is needed to continue this work on the identification of early predictors and critical factors in the development of delinquency. There is also a need to cross-validate these findings in different geographic regions and with different groups of youth, of both sexes, inasmuch as the predictive efficiency of these variables may vary somewhat. Furthermore, it is important to identify factors that prevent the development of delinquency in those youths who are at high risk.

Prediction and prevention are the most desirable ways to deal with delinquency. Despite the fact that evaluations of treatment programs have generally yielded inconsistent and discouraging results, there is no evidence that increased incarceration is the most effective way to deal with delinquency.

Treatment efforts must recognize and incorporate the heterogeneity of delinquents. Again, there is no single best treatment for all delinquents. The few studies that report successful treatment programs take into account the differential needs of the youngsters, tailoring treatment programs accordingly. We must ask which treatments best fit which types of youths at different points in their lives and under varying environmental circumstances. The identification of similar types in the widely divergent classification schemes is encouraging and exciting. Yet, if these are to become clinically useful typologies, there is much work to be done to develop consistent criteria, to incorporate these into treatment programs, and to evaluate these typologies in scientifically sound ways.

Policy makers are increasingly utilizing information from behavioral and social science research. For example, over 5 million dollars was recently designated by the Office of Juvenile Justice and Delinquency Prevention to direct prosecutorial efforts at segments of the delinquent population, specifically juvenile gangs and habitual offenders. This concentration on particular elements within the larger delinquent population is based on the research finding that small numbers of delinquents are responsible for a disproportionate amount of crime.

Despite the lack of demonstrable success in prevention and treatment programs to date, society remains reluctant to fall back on purely retributive sanctions for juvenile offenders. Treatment efforts continue, and research on prediction and primary prevention of delinquency indicates that there may be cause for qualified optimism.

REFERENCES

1. US DEPARTMENT OF JUSTICE, FEDERAL BUREAU OF INVESTIGATION: *Uniform Crime Reports for the United States, 1979.* US Government Printing Office, Washington, DC, 1980.

2. WOLFGANG, M, FIGLIO, RM, SELLIN, T: *Delinquency in a Birth Cohort.* University of Chicago Press, Chicago, 1972.

3. ELLIOTT, DS AND VOSS, HL: *Delinquency and Dropout.* DC Heath, Lexington, MA, 1974.

4. WILLIAMS, JR AND GOLD, M: *From delinquent behavior to official delinquency.* Social Problems 20:209, 1972.

5. PETRIE, A: *Individuality in Pain and Suffering.* University of Chicago Press, Chicago, 1967.

6. ZUCKERMAN, M: *Sensation seeking and psychopathy.* In HARE, RD AND SCHALLING, D (EDS): *Psychopathic Behaviour.* John Wiley & Sons, New York, 1978.

7. HARE, RD, AND SCHALLING, D (EDS): *Psychopathic Behavior.* John Wiley & Sons, New York, 1978.

8. LEWIS, DO (ED): *Vulnerabilities to Delinquency.* Spectrum Publications, Jamaica, NY, 1981.

9. PENNER, MJ; *The role of selected health problems in the causation of juvenile delinquency.* Adolescence 17:347, 1982.

10. MEDNICK, SA AND VOLAVKA, J: *Biology and crime.* In MORRIS, N AND TONRY, M (EDS): *Crime and Justice: An Annual Review of Research,* Vol 2. University of Chicago Press, Chicago, 1980.

11. ELLIS, L: *Genetics and criminal behavior.* Criminology 20:43, 1982.

12. CHRISTIANSEN, KO: *The genesis of aggressive criminality: Implications of a study of crime in a Danish twin sample.* In DEWIT, J AND HARTRUP, WW (EDS): *Determinants and Origins of Aggressive Behavior.* Mouton, The Hague, 1974.

13. DALGARD, OS AND KRINGLEN, E: *A Norwegian twin study of criminality.* British Journal of Criminology 16:213, 1976.

14. HUTCHINGS, B AND MEDNICK, SA: *Registered criminality in the adoptive and biological parents of registered male criminal adoptees.* In MEDNICK, SA, SCHULSINGER, F, HIGGINS, J, BELL, B (EDS): *Genetics, Environment and Psychopathology.* North Holland/Elsevier, Amsterdam, 1974.

15. CROWE, RR: *An adoption study of anti-social personality.* Arch Gen Psychiatry 31:785, 1974.

16. AICHHORN, A: *Wayward Youth.* Viking Press, New York, 1936.

17. KONOPKA, G: *The Adolescent Girl in Conflict.* Prentice-Hall, Englewood Cliffs, NJ, 1966.

18. BANDURA, A: *The social learning perspective: Mechanisms of aggression.* In TOCH, H (ED): *Psychology of Crime and Criminal Justice.* Holt, Rinehart, & Winston, New York, 1979.

19. HIRSCHI, T: *Causes of Delinquency.* University of California Press, Berkeley, CA, 1969.

20. COHEN, AK: *Delinquent Boys.* Free Press, New York, 1955.

21. CLOWARD, RA AND OHLIN, LE: *Delinquency and Opportunity.* Free Press, New York, 1960.

22. SUTHERLAND, EH: *Principles of Criminology,* ed 4. JB Lippincott, Philadelphia, 1947.

23. MERTON, R: *Social structure and anomie.* American Sociological Review 3:672, 1938.

24. ELLIOTT, DS: *Diversion: A Study of Alternative Processing Practices.* Behavioral Research Institute, Boulder, CO, 1978.

25. HEPBURN, JR: *The impact of police intervention upon juvenile delinquents.* Criminology 15:235, 1977.

26. WIDOM, CS, KATKIN, FS, STEWART, AJ, FONDACARO, M: *Multivariate analysis of personality and motivation in female delinquents.* Journal of Research in Crime and Delinquency 20:277, 1983.

27. US FEDERAL BUREAU OF INVESTIGATION: *Uniform Crime Report of the United States, 1981.* US Government Printing Office, Washington, DC, 1982.

28. JENSEN, GF AND EVE, R: *Sex differences in delinquency.* Criminology 13:427, 1976.

29. CERNKOVICH, SA AND GIORDANO, PC: *A comparative analysis of male and female delinquency.* Sociological Quarterly 20:131, 1979.

30. GOLD, M: *Delinquency Behavior in an American City.* Wadsworth, Belmont, CA, 1970.

31. HINDELANG, MJ: *Age, sex, and versatility of delinquent involvements.* Social Problems 18:522, 1971.

32. SHOVER, N AND NORLAND, S: *Sex roles and criminality: Science or conventional wisdom?* Sex Roles 4:111, 1978.

33. CANTER, RJ: *Sex differences in self-report delinquency.* Criminology 20:373, 1982.

34. GOLD, M AND REIMER, DJ: *Changing Patterns of Delinquent Behavior Among Americans 13 to 16 Years Old, 1967-1972. Report no. 1 of the National Survey of Youth, 1972.* Institute for Social Research, University of Michigan, Ann Arbor, MI, 1972.

35. WIDOM, CS: *Sex roles, criminality, and psychopathology.* In WIDOM, CS (ED): *Sex Roles and Psychopathology.* Plenum, New York, 1984.

36. MOFFITT, TE, GABRIELLI, WF, MEDNICK, SA, SCHULSINGER, F: *Socioeconomic status, IQ, and delinquency.* J Abnorm Psychology 90:152, 1981.

37. AMERICAN PSYCHIATRIC ASSOCIATION: *Diagnostic and Statistical Manual of Mental Disorders,* ed 3. American Psychiatric Association, Washington, DC, 1980.

38. MENDELSON, W, JOHNSON, N, STEWART, MA: *Hyperactive children as teenagers.* J Nerv Ment Dis 153:273, 1971.

39. QUITLAN, F AND KLEIN, D: *Two behavioral syndromes in young adults related to possible minimal brain dysfunction.* J Psychiatr Res 7:131, 1969.

40. SHELLEY, E AND RIESTER, A: *Syndrome of minimal brain damage in young adults.* Diseases of the Nervous System 33:335, 1972.

41. MORRISON, JR AND STEWART, MA: *A family study of the hyperactive child syndrome.* Biol Psychiatry 3:189, 1971.

42. CANTWELL, DP: *Psychiatric illness in families of hyperactive children.* Arch Gen Psychiatry 27:414, 1972.

43. LANE, BA: *The relationship of learning disabilities to juvenile delinquency: Current status.* Journal of Learning Disability 13:425, 1980.

44. BRODER, PK, DUNIVANT, N, SMITH, EC, SUTTON, LP: *Further observations on the link between learning disabilities and juvenile delinquency.* National Center for State Courts Publications Dept., Williamsburg, VA, 1980.

45. WOLFF, PH, WABER, D, BAUERMEISTER, M, COHEN, C, FERBER, R: *The neuropsychological status of adolescent delinquent boys.* J Child Psychol Psychiatry 23:267, 1982.

46. FRANK, S AND QUINLAN, DM: *Ego development and female delinquency: A cognitive-developmental approach.* J Abnorm Psychology 85:505, 1976.

47. LUND, NL AND SALARY, HM: *Measured self-concept in adjudicated juvenile offenders.* Adolescence 15:65, 1980.

48. TITTLE, CR, VILLEMEZ, WJ, SMITH, DA: *The myth of social class and criminality: An empirical assessment of the empirical evidence.* American Sociological Review 43:643, 1978.

49. ELLIOTT, DS AND AGETON, SS: *Reconciling race and class differences in self-reported and official estimates of delinquency.* American Sociological Review 45:95, 1980.

50. RUTTER, M AND GILLER, H: *Juvenile delinquency: Trends and perspectives.* Home Office Research Bulletin 13:26, 1982.

51. LEWIS, DO, BALLA, DA, SHANOK, SS, SNELL, L: *Delinquency, parental psychopathology, and parental criminality.* J Am Acad Child Psychiatry 15:665, 1976.

52. HETHERINGTON, EM AND MARTIN, B: *Family interaction.* In QUAY, HC AND WERRY, JS (EDS): *Psychopathological Disorders of Childhood.* John Wiley & Sons, New York, 1979.

53. FARRINGTON, DP: *The family backgrounds of aggressive youths.* In HERSOV, L, BERGER, M, SHAFFER, D (EDS): *Aggression and Anti-Social Behavior in Childhood and Adolescence.* Pergamon Press, Oxford, 1978.

54. McCORD, J, McCORD, W, HOWARD, A: *Family interaction as antecedent to the direction of male aggressiveness.* Journal of Abnormal and Social Psychology 66:239, 1963.

55. LOEBER, R AND DISHION, T: *Early predictors of male delinquency: A review.* Psychol Bull 94:68, 1983.

56. WADSWORTH, M: *Roots of Delinquency—Infancy, Adolescence and Crime.* Martin Robertson, London, 1979.

57. HENNESSEY, M, RICHARDS, PJ, BERK, RA: *Broken homes and middle-class delinquency.* Criminology 15:505, 1978.

58. DATESMAN, SK AND SCARPITTI, FR: *Female delinquency and broken homes: A reassessment.* Criminology 13:33, 1975.

59. AUSTIN, RL: *Race, father-absence and female delinquency.* Criminology 15:487, 1978.

60. WILKINSON, K: *Broken home and delinquent behavior—An alternative interpretation of contradictory findings.* In HIRSCHI, T AND GOTTFREDSON, M (EDS): *Understanding Crime.* Sage, Beverly Hills, CA, 1980.

61. ALFARO, JD: *Report on the relationship between child abuse and neglect and later socially deviant behavior.* In HUNNER, RJ AND WALKER, YE (EDS): *Exploring the Relationship Between Child Abuse and Delinquency.* Allanheld, Osmun, & Co., Montclair, NJ, 1981.

62. FREASE, DE: *Delinquency, social class, and the schools.* Sociology and Social Research 57:443, 1973.

63. JENSEN, GF: *Race, achievement, and delinquency: A further look at delinquency in a birth cohort.* Am J Soc 82:379, 1976.

64. POLLITT, E, GREENFIELD, D, LEIBEL, R: *Behavioral effects of iron deficiency among preschool children in Cambridge, Mass.* Fed Proc 37:487, 1978.

65. SCHAUSS, A: *Diet, Crime and Delinquency.* Parker House, Berkeley, CA, 1980.

66. BURSIK, RJ AND WEBB, J: *Community change and patterns of delinquency.* Am J Soc 88:24, 1982.

67. JANKOVIC, J, GREEN, RK, CRONK, SD (EDS): *Juvenile Justice in Rural America.* University of Tennessee School of Social Work, Knoxville, TN, 1980.

68. WARREN, MQ: *Intervention with juvenile delinquents*. In ROSENHEIM, M (ED): *Pursuing Justice for the Child*. University of Chicago Press, Chicago, 1976.

69. SULLIVAN, C, GRANT, MQ, GRANT, JD: *The development of interpersonal maturity: Applications to delinquency*. Psychiatry 20:373, 1957.

70. WARREN, M: *Correctional treatment and coercion: The differential effectiveness perspective*. Criminal Justice and Behavior 4:355, 1978.

71. JENKINS, R: *Classification of behavior problems of children*. Am J Psychiatry 125:1032, 1969.

72. QUAY, H AND PARSONS, L: *The Differential Behavioral Classification of the Juvenile Offender*. US Bureau of Prisons, 1970.

73. HENN, FA, BARDWELL, R, JENKINS, RL: *Juvenile delinquents revisited*. Arch Gen Psychiatry 37:1160, 1980.

74. KASHANI, JH, HORWITZ, E, DANIEL, AE: *Diagnostic classification of 120 delinquent boys*. Bull Am Acad Psychiatry Law 10:51, 1982.

75. BLACKBURN, R: *Personality types among abnormal homicides*. British Journal of Criminology 11:14, 1971.

76. BUTLER, EW AND ADAMS, SN: *Typologies of delinquent girls: Some alternative approaches*. Social Forces 44:401, 1966.

77. WIDOM, CS: *An empirical classification of female offenders*. Criminal Justice and Behavior. 5:35, 1978.

78. US DEPARTMENT OF JUSTICE, OFFICE OF JUVENILE JUSTICE AND DELINQUENCY PREVENTION: *Program Announcement: Diversion of Youth from the Juvenile Justice System*. US Law Enforcement Assistance Administration, Washington, DC, 1976.

79. US DEPARTMENT OF JUSTICE, OFFICE OF JUVENILE JUSTICE AND DELINQUENCY PREVENTION: *Children in Custody: Advance Report on the 1979 Census of Public Juvenile Facilities*. US Department of Justice, Washington, DC, 1980.

80. CARLSON, K: *American Prisons and Jails, Volume 2, Population Trends and Projections*. US Government Printing Office, Washington, DC, 1980.

81. THOMAS, CW: *Are status offenders really so different?* Crime and Delinquency 22:438, 1976.

82. WEIS, JG: *Jurisdiction and the Elusive Status Offender—A Comparison of Involvement in Delinquent Behavior and Status Offenses*. National Center for the Assessment of Delinquent Behavior and Its Prevention, Center for Law and Justice, Washington, DC, 1980.

83. KOBRIN, S AND KLEIN, MW: *Final Report: National Evaluation of the Program for the Deinstitutionalization of Status Offenders*. National Institute of Juvenile Justice and Delinquency Prevention, Washington, DC, 1981.

84. RUTHERFORD, A AND McDERMOTT, R: *National Evaluation Program. Juvenile Diversion: Phase I Summary Report*. National Institute of Law Enforcement and Criminal Justice, Washington, DC, 1976.

85. PALMER, T AND LEWIS, RV: *Evaluation of Juvenile Diversion*. Oelgeschlager, Gunn, and Hain, Cambridge, MA, 1980.

86. COATES, RB, MILLER, AD, OHLIN, LE: *Diversity in a Youth Correctional System: Handling Delinquents in Massachusetts*. Ballinger, Cambridge, MA, 1978.

87. SPERGEL, IA, REAMER, FG, LYNCH, JP: *Deinstitutionalization of status offenders—individual outcome and system effects*. Journal of Research in Crime and Delinquency 18:4, 1981.

88. PALMER, T: *California's community treatment program for delinquent adolescents*. Journal of Research in Crime and Delinquency 8:74, 1971.

89. LERMAN, P: *Community Treatment and Social Control*. University of Chicago Press, Chicago, 1975.

90. JENSEN, GF AND ROJEK, DG: *Delinquency: A Sociological View*. DC Heath, Lexington, MA, 1980.

91. Fo, WSO and O'Donnell, CR: *The buddy system: Effect of community intervention of delinquent offenses.* Behavior Therapy 6:522, 1975.

92. Bullington, B, Sprowls, J, Katkin, D, Phillips, M: *A critique of diversionary juvenile justice.* Crime and Delinquency 24:59, 1978.

93. Levitt, EL: *Research on psychotherapy with children.* In Bergin, A and Garfield, SL (eds): *Handbook of Psychotherapy and Behavior Change.* John Wiley & Sons, New York, 1971.

94. Davidson, WS: *The juvenile justice system.* In Nietzel, MT, Winett, RA, Mac-Donald, ML, Davidson, WS (eds): *Behavioral Approaches to Community Psychology.* Pergamon, New York, 1977.

95. McCord, W and McCord, J: *A follow-up report on the Cambridge—Somerville youth study.* Annals of the American Academy of Political and Social Sciences 322:89, 1959.

96. McCord, J: *A thirty-year follow-up of treatment effects.* Am Psychol 33:284, 1978.

97. Adams, S: *Interaction between individual interview therapy and treatment amenability in older youth authority wards.* In Adams, S: *Inquiries Concerning Kinds of Treatment for Kinds of Delinquents.* Board of Corrections, Sacramento, CA, 1961.

98. Grant, J and Grant, M: *A group dynamics approach to treatment of nonconformists in the Navy.* Annals of the American Academy of Political and Social Sciences 322:126, 1959.

99. Warren, M: *Classification as an aid to efficient management and effective treatment.* Journal of Criminal Law, Criminology, and Police Science 62:239, 1971.

100. Davidson, WS and Seidman, E: *Studies of behavior modification and juvenile delinquency: A review, methodological critique and social perspective.* Psychol Bull 81:998, 1974.

101. Braukmann, CJ, Fixsen, DL, Kirigin, KA, Phillips, EA, Phillips, EL, Wolf, MM: *Achievement Place: The training and certification of teaching-parents.* In Wood, WS (ed): *Issues in Evaluating Behavior Modification.* Research Press, Champaign, IL, 1975.

102. Jesness, C, Derisi, W, McCormick, P, Wedge, R: *The Youth Center Research Project.* California Youth Authority, Sacramento, CA, 1972.

103. Kazdin, AE and Bootzin, RR: *The token economy: An evaluative review.* J Appl Behav Anal 5:343, 1972.

104. Kazdin, AE: *The failure of some patients to respond to token programs.* J Behav Ther Exp Psychiatry 4:7, 1973.

105. Sarason, IG: *A cognitive social learning approach to juvenile delinquency.* In Hare, RD and Schalling, D: *Psychopathic Behaviour: Approaches to Research.* John Wiley & Sons, Chichester, England, 1978.

106. Alexander, JF and Parsons, BV: *Short-term behavioral intervention with delinquent families: Impact on family process and recidivism.* J Abnorm Psychology 81:219, 1973.

107. Braukmann, CJ, Kirigin, KA, Wolf, MM: *Group home treatment research: Social learning and social control perspectives.* In Hirschi, T and Gottfredson, M (eds): *Understanding Crime: Current Theory and Research.* Sage Publications, Beverly Hills, CA, 1980.

108. Kirigin, KA, Braukmann, CJ, Atwater, JD, Wolf, MM: *An evaluation of teaching-family (Achievement Place) group homes for juvenile offenders.* J Appl Behav Anal 15:1, 1982.

109. Wolfgang, M: *Crime in a birth cohort.* Proceedings of the American Philosophical Society 117:404, 1973.

110. Wolfgang, M: *Crime in a birth cohort.* In Hood, R (ed): *Crime, Criminology and Public Policy.* Heinemann, London, 1974.

111. Hamparian, DM, Schuster, R, Dinitz, S, Conrad, JP: *The Violent Few.* DC Heath, Lexington, MA, 1978.

112. WEST, DJ AND FARRINGTON, DP: *The Delinquent Way of Life.* Heinemann, London, 1977.

113. OLWEUS, D: *Stability of aggressive reaction patterns in males: A review.* Psychol Bull 86:852, 1979.

114. SPIVACK, G AND SWIFT, M: *"High risk" classroom behaviors in kindergarten and first grade.* Am J Community Psychol 5:385, 1977.

115. ROBINS, LN AND RATCLIFF, KS: *Risk factors in the continuation of childhood antisocial behavior into adulthood.* International Journal of Mental Health 7:96, 1979.

116. WEST, DJ AND FARRINGTON, DP: *Who Becomes Delinquent?* Heinemann, London, 1973.

117. PATTERSON, GR, CHAMBERLAIN, P, REID, JB: *A comparative evaluation of a parent-training program.* Behavior Therapy 13:638, 1982.

118. SHURE, MB AND SPIVACK, G: *Interpersonal problem-solving in young children: A cognitive approach to prevention.* Am J Community Psychol 10:341, 1982.

PART 4
SEXUALLY RELATED OFFENSES

This section examines sexually related offenses, one of the most troubling areas of criminal law and a constant source of public disquiet and fear.

The trend of the law has been to concentrate upon crimes of sexual violence and to withdraw attention to socially deviant conduct that involves consenting adults and no violence. Most of the coverage in this part follows this trend. Three of the four chapters deal with violence; the remaining chapter examines male sexual exhibitionism, still a disturbing public offense, which may or may not be a precursor of later more serious and violent conduct.

Chapter 13 reviews generally the subject of sexually related violence. It begins with a classification of sexually aggressive men. (The authors point out that sexually aggressive crimes are rare in women; when so charged, the women are usually alleged to be accomplices to men, acting to lure the victim into proximity to the primary offenders.) The male offenders are grouped in three categories: those acting out of psychotic disorders; those who are essentially antisocial personalities and with whom the sexually related offense is only incidental to other crimes; and the largest group, the paraphiliacs, for whom sexual motivation is the predominant theme of their violence. The latter grouping is consistent with the terminology of the new diagnostic manual of the American Psychiatric Association. Conduct in this grouping includes frottage, sadism, masochism, bestiality, pedophilia, and rape. The authors describe current techniques of psychophysiological assessment and their implications for criminal investigation and interrogation. Also examined are a range of ethical issues presented to forensic evaluators and clinicians utilizing these techniques.

Chapters 14 and 15 deal with the victims of the more serious sexually aggressive crimes: sexual abuse of children and aggressive rape offenses against women. The chapter on child sexual abuse by Drs. Becker and Shah is a particularly successful collaboration. It offers useful material on the characteristics of victims of these crimes. Indicators of child abuse may be manifested in personal histories, observations, and interviews by trained mental health professionals. A complete physical examination of the child is essential. If any of the listed signs and symptoms are found, sexual abuse should be strongly suspected. The authors provide suggestions on interviewing potential victims, their immediate families, and extrafamilial persons of relevance to the investigation and evaluation.

The chapter contains thoughtful commentary on the effects upon the child victim of participation in criminal investigation and trial of child molesters and child rapists. Law enforcement personnel and the courts are concerned with needed protection for the child, and yet, at the same time, they are required to conduct a thorough and unbiased investigation of the allegations and to assure a fair trial for any defendant charged with the crime. These are not interests easily balanced. Suggestions are made to mental health professionals to avoid, or at least to minimize, the further trauma and embarrassment of the child victim during the criminal trial process and investigation, especially in any required appearance at the trial as a complaining witness.

The next chapter, that on the rape experience, is an updating of a very important chapter prepared for the previous text, *Modern Legal Medicine, Psychiatry, and Forensic Science.* The earlier book collected several chapters on rape and rape-death investigation and studies of both the offenders and the victims of the crime. Most of these chapters were investigational in nature and were concerned with forensic pathology and other forensic scientific techniques. These chapters were not suitable for this new text, with the exception of this contribution by Dr. Carol Nadelson and her colleagues, Drs. Notman and Carmen. The authors have retained for this text their emphasis on the total experience of the woman who is the victim of a rape offense.

The authors place particular stress on the findings of research in this field indicating that rape is essentially a crime of violence, not the result of sexual passion. The crime is opportunistic arising out of many environmental factors. Until these factors are understood, neither the crime nor its effect upon the victim can be understood.

The legal reforms in this field in the past 10 years since the adoption of recommendations of the American Bar Association in 1975 are reviewed in the chapter. The changes were designed to reduce the trauma and stress of the criminal process on the victim and to protect her privacy. Also, the changes redefined the crime and associated punishment into various classes of offense, usually dependent upon the age of the victim and the degree of force and coercion involved, in order to overcome widespread reluctance of juries to convict in this field.

Despite the changes in the law, however, the authors report that in the 1980s a distressingly large percentage of rapes still are unreported and that rape crimes that are investigated and tried still result in convictions in only a minority of instances.

The last chapter in this section on sexual offenses is an entirely new examination of issues concerning male genital exhibitionism. The authors are Dr. Park Dietz and his colleagues Drs. Cox and Wegener at the University of Virginia, another psychiatry-psychology collaboration. Their efforts have produced a comprehensive review of a subject largely ignored in recent years by researchers specializing in the forensic mental health field. Like other sexual offenders, exhibitionists seem to have an early onset in adolescence (11 to 15 years of age) or in early adulthood (21 to 24 years of age). Various theories have been offered to define the disorder—none of them satisfactory—ranging from psychodynamic explanations of fixation on castration anxieties (relieved temporarily by the exposure and reaction of observers) to biological abnormalities of the brain, endocrine hormonal dysfunction, and hereditary characteristics leading to such repeated deviant behavior. The authors also review treatment technique and research evaluations of effectiveness of treatment with this group of offenders. Their contribution to this much-neglected aspect of sexual offenses should prove particularly valuable in forensic practice.

CHAPTER 13

SEXUALLY AGGRESSIVE BEHAVIOR*

Gene G. Abel, M.D.
Joanne-L. Rouleau, Ph.D.
Jerry Cunningham-Rathner, B.A.

Human sexual behavior has shown considerable variation over centuries, both between and within different cultures. When such behavior is so deviant from the cultural norm that it seriously offends its members, legal sanctions are placed against that behavior and it is labeled a crime. Sexual deviations may vary from highly private sexual behaviors generally conducted outside of public awareness (for example, fetishism) to sexual behaviors that occur in public but are considered nonthreatening to others (for example, transvestism) to sexual behaviors that are considered damaging to the victims because they are carried out against the victim's will (for example, forcible rape). This chapter will focus on sexually aggressive behaviors that involve bodily touching and are carried out against the will of the victim. It is this type of behavior that is most likely to disturb the community and to be prosecuted in criminal courts. Although other sexually related offenses may produce emotional anguish (voyeurism, obscene telephone calls, and so forth), they are considered less dangerous and are classified as minor criminal offenses.

A variety of theoretical orientations have attempted to explain how deviant sexual behavior develops and is maintained. Psychodynamic theory views sex offenses as an outcome of the offender's unconscious conflicts about sexuality (castration anxiety).[1] Pastoral counseling views sex offenses as resulting from the breakdown of moral control.[2] A variety of programs see the behavior as multicausal, requiring motivation of the offender to realize that he or she has a problem and to use various self-control methods to prevent recommission of the crime.[3-5] Biological approaches generally have viewed deviant behavior as

* Portions of this chapter were supported by Grant MH 36347, entitled "The Treatment of Child Molesters," awarded to Dr. Abel by the NIMH Center for Studies of Crime and Delinquency.

controllable by reducing the offender's sex drive through surgical or chemical castration.[6-9] Although each of these theoretical orientations offers possible suggestions for our understanding of sex offenders, none has provided controlled studies demonstrating their validity, and a few deal with unobservable phenomena that make them nearly impossible to evaluate.

In recent years a behavioral approach has been used to evaluate sexual aggressive behavior. This theoretical orientation based on social learning theory[10] has not only conceptualized how deviant arousal develops and is maintained,[11] but has also developed an objective system to determine the treatment needs of sex offenders and to measure whether any particular offender has successfully responded to treatment.[12-19] This chapter will focus predominantly on the behavioral orientation because it appears most easily to explain sexually aggressive behavior and because objective means of evaluating treatment needs and response to treatment are available and are easily measurable.

CATEGORIZATION OF SEXUALLY AGGRESSIVE MEN

Sexual offenses perpetrated against the will of others are almost entirely committed by males. When women are charged with such crimes (5 percent of individuals charged with rape in New York State are women), it is usually as accomplices (they lure the potential victim into the proximity of the male[s] who forces himself on the victim). When women are charged with forcing themselves on others, it is treated as a medical curiosity.[20,21]

Within the group of male sex offenders, it is helpful to separate three subgroups, those with major psychiatric diseases (psychoses); those with personality disorders (primarily antisocial personalities); and those responsible for the majority of repetitive sex crimes, the paraphiliacs.

Men who are sexually aggressive because of underlying psychoses constitute less than 5 percent of individuals charged with such crimes. They commit sex crimes as a result of their psychotic illness (generally schizophrenia, manic-depressive disease, or organic brain syndromes). Their sexually aggressive behavior results from their poor impulse control, which in turn stems from their psychotic illness. By careful psychological and psychiatric examination, these individuals are easily separated from men who commit sexual aggression. Their psychosis is usually quite apparent, and their deviant sexual behavior stands out because of its peculiar, idiosyncratic nature. Their sexually aggressive behavior is usually not long-standing or repetitive, and the aggressive act itself frequently appears to serve no positive function for the offender.

Case Example

> A young man with paranoid delusions, social withdrawal, and a thought disorder was hospitalized at age 18 for one year. Diagnosed as having paranoid schizophrenia, he was treated with neuroleptics and released to outpatient day-care treatment. Three months prior to his referral, at age 24, he began socializing less, had greater difficulty concentrating, and felt detached from his environment. Twelve days before his referral, he had seen a 22-year-old woman to whom he was attracted but with whom he was not acquainted. Frightened of social interactions and lacking dating

skills, he ran up to the woman on the street, felt her breasts, put his arms around her, and attempted to embrace her. He grabbed the woman in public and made no attempt to conceal his behavior or to escape. During a psychiatric interview he reported that in the last few days he had been having strong sexual thoughts and felt that by fondling the woman's breasts and putting his arms around her, she would realize that he wanted to date her and a romance would ensue. He was startled when he was arrested instead. He denied a lengthy history of thoughts of approaching women; had no history of previous sexually aggressive behavior; and, on mental status examination, demonstrated a thought disorder and the flattening of affect associated with schizophrenia.

The treatment for individuals whose sexually aggressive behavior results from a psychotic disorder must be focused on the primary psychiatric disease. Generally, this involves the use of neuroleptics (major tranquilizers) to assist the offender in controlling urges, including sexual urges. Additional treatment for control of the sexually aggressive behavior is usually not necessary, because control improves as the psychosis subsides.

The second category of individuals committing sexually aggressive behaviors are men with antisocial personalities. These individuals typically have lengthy histories of poor impulse control and antisocial acts since their early teen years. They have marked difficulties in their social relationships, have been disruptive and truant in school, form few lasting friendships, feel minimal guilt and, as a result, often commit acts that are against community standards and the law. (See also chapter 17 for a more general analysis of antisocial personality disorder.) The hallmark of this category of sex offender is the pervasiveness of the antisocial behavior. Moreover, the person's opportunistic nature leads to the committing of sexually aggressive crimes during the course of other antisocial acts (for example, burglary and robbery).

Case Example

A 22-year-old man had a lengthy history of multiple arrests for breaking and entering of property, car theft, and robbery. He had been married four times but refused to pay child support for any of his three children. Recently he had burglarized a woman's apartment. Armed with a knife, he asked for her money and other valuables, telling her that if she complied, she would not be hurt. Shortly before leaving the apartment, he tied her up and raped her. During a psychiatric interview following his arrest, he denied prior fantasies or any history of rape. He indicated that he had raped the woman because she was there in the apartment, and as long as he was committing the burglary, he felt there was no reason not to rape her inasmuch as he was already in the victim's apartment.

Antisocial individuals do not have ongoing urges to commit sexual crimes. As noted above, their sexually aggressive acts are usually committed within the context of some other antisocial behavior. Approximately 29 percent of men charged with rape have antisocial personalities; however, if one examines a large number of antisocial individuals, a much smaller proportion would be found to have committed rape. Furthermore, the number of sexually aggressive acts per antisocial individual is much smaller than the number of such acts committed by the third category of sexual offender, the paraphiliac.

The paraphiliac will be the major focus of this chapter. Paraphiliacs (formerly called sexual deviates) stand out from psychotic and antisocial personalities because of their characteristic compulsive thoughts and urges to carry out sexually aggressive behaviors. These individuals infrequently get involved in antisocial behaviors outside the sexual sphere. From an early age (11 to 12 years), they develop specific interests in various deviant sexual behaviors. Concealing these thoughts from others, they ruminate and fantasize about them during masturbation and thereby develop even stronger interests in the deviant themes.[11] As their deviant sexual interest increases, their desire to act on the deviant urges also increases. Most paraphiliacs attempt to control their urges; however, the deviant fantasies continue, their control breaks down, and they eventually act on their deviant urges. After committing the deviant behavior, most offenders will temporarily feel uncomfortable or guilty and therefore gain some control over their urges. However, as time passes, the guilt dissipates, their sexual urges increase, and the cycle starts again.

Paraphiliacs engage in a variety of deviant sexual behaviors that may or may not involve actual physical contact with the victim. Early attempts at classification and categorization have inappropriately depicted paraphiliacs as falling into discrete groups with minimal overlap between them. However, there actually is frequent overlapping of paraphilic behaviors; for example, exhibitionists who expose themselves but also window peep, frotteurs who may also have a clothes fetish and make obscene phone calls, pedophiles who are aroused to nonsadistic as well as sadistic sexual acts with children, and rapists who rape children as well as adults.

From a group of 232 child molesters seen in our clinic, 29.7 percent also were exposing themselves to children and to adults, 16.8 percent were involved in rape, 13.8 percent were involved in voyeurism, and 8.6 percent were involved in frottage. Of 89 rapists, 50.6 percent were involved also in child molestation, 29.2 percent were exhibitionists, 20.2 percent were voyeurs, 11.2 percent were sadists, 12.4 percent were frotteurs.[22] These findings highlight the importance of evaluating the sex offender not only for the crime for which he is charged but also for other paraphilic interests or behaviors. The categories of paraphilias in which sexually aggressive behaviors are more likely to occur include those described below.

Exhibitionism

The exhibitionist becomes aroused by exposing his penis to others (usually females) from a distance. The degree of aggressiveness used during such exposures may vary from exposing himself to targets who are not even looking at the offender to holding the victim to prevent her escape, while exposing himself to her. As the following case demonstrates, there may be other things occurring beyond the observable indecent exposure.

Case Example

A 16-year-old boy was referred for treatment following two arrests for exposing himself to 10-year-old girls. The patient reported that since age 13 he had been masturbating to thoughts of surprising or shocking 8- to-

10-year-old girls by exposing himself to them. Although usually able to control the impulse to expose himself, on seven occasions his control had broken down. In the laboratory (see section on psychophysiologic assessment below) he not only had shown arousal to descriptions of exposing himself but also had 60 percent to 80 percent full erections to descriptions of having intercourse with 8- to 10-year-old girls. When confronted with these results, he admitted that over the last 7 months he had been having strong urges not only to expose himself but to have intercourse with the young girls. Aware that this attraction to very young girls was abnormal, he concealed his interests from others, knowing that others would disapprove of such thoughts. He did not know whether effective treatment was available for his problem.

Frottage

Frotteurs have specific preferences for touching victims' genital areas while in crowded places. Touching is usually done with their hands or penis, and the frottage behavior generally occurs where crowding together or personal contact is commonplace (subway trains, buses, elevators).

Case Example

A male business executive had touched over 500 women (all unknown to him) while riding the subway. He had never touched women unknown to him outside the subway. His job as an executive caused him to travel the subways at least twice a day. Because he usually ejaculated during his frottage activities, he had learned to put cellophane around his penis so that his business suit would not be stained when he ejaculated and he could proceed to work. He would generally set aside an extra 30 minutes to travel to work on the days he planned to carry out his frottage behavior. While waiting on the subway platform he would remain about 6 feet behind the crowd that was standing near the train tracks, and he would move parallel to the tracks, looking for a woman who especially appealed to him. Having identified her he would position himself directly behind her as the train pulled into the station. He would then put his forearms parallel to the ground and move in behind her, preventing anyone from getting between him and the potential victim. As the mass of commuters moved into the train, he would keep his arms up and wait until the subway doors had closed before beginning to touch her. When the train doors closed, he would fantasize that he and his victim had an ongoing, close sexual relationship and would begin to fondle the victim's buttocks or vaginal area. The woman's escape would be prevented by the compressed mass of commuters. However, when the train was not absolutely packed, he would put his arms around the woman's waist and hold her next to him while pushing his penis against her buttocks until he ejaculated. He would hold and continue to fondle his victim until the train arrived at the next platform. As the doors opened he would leave the train, cross quickly over to the other platform, board the train going in the opposite direction to begin the behavior again. This cycle would continue until he had victimized four to six women, or until he ejaculated.

Contrary to the attitude that such crimes are benign, many women are terrified during the encounter, fearing that if they fight back, something dreadful might happen, such as being knifed or otherwise physically assaulted. As a result of such fears (and anticipating that the police would not take the encounter seriously), the offense is not reported and the offender continues to victimize.

Pedophilia and Incest

Pedophilia and incest appear to be among the most serious sexual crimes in the United States because of their high frequency. It is estimated that the rate of rape for girls less than 17 years old is over 150 victims per 100,000 girls at risk. This rate is approximately four times greater than the risk of rape for adults.[23] By the time he reaches adulthood, the average pedophile or incest offender has attempted over 25 child molestations. The amount of violence used during child molestation is especially high in paraphiliacs who select children unknown to them. DeFrancis[23] reports that 50 percent of child molestation reported to child protection agencies involves the use of physical force. Christie, Marshall, and Lanthier[24] report that when emergency room records, court testimony, and investigative officers' reports are examined in detail, child molesters are found to have produced as much visible physical injury to their victims as rapists, with 39 percent of such victims having visible injury.

Case Example

A 16-year-old boy was arrested for child molestation. He and his sister had been babysitting a 4-year-old girl who was later found to have vaginal bleeding. During his clinical interview he adamantly denied any involvement with the child. Psychophysiologic assessment (a method described below) confirmed, however, that he showed sexual arousal to young girls; in addition, he showed significant sadomasochistic arousal. When confronted by this objective evidence he admitted his involvement in child molestation and expressed a desire for help to control his arousal to sadomasochistic stimuli.

Rape

This is the paraphilia usually thought of when references are made to serious sexual aggression. Texts on forensic psychiatry have viewed rapists as primarily antisocial personalities. However, in recent years, psychophysiologic studies and interviews with rapists[12,14,25-28] have revealed that many of them have a specific sexual preference for aggressive acts against their victims, and they rape in order to satisfy their sexual arousal.

Case Example

A young man was 18 years old when arrested for the first time and charged with the rape of a 63-year-old woman and a 13-year-old girl. He reported that for the past 3 years, he had ongoing thoughts of rape. Furthermore, if given the choice of raping his victim or having consensual sexual intercourse, he clearly preferred rape because of the greater sexual excitement it produced. His history was replete with evidence that his statement was indeed correct. Even when he had a sexual partner who was very amenable to having intercourse with him, he would frequently use force to pin her down and to cause her pain during intercourse.

It appeared that the age and attractiveness of his victim had little to do with his decision to rape. When he experienced strong sexual urges he would go to a specific geographic location from which he knew how to exit (for example, a park). His plan would be to rape any available victim in that area, irrespective of age or attractiveness. Psychophysiologic assessment of his sexual arousal preferences confirmed that he was minimally aroused to mutually consenting intercourse but was highly aroused to raping a potential victim.[4]

Sadism

Sadists are probably the most dangerous of the paraphiliacs. They are specifically attracted to violence perpetrated against their victims. In some cases, sadists have no sexual arousal to nonaggressive interactions with willing partners but instead require the use of force and suffering of the victim in order to become sexually aroused.

Case Example

The patient was 31 years of age and had a lengthy history of sexual arousal to adolescent girls 13 to 15 years of age. In a rather predatory fashion, he would frequent bus stations in neighboring cities, seeking out adolescent runaway girls, hoping they were in need of money, a place to stay, or drugs. He would start conversations with them and talk about his access to marijuana and other drugs. If the girls indicated any interest, he would give them some marijuana and offer them a ride to wherever they wanted to go. He would then drive them away from the bus station to some deserted building under the guise of getting some more drugs. Once inside the deserted building he would force anal intercourse on them, becoming especially aroused when this was done on cement floors where the victim's pain was intensified. In spite of over 15 such sadistic assaults, he had never been arrested and had been questioned on only one occasion. His selection of runaway adolescents and his involving them in drug-related behaviors apparently had minimized the likelihood of the crimes being reported.

THE PARAPHILIAC OFFENDER

Until recently our knowledge of paraphilic personalities has been limited by the source of information, namely, prison populations. Obtaining information from paraphilic persons who are incarcerated provides an inaccurate image of the paraphilic personality. Many individuals are in jail because they were inept enough to be apprehended, lacked financial resources to present a strong defense at their trial, or the brutality of their crime made incarceration more probable. A greater impediment to reporting accurate information is that incarcerated individuals are justifiably reluctant to describe their true deviant arousal and behavior because they could lead to further charges, could reduce the likelihood of their being considered for parole, and could prolong their incarceration.

To circumvent these problems, the characteristics of paraphilic personalities described in this section have been obtained from individuals whose confidentiality was extensively protected. The subjects were all outpatients seen by the authors at three separate treatment programs at medical centers in Mississippi, Tennessee, and New York. Subjects' names were not identified in the chart; instead, they were given identification numbers, the key of which was held outside the United States. Participants were also instructed not to provide specifics of any particular sex crime they committed so that identification with a particular crime would not be possible. The interviewers filtered information provided by the paraphiliac subject, excluding from the chart any information that might identify the subject as being involved in a specific crime. Most of the information was collected under a Certificate of Confidentiality from the federal government, which precludes anyone outside the research project from gaining access to clinical records (this certificate is provided by the Secretary of Health and Human Services under Section 303 (a) of the Public Health Service Act §42 U.S.C. 242a (a). During the 11-year period of collecting this data there was no known breach of confidentiality; no subpoena of records was ever received; and, in the authors' opinion, the paraphiliac subjects providing this information appeared open in their discussion of their true deviant behaviors. The information derived from patients was collected with provision of the above safeguards of confidentiality.

Sources of Referral

The 194 persons entering treatment in our program were referred from a variety of sources as indicated below:

Health/mental health professionals	27.8 percent
Lawyers and/or legal aid agencies	19.6 percent
Probation or parole agencies	13.4 percent
Hospitals/mental health clinics	8.2 percent
Family or friends	6.7 percent
Via the media (resulting from staff appearances on radio, television, and news items about the program)	6.2 percent
Courts	5.7 percent
Self-referrals	5.7 percent
Child-protective agencies	3.1 percent
Other sources	3.6 percent

Early Age of Onset

One of the striking findings of our research was the early age of onset of paraphilic sexual arousal. Over 50 percent of the various categories of paraphiliacs had developed their deviant arousal pattern prior to age 18. Table 1 shows

TABLE 1. Onset of Sexual Arousal to Paraphilic Stimuli by Age

| | CUMULATIVE % OF PARAPHILIACS WITH AROUSAL BY AGE (N = 411) | | | | | | |
| | AGE | | | | | | |
PRIMARY PARAPHILIAC CATEGORY	13	14	15	16	17	18	19
Rapist	14%	25%	29%	36%	40%	51%	56%
Heterosexual pedophilia	16	23	31	35	37	42	45
All paraphilias	24	31	40	47	50	56	60
Exhibitionist	26	34	41	50	54	62	66
Homosexual pedophilia	30	42	53	60	63	70	75

the distribution of various paraphiliacs who had developed their arousal at different teenage years.

These data demonstrate that paraphilic arousal begins at a rather early age, especially for homosexual pedophiles (where the targets are boys) and exhibitionists. If we are to prevent individuals from developing into hard-core, chronic offenders, we must provide assessment and treatment programs to individuals when they first develop paraphilic arousal; for 50 percent of paraphiliacs this would be during their teenage years.

Further support for preventive treatment of paraphilic persons at an early age comes from a comparison of the number of crimes attempted or committed when paraphiliac subjects were young versus the number of such acts at the time of their referral for treatment as adults. Examination of the records of 20 paraphiliac patients seen prior to age 18 revealed that on the average they had attempted or had completed 7.7 sexual crimes per offender against an average of 6.75 victims. A second group of 240 offenders who also had onsets of deviant sexual arousal prior to age 18 but who were not seen until later in their adult life (mean age was 34.4 years) on the average had attempted or had completed 581 deviant acts per offender against an average of 380 victims.

When paraphilic persons develop their deviant arousal at an early age and continue with that arousal throughout their lives, the above data indicate that there is at least a 70-fold increase in the number of crimes committed. These findings underscore the great need to attend to paraphiliac offenders early in their deviant careers. In order to curtail their subsequent deviant behavior and to reduce drastically victimization.

Multiple Paraphilias per Offender

Much of the older clinical and research literature on paraphiliac subjects suggests that single paraphilic arousal patterns are the rule, with multiple deviations only infrequently being found in the same offender. More recent research reveals quite the contrary. Over 50 percent of the paraphiliac patients seen in our studies had multiple diagnoses that overlapped a variety of paraphilias.

Table 2 shows the paraphilic arousal pattern that developed first for 411 individuals who were diagnosed either as child molesters or as rapists as adults. Although 75 percent of child molesters first developed pedophilic interests, 13 percent initially were exhibitionists, 3 percent were rapists, and 3 percent were voyeurs. Of the rapists, 44 percent were first aroused to rape, but 26 percent began as pedophiles, 9 percent as voyeurs, 8 percent as exhibitionists, 6 percent

TABLE 2 The Initial Paraphilic Behavior of Child Molesters and/or Rapists [N = 411]

FIRST PARAPHILIA	CHILD MOLESTERS	RAPISTS
Pedophilia	75.0%	25.8%
Rape	3.4	43.8
Exhibitionism	12.9	7.9
Transvestism	1.3	1.1
Fetishism	1.3	2.2
Voyeurism	3.0	9.0
Sadism	0.4	1.1
Masochism	0.9	1.1
Obscene telephone calls	0.4	0
Frottage	1.3	5.6
Bestiality	0	1.1
Arousal to odors	0	1.1

as frotteurs, and the remaining rapists showed a variety of other paraphilic arousal patterns.

These findings suggest that when an individual is found to have one category of paraphilic arousal, he should also be questioned extensively about other categories of deviant sexual interest.

Denial of Paraphilic Arousal

Mental health professionals are often handicapped in their attempts to work with paraphiliac patients because of the tremendous conscious and unconscious concealment manifested by some individuals. The usual neurotic patient comes to the therapist because of his or her discomfort with neurotic symptoms. The neurotic patient freely and openly provides extensive details of the symptoms to assist the therapist in developing an effective treatment program. The paraphiliac patient, by contrast, has usually spent a lifetime consciously concealing his deviant behavior. Knowing society's attitudes toward exhibitionists, rapists, or child molesters, he is acutely aware that reporting the truth about his interests would be met by severe social condemnation and sanctions, including loss of job, arrest, family upheaval, and large financial expenses. Concealment of his deviant arousal and associated conduct has usually served him well and arrests have been infrequent. When such an individual is forced to be interviewed by a mental health professional, often with the threat of arrest and potential incarceration resulting from his identification as a paraphiliac offender (and especially when unprotected by any system of confidentiality), he is most likely to fall back on the most commonly used defense: conscious or unconscious denial.

Case Example

The patient was referred by his attorney for assessment. He was accused of child molestation by his estranged wife. His lawyer, who had been a district attorney for a number of years, indicated that from experience with many men whom he had interviewed during the course of his professional career, he was certain that the patient was being falsely accused by a malicious ex-wife. The attorney felt that the ex-wife was attempting to besmirch his client's character and to blackmail him for larger alimony payments. The patient reported that his former wife had threatened to have his children accuse him of child molestation if he refused to increase his annual support payments by $5000. He also reported that she had sent him a letter detailing this arrangement, a letter which he had in his safety deposit box and was willing to show the interviewer at the next visit.

Psychophysiologic assessment of the patient's sexual arousal patterns, however, demonstrated clear pedophilic arousal. When assured of the confidentiality of his records, the patient admitted that he had fabricated the story about his ex-wife. In actuality, he had been involved sexually with three of his children, two of these for over 5 years. Prior to the assessment, he had adamantly denied any paraphilic behavior and appeared to show a genuine concern for his financially troubled ex-wife. The patient was then asked what he wanted communicated to his lawyer. He decided that this new information should be disclosed to his lawyer, who was flabbergasted that such a revelation was possible via psychophysiologic assessment in such a short time. We then advanced a letter to the patient indicating our willingness to accept him in our outpatient treatment program. At the time of his trial the patient maintained his innocence to the charge of child molestation but was found guilty and sentenced to jail.

This case illustrates some of the dilemmas of our evaluation/treatment system and interactions with the criminal justice system. First, the validity of psychophysiologic assessment is greatest when the patient shows erection responses to deviant stimuli (rather than an absence of arousal). Unfortunately, this always works against the patient, identifying deviant arousal that he verbally denies. Secondly, as the patient attempts to conceal his deviant behavior from others, he avoids working with others to bring about his own treatment and, instead, denies any need for treatment to the court. The net effect is that a jury or judge must approach the case in terms of determining guilt or innocence. If found not guilty, the patient will obviously be reluctant to seek treatment for a problem that he denies having. Hence, he is less likely to seek out treatment if acquitted.

Finally, if the mental health worker were to violate the patient's confidence and reveal to the court that the person was a paraphiliac, some serious and troubling confidentiality problems would be raised and the worker would take on the role of an investigator for the court. Clearly, many referrals to the worker would cease if confidentiality could not be assured to patients.[29]

Because of the frequent use of conscious and unconscious denial by paraphiliac persons, mental health professionals, legal counsel, child protection agents, and criminal justice personnel must rely on multiple sources of information if an accurate assessment is to be obtained. This is especially critical if the evaluator is unaccustomed to working with sexual offenders. The problem of denial is further compounded by the fact that sex offenses typically occur only between the offender and the victim, and thus corroborating information is usually unavailable. When pedophilia or incest are involved, corroboration is even more difficult because of the young child's inability to conceptualize, to formulate, and to recount the experiences adequately. In recent years, the psychophysiologic assessment procedure described later has provided a new means of assessing the paraphiliac individual.

Evaluating Paraphiliac Offenders

Everyone involved in the alleged offender's case wants to know if the person is a true paraphilic personality. Both prosecution and defense attorneys seek corroborating information or expert opinions on behalf of their respective positions in court. The person's family wants to know because the truth will determine how they will respond to the defendant. The therapist wants to know in order to determine if treatment is indicated and, if so, where the treatment should focus.

The problem in gaining such information is that paraphiliac persons sometimes either cannot or will not report the extent of their actual sexual interests. Some paraphiliac individuals who are anxious to receive treatment report the extent of their sexual arousal, its duration, its quality and quantity. Other paraphiliac persons adamantly deny any deviant arousal whatsoever, in spite of overwhelming evidence of their paraphilic interests and behaviors.

Traditionally, therapists have relied upon the clinical interview and the relationship between therapist and patient as a means of getting to the truth. Unfortunately, the necessary ongoing interviews to establish a trusting relationship are time-consuming, exceedingly costly, and often ineffective at helping the paraphiliac patient reveal his true sexual interests and the extent of past deviant behavior.

Psychophysiologic Assessment of Sexual Arousal

For a number of years, psychophysiologic assessment has been used to evaluate the sexual arousal patterns of persons who are possible paraphiliacs. Zuckerman's[30] extensive review of assessment methodology concludes that direct measurement of the patient's penis size (penile tumescence) in response to various sexual stimuli is the most valid means of determining sexual interests. Based on the pioneering work of Freund,[31] a number of evaluation and treatment centers have been using psychophysiologic methods involving these penile measurements to assess sexual arousal in sex offenders. This technique involves the patient wearing a circumferential, penile transducer that very accurately measures the extent of his erection. While wearing the transducer alone in the laboratory, the patient either hears via audiotape or is shown via 35 mm slides or videotape various sexual stimuli depicting specific paraphilic behaviors. The patient's penile tumescence responses to these deviant stimuli are then compared with his responses to nondeviant (more socially acceptable) sexual stimuli, in order to identify and to quantify the extent of deviant arousal. Numerous studies have reported the use of this methodology with a variety of paraphiliac populations,[12,14,25-27,32-35] and it is now possible to measure an individual's interests in almost all types of paraphilic behavior.

With these technological advancements have also come a variety of methodological and ethical concerns. One major problem is that it is possible to identify interests outside the patient's awareness by measuring arousal responses of less than 10 percent of full erection. This degree of measurement sensitivity complicates the ability of the offender to give consent to such assessment, because he is unaware of the response being measured. However, information about the sensitivity of the measurement is provided and explained to each patient before his informed consent is obtained. A second difficulty is that it is possible for the offender to control his larger erection responses (those greater than 10 percent of a full erection).[36-39] If the examiner takes greater steps to identify such faking, it is likely that the helping relationship between the patient and the examiner will break down, and subsequent treatment can become more problematic.[40] We have taken what we believe to be a first step in unraveling this complicated issue of the validity of psychophysiologic assessment by working with nonincarcerated patients with whom confidentiality was assured, and we validated psychophysiologic assessment results only by positive assurance from the patient that a specific paraphilic arousal existed.

Ninety consecutive referrals (80 adult and 10 adolescent) were evaluated using clinical interviews, paper-and-pencil testing, and psychophysiologic assessment.[41] In 45.5 percent of these cases, the patient's self-reporting of paraphilic interests was fully consistent with the psychophysiologic measures (his erection response). In the remaining 55.5 percent of the cases, however, the patients denied specific paraphilic arousal while the psychophysiologic assessment confirmed its presence. These patients were then confronted with their physiologic recordings. Their penile recordings were described to them in detail; the clearly visible erection responses on chart paper were pointed out to them, along with exactly what type of paraphilic stimuli they were shown at the time of those arousal responses. In 62.2 percent of the cases in which patients had denied any deviant interests, the individuals changed their stories and confirmed their paraphilic sexual interests when confronted with the psychophysiologic recordings. These results suggest that in spite of the various limitations of psychophysiologic assessment, a very high percentage of patients will admit to previously unrevealed paraphilic interests and behavior when confronted with their erection responses to paraphilic stimuli. If this confrontation methodology were the only way in which psychophysiologic assessment could be used, it would still be a very valuable help in our understanding of paraphiliacs. What is needed, however, is research to determine how and under what conditions psychophysiologic assessment can be used (1) to evaluate the treatment needs of paraphiliacs, (2) to motivate them for treatment, and (3) to evaluate their response to treatment.

As psychophysiologic assessment has become more accurate at determining an individual's deviant interests, many ethical concerns have also arisen. Can an offender give informed consent when the measurement is beyond his awareness? If the assessment identifies dangerous arousal patterns previously unknown, who (if anyone) should be told, and how will such situations be monitored? If an offender "does his time" and completes a course of treatment but still has an obvious dangerous arousal pattern, what does it mean regarding release and continuation of the treatment program? As forensic mental health services become aware of the positive deviant arousal patterns that can be measured, how might various agents and agencies of the criminal justice system use such information with respect to sentencing and conditional release decisions regarding the patient?

Currently, in addition to using extensive informed consent procedures, we present such ethical issues to an external governing board for our clinic. The board is composed of other professionals (lawyers, police, psychiatrists, psychologists, ministers), representatives of the public and of the consumer sectors (in this case, sex offenders).[29] Decisions made by such a governing board are more likely to reflect community standards than are decisions made by any single individual.

Behavioral Characteristics

Earlier conceptualizations of paraphilias focused almost exclusively on their deviant arousal patterns to the exclusion of other behavioral excesses or deficits seen in this population. These other problems include cognitive distortions regarding the paraphilic behavior and its impact on others, deficits in social and assertive skills, and marked limitations in sexual knowledge.

COGNITIVE DISTORTIONS

When a paraphiliac person first begins to commit sexual offenses (engages in behavior that is against the law, against the social mores of his community, and in violation of his religious or personal notions of right and wrong), he will frequently become uncomfortable, anxious, and feel guilty or depressed. Reinforced by the pleasure of the sexual activity, almost all paraphiliac individuals begin to modify their cognitions or belief systems in order to support and to justify their deviant behavior.[10] Supported by these cognitive distortions and rationalizations, the person's anxiety, guilt, and depression are reduced in frequency and intensity, thereby helping reinforce and increase his deviant behavior. As the paraphiliac person uses these distortions to justify and to rationalize his behavior, the distortions become more ingrained; and the guilt, anxiety, and related inhibitions become less effective in controlling his behavior. Any thorough assessment of the paraphiliac patient must, therefore, examine these cognitive distortions, and therapy needs to be directed toward confronting and challenging their reality base.

Although a thorough listing of cognitive distortions is beyond the scope of this chapter, a few of the more common ones for each category of sexual aggressive behaviors are listed below.

Exhibitionism

"My penis is unique and different from the penises of other men and therefore others should see it." "If a woman looks at my penis as I expose myself, she is really wanting to have intercourse with me." "If a woman appears frightened or shocked to see my penis, it is because she is overwhelmed by her sexual attraction to me." "I can tell if exposing myself to others is going to have a negative impact on them now and in the future." "If someone looks at my penis and is startled, surprised, angry, smiles, or has no reaction whatsoever, it means that (s)he wants to look at my penis."

Frottage

"Since I am infrequently arrested for frottage, it is proof that I will not be arrested in the future for touching others." "I have seen other men touch women on the subway, so I am justified in touching women." "If I touch a woman on the bus and she does not yell or scream, it means that she is really enjoying the experience and wants me to continue to touch her." "When I touch a woman on the bus, it will be a good way of establishing a relationship with her that will eventually lead to sexual intercourse." "I can tell if my touching someone on the subway is harming them now or in the future."

Pedophilia and Incest

"Children know all about sexual behavior between adults and children; children are informed and can give consent." "Children know the repercussions to them should others learn of their sexual encounters with adults." "Children are on an equal power base with adults and can therefore give consent for sex with an adult." "A child feels no pressure to do what his or her father (uncle, grandfather) says, and incest is something they can decide about having or not having." "If a child has been voluntarily sexual with another child, it is okay for an adult to have sex with that child inasmuch as it is the same thing." "All things that children want to do are good for them, and, therefore, they should be allowed to do them." "A sexual experience between a boy and an adult will not predispose that boy to become a child molester in the future." "I cannot harm a child unless I use force during a sexual encounter." "My son or daughter would know that if they said no to my sexual offers, there would be no repercussions to them." "My children know that if others find out about their sexual experience with me, there will be no repercussions to the family or to them." "I can control what others will say or do if they learn of my sexual involvement with my own child."

Rape

"If a woman goes to a bar, it means she wants to have intercourse with any man there." "Unless a woman physically resists a man throughout any attempt at making love to her, it is not rape." "Women in our culture find it difficult to initiate sex, so they wait for the man to force himself on them, so they won't feel guilty for agreeing to have sex." "Rape is so common that a woman isn't particularly harmed if she is raped." "Women want to be sexual objects." "When women say no to sexual advances, they frequently mean yes."

Sadism

"A sexual assault is justified if a woman is drunk, on drugs, a runaway, of a lower socioeconomic group, or lives in a large city." "My sexual enjoyment is all important." "If my spouse stays with me after I force myself on her, it means that such force doesn't disturb her or cause her much harm." "Pain inflicted on someone else is erotic to them."

A note of caution must be added here. There is no evidence that the paraphiliac person's cognitive distortions are responsible for the paraphilic behavior. Rather, as noted earlier, these distortions develop like rationalizations in that they help explain and justify the deviant behaviors. The important point to note here is that the maintenance of such cognitive distortions **after** a course of treatment frequently means that recidivism is very likely. The importance of probing for cognitive distortions is that often the paraphiliac is unaware of the inappropriateness of these beliefs or about the importance of correcting them in the interest of preventing future deviant behavior.

Case Example

The patient was a 37-year-old child psychiatrist who had recently been charged with molestation of young boys. As a psychiatrist for a school system, he had arranged for consultation with various boys whom he found particularly attractive. During the course of his supposed therapy he became sexually involved with the youngsters. In addition to the criminal charges, his medical license was being challenged for revocation. In a meeting before the licensing board, he was asked if his behavior with these boys had been harmful to them. He replied that although he had been sexually involved with a number of boys younger than 13 years of age, he had not harmed them because he had been attentive to any possible injury to them, had watched their responses to him, and had determined—given his training—that nothing he had done had harmed them. He did admit that the eventual result of his arrest was harmful to the boys because of society's response to his having been involved with them sexually. The anger manifested by the boys' parents, the questioning of the boys by school authorities, and the disruption in the boys' schooling occasioned by the events surrounding the criminal charges were, in his estimation, the major contributors to the boys' having suffered any adverse experience.

What was amazing in this case was how tenaciously the patient held on to his cognitive distortions despite their marked conflict with the views of the licensing board. The patient lacked the understanding that he could not control the attitudes of others about child molestation nor society's reactions to learning of his paraphilic behavior. To hold such beliefs so tenaciously in front of a board that would probably terminate his license to practice his chosen profession demonstrates how resistant these cognitive distortions are and how clearly they can be observed in the paraphiliac. The resistance to change in the paraphiliac's cognitions can serve as an important sign to a clinical evaluator regarding the paraphiliac's arousal patterns and his potential for continued deviant behavior.

INSUFFICIENT AROUSAL TO NONDEVIANT STIMULI

An individual's sexual behavior flows from his arousal pattern. If aroused to adult females, an individual is likely to fantasize about females and act to bring himself into proximity to women so that sexual interactions are more likely to occur. Many paraphiliac persons, including about 15 percent of pedophiles, have no arousal to stimuli other than those associated with young children. Even if therapy were effective at eliminating their arousal to young children, they would **not** automatically develop sexual arousal to adult partners. Without arousal to adults, they would be less likely to make efforts to involve themselves with potential adult sexual partners. The eventual outcome of having no alternate nondeviant sexual outlet is an increased likelihood of relapse and recidivism. The assessment of this type of deficit can be made during the clinical interview and confirmed with psychophysiologic measurement.

A number of specific treatments are available for generating nondeviant sexual arousal in such individuals.[42]

SOCIAL SKILLS DEFICITS

Many paraphiliac persons have adequate sexual arousal to adult partners but still lack the social skills necessary to approach, to talk with, and eventually to develop a relationship with an adult partner. Most people acquire appropriate social skills during the socialization process, as we observe others' social interactions, model others' behavior, practice these skills, and eventually become effective at talking with others. Some paraphiliac persons (in our sample, 41 percent of child molesters and 47 percent of rapists) failed to learn appropriate social skills, and as a result they felt anxious and uncomfortable with potential partners and were clumsy as they attempted social interactions with them. The importance of social skills deficits should be obvious: If the offenders cannot develop normal sociosexual relationships with appropriate adult partners, they are more likely to focus on their paraphilic arousal and to engage in deviant sexual behaviors.

The most effective means of assessing whether a paraphiliac patient does or does not have appropriate social skills is to ask him to role play situations in which he has to demonstrate appropriate skills (for example, initiating conversation, maintaining the flow of conversation, maintaining eye contact, asking open-ended questions, and so forth). The therapist can then observe and assess the paraphiliac patient's behavior.[43] If the paraphiliac person's social skills are seriously deficient, appropriate training is clearly indicated.

ASSERTIVENESS SKILLS DEFICITS

One of the most common behavioral deficits in our society is in personal assertiveness—or letting others know what it is that we want, telling others how we feel (both positive and negative feelings), and appropriately asking others for behavior changes. Deficits in assertiveness skills manifest themselves in two ways: passivity and hyperaggressiveness. Although deficits in assertiveness are seen potentially in all types of paraphiliac individuals, they are especially obvious in rapists and pedophiles. Fifty-one percent of our sample of rapists had below-average assertiveness skills, and 45 percent of child molesters displayed similar problems.

Rapists frequently appear to commit the crime because of their inability to assert themselves with some other woman.[15]

Case Example

The patient was 28 years of age and being evaluated following his release after four years of incarceration for rape. Five years earlier, and much to his chagrin, his relationship of two years with a woman had broken up. He was angry with her, and shortly after the breakup, found himself in the park where they had first made love. By chance, he encountered a young woman in the park by herself, sexually assaulted her, and escaped from the scene. One year later he was seen by the victim and identified to police. He admitted his crime and was convicted. It was only in retrospect that he realized the relationship between his break-up with his girl friend and his attack on an unknown woman in a park he and his girl friend had often frequented.

Pedophiles also have specific assertiveness deficits, especially in their relationships with children. Because some pedophiles establish ongoing relationships with the same children and give money or other reinforcers following sexual activity with them, the children learn that by approaching the pedophile, they will be rewarded. Consequently, some children continue to approach the pedophile, and many pedophiles find it nearly impossible to turn down these approaches. Their inability to assert themselves and to say no to the child becomes a potentially dangerous situation for the pedophile because these approaches may lead to deviant behavior and arrest.

The assessment of appropriate assertiveness skills is similar to assessing other social skills. The paraphiliac patient is asked to role play, asserting himself in a variety of common situations. As he practices his assertiveness skills, the therapist can directly observe whether the paraphiliac is able to display appropriate responses. If deficits are apparent, assertiveness training needs to be initiated.

DEFICITS OF SEXUAL KNOWLEDGE AND DYSFUNCTION

Some paraphiliac individuals have limited sexual knowledge or suffer from specific sexual dysfunctions that interfere with their carrying out socially acceptable sexual activities. This is especially the case with many adolescent offenders in which rigid, controlling parents feel uncomfortable about communicating and discussing matters pertaining to sex with their children. As the adolescent experiments with various sexual activities, he is likely to attempt some inappropriate behavior. Because his parents have taught him not to talk about sex, he may continue his inappropriate behavior without discussing it with others who might correct it. As the deviant behavior continues over time and is further reinforced, the paraphilias become more powerful and treatment is more difficult.

Assessment of lack of sexual knowledge and of sexual dysfunction can be accomplished by clinical interview or standard sex information questionnaires. Appropriate intervention is accomplished by sex education or sexual dysfunction treatment.

Treatment and Recidivism

Treatment of paraphiliac patients flows naturally from the observation of behavioral excesses and deficits developed during clinical evaluation. The principal treatment component needed by all paraphiliac patients is intervention to eliminate paraphilic arousal. Aside from this, some will need treatment to eliminate their cognitive distortions, help them develop arousal to adult partners, learn effective social skills, develop new assertiveness skills, and/or specific sex education, and/or sex dysfunction treatment to eliminate sexual deficits.

The following case exemplifies how treatment must be tailored to fit the specific needs of the offender.

Case Example

The patient was 36 years of age and had been arrested four times for rape. History revealed that at age 10 he had begun to steal female garments and would masturbate while holding the clothes (a fetish). About the same time he also began lifting girls' skirts in school. By age 12 he had become more aggressive in his behavior: following, pushing, or grabbing girls in the neighborhood and looking under their skirts. He also began making obscene phone calls. At age 14 he followed an adult female, pushed her into her apartment, but did not sexually attack her. At this time he also began window peeping, a behavior that continued for approximately 1 year. By age 18, his behavior had become well established, thoughts of attacking women were permeating his masturbatory fantasies, and at this age he was arrested for the first time after following a young woman into an elevator and slapping her around. Although the patient's intent was sexual in nature (he became aroused by slapping the victim), superficially his behavior looked like a simple assault and battery. As a result, the patient was not incarcerated. At age 25 he married, and at age 26 his most aggressive behavior began: forcing females to fellate him. His usual pattern was to go out in the late evening wearing a mask and carrying a knife. He would approach adult females who were alone, threaten them with the knife, force them to fellate him, and then flee. As he engaged in such behavior more frequently, his arousal was further strengthened, since he usually fantasized about forcing oral sex on a female while he masturbated to an orgasm. His behavior accelerated to one or two attacks per week, and approximately 1½ years later he was arrested, charged with rape, found guilty, and sentenced to a prison term.

Following incarceration he was required to seek therapy and to continue in dynamically oriented individual therapy for 5 years. Shortly after release from prison, his wife divorced him because of his arrest and conviction. By age 34, he had begun to have sexual interest in young girls and boys and had had two sexual experiences with 8- and 9-year-old girls and had propositioned a 14-year-old boy. His involvement with young children appears to have emanated directly from his difficulty in performing sexually with adults; he would have difficulties in getting erections (unless forcing oral sex on the female) and also would have premature ejaculation. He began dating but had marked difficulties and became more and more frustrated. When evaluated at age 36, he reported a 1-year history of driving around at night, once again looking for women. He admitted to grabbing women, squeezing their breasts, and pushing them to the ground, but he denied forcing oral sex on them. During the course of his assessment, it was learned that he had again purchased a knife and ski mask. By the time he was seen initially, he had attempted to force oral sex on over 300 women and had completed this victimization on over 200 women. His clinical interview revealed that in spite of having been aroused to fetish objects, having made obscene phone calls, having window peeped, and having been aroused by both young girls and young boys, when seen at age 36 the only persistent arousal was his ongoing urges to force oral sex on adult women.

With such an aggressive, chronic, behavioral pattern displaying very poor control, treatment needs to focus first on eliminating the offender's interest in the deviant behavior (forcing oral sex on adult partners). Dynamically oriented psychotherapy was used to help the offender understand the developmental roots of his deviant behavior. This form of treatment, however, has demonstrated only limited success, requires extensive treatment contacts over long periods of time, and could not be expected to reduce swiftly an individual's current deviant behavior. The use of antiandrogens has proven moderately effective at reducing deviant arousal on a fairly prompt and short-term basis, but unfortunately its long-term effectiveness has shown relapse in 65 percent of cases.[9] However, in spite of their long-term limitations, antiandrogens were used as a treatment alternative with the above-mentioned patient until treatment to specifically eliminate his particular deviant interests could be implemented. Finally, implementation of satiation and covert sensitization procedures—two treatments to eliminate the patient's major deviant interest (forced oral sex)—were begun.

SATIATION

Satiation is a training technique in which the patient repeatedly uses his deviant fantasy at a time when it cannot be erotic for him.[27,44,45] Following orgasm, the offender repeatedly verbalizes his strongest deviant interest to the point of boredom, then to aversiveness, and finally to disgust at having to ruminate or to think about the deviant behavior. Compliance with the treatment is insured by having the offender audiotape his satiation sessions so that the therapist can spot-check the tapes and teach the patient to use the satiation procedure most effectively.

COVERT SENSITIZATION

Covert sensitization is a technique in which the patient is taught how to disrupt the early thoughts or antecedent behaviors in the chain of events that leads to and culminates in the commissions of his crimes. Deviant sexual behaviors are usually the product of a lengthy chain of events. For this last case example provided above, the chain would begin with difficulties on the job, feeling as if he were being picked on, being bored, deciding to go for a ride in his car, driving to the usual area in which he attacked women, recalling previous experiences of assaulting women, feeling sexually aroused and beginning to masturbate in his car while watching women walk by, deciding to leave his car to get closer to the women he was watching, taking out his knife and ski mask and preparing himself for attack, and finally actually attacking a woman. Covert sensitization teaches the offender how to recognize all (especially the early) elements of this chain, how to disrupt any of the behaviors in the chain, and to anticipate the negative consequences of continuing to pursue the behaviors in the chain. In this case, and in the safety of the therapist's office, the patient fantasizes the early steps in the chain until he gets them clear; for example, thinking about how hurt he is by problems at work, feeling sexually frustrated because he is not dating, and deciding to drive around a little in his car. Once such images are clear, he then switches to thoughts of the most highly aversive consequences to his continuing the behavior, such as images of being attacked and raped while serving a prison term, his parents being beaten up by relatives of his victim as a means of retaliation, being arrested in front of his fellow employees while it is made public that he attacks women, and so forth. The patient then practices the sequences, so that any thoughts of the chain of behaviors leading to assaulting women are immediately recognized by the patient and disrupted by recalling highly aversive images.[15]

As the patient carries out the satiation and covert sensitization treatments, his use of deviant fantasies during masturbation lessens so that within a relatively short amount of time he is feeling remarkably better regarding his ability to control his deviant behavior. Although he has learned to gain control over his deviant sexual behavior, he still has marked difficulties relating to adult partners in nondeviant areas, primarily because of his poor social skills and specific sexual dysfunctions (intermittent impotence and premature ejaculation). As he continues masturbatory satiation and covert sensitization, social skills training is also provided. Skills training involves modeling for or role playing with the patient various social situations in which he must interact with a potential date. Starting with the simplest of skills (e.g., maintaining eye contact, determining common interests with potential partners, initiating nonthreatening comments, asking questions that are easy for the average adult to reply to, and so forth), he then progresses to more complicated skills such as maintaining the flow of conversation and assessing the social interests of other adults. Care is taken to use social situations from the patient's real life experiences for the role playing. This insures that the skills being taught are relevant to the particular needs of the patient. When the offender lacks even primitive interpersonal and heterosocial skills, the therapist models such social behaviors for him. The patient then tries to duplicate the therapist's performance and is socially reinforced for the acquisition of good skills. The social skills training for this particular patient was completed over a period of 6 to 8 months and helped him in his attempts to approach adult females.

Approximately 1½ years after starting this therapy, the patient became involved with an adult female, started dating on a regular basis, but became more and more concerned about his sexual performance. Sex education and specific training in how to deal with his intermittent impotence and premature ejaculation were then added to his treatment. This culminated in joint therapy with the patient and a new girl friend.

Two years after completion of treatment the patient is now married, has a 1-year-old child, has a very pleasant and enjoyable sexual life with his wife, and finds it peculiar to look back on his previous deviant sexual behavior (which he now sees as bizarre). The therapist continues intermittent follow-up contacts and questions the patient about any possible urges or fantasies about committing any of his previous sex offenses.

In this particular case, treatment was not necessary to help the patient acquire arousal to adult partners, since such sexual interest was already present. Therapy, however, did have to focus on his specific sexual dysfunctions: intermittent impotence and premature ejaculation. Assertiveness skills were evaluated in this particular patient but were not found to be lacking and hence assertiveness training was not implemented. As in any form of therapy for sex offenders, it is critical to evaluate the potential treatment needs of any patient prior to instituting treatment and to repeat these measures during and following treatment to insure that treatment has indeed been effective. For this reason psychophysiologic assessment on this patient was conducted prior to treatment, during treatment, and after treatment to insure that his high arousal to aggressive themes toward adult women was no longer present after treatment was completed. Should high deviant arousal persist, the therapist would obviously see that the treatment had not been effective and would implement another form of therapy to reduce deviant arousal.[15]

TREATMENT EFFECTIVENESS

The major issue in treating paraphiliac patients is the effectiveness of such interventions. Evaluating the effectiveness of any therapy is difficult, but evaluating the effectiveness of treatment for sex offenders has some major obstacles. To determine if a sex offender will repeat his deviant behavior after treatment demands that that offender be physically in an environment where reoffending is possible. For offenders treated in a prison setting, it is extremely difficult to evaluate recidivism because they are not in a free environment where they might have opportunities to engage in the deviant acts. Another dilemma is present when the therapist or clinician who is determining recidivism works for the criminal justice system (such as staff or consultant to probation, prison, or parole departments). In such circumstances the person under supervision is understandably reluctant to report any deviant arousal or offensive behavior for fear that this may jeopardize his probation or parole. As a result, relapse rates determined from projects under the supervision of the criminal justice system typically report low levels of recidivism.[46] In these circumstances the reported recidivism rates appear to be influenced more by who determined them rather than by any treatment intervention.

Another alternative is to conduct treatment outcome studies under circumstances in which confidentiality is assured. Such a study has been underway at the New York State Psychiatric Institute in New York City where 199 sex offenders are being treated. At the present time 125 of the 199 offenders have completed the 8-month outpatient treatment. Of those who have completed treatment, 98.9 report committing no further sex crimes. Preliminary data indicate that of those who have had the opportunity to be seen 6 months after completion of treatment (a total of 107 offenders at present), 96 (or 90 percent) report committing no further sex crimes. Of those who have had the opportunity to complete a 1-year period of follow-up (98), 82 percent (80 paraphiliac persons) report no longer being involved in deviant sexual behavior. Recidivism, when it did occur in child molesters completing treatment, almost exclusively involved homosexual pedophiles (men whose arousal was to young or adolescent boys). Incest offenders and heterosexual pedophiles had exceedingly low recidivism rates. These results suggest that a relatively inexpensive therapy intervention (1½ hours of therapy per week for 30 weeks) can be quite successful with outpatient offenders who have voluntarily sought treatment. Whether such a treatment intervention would be equally effective with offenders required to receive treatment has yet to be determined.

Conclusions

Major changes have occurred in our knowledge regarding paraphiliac offenders. New findings reveal that the extent of the paraphiliac person's crimes is much greater than previously believed. It is also apparent that paraphilic arousal begins at a very early age; over 50 percent of such individuals develop their arousal prior to 18 years of age. This suggests that prevention efforts should focus on those young individuals developing deviant patterns of sexual arousal at an early age, in order to prevent serious or chronic sexually offensive behaviors. New psychophysiologic and related assessment methods that have been described here can identify deviant arousal patterns and objectively categorize the behavioral excesses and behavioral deficits associated with paraphiliac behavior. Once these patterns are identified, it is possible to implement treatment to help the sex offender bring his behavioral excesses or deficits into a normal range. A major problem facing the field at present is to develop a system by which the effectiveness of treatment can be more accurately evaluated. At present, tentative results of treatment outcome studies suggest that current treatment can effectively help the sex offender control his deviant behavior.

REFERENCES

1. SALZMAN, L: *The psychodynamic approach to sex deviation*. In RESNIK, H AND WOLF-GANG, M (EDS): *Sexual Behaviors*. Little, Brown & Co., Boston, 1972.

2. OATES, WE: *Religious attitudes and pastoral counseling*. In RESNIK, H AND WOLFGANG, M (EDS): *Sexual Behaviors*. Little, Brown & Co, Boston, 1972.

3. BOOZER, G: *Offender Treatment: Programming* (Workshop). Presented at the Sixth Alabama Symposium on Justice and the Behavioral Sciences, University of Alabama, January 1975.

4. HENDRICKS, L: *Some effective change-inducing mechanisms in operation in the specialized treatment programs for the sex offender*. State of Washington, Department of Social and Health Services, Western Washington State Hospital, Fort Steilacoom, Washington, April 1975.

5. MACDONALD, S: *Rape offenders and their victims*. Charles C Thomas, Springfield, IL, 1974.

6. BANCROFT, JA, TENNENT, G, LOUCAS, K, CASS, J: *The control of deviant sexual behavior by drugs: Behavioral changes following estrogens and antiandrogens*. Br J Psychiatry 25:310-315, 1974.

7. LANGEVIN, R, PAITICH, D, HUCKER, S, NEWMAN, S, RAMSAY, G, POPE, S, GELLER, G, ANDERSON, C: *The effects of assertiveness training, provera and sex of therapist in the treatment of genital exhibitionism*. J Behav Therapy and Exp Psychiatry 10:275-282, 1979.

8. SPODAK, MF, FALCK, ZA, RAPPEPORT, JR: *The hormonal treatment of paraphiliacs with Depo-provera*. Criminal Justice and Behavior 5:304-314, 1978.

9. BERLIN, FS AND MEINECKE, C: *Treatment of sex offenders with antiandrogenic medication: Conceptualization, review of treatment modalities, and preliminary findings*. Am J Psychiatry 138:601-607, 1981.

10. BANDURA, A: *Aggression: A social learning analysis*. Prentice-Hall, Englewood Cliffs, NJ, 1973.

11. ABEL, GG AND BLANCHARD, EB: *The role of fantasy in the treatment of sexual deviation*. Arch Gen Psychiatry 30:467-475, 1974.

12. ABEL, GG, BLANCHARD, EB, BARLOW, DH, MAVISSAKALIAN, M: *Identifying specific erotic cues in sexual deviation by audio-taped descriptions*. J Appl Behav Anal 8:247-260, 1975.

13. BARLOW, DH, ABEL, GG: *Sexual deviation*. In CRAIGHEAD, E, KAZDIN, A, MAHONEY, M (EDS): *Behavior Modification: Principles, Issues and Applications*. Houghton Mifflin, Boston, 1976.

14. ABEL, GG, BARLOW, DH, BLANCHARD, EB, GUILD, D: *The components of rapists' sexual arousal*. Arch Gen Psychiatry 34:895-903, 1977.

15. ABEL, GG, BLANCHARD, EB, BECKER, JV: *An integrated treatment program for rapists*. In RADA, R (ED): *Clinical Aspects of the Rapists*. Grune & Stratton, New York, 1977.

16. MARSHALL, WL, MCKNIGHT, RD: *An integrated treatment program for sexual offenders*. Canadian Psychiatric Association Journal 20:133-138, 1975.

17. COLSON, CE: *Olfactory aversion therapy for homosexual behavior*. J Behav Therapy Exp Psychology 3:185-187, 1972.

18. DAVIDSON, G: *Elimination of a sadistic fantasy by a client-controlled counter-conditioning technique: A case study*. J Abnorm Psychology 73:84-90, 1968.

19. LAWS, DR: *Treatment of bisexual pedophiles by a biofeedback assisted self-control procedure*. Behav Res Therapy 18:207-211, 1980.

20. FREUND, K: *Assessment of pedophilia*. In COOK, M AND HOWELLS, K (EDS): *Adult Sexual Interest in Children*. Academic Press, New York, 1981.

21. SARREL, P AND MASTERS, WH: *Sexual molestation of men by women*. Archives of Sexual Behavior 11:117-131, 1982.

22. ABEL, GG, MITTELMAN, MS, BECKER, JV: *Sexual Offenders: Results of Assessment and Recommendations for Treatment* (in press).

23. DeFRANCIS, V: *Protecting the child victim of sex crimes committed by adults.* American Humane Association, Denver, 1969.

24. CHRISTIE, M, MARSHALL, WL, LANTHIER, RD: *A descriptive study of incarcerated rapists and pedophiles.* Unpublished manuscript, 1978.

25. ABEL, GG, BLANCHARD, EB, BECKER, JV, DJENDEREDJIAN, A: *Differentiating sexual aggressives with penile measures.* Criminal Justice and Behavior 5:315-332, 1978.

26. ABEL, GG, BECKER, JV, SKINNER, LJ: *Aggressive behavior and sex.* Psychiatric Clinics of North America 3, 1980.

27. ABEL, GG, BECKER, JV, SKINNER, LJ: *Treatment of the Violent Sex Offender.* In ROTH, LH (ED): *Clinical Treatment of the Violent Person.* Crime and Delinquency; a monograph series, NIMH, 1983.

28. BARBAREE, HE, MARSHALL, WL, LANTHIER, RD: *Deviant sexual arousal in rapists.* Behav Res Therapy 17:215-222, 1979.

29. BECKER, JV AND ABEL, GG: *Preservation of client's rights: Sexual abuse victims and sexual offenders.* In HANNAH, T, CLARK, H, CHRISTIAN, W (EDS): *Preservation of Client's Rights.* The Free Press/Macmillian, New York, 1981.

30. ZUCKERMAN, M: *Physiological measures of sexual arousal in the human.* Psychol Bull 75:279-329, 1971.

31. FREUND, K: *Erotic preference in pedophilia.* Behav Res Therapy 5:339-348, 1967.

32. ABEL, GG, BLANCHARD, EB, BARLOW, DH: *Measurement of sexual arousal in several paraphilias: The effects of stimulus modality, instructional set and stimulus content.* Behav Res Therapy 19:25-33, 1981.

33. BANCROFT, J AND MATTHEWS: A: *Automatic correlates of penile erection.* Journal of Psychosomatic Research 15:159-167, 1971.

34. FREUND, K: *A laboratory method for diagnosing predominance of homo or hetero erotic interest in the male.* Behav Res Therapy 1:85-93, 1963.

35. LAWS, DR, MEYER, J, HOLMER, ML: *Reduction of sadistic sexual arousal by olfactory aversion: A case study.* Behav Res Therapy 16:281-285, 1978.

36. LAWS, DR AND RUBIN, HB: *Instructional control of an autonomic sexual response.* J Appl Behav Anal 2:93-99, 1969.

37. HENSON, DE AND RUBIN, HB: *Voluntary control of eroticism.* J Appl Behav Anal 4:37-44, 1971.

38. QUINSEY, VL AND CARRIGAN, WF: *Penile responses to visual stimuli: Instructional control with and without auditory sexual fantasy correlates.* Criminal Justice and Behavior 5:333-342, 1978.

39. WYDNA, A, MARSHALL, WL, BARBAREE, HE, EARLS, CM: *Control of sexual arousal by rapists and non-rapists.* Paper presented at 42nd Annual Convention of the Canadian Psychological Association, Toronto, June 1981.

40. LAWS, DR AND HOLMAN, ML: *Sexual response faking by pedophiles.* Criminal Justice and Behavior 5:343-356, 1978.

41. ABEL, GG: *Violent Sexual Behavior.* Paper presented at Clarke Institute of Psychiatry, Clinical Criminology; Current Concepts, April 1983.

42. ABEL, GG AND BLANCHARD, EB: *The measurement and generation of sexual arousal in male sexual deviates.* In HERSEN, M, EISLER, R, MILLER, PM (EDS): *Progress in Behavior Modification,* Vol 2. Academic Press, New York; 1976, pp 99-136.

43. BARLOW, DH, ABEL, GG, BLANCHARD, EB, BRISTOW, A, YOUNG, LA: *Heterosocial skills checklist for males.* Behavior Therapy 8:229-239, 1977.

44. MARSHALL, WL: *The modification of sexual fantasies: A combined treatment approach to the reduction of deviant sexual behavior.* Behav Res Therapy 11:557-564, 1973.

45. MARSHALL, WL AND BARBAREE, HE: *The reduction of deviant arousal: Satiation treatment for sexual aggressors.* Criminal Justice and Behavior 5:294-303, 1978.

46. ABEL, GG, BLANCHARD, EB, BECKER, JV: *Psychological treatment of rapists.* In WALKER, MJ AND BRODSKY, SL (EDS): *Sexual Assault: The Victim and the Rapist.* Lexington Books, Lexington, MA, 1976.

CHAPTER 14
THE SEXUALLY ABUSED CHILD

Judith V. Becker, Ph.D.
Saleem A. Shah, Ph.D.

Every society has norms for the regulation of conduct in order to prevent conflicts and to maintain order, stability, and social cohension. Among the conduct that is subject to regulations is, of course, sexual behavior. Various laws that circumscribe and define the bounds of permissible sexual conduct reflect the values and norms of that society. And, as in the case of conduct that inflicts bodily harm on others, prohibitions on sexual activity between adults and children appear to be fairly universal.

This chapter addresses a number of issues and related clinical concerns pertaining to sexually abused children. The discussion begins with brief references to relevant legal definitions and criminal statutes proscribing such behaviors and to relevant categories of the third edition of the *Diagnostic and Statistical Manual* of the American Psychiatric Association *(DSM III)*.[1] The next two sections provide information about the incidence and prevalence of child sexual abuse and about the patterns of behavior by children that are suggestive of their possible sexual victimization. The discussion then turns to a number of clinical concerns about interviewing, evaluating, and treating child victims of sexual abuse.

LEGAL DEFINITIONS

Criminal statutes covering various forms of sexual abuse of children tend to vary somewhat from state to state. However, the major relevant laws are to be found in the criminal or penal codes, and a few related offensive behaviors may also be covered by statutes pertaining to child abuse more generally. In the main, sexual abuse is considered to have been committed when an adult engages in various sexual acts involving children. Although the term "child" is usually defined by the relevant statutes, it generally refers to a person under the age of 14 years. Moreover, the vast majority of states have affixed the legal "age of nonconsent" at under 16 years; however, some slight variations will be found in that the specified age may be 17 or even 18 years in some instances. With regard to sexually abusive behavior involving children, the laws proscribing such acts typically refer to the adult's use of the child for his or her own sexual gratification and stimulation, or even for the sexual arousal and stimulation of the child.

A very useful source of information about criminal statutes involving sexual offenses against children is the monograph developed by the American Bar Association's National Legal Resource Center for Child Advocacy and Protection.[2] This publication provides a state-by-state breakdown of the relevant laws and also contains a discussion and analysis of the major problem areas and recent trends in the laws.

Numerous changes have occurred in child sexual abuse laws over the years, with the general trend being to provide more specific definitions of the proscribed deviant acts. Several states have developed a tiered structure of criminal offenses with graduated penalties based on the age of the victim and sometimes also the age of the offender. The specific statutory terms frequently used to describe various prohibited sexual acts involving children include the following: sexual assault or abuse; contributing to the delinquency of a minor; indecent liberties with a child; carnal knowledge of a child; lewd, lascivious, or perverted acts with a child; child molestation, rape, and sodomy.

Although all 50 states now have laws forbidding various types of adult-child sexual activity,[2] we shall refer to the New York State (NYS) penal laws[3] to illustrate the major legal definitions and statutes pertaining to sexual offenses involving children.

Article 130 of the NYS penal code deals with sex offenses and provides definitions of key terms such as "deviate sexual intercourse" (which covers what most other states subsume under "sodomy") and "sexual contact." In New York State, persons are deemed **legally incapable of consent** when they are less than 17 years old, or mentally defective, or mentally incapacitated, or physically helpless (Section 130.05).

Sexual misconduct covers males who engage in "sexual intercourse with a female without her consent," or who engage in "deviate sexual intercourse with another person without the latter's consent" (Section 130.20).

Three degrees of **rape** are specified when a male engages in sexual intercourse with a minor female. **Rape in the third degree** covers sexual intercourse between a female less than 17 years old and a male 21 years or older; **rape in the second degree** is involved when a male 18 years or older engages in sexual intercourse with a female less than 14 years; and **rape in the first degree** is involved when the victim is less than 11 years old (sections 130.25, 130.30 and 130.35, respectively). The seriousness of the crime and the associated penalties increase in proportion to the youthfulness of the victim.

Similarly, the NYS penal code provides three degrees for the offense of **sodomy** (which involves "deviate sexual intercourse"), depending upon the age of the victims and considering also the age of the offender (Sections 130.40, 130.45, and 130.50). Three degrees of **sexual abuse** are also specified (Sections 130.55, 130.60, and 130.65).* More recently, the crime of **aggravated sexual abuse** (Section 130.70) has been added and is classified as a Class B felony.

---

* As defined in the NYS penal code, sexual abuse involves any nonconsensual "sexual contact" (any salacious "touching" of a person's sexual or other intimate parts). Indecent exposures, gestures, or proposals are covered by other criminal statutes.

Other sections of the NYS penal code cover the offense of **incest** (Section 255.25) and also proscribe **endangering the welfare of a child** (Section 260.10). With regard to incest, the statute provides that

> A person is guilty of incest when he marries or engages in sexual intercourse with a person whom he knows to be related to him, either legitimately or illegitimately, as an ancestor, descendant, brother or sister of either the whole or the half blood, uncle, aunt, nephew or niece.[4]

Thus, the essential feature of the crime of incest is not sexual intercourse, but intercourse with a relative within the prescribed line of consanguinity indicated in the statute. (It should be noted that the male nouns and pronouns in the above laws are used in their generic meaning.)

PSYCHIATRIC DEFINITIONS

Under the broad category of psychosexual disorders, *DSM III*[1] classifies various **paraphilias;** that is, disorders with the essential feature that "unusual or bizarre imagery or acts are necessary for sexual excitement."[5] (In the second edition of the manual [*DSM II*],[6] these disorders were referred to as sexual deviations.) *DSM III* points out that the term paraphilias is preferred "because it correctly emphasizes that the deviation (para) is in that to which the individual is attracted (philia)."[7]

Among the specific paraphilias listed in *DSM III* is **pedophilia,** "the essential feature of which is the act or fantasy of engaging in sexual activity with prepubertal children as a **repeatedly preferred** or **exclusive** method of achieving sexual excitement"[8] (emphasis added). (Attention should be called, however, to the studies reported in the preceding chapter indicating not-infrequent overlaps of other sexual deviancy with pedophilia.) Pedophiles could further be classified in reference to their victims' sex (heterosexually or homosexually oriented), age (whether involving prepubescent or pubescent children), and family relationship and degree of consanguinity (that is, incest or other intrafamilial contacts).

It should be pointed out, however, that there is no direct or necessary relationship between the various criminal offenses noted earlier and a psychiatric diagnosis such as pedophilia. As the emphasized words in the above quoted definition of pedophilia should indicate, not all acts of sexual abuse, rape, or sodomy necessarily involve persons with a diagnosable psychiatric disorder. For example, *DSM III* notes that isolated sexual acts with children that may be precipitated by marital discord, recent loss, or intense loneliness—although certainly constituting violations of relevant criminal statutes—would **not** necessarily warrant this psychiatric diagnosis.[9]

THE INCIDENCE AND PREVALANCE OF CHILD SEXUAL ABUSE

Given the problems that already exist with regard to estimating the frequency of child sexual abuse, it seems essential that one try to be as clear as possible about the terms used in referring to the estimated frequencies. Thus, **incidence** refers to various indicators (whether official crime statistics or various victimization surveys) of the number of persons who were victims of certain offenses during a particular time period; for example, during the past year. **Prevalance,** on the other hand, refers to estimates of the number of persons who have **ever during their lives** been victims of certain offenses. It is, therefore, important that estimates of incidence and prevalence not be used interchangeably nor be otherwise confounded.

The national incidence of child sexual abuse is unknown. However, various estimates have been made, and studies indicate that the phenomenon is much more common than is generally believed; it affects literally millions of children, and hence it must be considered to be a serious social problem.

The classic study by Kinsey and colleagues[10] surveyed a large sample of white American females (N = 5940) to learn about their sexual experiences, including sexual contacts with adults during their childhood. The experiences covered in the study ranged from nonphysical events, such as exhibitionism, to forced sexual intercourse. The results indicated that fully 24 percent of the adult females surveyed had been childhood victims of various types of sexual contact with adult males. Landis[11] studied a sample of 1800 university students, mainly from urban families, and found that 500 reported having been child victims of sexual abuse by adults. Of those reporting such experiences, 360 were women (35 percent of all the women questioned) and 140 were men (30 percent of the men questioned). Similarly, in a retrospective study of 12,000 college-age females, Gagnon[12] found that 28 percent reported sexual experience with an adult before they were 13 years old. And, following her review of the five studies of child sexual abuse that had been reported since 1940, Herman[13] concluded that about one fifth to one third of women had reported a childhood sexual encounter with an adult male, and 1 percent had reported a sexual experience with her father or stepfather.

Finkelhor[4,15] surveyed 796 undergraduates at six New England colleges and universities and found that 19 percent of the women reported experiences of childhood sexual victimization. Of all the women who reported such experiences, 40 percent indicated encounters in which touching or manipulation of the genitals had occurred; 20 percent had been victims of exhibitionism. Only a few of the reported incidents had involved sexual penetration or intercourse, but more than half of the victimizations had involved some use of force. In fully 75 percent of the incidents the offenders were known to the victims. Finkelhor[14] has estimated that the general prevalence of father-daughter incest was about 1 percent. He emphasizes that, although this figure may appear to be very small, "if it is an accurate estimate, it means that approximately three quarters of a million women 18 years and over in the general population have had such an experience, and that another 16,000 cases are added each year from among the group of girls aged 5 to 17."[16]

In a recent article, Koss[17] refers to a survey of adult women that was done by D.E.H. Russell in San Francisco which included questions about childhood sexual abuse experiences. Russell distinguished between extrafamilial and intrafamilial cases of child sexual abuse, and the acts encompassed ranged from petting (touching of breasts or genitals or attempts at such touching) to rape before the victim was 14 years, and completed or attempted forcible rape experiences between the ages of 14 and 17 years. Russell found that by the age of 14 years, 20 percent of the women had experienced extrafamilial sexual abuse; and by 18 years, 31 percent of the sample had had at least one such sexually abusive experience. Only 15 percent of the perpetrators were complete strangers, and 53 percent of the incidents were classified as very serious (from acts involving forced penile-vaginal penetration to those involving nonforced attempted fellation, cunnilingus, anilinction, and anal intercourse). With respect to intrafamilial sexual abuse (defined as any kind of exploitative sexual contact that occurred between relatives, no matter how distant the relationship, before the victim was 18 years old), 12 percent of the respondents had experienced such abuse prior to age 14, and 16 percent by age 18 years. Fathers and uncles were reported as the major perpetrators, and 23 percent of the experiences were classified by Russell as very serious. Father-daughter incest was reported by 4.6 percent of the respondents. Experiences between siblings that the women reported as being consensual were regarded as nonexploitative and were not included in the figures reported above.

The National Center on Child Abuse and Neglect (US Department of Health and Human Services) points out that child sexual abuse is not limited by racial, ethnic, or socioeconomic boundaries but is found in all strata of society. In its report, the center lists varying figures for the incidence of child sexual abuse, ranging from 800 to 1000 per million; there are 500,000 cases per year for girls under 14 years of age, alone.[18]

In sum, regardless of the definition and study samples that have been used by various researchers, it seems clear that childhood sexual abuse is much more common than has generally been thought. Yet only 2 percent of the intrafamilial and about 6 percent of the extrafamilial cases of child sexual abuse are ever reported to the police.[17] If both extrafamilial and intrafamilial cases are combined, Russell's study indicates that 28 percent of the women respondents had been sexually victimized before age 14 and that 38 percent had been victimized by the time they reached 18 years. Moreover, it should be noted that some of the aforementioned studies have not included relevant information about child sexual abuse experienced by male persons. DeFrancis[19] has reported an incidence of 10 female victimizations for every 1 male victimization of childhood sexual abuse. However, Gibbens and Prince[20] in their study in England found that 71 percent of their random sample of child victims were girls, and 29 percent were boys.

It would appear, then, that despite the relatively high frequency of the phenomenon of child sexual abuse, our society has not invested very much by way of resources for the identification, treatment, and prevention of this problem. In part, this may be explained by the fact that the seriousness of the problem has traditionally been underestimated; moreover, the topic of child sexual abuse remains enshrouded in myths and misinformation. For example, many people believe that child sexual abuse is both infrequent and is limited particularly to certain groups (the poor and socially disadvantaged) or to certain geographic areas (for example, rural Appalachia).

Many people also seem to believe in the "Lolita" notion of childhood sexuality, which views children as sexually precocious and oftentimes even provocative. The general notion appears to originate in faulty perceptions and interpretations of children's behavior, possibly facilitated by some aspects of psychoanalytic theories and speculations about childhood sexuality. For example, if a 6-year-old girl approaches a man, sits on his lap, and puts her arms around him, this behavior does not mean that the child is intitiating a sexual encounter. A more accurate appraisal of such behavior would be that the child has seen her mother or other female relatives engage in similar behavior and hence is merely imitating it. Also, the child could simply be seeking attention and affection—**not** sexual interaction. And, if the child agrees to "go along" with some sexual activities suggested by the adult, this does not mean that the child wants to or that he or she even understands the nature, implications, or the likely injurious consequences of such acts. Rather, the child may simply comply to the requests or demands of an adult who has authority over the child.

Indeed, it is precisely because of societal concerns about protecting children and safeguarding their welfare that for centuries our legal system has very explicitly recognized a "lack of consent" when children are below certain ages. And, even when the legal reference to "child" pertains to persons below the age of 14 years, statutory provisions for **legal incapacity** to give consent go to age 16, 17 (as in the case of New York State), or even 18 years.

CHARACTERISTICS OF VICTIMS

It has been noted earlier that girls are clearly at greater risk for childhood sexual abuse than boys. Moreover, even though children of almost all ages have been subjected to such abuse (victims have been as young as 4 months old[18]), Kinsey and colleagues[10] and Gagnon[12] found that the ages of greatest vulnerability were 9 to 12 years; Landis[11] reported two periods of increased risk: ages 7 to 10 and ages 13 to 14. The average age range appears to be between 11 and 14 years.[18]

In general, then, all children are potential victims, regardless of their age, race, ethnicity, and the socioeconomic status of the family. The sexual behaviors involved in such abuse can range from an adult male exposing his penis to a child, to fondling; and to digital, oral, vaginal, or anal penetration of the child. Sgroi and associates[21] have reported that perpetrators may escalate the nature of the sexual interaction, beginning with fondling and in some cases going on to sexual intercourse.

Perpetrators of child sexual abuse may also use varying degrees of coercion, from bribing the child with gifts and other tangible rewards to intimidation and threats of serious physical harm to the child, or to members of his or her family, should the sexual molestation be disclosed. When the offender is either a relative or family friend, he often plays on the child's loyalty. The child may be initiated into sexual interactions under the guise of a "special game" that other family members would be jealous or upset about if they were to be told about it. And, when the child feels uncomfortable about the behavior or complains, the adult will admonish the child "not to tell" under penalty of being sent away to a foster home. The offender may also play on the child's feelings by warning that he (the perpetrator) will be sent away from the family, or might even be imprisoned, if the child were to disclose the abuse. Thus, the child is placed under further emotional stress and is made to feel responsible for the sexual interaction and/or the consequences that might result from disclosure.

Behaviors Indicative of Possible Child Sexual Abuse

In her extremely useful *Handbook of Clinical Interventions in Child Sexual Abuse*, Sgroi[22] mentions 20 behavioral indicators of possible sexual abuse. These indicators have been grouped into broader categories below. Observation of these behaviors in children should alert mental health and other professionals to look into the situation more carefully to ascertain the possible existence of child sexual abuse.

Overly compliant behavior is frequently manifested by children who are experiencing ongoing sexual abuse by a family member. The perpetrator controls not only the child's body but also other aspects of the child's behavior. If the father or father-surrogate is involved, he will frequently become very restrictive of the child when he or she reaches adolescence and will be inclined to prohibit the youngster from dating and engaging in other social activities of the peer group.

Acting out aggressive behavior is seen more frequently in male victims of childhood sexual abuse. Boys who have been so victimized are at risk for becoming sex offenders themselves when they reach adolescence and adulthood.

Withdrawal is another behavioral indicator. The child may withdraw into a fantasy world that provides the safety and security missing in real life.

Difficulties in school are often a manifestation associated with this type of victimization. The educational performance may be characterized by difficulties in concentration and/or by a sudden drop in the child's school performance.

Failure to participate in school and other social activities is another consequence noted in children experiencing ongoing victimization. In cases of incest, the perpetrator tries to restrict the child's activities out of jealousy, fear of losing control of the child, and fear of disclosure.

Depressed mood and feelings of helplessness might be displayed; at times these symptoms may even attain the proportion of clinical depression and be accompanied by suicidal feelings.

Sleep disturbances characterized by difficulties in falling asleep, waking up during the night, having nightmares, or related nocturnal fears should be matters of concern. Children who are or have been victims of nocturnal intrafamilial sexual abuse may try to avoid going to bed in order to escape the feared abuse.

Pseudomature behavior may be displayed by children who are placed in the role of an adult (for example, the female child being placed in the role of the wife) and made to assume a level of maturity and sophistication uncharacteristic for that age.

Hints about sexual activity might be displayed. Children may "act out" their victimization either in doll play or in interactions with their peers. For example, a 3-year-old girl evaluated by Becker was first suspected of having been abused when her mother noticed her rubbing a doll between the legs. When the mother asked what the child was doing, the girl replied that her Uncle Jim did this to her when he came to visit the family.

Age-inappropriate behavior is sometimes displayed by children who have been sexually abused. For example, the female child's behavior toward males might reflect either unusual fear or even seductiveness.

Spending a lot of time away from home is another behavioral pattern that has been noted in children who are victims of intrafamilial sexual abuse. These children may look for every opportunity to escape from the home and to be away from the perpetrator. Consequently, these children may use school as a legitimate place in which to escape; they may regularly arrive quite early for school and leave late. They may also become uncharacteristically active in numerous extracurricular activities in order to reduce the amount of time they spend at home.

Running away from home is a fairly common reaction of adolescent females who are the victims of abuse in the family generally and also if they were victims of intrafamilial sexual abuse.

Avoidance of adults and distrust of them is another behavioral pattern sometimes associated with the experience of sexual abuse by children. Children are taught to obey and to trust adults; but when the child experiences sexual or other forms of abuse, there may be a feeling of betrayal and the sense that adults cannot be trusted. It is not uncommon, for example, for victims of incest to continually find themselves, in later years, in rather dysfunctional relationships and to become involved in a series of failed relationships because of their impaired ability to trust and related psychological sequelae of sexual victimization.

It must be emphasized that the foregoing indicators are based on clinical experience and are worthy of the attention and concern of mental health and other professionals. These indicators suggest some increased likelihood of—**not** certainty of—child sexual abuse. Thus, clinicians should be supportive of the child while attempts are made to evaluate more carefully the possible or suspected abuse and to validate or to rule out the possibility.

Sgroi also emphasizes that the child should receive a complete medical evaluation, and if any of the following signs or symptoms are present, sexual abuse should be suspected strongly:

1. Any damage to the genital or rectal tissues. Children may show soft tissue injury or lacerations in the urethral, genital, or rectal openings if penetration was effected.

2. The presence of a foreign object in the genital, rectal, or urethral openings. Some perpetrators will place objects in the child's orifices; or, on occasion, a young child modeling the behavior of the assailant will place such objects in his or her own bodily orifices.

3. Any trauma to the body—including soft tissue damage to the child's buttocks, thighs, or lower abdomen—should be questioned.

4. The presence of any sexually transmitted disease (herpes, syphilis, gonorrhea, and so forth, especially in very young children, should raise serious concern about possible child sexual abuse).

5. Pregnancy in an adolescent should be investigated to determine if sexual abuse might have been involved.

Other physical symptoms frequently seen in cases of child and adolescent sexual abuse include recurring headaches, stomach ailments, and infections of the urinary tract.

Although the foregoing list of behavioral indicators and physical signs and symptoms is not meant to be exhaustive, it should offer some useful guidelines for mental health and other professionals working with children who are suspected of having been sexually abused.

INTERVIEWING CHILD VICTIMS

It has often been observed that children and adolescents who have been evaluated by mental health professionals, and especially those who have participated in criminal justice proceedings resulting from their experience of sexual abuse, feel psychologically or emotionally victimized by these procedures. Some of these feelings and reactions could well relate to the attitudes, manner, and perceived insensitivity of the criminal justice and mental health personnel. It is very important, therefore, that mental health and other professionals working with such children be particularly alert and sensitive to the feelings and vulnerabilities of youngsters who have been sexually victimized.

Moreover, criminal justice and mental health professionals should never ignore or take lightly a child's disclosure of sexual abuse or any comments regarding such abuse. Professionals have often been surprised to learn that what was thought to be a groundless allegation was later substantiated. Moreover, even in those cases in which the allegation proves to be false, the mere fact that the allegation was made would indicate that the child or adolescent is experiencing psychological problems and needs help. Indeed, the allegation might well serve as the functional equivalent of a "cry for help."

Eight useful guidelines for mental health and other professionals who interview sexually abused children are recommended.[22]

1. The interviewer should not assume that the particular report of abuse was the first such instance. More often than not, especially in cases of intrafamilial sexual abuse, the behavior may have been going on for weeks, months, or even years. In such cases, it is unusual for the perpetrator to molest the child only on a single occasion; often there may also be some escalation of the abusive behavior. And, because the child victims have typically been admonished by the perpetrator to keep the molestation secret, the interviewer is unlikely to get an accurate and complete picture of the abusive behavior if the questions are limited simply to the reported instance. If the child knows that the interviewer does not assume that there was just one occurrence, he or she may be able to discuss more readily the range of abusive incidents that might have been experienced. More specifically, interviewers should determine (a) how the abuse began; (b) the relationship of the perpetrator to the child; (c) the specific sexual behaviors involved; (d) where the abuse occurred; (e) the nature and degree of coercion, enticement, force, or intimidation that may have been used; (f) the duration of the abuse; and (g) whether the child has told anyone else about the abuse and that person's reactions.

2. To reduce their feelings of alienation, it is helpful to inform the children that others have also experienced the same or similar problems and that the interviewer has knowledge and expertise in this area. It is important that the children be made aware that they are not the first persons to have had such experiences or that their victimization was an entirely rare event. Because these children often feel very alone in their plight, they should be provided plenty of reassurance and support and may be informed that the interviewer will work closely with them to be of assistance.

3. The setting in which the children are interviewed can be extremely important in terms of their level of comfort. Whenever possible, the children should be interviewed in a neutral setting; for example, the interviewer's office. If interviewed in their own homes and that is where the abusive behaviors took place and also involved a member of the family, the children might feel pressured not to disclose very much. They may fear that other family members may be able to hear what is being discussed. Thus, the child might be asked where he or she would feel more comfortable in talking about the incident, and every effort should be made to accommodate the child's request or preference. Moreover, whenever possible, the child should be interviewed alone. If, however, the child is uncomfortable or unwilling to be interviewed alone and wishes

another person to be present, the child's feelings in this regard and also the choice of the support person should be respected.

4. It is important that the interviewers be familiar with the language and vocabulary used by children when describing the sexual behaviors that occurred. Because many children are unfamiliar with standard sexual terms, interviewers should be careful to use general descriptions of body parts and/or sexual activities, rather than relying on technical terminology. In this regard, anatomically correct dolls or drawings can be used to facilitate clear communications about and discussion of the sexual acts involved.

5. Children do not have the same sense of time as adults. Consequently, interviewers must be aware of the child's sense of time and make use of special events to pinpoint particular incidents. For example, in trying to determine exactly when the abusive behavior first started or a particular incident took place, one might ask the child if it occurred before or after his or her birthday, before the school session started, during the summer vacation period, before or after Christmas or other appropriate holiday or special occasion. Associating the events with certain times that a child readily remembers will help pinpoint the occurrence.

6. In recalling and describing the sexual abuse, children may well confuse a few details or appear to contradict themselves. Such discrepancies may lead the interviewers to consider the case as being unfounded, when in fact the discrepancies may well relate simply to the child's confusion about certain temporal sequences of particular events. It is advisable, therefore, that clinicians try to have multiple interviews with the children in order not to strain their attention span, to reduce the stress of the interviews, and also to obtain more precise and correct reports regarding the sequence of events.

7. Inasmuch as the sexual abuse in question could have extended from a period of a few weeks to several years, it is important for the interviewers to obtain information regarding the duration and extent of the abuse. Interviewers must also be sensitive to the fact that pressure may have been placed on the child **not** to disclose the extensiveness of the abuse.

8. To facilitate the obtaining of an accurate history and to reduce as much as possible the pressure and stress on the children, it is most important that they be made to feel as comfortable as possible and for the interviewer to defuse the anxiety that the children may feel in the interview situations. It should also be noted that not every mental health or other professional will be able to interview or to serve as an effective therapist for children who have suffered sexual abuse. If the professional is uncomfortable in taking history from such children or in treating such youngsters, it would be in the child's best interest to refer him or her to a colleague. Otherwise, the clinician's discomfort is likely to be "picked up" by the child and will tend to constrain the information the child feels able to disclose. The more trust the child has in the interviewer, the more at ease the child is during the interview and the better able the child will be to communicate what happened.

Procedures in Cases of Intrafamilial Sexual Abuse

If a child has been the victim of incest, the professional must also assess the family, determine the impact of the sexual abuse on the family unit, and determine how safe it is for the child to be returned to the home. In the initial meeting with the parent(s), the interviewer should be prepared for one or both the parents to deny that the child was actually abused, or for the parents to blame the child for the abuse. If the parents blame the child, it is important that the mental health professional explain to them that the child cannot be expected to understand the nature, implications, and consequences of the sexual activity, as must be expected of the adult involved. Moreover, children below certain ages cannot give "consent" for sexual relations. If both parents are quite united and seem determined to place the blame for the sexual abuse on the child, the professional must then determine how safe it would be for the child to remain in the home. The child could be at risk for continued sexual or other abuse (for example, punishment for disclosing the sexual abuse). And, if the disclosure and other related reactions from social, mental health, or criminal justice agencies help stop the sexual abuse, the child may still be under considerable pressure from the perpetrator as well as from the other parent to withdraw the complaint or to deny that the abuse actually occurred. Consequently, it may become necessary to effect some type of separation (removing either the offender or the child from the family) until the matter can be evaluated further or until other suitable disposition can be made. Although the removal of the offender is the generally preferred type of separation, the child should be removed without any hesitation if there is reason to be concerned about his or her immediate safety. If the child has a reliable and concerned ally in the family (for example, the nonabusing parent or another adult relative), and if that relative can be depended on not to leave the child alone with the perpetrator, and if the perpetrator also agrees to become involved in treatment, then no one may need to leave the home. It is important to involve the victim as much as possible in the above decision making. For example, the child should be asked whether he or she would feel more comfortable in being returned to the home or would prefer to be placed with some relatives or close friends.

The assessment interview should also obtain information from the family about their response to and knowledge of the sexual abuse, ascertain the strength and direction of emotional ties within the family, and identify the extended family members and relatives who may be important to the family and who could serve as a support system for the child. Sgroi[22] has offered some very useful suggestions for assessing the contribution an adult family member can make in helping a child victim recover from the abusive experience.

Procedures in Cases of Extrafamilial Sexual Abuse

The response of the parent(s) to the abuse of their child is crucial, and their feelings and reactions must be dealt with regardless of whether the perpetrator is a relative, an acquaintance, or a total stranger. Burgess and Holmstrom[23] found that parents of child victims often experience an acute phase of disorganization and a longer-term reorganization phase in reaction to the molestation of their child. Mann[24] interviewed 122 teenagers who had been sexually abused and compared the reactions of the victims with those of their parents. He found that 50 percent of the parents expressed fear for the child's safety after the assault. More parents (69 percent) than adolescents (45 percent) expressed anger at the assailant, mentioned retaliatory actions, or demanded that the perpetrator be prosecuted. Surprisingly, fully 41 percent of the parents actually blamed their children for the occurrence of the assault. About 60 percent of the parents expressed deep concerns about the child's future emotional development and were particularly concerned whether the children would develop sexual problems in the future. The abused children reported that their parents had become overreactive, overprotective, and overrestrictive with them following the abuse incident. They also spoke of having to deal with parental feelings of anger and rejection.

The above and related findings underscore the need for mental health and other professionals to seek the active cooperation and involvement of the parents and other family members. Providing parents and family members with counseling and other support in coping more effectively with the event will thereby enable them to provide greater help to the victim of the sexual abuse.

THE IMPACT OF SEXUAL VICTIMIZATION

Children can experience both short-term and long-term psychological sequelae associated with their sexual abuse experience. Although there are numerous observations of the reactions of children and adolescents to sexual abuse, few researchers and clinicians have attempted to document the sequelae by using standardized assessment instruments and appropriate comparison groups. Consequently, much of what is known about the effects of sexual abuse is based on case reports and retrospective self-reports of persons interviewed or surveyed as adults about their childhood experiences of sexual abuse. (For a recent review of empirical rape research, reactions and responses of victims during various stages of recovery following the attack, and a discussion of some methodological and theoretical issues, see Ellis.[25] See also the more general descriptions of rape victims, particularly of adult women, in chapter 15.)

Short-Term Effects

Gibbens and Prince[20] compared a selected "court sample" of child victims who were involved in criminal proceedings with a random sample of child victims of sexual abuse. They found that 72 percent of the court sample had behavior problems and other overt psychological disturbances, as compared with 53 percent of the victims in the random sample who had not been involved in criminal and court proceedings. Moreover, recovery from these psychological effects was slower and more difficult for children who had been involved in court proceedings.

Similarly, Rogers and Weiss[26] reported that one third of their sample of child victims experienced nightmares, phobias, and compulsive behaviors following the sexual abuse. Burton[27] reported that victimized children were more depressed than a control group of nonvictimized children.

One of the most comprehensive studies conducted thus far was done by DeFrancis,[19] and his sample consisted of 263 children. Sixty-six percent of the children were found to be emotionally disturbed (14 percent were severely disturbed, 19 percent moderately so, and 33 percent mildly disturbed), but 21 percent did not manifest any emotional disturbance, and no information was available for 13 percent of the cases. DeFrancis reported that 20 percent of the children developed anxiety reactions after the assault. A majority of the children

(60 percent) also had difficulties with their school adjustment and functioning; in 16 percent of these cases the school problems clearly had developed following the sexual abuse.

Burgess and Holmstrom[23] found that the majority of the children they studied had difficulty returning to school; the children were quite sensitive to peer group reactions to their victimization.

In summary, then, acute reactions seen in both children and adolescents include withdrawal, anxiety symptoms, school problems, feelings of guilt, psychosomatic problems, aggressive and antisocial behaviors (mainly among boys), insomnia, depression, and problems with their body image. (See also the earlier section on behaviors indicative of possible child sexual abuse.)

Long-Term Effects

The studies that have been conducted thus far to evaluate the long-term effects of childhood sexual victimization indicate somewhat equivocal results. Such findings could well relate to factors such as differences in the samples of children studied, the research design and procedures, and the nature of the assessment procedures.

Bender and Grugett[28] conducted a follow-up, ranging from 11 to 16 years after the victimization, of a sample of sexually abused children and found that 35 percent were experiencing emotional problems. However, these investigators felt that the problems were, in general, not assault related. Gagnon[12] reported that only 5 percent of the 333 child victims who were interviewed when they were adults reported serious psychological problems. As adults, these persons felt that they had been "severely damaged." Some of these cases included involvement in prostitution and criminal or mental hospitalization experiences. Landis,[11] in his retrospective study of 360 adults who had been molested as children, found that only 3.7 percent felt that the childhood sexual victimization had permanently affected their lives.

Thus, the majority of the studies to date do not report long-term deleterious effects of childhood sexual abuses. However, these findings must understandably be viewed with caution because of various limitations in the design of the research; for example, the majority of the studies did not have suitable comparison groups of nonvictimized children, and the studies were retrospective in nature and typically relied on self-reports and self-assessments of short-term and long-term effects.

Considering the various studies that have been discussed in this chapter, as well as related clinical experience, rather complex relationships between many sets of variables are clearly involved. Whether a child develops various emotional and psychological sequelae appears to be related to such factors as the age of the victim, prior sexual experience, the type and seriousness of the sexual assault, the amount of coercion and force used against the victim, the developmental stage of the victim, the duration of the victimization period, the relationship of the offender to the victim, the reactions of significant others to the incident, and whether the child received any treament following the victimization experience.

In sum, although the majority of children do experience various psychological symptoms immediately following the sexual abuse, clear information is lacking with respect to the long-term effects because well-designed prospective follow-up studies have not been conducted. A very small percentage of the victims do report serious and long-term damaging effects.

Lacking the needed prospective longitudinal studies, there are some difficult methodological problems in trying to establish clear causal relationships between the sexual abuse and the constellation of related problems and consequences. However, several sets of variables and categories of trauma have been discussed.[29] For example, one must keep in mind the possibility that **prior emotional and personality problems** in the victims may to some extent affect the vulnerability of the child for later problems and complications. Another set of stressors will obviously be associated with the nature of the **crime trauma** itself; that is, the psychological effects directly resulting from the sexual victimization. It has been suggested, for example, that the degree and seriousness of the sexual molestation has a direct and positive relationship with the seriousness of the resulting physical and psychological injury to the victims.[11,12] There is also the **environmental reaction trauma,** namely, the psychological ill-effects associated with the reactions, attitudes, opinions, and related responses of various significant others in the victim's life, as well as the reactions of officials in various medical, social, legal, and other agencies that might be involved. Finally, on the basis of what is known about the experiences of adult sex crime victims with the legal (especially the criminal justice) process, we must also consider what has been referred to as the **legal process trauma.** This refers to the series of experiences that victims of sexual crimes face in terms of numerous and repeated interrogations with various strangers in the medical, law enforcement, prosecutorial, and other agencies; involvement in various stages of the formal criminal process (preliminary hearing and, in the case of felonies, possible appearance before a grand jury); and the eventual trial. In light of the considerable extant literature about the experiences of adult female victims of rape (see, for example, Berger[30] and Bohmer and Blumberg[31]), one would expect that the stress and associated trauma would be at least as great—possibly even greater—for child victims of sexual assault.

THE VICTIM AND THE CRIMINAL JUSTICE PROCESS

A sizable literature has developed describing and commenting upon the special problems that are posed for victims in the criminal prosecution of certain sexual crimes, such as rape. A fairly common tactic of defense attorneys is to try to place "on trial," as it were, the character, reputation, and prior sexual history of the rape victim.[30-32] Moreover, Libai[29] has noted that although the problems of juvenile offenders have received general recognition in Anglo-American countries, the special needs and problems of juveniles who are victims of sexual offenders typically have not. The plight of the child victims remains generally neglected. Ordway[33] concluded, "Unfortunately, current legal procedures devised to protect the child and to punish or rehabilitate the adult perpetrator actually punish the child and leave the problem unresolved."

In addition to the usual stresses and associated **legal process trauma,** there are a number of psychological and mental health concerns with regard to the role of the child as a key witness in the legal process and the role of mental health and legal professionals in the prevention and amelioration of possible deleterious effects of the legal process on the child and the family.

SEXUALLY RELATED OFFENSES

Legal Issues and Concerns

In the adversary process that governs the prosecution of criminal cases in the United States, various constitutional protections must be afforded to the defendant (for example, the Sixth Amendment rights to a speedy trial, trial before an impartial jury, to be confronted with the witnesses against him, to have compulsory process for obtaining witnesses in his favor, and to have the assistance of defense counsel). There are, therefore, clear constraints on the lengths to which criminal procedures can be modified to protect the interests of the child victims, while still adequately safeguarding the rights of the criminal defendant. The balancing and reconciliation of these competing and even conflicting societal values pose a continuing challenge for our legal system. We have already noted the series of experiences associated with the legal process trauma. In addition, there are often competing pressures from the child's family to seek prosecution and punishment of the alleged offender while trying also to protect the interests of the child. Such conflicting concerns may well complicate the prosecution of such cases and push toward plea negotiations.[29] Moreover, in cases of intrafamilial child sexual abuse, one might expect that there would be further conflicts and complications; for example, divided loyalties among the family members with regard to concerns for the best interests of the victim, the interests of the offender (in incest cases most typically the father or stepfather), as well as overall concerns for the integrity of the family unit.

We should also note very briefly the issue of the child victim's competency to serve as a witness. The legal concern here is whether the child has sufficient intelligence and ability to give reliable testimony that could be of assistance to the triers of fact.[34,35] Although many state statutes indicate that children below a certain age (10, 11, or 12 years) are presumed not to be competent witnesses, this presumption can be rebutted when the child has sufficient intelligence and capacity to provide relevant and useful information. However, appellate courts of most states have held that 4 years of age is about the absolute minimum at which children will be considered competent to testify.[35] (We shall discuss psychological knowledge and research relevant to this issue later in this section.)

In his comprehensive article, Libai[29] has described several efforts that have been made in some Scandinavian countries, Israel, and in many United States jurisdictions to give special attention to the needs of child victims of sexual abuse. For example, use of specially trained police officers in designated youth or juvenile divisions, specially trained prosecutorial staff, the use of special youth interrogators (in Israel) to interview the children and to tape record the sessions for later use and to avoid repetitions of such interrogations by other criminal justice or related functionaries.

Ordway[33] has proposed that incest victims should not have to testify personally at the trial. Instead, the victims' testimony should be replaced with tape-recorded pretrial examinations conducted by a special expert,* supplemented by the in-court testimony of the examining expert. A number of extensions and modifications of Ordway's basic proposal could easily be conceived

---

* This expert could be a specially trained social services worker with qualifications to deal with victims and families in cases of sexual abuse, and also having requisite knowledge of and familiarity with legal standards, procedures, and practices.

in order to safeguard quite adequately the defendant's Sixth Amendment rights with regard to the confrontation clause. For example, the direct and cross-examination of the child, if deemed essential, could take place in the informal setting of the judge's chambers, preferably with the presence and participation of appropriate experts to assist in the questioning and to advise the judge concerning the protection of the child in that situation. Serious consideration should be given also to the enactment of appropriate "shield" statutes for child victims of sexual abuse, as has been done in many jurisdictions to protect rape victims from intrusive and harassing questions by defense attorneys.[32]

Mental Health Issues and Concerns

Two sets of concerns will briefly be discussed: (1) considerations pertaining to the role of the child victim as a key witness in the criminal process, and (2) efforts to prevent and to ameliorate stress and trauma for the child and the family.

THE CHILD VICTIM AS A WITNESS

If the family and/or the criminal justice authorities have decided to prosecute the perpetrator, the legal and mental health professionals involved in the case should be aware of certain developmental characteristics that may affect the child's ability to give reliable testimony. There is much psychological knowledge and research in the child development area that is very relevant here.[36-40] Some of the experimental research on cognitive development and memory processes provides information that questions some longstanding legal assumptions and beliefs. For example, on certain recognition memory tasks, children as young as age 4 to 5 years are able to perform generally as well as most adults; problems of suggestibility may not be quite as great as has generally been assumed; and given simple and supportive questions, even young children have sufficient information retrieval capabilities to respond adequately to the recall demands of testimony. It is known, however, that young children do have difficulty in understanding the concepts of time, distances, and space. They are also likely to have some difficulty in conceptualizing complex events and thus, quite possibly, of describing them reliably. However, for certain simple eyewitness and related descriptions of events, young children have done about as well as adults in certain laboratory experiments.[38] In cases of sexual abuse, children can be expected to give accurate descriptions of what happened, **provided** the questions are direct and use language and terms that are familiar to the child.[36] It is necessary, we might add, to make certain that the appearance of incompetence given by the child is **not** directly related to the nature of the questioning and examination. That is, if difficult or technical terms are used and the questions are long and complex, determinations of the child's competence to testify could well be confounded by the poor interviewing skills of the adult. (See the earlier section on interviewing child victims.) A separate, albeit related, issue is whether the child will be able to maintain the aforementioned skills in the face of psychological stress and the perceived and real pressures from adult authority figures in the trial situation to shape the child's responses in particular directions. Appropriate mental health expert testimony can be of assistance on this issue.

THE PREVENTION AND AMELIORATION OF STRESS AND TRAUMA

There is much that can and should be done to inform the child and the family *inform* about the various stages of the criminal process; the usual inefficiencies of bureaucratic organizations; the seemingly glacial speed with which the case will appear to progress; and the predictable delays, postponements, and other likely complications. Such prior information and preparation can reduce appreciably the frustration, annoyance, and related stress associated with involvement with the legal process. Unfortunately, busy and harried prosecutors typically do not take the time to explain the above matters to the child or the family, nor even to prepare the child more carefully for court appearances (see Bohmer and Blumberg[31]). Hence, counselors associated with various victim assistance groups, knowledgeable mental health professionals, and other appropriate persons will need to fill this gap. Similarly, it would be most desirable to take the child and appropriate members of the family to see the courtroom ahead of time to learn where the key cast of characters will be seated and where in the audience section the family members will be located, to provide information about courtroom decorum and rules, and to answer any questions. These procedures, it will be noted, are much like the presurgery stress prevention and reduction measures increasingly used with children in the medical context.

In addition, although not exactly the "victim's attorney," prosecutors should spend more than the usual amount of time to go over the child's testimony, to rehearse and to role play the major questions to make sure the child understands them, and to prepare—not to coach—the child for the trial.

In sum, legal as well as mental health professionals involved in the case can do much in order to prevent, to reduce, and to ameliorate much of the stress and trauma that child victims of sexual abuse (and their families) are likely to experience in their interactions with the criminal justice process. Lacking such assistance, as has rather aptly been noted, the defendant's trial is very likely to be an additional tribulation for the child victim.[30]

TREATMENT

In this section we shall highlight a few of the major issues, approaches, and developments concerning the treatment of child victims of sexual abuse and related work with their families.

Sgroi and colleagues[21] have identified 10 major problem areas and symptoms in working with sexually abused children: (1) The "damaged goods" syndrome; (2) feelings of guilt; (3) fears and phobic symptoms; (4) depression; (5) low self-esteem and poor social skills; (6) repressed anger and hostility; (7) impaired ability to trust people, especially adults; (8) blurred role boundaries and role confusion; (9) pseudomaturity coupled with a failure to accomplish age-appropriate development tasks; and (10) problems regarding self-mastery and control over one's life.

These investigators note that the first five problem areas are likely to affect all children who have been sexually abused, whereas the remaining problems are more likely to affect children who have been victims of intrafamilial sexual abuse.

The great majority of abused children experience a feeling of being "damaged goods" in one form or another. Many feel directly damaged because of the sexual experience; other children feel damaged because of the negative social responses toward persons who have been sexually molested—much like the reactions to women who have been raped. The reactions of the community serve to reinforce the child's feelings of having been damaged. A key role of treatment agents as well as of other significant persons in the child's family and support system is to respond to the child positively and thereby to remove the negative self-perception and feelings discussed above.

Most sexually abused children and adolescents experience much guilt following their victimization experience. The guilt appears to be related to the feeling that they are somehow responsible for their abuse, and/or to their disclosure of the abuse, and/or to various disruptions and crises that occur in the family following the disclosure. Understandably, the same dynamics that helped various family members to remain unaware of or to avoid dealing with the intrafamilial abuse may also function to impute (overtly or covertly) some blame or responsibility to the child for the crisis that certainly erupts in the family upon disclosure. A major treatment goal, therefore, is to help the child as well as the other family members to see that the victim could scarcely be viewed as responsible neither for the sexual abuse at the hands of some adult nor for the crises and consequences that result from the **adult's** molestation.

The development of various fears and phobias is fairly frequent among child victims of sexual abuse. Indeed, many of these fears are quite realistic in terms of what the child has actually experienced—especially in cases of intra-familial abuse. The therapeutic objectives for these problems would focus on enabling the child to discuss the various fears, in order for the child to begin to see that following the disclosure and various interventions those experiences are not likely to occur. A variety of available therapeutic approaches that have been used for treatment anxiety, phobia, and related disorders can be utilized in working with these children.[25,41-46] Similarly, the fairly common depressive mood and clinical depression can be treated with various psychotherapeutic and especially cognitive behavioral approaches;[47,48] and, when these interventions are not sufficient, medication and/or brief hospitalization may have to be considered.

As noted earlier in this chapter, when intrafamilial sexual abuse has been involved, the perpetrator often tends to restrict the child's interactions with peers and participation in other related social activities. Not surprisingly, therefore, the child often displays inadequate social skills and concomitant low self-esteem. This pattern is more striking in cases in which the abuse has occurred over some period of time. Given the specific, albeit interrelated, pattern of problems and symptoms, therapists can draw upon a variety of interventions; for example, social-skills training implemented through instructions, modeling, and behavioral rehearsals; encouraging and facilitating the child's involvement with extracurricular activities and gradually increased interaction with peers in order to improve social skills, self-confidence, and self-esteem.

Sexually abused children often display feelings of anger and hostility over the abuse itself, and/or over the fact that other family members did not provide sufficient protection, and/or concerning the manner in which they were treated following disclosure of the abuse. Such feelings are normal, understandable, and, in fact, appear to be healthy aspects of the recovery process. Assertiveness training can facilitate appropriate discharge and handling of the anger and related feelings.

Sexually abused children, particularly victims of incest, frequently develop an inability to trust adults. These sequelae can be fairly severe and long-term and may well require much time and effort to overcome. In the absence of appropriate treatment, as well as related help and support from family and significant others, victims of incest are at risk for a variety of psychological and social problems.

It was noted earlier that pseudomature patterns of behavior may be displayed by victims of intrafamilial sexual abuse because the children are often placed in an adult and pseudospousal role. Therapeutic interventions for these problems will entail providing the child with instruction and information about age-appropriate behaviors, working closely with the child's parent or parent-surrogates to encourage and to reinforce appropriate developmental roles and behaviors, and providing increased opportunities for the child to learn such age-appropriate behaviors in interactions with peers.

Because the perpetrator controlled the child's body for purposes of sexual abuse, the victims frequently experience a sense of loss of control, helplessness, and a loss of their sense of self-mastery. Accordingly, the therapeutic program would involve family members who could help the child or adolescent have increasing opportunities to assume responsibility for aspects of his or her behavior and related decision making. The therapist can use modeling, role playing, and family therapy for such purposes.

The traditional model for the counseling and treatment of sexual assault victims is primarily psychotherapeutic. Unfortunately, such approaches are not very suitable for working with young children who have limited communication skills. Thus, various forms of play therapy might be more useful in working with younger children; and psychotherapy and various cognitive behavioral approaches could be used quite effectively with older children and adolescents. To date, however, no controlled group outcome studies have been reported that have evaluated the effectiveness of some of the major therapeutic approaches for working with sexually abused children.

Burgess and colleagues[49] have advocated the use of play therapy as particularly useful with young children and also with some junior-high-school-age youngsters. The use of age-related toys or other materials provides the child with opportunities to communicate and to express feelings through play. Stember[50] has recommended the use of art therapy as an effective means by which child victims are enabled to express many of the emotions they are unable or unwilling to verbalize. Similarly, Naitove[51] has suggested that, in addition to the use of art therapy, children can also express their feelings through dance, drama, and poetry.

A variety of behavioral techniques can be directed at alleviating a number of specific problems manifested by victims of child molestation, such as various fears and phobias, eating problems, and self-destructive behaviors.[41-46] Becker and colleagues[52] have reported on the use of behavioral techniques in the treatment of a 4-year-old victim of sexual assault. Behavioral techniques are particularly useful in working with children who are too young or who lack the necessary verbal skills for other treatment approaches.

Family therapy is the recommended treatment in cases of incest, because generally all family members have played either a direct or an indirect role in allowing the abuse to take place—especially if the abuse has continued over some period of time.[22,53] Sgroi[22] has pointed out several treatment issues for family therapy with incest cases—for example, the abuse of power, the isolation and insularity of the family, fear of authority, patterns of poor familial communications, denial of family problems, blurred role boundaries, and inadequate parental controls and limit setting. The success of family therapy depends, of course, on the commitment and combined efforts of all family members.

Dixen and Jenkins[54] have provided a useful review of a variety of treatment approaches for incestuous child sexual abuse, and Giarretto[55] has provided a good description of the Child Sexual Abuse Treatment Program of Santa Clara County, California.

CONCLUSION

The sexual victimization of children is a serious and longstanding problem that only in recent years has begun to receive the public and professional attention that it requires. Much like the phenomenon of family violence (see chapter 10), the problems of child sexual abuse have also remained hidden in our societal closet, so to speak. Understandably, therefore, we still lack precise information about the incidence and prevalence of the phenomenon; and there are no well-designed prospective longitudinal studies that can provide clearer understanding of the long-term effects on the child victims and, in cases of intrafamilial abuse, on the family unit. Similarly, there is precious little by way of controlled and methodologically sound research evaluating the relative and comparative efficacy of the various treatment approaches that are being used.

As this chapter has indicated, however, enough is already known about the nature and seriousness of the problems to justify markedly increased efforts to reduce as much as we can such victimization of children and also to prevent and to ameliorate the impact of such experiences on the victims. To this end, more effective treatment of sex offenders is essential, because it **is** known that rather high rates of offending behaviors (often with multiple victims) may be involved—even though the vast majority of these incidents do **not** come to official attention (see, for example, chapter 13). In addition, it is essential that in the rearing of children much greater emphasis be placed on teaching them about potential problems and how to avoid them; also, children need to know that they have the right to control their bodies and that other people do not have the right to take various liberties with them.

Increased attention should also be given to primary prevention endeavors. In this regard, it seems essential that we address certain deeply rooted and longstanding manifestations of cultural norms and attitudes that tend to demean and to exploit female persons. It is important that boys not be reared and socialized to expect and to assume positions of power and control over women and that girls be taught that they do not have to acquiesce to such power and any associated sexual exploitation. Such demeaning and exploitative attitudes toward girls and women are manifested in rather stark and extreme form in antifemale and violent pornography that appears to have increased both in the numbers of such items (books, magazines, films) and in the brutality and violence depicted (see Vivar[56] and Hommel[57]). These and related materials serve to maintain and even to reinforce the aforementioned attitudes and thereby to facilitate exploitative and abusive sexual behaviors. Hommel[57] indicates that in the United States there are over 250 pornographic publications (one is called

Little Girls) devoted entirely to children and adolescents and catering to adults with pedophilic interests.

Clearly, it seems to us, concerns about First Amendment rights and "protected speech" need to be balanced more carefully against the harm to our societal values generally and to the millions of victims of child sexual abuse more specifically.

REFERENCES

1. AMERICAN PSYCHIATRIC ASSOCIATION: *Diagnostic and Statistical Manual of Mental Disorders,* ed 3 *(DSM III).* American Psychiatric Association, Washington, DC, 1980.
2. AMERICAN BAR ASSOCIATION: *Child Sexual Abuse and the Law.* National Legal Resource Center for Child Advocacy and Protection, Washington, DC, 1982.
3. *McKinney's Consolidated Laws of New York, Annotated: Penal Law, Book 39.* West Publishing, St Paul, MN, 1975.
4. Op cit, n 3, p 397.
5. Op cit, n 1, p 271.
6. AMERICAN PSYCHIATRIC ASSOCIATION: *Diagnostic and Statistical Manual of Mental Disorders,* ed 2 *(DSM II).* American Psychiatric Association, Washington, DC, 1968.
7. Op cit, n 1, p 267.
8. Op cit, n 1, p 271.
9. Op cit, n 1, p 271.
10. KINSEY, AC, POMEROY, WB, MARTIN, CE, GEBHARD, PH: *Sexual Behavior in the Human Female.* WB Saunders, Philadelphia, 1953.
11. LANDIS, JT: *Experiences of 500 children with adult sexual deviations.* Psychiat Quart (Suppl) 30:91, 1956.
12. GAGNON, JH: *Female Child Victims of Sex Offenses.* Social Problems 13:176, 1965.
13. HERMAN, J: *Father-Daughter Incest.* Harvard University Press, Cambridge, MA, 1981.
14. FINKELHOR, D: *Sexually Victimized Children.* Free Press, New York, 1979.
15. FINKELHOR, D: *Risk factors in the sexual victimization of children.* Child Abuse and Neglect 4:265, 1980.
16. Op cit, n 14, p 88.
17. KOSS, MP: *The scope of rape: Implications for the clinical treatment of victims.* The Clinical Psychologist 36:88, 1983.
18. *Child Sexual Abuse.* US Department of Health and Human Services, National Center on Child Abuse Neglect, Washington, DC, 1981.
19. DEFRANCIS, V: *Protecting the Child Victim of Sex Crimes Committed by Adults.* American Humane Association, Denver, 1969.
20. GIBBENS, TCH AND PRINCE, J: *Child Victims of Sex Offenses.* Institute for the Study and Treatment of Delinquency, London, 1963.
21. SGROI, SM, BLICK, LC, PORTER, GS: *Validation of child sexual abuse.* In SGROI, SM (ED): *Handbook of Clinical Intervention in Child Sexual Abuse.* Lexington Books, Lexington, MA, 1982.
22. SGROI, SM (ED): *Handbook of Clinical Intervention in Child Sexual Abuse.* Lexington Books, Lexington, MA, 1982.
23. BURGESS, AW AND HOLMSTROM, LL: *Rape: Victims of Crisis.* Robert J Brady, Bowie, MD, 1974.
24. MANN, EM: *Self-reported stresses of adolescent rape victims.* J Adolescent Health Care 2:29, 1981.

25. Ellis, EM: *A review of empirical rape research: Victim reactions and response to treatment.* Clin Psychol Review 3:473, 1983.

26. Rogers, E and Weiss, J: *Study of sex crimes against children.* In Bowman, K (ed): *California Sexual Deviation Research.* Assembly of the State of California, Sacramento, 1953.

27. Burton, L: *Vulnerable Children.* Schocken Books, New York, 1968.

28. Bender, L and Grugett, AE: *A follow-up report on children who had atypical sexual experiences.* Am J Orthopsychiatry 22:825, 1952.

29. Libai, D: *The protection of the child victim of a sexual offense in the criminal justice system.* Wayne Law Review 15:977, 1969.

30. Berger, V: *Man's trial, woman's tribulation: Rape cases in the courtroom.* Columbia Law Review 77:1, 1977.

31. Bohmer, C and Blumberg, A: *Twice traumatized: The rape victim and the court.* Judicature 58:390, 1975.

32. Tanford, JA and Bocchino, AJ: *Rape victim shield laws and the Sixth Amendment.* University of Pennsylvania Law Review 128:544, 1980.

33. Ordway, DP: *Parent-child incest: Proof at trial without testimony in court by the victim.* University of Michigan Journal of Law Reform 15:131, 1981.

34. *The competence of children as witnesses.* Virginia Law Review 39:358, 1953.

35. Stafford, CF: *The child as a witness.* Washington Law Review 37:303, 1962.

36. Melton, GB: *Children's competency to testify.* Law and Human Behavior 5:73, 1981.

37. Levin, L: *The development of time concepts in young children: Reasoning about duration.* Child Development 48:435, 1977.

38. Marin, BV, Holmes, DL, Guth, M, Kovac, P: *The potential of children as eyewitnesses: A comparison of children and adults on eyewitness tasks.* Law and Human Behavior 3:295, 1979.

39. Perlmutter, M and Myers, NA: *Young children's coding and storage of visual and verbal material.* Child Development 46:215, 1975.

40. Perlmutter, M and Ricks, M: *Recall in preschool children.* J Experimental Child Psychology 27:423, 1979

41. Kilpatrick, DG and Veronen, LJ: *Treatment for rape-related problems: Crisis intervention is not enough.* In Cohen, LH, Clairborn, W, Specter, G (eds): *Crisis Intervention.* Human Sciences Press, New York, 1983.

42. Meichenbaum, DH: *Cognitive-Behavior Modification.* Plenum, New York, 1977.

43. Meichenbaum, DH and Jaremko, M (eds): *Stress Reduction and Prevention.* Plenum, New York, 1983.

44. Veronen, LJ and Kilpatrick, DG: *Stress management for rape victims.* In Meichenbaum, DH and Jaremko, M (eds): *Stress Reduction and Prevention.* Plenum, New York, 1983.

45. Vernon, LJ and Best, CL: *Assessment and treatment of rape-induced fear and anxiety.* The Clinical Psychologist 36:99, 1983.

46. Becker, JV and Skinner, LJ: *Behavioral treatment of sexual dysfunctions in sexual assault survivors.* In Stuart, IR and Greer, JG (eds): *Victims of Sexual Aggression: Treatment of Men, Women and Children.* Van Nostrand Reinhold, New York, 1983.

47. Beck, AT, Rush, AJ, Shaw, BF, Emery, G: *Cognitive Therapy with Depression.* Guilford Press, New York, 1979.

48. Frank, E and Stewart, BD: *Treatment of depression in victims of rape.* The Clinical Psychologist 36:95, 1983.

49. Burgess, AW, Holmstrom, LL, McCausland, MP: *Counseling young victims and their families.* In Burgess, AW, Groth, AN, Holmstrom, LL, Sgroi, SM (eds): *Sexual Assault of Children and Adolescents.* Lexington Books, Lexington, MA, 1978.

50. STEMBER, CJ: *Art therapy: A new use in the diagnosis and treatment of sexually abused children.* In McFARLANE, K (ED): *Sexual Abuse of Children and Adolescents: Selected Readings.* National Center on Child Abuse and Neglect, Washington, DC, 1980.

51. NAITOVE, CE: *Art therapy with sexually abused children.* In SGROI, SM (ED): *Handbook of Clinical Intervention in Child Sexual Abuse.* Lexington Books, Lexington, MA, 1982.

52. BECKER, JV, SKINNER, LJ, ABEL, GG: *Treatment of a four-year-old victim of incest.* Am J Family Therapy 10:41, 1982.

53. GIARRETTO, H, GIARRETTO, A, SGROI, SM: *Coordinated community treatment of incest.* In BURGESS, AW, GROTH, AN, HOLMSTROM, LL, SGROI, SM (EDS): *Sexual Assault of Children and Adolescents.* Lexington Books, Lexington, MA, 1978.

54. DIXEN, J AND JENKINS, JO: *Incestuous child sexual abuse: A review of treatment strategies.* Clin Psychology Review 1:211, 1981.

55. GIARRETTO, H: *A comprehensive child sexual abuse treatment program.* Child Abuse and Neglect 6:263, 1982.

56. VIVAR, MA: *The new anti-female violent pornography: Is moral condemnation the only justifiable response?* Law and Psychology Review 7:53, 1982.

57. HOMMEL, T: *Images of women in pornography and media.* New York University Review of Law and Social Change VIII:207, 1978-1979. (See also this entire issue, devoted to a colloquium entitled "Violent Pornography: Degradation of Women Versus Right of Free Speech.")

CHAPTER 15

THE RAPE VICTIM AND THE RAPE EXPERIENCE

Carol C. Nadelson, M.D.
Malkah T. Notman, M.D.
Elaine (Hilberman) Carmen, M.D.

DEFINITION OF THE CRIME

Rape has been defined as the act of taking anything by force.[1] Most statutes in the United States define rape as carnal knowledge of a person against the will of the person.[2] Two elements are necessary to constitute the crime: (1) sexual intercourse, and (2) failure to seek or to obtain the consent of the victim. Neither complete penetration of the vagina by the penis nor emission of seminal fluid is necessary. Most rapes include force or violence applied to the victim in order to accomplish the act, but acquiescence can be obtained by verbal threat or other circumstances indicating lack of consent.

The response of the rape victim is variable, depending on the circumstances, the setting where the action takes place, and her own personal response. She may fight back quickly when taken by surprise in an attack accompanied by threat of death or mutilation, or she may react more slowly and with disbelief in the forceful intentions of the man who continues to insist on sexual intercourse in the midst of a social encounter in which sexual contact is unexpected and unagreed upon by the woman. In the latter situation, nonconsent is often overlooked or misinterpreted by assuming that certain social situations imply a willingness for a sexual relationship.[3]

The Uniform Crime Reports of the Federal Bureau of Investigation reveal an estimated total of more than 81,500 rapes in 1981. This represented a 29 percent increase over the total in 1977.[4] Comparative statistics indicate that rape is the fastest growing of the violent crimes. Although better reporting may account for part of the increase, the actual incidence of the crime continues to be underestimated. An interview survey of a random sample of 930 women in San Francisco concluded that there is a 46 percent probability that a woman will be the victim of a rape or attempted rape in her lifetime.[5]

THE RAPE VICTIM'S EXPERIENCE

Burgess and Holmstrom[6] have divided rape victims into three groups: (1) victims of forcible, completed, or attempted rape; (2) victims who were an accessory due to their inability to consent; and (3) victims of sexually stressful situations in which the encounter went beyond the expectations and ability of the victim to exercise control. In this chapter we will explore primarily the first category, recognizing that the lines drawn between the categories are often unclear. Despite differences in circumstances, the intrapsychic experiences of rape victims in all groups have features in common.

The rape victim has usually had an overwhelmingly frightening experience in which she feared for her life.[7] Generally the experience results in feelings of helplessness and intensifies conflicts about dependence and independence. It generates self-criticism and guilt which devalue her as a victim, and it may interfere with trusting relationships, particularly with men. Other important consequences of the situation are a sense of shame, difficulty handling anger and aggression, and persistent feelings of vulnerability. Each rape victim responds in her own way, depending on her age, life situation, the circumstances of the rape, her specific personality style, and the responses of those from whom she seeks support.[8]

THE MYTHOLOGY OF RAPE

The mythology which surrounds rape has been developed, perpetuated, and reinforced by a number of attitudes and values which are reflected in both the medical and legal systems. A few of these myths are discussed below.[7]

1. Women can't be raped unless they want to be. A corollary of this might be that women enjoy rape, or that they at least unconsciously want it; therefore, there is no such thing as rape.
2. The rapist is a sexually unfilled and/or disturbed man carried away by a sudden, uncontrollable rage.
3. Rapists are always strangers to victims.
4. Rape occurs primarily on the street, and as as long as a woman stays home, she's safe.
5. Most rapes involve black men raping white women.
6. Women are raped because they ask for it by dressing seductively and walking provocatively; thus only "bad" women are raped.

The first of these myths represents a serious misperception of the situation, as well as of the concept of the unconscious. The prevalence of conscious or unconscious rape fantasies hardly makes every woman a willing victim and every man a rapist. The fantasy does not remotely capture the actual violence or degradation of the experience. Although fantasies in which rape plays a part are frequent, the rape victim in a real situation knows that she is submitting because there is no choice without real danger to her person or to her life.

Although definitive data are lacking, there are studies that shed light on a few of the other myths involving rape. In 1971, Amir[9] published data that encompassed all cases of rape, not including incest or statutory rape, listed by the police in 1958 and 1960 in the city of Philadelphia. The data included 646 victims and 1291 offenders. Three-quarters of the rapes involved one or two assailants (single rape, 57 percent; pair rape, 16 percent); group rape (three or more assailants) was the pattern in 27 percent. Of the total number of incidents, 71 percent were planned in advance, and only 16 percent could be considered as resulting from an uncontrollable impulse. Group rapes were planned in 90 percent of cases, and single and two-assailant rapes in 58 percent of cases. Thus the "uncontrollable urge" theory of rape is challenged.

The myth that staying at home is safe fails to recognize that 56 percent of rapes in the Amir study occurred in the victim's residence, and the remainder were divided among automobiles, outdoors, and other indoor places. Moreover, in only half of the cases was the rapist a stranger to the victim; the remainder included casual acquaintances, neighbors, boyfriends, family friends, and relatives. Indeed, a recent study concluded that the number of victims who know their assailants is probably higher than 50 percent.[10] Husbands were not included in these statistics because, until quite recently, a sexual act between husband and wife was not considered rape under American law.

Hayman and Lanza[11] report on 1223 cases in which the age of the victim ranged from 15 months to 82 years. Twelve percent were victims under 12, 25 percent were between 13 and 17, 32 percent were between 18 and 24, and 30 percent were over 25. The rapists were almost all less than 30 years of age. The majority of reported rapes involved rapists and victims of the same race. Earlier studies suggested a high proportion of black rape, but the significance of this is unclear. It is possible that black rapists are more likely to be reported and apprehended and that white rape may be grossly underreported or less aggressively pursued when reported. A Denver study[12] is an exception in that the percentage of victims by race was similar to the at-large population; that is, 71 percent white, 15 percent black, 11 percent chicano.

More recent studies lend support to the view that rape is a crime of opportunity.[13] Rape is largely an intraracial event and is ecologically bound, occurring as it does between members of the same race, economic class, and geographic neighborhood.[9] Rape is most likely to occur in areas with higher unemployment rates and lower median incomes and in areas where there are higher numbers of unemployed youths between the ages of 14 and 21 years.[10]

In Amir's study, physical force was present in 86 percent of cases, the remainder involved various degrees of nonphysical force such as coercion or intimidation with or without weapons. Amir characterizes physical force in the following way:

Roughness (holding, pushing around)	29 percent
Nonbrutal beating (slapping)	25 percent
Brutal beating	20 percent
Choking and gagging	12 percent

These statistics do not include rape that ends in death. This group is reported in the homicide statistics rather than in rape statistics. Thus, in one third of the cases in which physical force occurred, extreme brutality was used.

In group rape there is evidently a higher frequency of both alcohol intake and prior criminal records, especially of sexual offenses. The assault is usually planned and is more brutal in terms of beatings and subjecting the victim to sexually humiliating practices in addition to the rape.

Victim behavior is described by Amir as submissive in 55 percent, with some degree of resistance in the remainder. At the time of the assault, the victim must decide whether she has a greater fear of the rape or of physical injury. Her actions will reflect her decision, usually without opportunity for thought. A dilemma is presented in that resistance increases the victim's chance of escape but also increases the likelihood of violence toward her should she not escape.

Perhaps the most significant finding of Amir's study is that rape occurs in a context of violence rather than of passion: "Rape is a deviant act, not because of the sexual act per se, but rather in the mode of the act, which implies aggression, whereby the sexual factor supplies the motive."[9] Mythology has it that most rapists are sexually perverted, but Amir suggests that rapists are a danger to the community not because they are necessarily sexually perverted but because of their violence and aggression. They often may appear to be "normal," but they tend to have criminal records of offenses committed with brutality and violence. In his series, rapists tend to be young members of low-class subcultures in which masculinity is expressed by displays of aggressiveness, which include sexual exploits against women. This is most evident in group rape, in which aggressive behavior is the result not of deviant sexuality but of participation in a group that condones the use of force in attaining goals.

Clearly, as extensive as Amir's study is, the sample may be limited to specific subgroups because of the possibility that other cases are not reported to the police. The reported incidence greatly underreflects the actual incidence of rape. It is estimated that between 50 and 90 percent of rape cases go unreported. The Federal Bureau of Investigation attributes underreporting to fear and/or embarrassment on the part of the victims. The woman is often afraid of being accused of provocation or active participation in the rape. She is fearful of the reactions of her husband, boyfriend, parents, or friends. In the case of a young victim, parents may wish to protect the child from the publicity and the legal ordeal. If the assailant is a close friend, relative, or employer, there are additional pressures not to report. Our own experience in Boston, working with the Beth Israel Hospital Rape Crisis Project, indicates that approximately 60 percent of women seeking medical aid reported the crime to the police.[14]

An examination of aspects of "victimhood" will help explain this underreporting. Weis and Borges[15] describe in some detail the process by which a person becomes a victim and, specifically, the way in which our cultural norms determine that women are "legitimate" victims for rape. People are socialized to equate aggressiveness with masculinity, and passivity with femininity. The relations between the sexes are often seen "as an instrumental exchange whereby female servility is the price of male protection." Women have tended to internalize the psychological characteristics of the victim. They often do not know how to use techniques of physical self-defense. They fear male strength and often accept the mythology that the typical rape situation involves a stranger in a dark alley and that it is up to women to avoid both dangerous and compromising situations. In general, "nice girls" are believed not to get into trouble or to be raped. A 1969 study by the National Commission on the Causes and Prevention of Violence reported that only 4.4 percent of rapes were victim-precipitated.[16] But guilt and self-blame are still high among victims. One study reported that 74 percent of victims blamed themselves behaviorally (for example, "I should not have walked down that street alone"), and 19 percent blamed themselves characterologically (for example, "I'm too naive").[16]

SEXUALLY RELATED OFFENSES

Males may perceive that aggressive conquest can be seen as an acceptable substitute for "masculine" failures in the economic and social spheres, so that aggressive and exploitative behavior toward women may become part of a mode of relating, and thus they may not conceive of such behavior as wrong or devious. The rapist may justify his behavior with the logic used for the legitimation of victims in general: She was in some way already inferior, and she asked for and deserved it. Weis and Borges[15] note that Amir himself uses this logic in his study. He characterized a group of cases as "victim-precipitated rape," yet 92.7 percent of rapes in this group were accompanied by violence, and 45.9 percent of the victims were raped by more than one offender who humiliated the victim in 61.5 percent of cases. The victim's behavior was resistive in 48.7 percent of cases. One might similarily imply that attractive bank tellers precipitate bank robberies.

LEGAL CONSIDERATIONS

Although we expect that hospitals and law enforcement agencies are legitimate places for reporting crime, Hilberman[7] notes that many people trust neither of these institutions, especially with regard to rape. Hospitals suffer from lack of personnel trained to work with rape victims, both in the crisis period and in follow-up, and from lack of consistent and clear procedures for evidence collection. In the absence of a formal policy and sufficient information about the treatment of victims in crisis, personal attitudes and fears prevail. Clinicians are often in conflict about their role, especially with regard to confidentiality. In addition, the prospect of a court appearance is intimidating. The legal system also suffers from lack of personnel identified and trained to work with rape victims. The victim who reports does not receive consistent treatment because of high rates of police turnover, rotating shifts, and personal attitudes. People equate reporting with prosecution and are fearful of harassment by law enforcement authorities to prosecute. Finally, reporting and prosecution are equated with the victim's life and past being made a matter of public record.

Unfortunately, there is considerable reality to the victim's fears, reflected in the attitudes about the victim that prevail in the criminal justice system and in the statutes about rape. The report of the Center for Women Policy Studies comments that "the credibility of the rape victim is questioned more than that of any other victim of crime."[17] Forcible rape is the only crime for which an "unfounded" rate is calculated. It is also the only violent crime for which corroboration is frequently required.

One of the consequences of the corroboration requirement in unwitnessed rapes is that it is the victim who essentially stands trial. The assumption that women will make false accusations against men leads to a focus on the victim's credibility rather than on the crime. This assumption has been pervasive in the literature on the law and raises serious questions about why these offenses are treated differently.

It is important to question this assumption from yet another perspective. What relevance does past behavior, social history, or mental make-up of a victim have in the determination of whether a crime was or was not committed? How accurate is a psychiatric report in predicting or deducing behavior?

Judge Hale's[18] statement that rape "is an accusation easily to be made and hard to be proved, and harder to be defended by the party accused" shows a lack of attention to the victim's experiences. The laws or court practices pertaining to rape trials may contribute to the unwillingness of the victim to report the crime to law enforcement agencies, much less agree to the ordeal of the trial. Wood[19] summarizes the complainant's ordeal and feels that the initial report becomes a traumatic event because of the requirement that an exquisitely detailed history of the rape be given and repeated to a variety of personnel connected with the subsequent investigation. Although attention has been focused recently on the importance of law enforcement sensitivity to the victim's mental state and to the management of victims in crisis, this is not the first priority of law enforcement agencies. Thus victim interrogation may be impersonal and unsupportive if not frankly disbelieving and hostile. In some interrogations, the victim is asked questions about how many orgasms she had during the rape, what fantasies she had, and inquiry about past sexual encounters—all of which appear to be irrelevant to the establishment of the occurrence of rape. Wood points out that the police have considerable discretion as to whether or not any action is taken. They may refuse to accept the complainant's charges or neglect to work on cases they feel are unsubstantiated. The acceptance of prevalent rape mythology makes it likely that these law enforcement personnel will often infer consent when none is given or assume victim precipitation in many situations.

When the complaint reaches trial, there are three major elements of the legal defense in a rape case:[18]

1. Lack of identification—that the man accused is not the perpetrator of the crime.
2. Lack of penetration—that a sexual act did not take place.
3. Consent—that the intercourse was consented to or voluntary on the part of the woman.

Independent corroboration of the victim's story may be presented by an eyewitness, by evidence acquired at the crime scene, and from the body of the victim or defendant. Because many rapes are not witnessed, circumstantial evidence is offered in most cases, including medical evidence and testimony, evidence of breaking and entering the complainant's residence, condition of clothing, bruises and scratches, emotional condition of the complainant, opportunity of the accused, conduct of the accused at the time of the arrest, presence of semen or blood in the clothing of the accused or of the victim, promptness of the victim's report to the police, and lack of motive to falsify. The complainant who attempts to restore a sense of control and cleanliness by bathing and changing clothes after the rape, who is too frightened to report immediately, or who presents a calm exterior may not be believed. The defense counsel can attack the case against the defendant by introducing evidence of the victim's mental illness, previous consensual intercourse with the same man, previous false accusations of rape, or an unchaste reputation. Supported by the myths about rape indicated earlier, many court cases seem to require evidence of a high degree of resistance by the victim, based on the belief that a healthy woman cannot be forcibly raped.

Recently, those studying victimology have recognized that resistance depends on the circumstances of the attack and the implications of continued resistance so that victim compliance is not a sign of consent but of futility.[20] The Report of the Center for Women Policy Studies comments on this issue.

SEXUALLY RELATED OFFENSES

When and how a woman should resist a rapist are under hot debate. . . . The few published studies of convicted rapists indicate that there are three or four different categories of offenders whose motives, methods, and reactions to resistance differ. Since rapists do not wear identifying labels, a woman cannot know which type she is confronting. . . .

An important element of any program on defense against rape should be emphasis of the right of the woman to submit. Although some people successfully resist robbery, others are killed in the attempt, so no one is counseled to fight a robber. Although there are different values at stake, the choice should still be the victim's. Even a person who wants to resist and is trained to fight may be unable to do so when confronted with a situation which she or he perceives as dangerous.[17]

In the law of rape, consent is considered an affirmative defense that must be pleaded and proved by the defense.[18] Otherwise, it is assumed that the woman did not consent to the intercourse. Nevertheless, after it is pleaded, the success of the consent defense depends practically on which version of the facts the jury believes. The defense must make its case believable and the victim's story unbelievable. This is often done through evidence of the complainant's general character or reputation for unchastity, the implication being that prior consensual intercourse—whether with the defendant or with someone else— implies consent to intercourse in this instance, even though force, violence, and verbal threats may have been admitted by the defendant or proved conclusively by the victim.

Many women feel that the trauma of a court proceeding is too great, especially if there is little reason to hope that the assailant will be punished for his crime. Not only has rape been the fastest growing of the index crimes against the person, but among these it has had the lowest proportion of cases closed by reason of arrest. In 1980, only 48 percent of the reported rapes led to an arrest. This figure can be put into perspective when we remember that between 40 percent and 50 percent of all rapes are never reported. In a study of 115 rape victims admitted to the emergency ward during a 1-year period, only nine of these cases led to conviction for rape or abuse of a child.[21]

Gates[22] cites a 1966 study of jury trials examining whether judges would have rendered the same verdicts as juries, and if not, what factors the judges thought influenced juries. In rape cases in which there was no extrinsic violence, one assailant, and no prior acquaintance of the victim and the assailant, the judge and jury would have reached the same conclusion in only 40 percent of cases. In the remaining 60 percent, the judge would have convicted when the jury acquitted. The judges concluded that in the absence of external evidence of violence, jurors ascribe to the complainant some contributory or precipitant behavior.

On the basis of jury decision, Hibey suggests:

The jury's assessment of the credibility of the witnesses and their evidence is not always rational. This phenomenon stems in large part from certain ideas jurors have about the crime of rape, some of which are believed with such ferocity that jury verdicts are often examples of outright nulli- fication—the ultimate and extreme exercise of the fact finder's preroga- tive.[18]

In addition to the complex social forces deterring reports of rape, the victim often has a set of internalized beliefs, stemming from her own socialization and self-perception, which decreases the likelihood of reporting.[7] She often believes that the rapist is perverted or "sick." When the actual experience does not coincide with this view, inasmuch as half of the assailants in rape cases are acquaintances—if not trusted friends—she is left to wonder about her own complicity in the event. She "knows" that "nice girls" don't get raped and that it is not possible to rape a woman against her will. This false belief further contributes to her silence and her reluctance to report the attack to the police, physicians, or friends.

The Prince George's County (Maryland) Task Force on Rape commented on the silence of the victim as follows:

> Rape and the investigation and treatment of the rape victim is a serious crime of assault on the body, but more grieviously on the psyche of a woman. All too often, she is treated at best as an object, a piece of evidence, and is made to relive the experience, must face the incredulity of the police, the impersonality of the hospital, and then must defend herself in court. Having been socialized to be passive, she is nevertheless expected to have put up a battle against her attacker. Her previous sexual experience can be used to impute her instability though the defendant's background often cannot be brought up against him. She does not have the benefit of a retained lawyer and sometimes the prosecutor does not have the time or perhaps the insight to prepare her beforehand for the ordeal of the trial. She suffers serious psychological stress afterward, largely due to the guilt and shame imposed by society. She may not recognize a need for professional help or she simply cannot afford it.[13]

Thus, as we have noted, there are multiple forces that act as deterrents to reporting, and it appears that it will be necessary to create a more sympathetic climate in order to allow the victim to identify herself as such to the hospital, law enforcement, and judicial systems. In 1975, the House of Delegates of the American Bar Association adopted a resolution[24] designed to protect the victim from unnecessary invasion of privacy and the consequent psychological trauma. The proposed changes in law and practice recommended the elimination of corroboration requirements which exceeded those applicable to other assaults, revision of the rules of evidence relating to cross-examination of the complaining witness, development of new procedures for police and prosecution in processing rape cases, and establishment of rape treatment and study centers to aid both the victim and the offender. Gates[22] and Wood[19] recommended a redefinition of rape to include oral and anal intercourse and a delineation of varieties of rape to be contingent on the degree of force or violence used. They suggested that the resistance standard be dependent on "reasonable fear" and whether victim resistance was reasonable to expect under the circumstances of the assault. Reduced or graded penalties as with a system of degrees for rape, in line with comparable violent crimes, should increase the likelihood of jury convictions. The impact of such changes should eliminate the present distinction between victims of rape and victims of other crimes. Most states have made changes in their rape statutes that incorporate some of these reforms. In a recent before-and-after study, Loh[25] compared the impact of common law and rape reform legislation on prosecution. He concluded that the main effects have been symbolic and educative rather than instrumental.

RAPE AS STRESS

The profound impact of the rape stress is best understood when rape is seen as a violent crime against the person, and not merely as a sexual encounter.[7] Victims of violent crimes generally experience crises which may be unrecognized. Bard and Ellison[20] describe the stresses confronting the victim and emphasize the extent of the personal violation as an important factor. Burglary, for example, is experienced as a violation of the self in that one's home and possessions are symbolic extensions of the self. When armed robbery occurs, stress is intensified by the encounter between the victim and the criminal. The violation is compounded by a coercive deprivation of independence and autonomy in which the victim surrenders his or her controls under the threat of violence. An actual physical assault, in addition to the robbery, further stresses the victim because injury to the body serves as concrete evidence of the forced surrender of autonomy. Rape, then, is an ultimate violation of self—short of homicide—with invasion of one's inner and most private space, as well as the loss of autonomy and control. Thus it is irrelevant to differentiate vaginal, anal, or oral intercourse when it is the self and not an orifice that has been invaded. The core meaning of rape is the same, whether the victim is a virgin, a prostitute, a housewife, or a lesbian.

Rape can be viewed as a crisis situation in which a traumatic external event breaks the balance between internal adaptive capacity and the environment. It is similar to other situations described in the literature on stress, including community disasters,[26] war,[27] and surgical procedures.[28] The unexpected nature of the catastrophe and the variability of the resources of the victim in coping with an experience that may be viewed as life-threatening are critical factors in all crisis situations.

Although there are variations related to cultural and personality style, descriptions of stress reactions generally define four stages, which vary in intensity and duration.[29] These responses are also found in rape victims.

1. First there is an anticipatory or threat phase in which some anxiety facilitates perception of potentially dangerous situations so that they can be avoided. Most people protect themselves with a combination of internal psychological mechanisms which enable them to maintain an illusion of invulnerability, with enough reality perception to be protected from real danger. Thus, in situations in which a potential stress is planned (for example, elective surgery), individuals can protect themselves by strengthening those mechanisms which will ward off feelings of helplessness.

2. The second phase is an impact phase in which varying degrees of disintegration may occur in a previously well-adapted person, depending on the degree of trauma and the adaptive capacity of the individual. During this phase, major physiologic reactions, including cardiovascular and sensorial shifts, may occur. The responses of people vary, from remaining calm to becoming confused, anxious, and even hyster-

ical. Most victims show variable but less extreme responses. They demonstrate restricted attention span and automatic or stereotyped behavior. This clinical picture is seen in rape victims as well as in other crisis victims.

3. The third phase is a posttraumatic or "recoil" phase in which emotional expression, self-awareness, memory, and behavioral control are gradually regained. Nevertheless, perspective may remain limited, and dependency feelings may increase. Individuals perceive adaptive and maladaptive responses in themselves and may question their own reactions. A positive or negative view of one's ability to cope may affect the course of resolution of the particular trauma and future capacity to respond to stress. Self-esteem may be enhanced or damaged during this phase.

4. A posttraumatic, reconstitution phase in which victims try to put their lives back together again follows. At this time, the loss of self-reassuring mechanisms, which had fostered a sense of invulnerability, may result in a decrease in self-esteem. The victim then blames herself for lack of perception or attention to danger. When individuals begin to question themselves, and then the ability of the group or of society to be protective, a resulting traumatic neurosis may develop. Such a neurosis is designed to protect the individual against further exposure to trauma, but it is psychologically costly, especially because it results in loss of self-esteem and of the ability to take risks or to be innovative in other situations.[30]

Sutherland and Scherl[31] have reported on three phases of response to rape:

1. **The acute reaction.** This is characterized by signs of acute distress which include shock, disbelief, emotional breakdown, and disruption of normal patterns of behavior and function. The victim is often unable to talk about what has happened and may have difficulty telling family and friends, or reporting to the hospital or police. Guilt may be prominent, with fears that poor judgment may have precipitated the rape. During this phase, there are concrete concerns that demand fairly immediate attention. These include whether to tell family, husband, friends, children, or others what happened, as well as the implications of telling or not telling them. The victim is often concerned about publicity, about the likelihood of pregnancy or venereal disease, about her responsibility or ability to report the crime, about being able to identify the rapist, and about the impact of possibly seeing the assailant again.

2. **Outward adjustment.** This begins within several days to some weeks after the rape with an apparent temporary resolution of the immediate anxiety-provoking issues. The victim often returns to her usual life patterns and attempts to behave as if all is well, reassuring both herself and those close to her. Denial of difficulty and suppression of feelings are prominent during this period. The impact of what has happened is often ignored.

3. **Integration and resolution.** Depression frequently occurs, although it may be mild. The victim often needs to talk about what has happened

in order to integrate the event with her self-image and to resolve her feelings about the rapist. The earlier attitude of tolerance and understanding of the rapist may be replaced by anger toward him. She may also wonder if she colluded in some unknown way with the rapist.

Burgess and Holmstrom[32] define a specific rape trauma syndrome in two stages: an immediate or acute response in which the victim's lifestyle is disrupted by the rape, and a long-term process in which the victim reorganizes herself. In addition, they comment on two types of acute response: "the expressed style," in which the victim is emotional and visibly upset; and the "controlled style," in which the victim may appear to be calm to the casual observer. The authors also comment on the prevalence of guilt and self-blame in the initial phase. They discuss a reorganizational phase which has elements in common with other stress reactions, although it varies with each individual. The primary acute reaction is related to the fear of physical injury, mutilation, and death. Mood swings are common, as are feelings of humiliation, guilt, shame, self-blame, and fear of another assault by the assailant.

There is often surprisingly little clinical evidence of rage in rape victims, compared with the outrage stimulated in others upon hearing of the rape. Feelings of anger and desire for revenge often appear somewhat later. A primary defense may be an attempt to avoid thinking about the rape, although this is difficult to do. The wish to undo the event may appear in fantasies of how the victim might have handled the situation differently.

A wide variety of physical and psychological reactions may occur during this time period, depending, in part, on the location and extent of the injuries sustained. Specific symptoms occur, such as sleep disturbance and loss of appetite. These should be differentiated from similar symptoms caused by treatment, including hormones administered to prevent pregnancy.[7] Like Sutherland and Scherl, these authors report that the acute phase may last from a few days to some weeks and is generally followed by a reorganizational process. The manifestations of this second stage depend on the victim's personality style, available support system, and the treatment she encounters from others. Changes in lifestyle are prominent, with impaired levels of function at work, home, and school. Some women may move to another residence, and others may be fearful of leaving their homes at all or may give up autonomy by returning to their families. Sleep disruptions often continue with vivid dreams and nightmares. Early dreams with re-enactments of the actual rape are frequent. These later progress to a point at which mastery of the rape may begin taking place, and the victim may apprehend the rapist or assailant in her dream. Phobias appear that seem specifically determined by the nature of the rape experience, such as fear of crowds or of being at home or of being outdoors, depending on the location of the assault. Sexual fears are common, with a decline of interest as well as withdrawal from a previous partner.

There are specific situations that increase the complexity of the reaction. The victim who is raped by a friend or a relative, an event more frequent with children and adolescents, has a greater psychological burden than would be true if the assailant were a stranger. She must also deal with issues of trust. The existence of psychological problems and/or maladaptive behavior patterns prior to the rape increases the likelihood of maladaptive coping patterns following the rape. Serious medical or psychiatric problems prior to, or as the result of, the rape may affect the outcome.[7]

LIFE-STAGE CONSIDERATIONS

Certain reactions relate directly to specific life stages. These reactions are described in the sections that follow.

The Single Young Woman

The single young woman between the ages of 17 and 24 years is the most frequently reported rape victim. She is inexperienced, and her relations with men have frequently been limited to family and friends. She has little sophistication, and she may easily become involved in an unwelcome sexual encounter. In this age group, rape victims frequently do have a prior acquaintance with the rapist. This may be the reason for a refusal to prosecute. She may reproach herself because she could have been more active in preventing the rape, and she experiences shame and guilt, regardless of the circumstances. These feelings, coupled with the victim's sense of vulnerability, may color her future relationships with men. This is especially true for the very young woman who may have had her first sexual experience in this context. The result can be a confusion of sexuality and violence.

The rape experience for a young single woman may revive concerns about separation and independence. She may feel inadequate to care for herself. Parents, friends, and relatives often respond by offering to take care of her again in an attempt to be supportive and reassuring. However, in doing this, they may foster regression and prevent mastery of the stress. Another problem for the younger rape victim is her perception of, and tolerance for, the gynecologic examination. Because she may have suffered physical trauma, is susceptible to venereal disease, and may become pregnant, a complete examination is indicated. It may be perceived, especially by an inexperienced or severely traumatized woman, as another rape. Thus, although she may be concerned about the intactness of her body, she will have difficulty with necessary procedures if they stimulate memories or reproduce in any way the original rape experience.

The Woman with Children

The woman with children must also deal with the problems of what, how, and when to tell them. If the event is known in the community, there are implications for her and her children. She is concerned about the trauma she may be inflicting as well as her image in their eyes. If she has a husband, she may be concerned about whether he can find her sexually attractive or even tolerate her. She may also have unexpected negative feelings toward her husband.

The Divorced or Separated Woman

The divorced or separated woman is in a particularly difficult position in that her credibility may be questioned because of her lifestyle. She, in turn, may experience the rape as a confirmation of her feelings of inadequacy. She is especially likely to feel guilty and may fail to obtain aid or to report the crime. Her ability to function independently is challenged. If she has children, she may worry about her ability to protect them and to care for them. Questions may be raised about her adequacy as a mother.

The Middle-aged Woman

The "middle-aged" woman is often in a period of reassessment of her life role, particularly in the face of changed relationships with her grown-up or already absent family members. Her husband may be in his own midlife crisis and may be less responsive to and supportive of her sexual and emotional needs. At this point the overwhelming experience of rape is particularly damaging. The myth that a middle-aged woman past her earlier, sexually most active period has less to lose than a younger woman is very much in error. It is difficult to quantify the self-devaluation and feelings in a woman who may be concerned about her sexual adequacy.

LONG-TERM CONSEQUENCES OF RAPE

It is difficult to predict all the long-term needs of the rape victim, because individual response patterns and circumstances differ so much. A few of the reactions that do appear clinically, often at a later date, are as follows:

1. Mistrust of men with consequent avoidance or hesitation to form relationships.
2. A variety of sexual disturbances, often presenting as sexual dysfunctions and marital conflicts.
3. Persistent phobic reactions.
4. Anxiety and depression, which may be precipitated by seemingly unrelated events that in some way bring back the original trauma.
5. Persistent anxiety and avoidance of gynecologic examinations or procedures.
6. Suicide or suicide attempts. Preliminary studies of female suicide attempters suggest the possibility of a relationship between an earlier rape experience and suicide attempts.

There is clinical evidence of a silent rape reaction in which an earlier rape is kept secret and after some investigation it appears that the event is still very much alive and unresolved.

Although it is apparent that a simple approach to the rape victim and her family cannot be provided, it is clear that crisis counseling, with follow-up for at least 1 to 2 years, may be necessary. In some circumstances the degree of trauma coupled with the previous developmental history of the victim may result in long-standing symptoms and even the development of a traumatic neurosis that requires intensive, long-term treatment.

COUNSELING ISSUES

There seems to be a consensus on three types of needs to be fulfilled in a counseling program: (1) crisis intervention to facilitate working through of the trauma and to diminish the likelihood of long-term psychopathologic consequences; (2) emotional support from whomever the victim comes in contact with during the crisis period; and (3) emotional support for family and friends of the victim.

There is some disagreement about the effectiveness of peer versus professional mental health counseling. Professionals often state that the trauma of rape is so serious that professional psychological help should immediately be made available. However, many feminists believe that it is detrimental to suggest to a victim that she needs professional help because it implies that her reaction is "sick," unless there is some indication that she cannot cope with the reality of the assault or its consequences. They believe that most victims need an empathetic listener and enough information to enable them to make realistic choices.

Rape crisis center counselors, who are generally volunteer lay people, usually state that they can assess their own limits and call upon professionals for advice and referral. Professionals often function in the training and supervision of lay counselors. The Center for Women Policy Studies recommends a coordinated and collaborative educational effort by physicians, hospitals, citizens, and criminal justice personnel as the most effective approach to training needs.[17] The psychiatrist or mental health professional can have both direct and consultative roles in all these educational endeavors.

The psychiatrist or mental health professional has many roles. In the emergency room setting, he or she functions in a consultative capacity with a variety of other specialty services, such as gynecology, pediatrics, nursing, and social work. A collaborative alliance must be established in the emergency room that will facilitate medical treatment, enable the victim to make a decision about legal involvement, and help the victim work toward crisis resolution. Consultative/liasion skills are crucial to the development of integrated programs which depend on an interdisciplinary team approach as the primary treatment modality.

The mental health professional can assist other staff members in the acquisition of skills necessary for taking an adequate history and assessing the victim's emotional state and ego functioning so that optimal treatment can be planned. It is useful to differentiate short-term crisis goals from long-term issues, which may require a psychiatric referral. The perspective of the psychiatrist in evaluating which victims might appropriately benefit from long-term intervention can be extremely important. Adequate case supervision with a focus on family dynamics and the life context in which the rape occurs should be a major concern of every treatment program. Immediate or long-term supervision is especially important in hospital settings, where counseling is often done by lay counselors or a variety of personnel functioning in training capacities.

Mental health professionals may be a referral resource for community agencies, crisis centers, and other physicians. They can be consulted when there is a maladaptive or delayed response to the crisis. Women already suffering from other emotional problems can be rape victims, and this experience may well intensify preexisting problems. The mental health professionals who are called upon must be knowledgeable not only in the special issues related to rape but also in terms of the clinical skills necessary to serve as consultants to other therapists, treatment-team members, and cooperating community agencies.[7]

The last decade has witnessed the spontaneous appearance of growing numbers of community-based rape crisis centers as part of a nationwide antirape movement.* These centers are largely staffed by volunteer, nonprofessional women, some of whom have been raped in the past or have been close to someone who was raped. Men are not usually accepted as volunteers in rape crisis programs. However, in some centers, men have been recruited to work with the significant men in the victim's life. Others have organized themselves to support the crisis program and to provide services to male friends and relatives of rape victims.

Most community rape crisis centers have similar goals, which include the following:

1. To provide supportive services to victims
2. To reform the institutions that deal with victims
3. To educate themselves and the public on rape-related issues
4. To reform the law

Direct services to victims are designed to meet the victim's needs for information, emotional support, and advocacy.[7] Many centers have 24-hour telephone hot lines that allow for immediate contact and support after a rape. Information is provided about local hospital and criminal justice procedures, and the victim is encouraged to make the necessary decisions about medical treatment, reporting to law enforcement, and communication with family and friends. Counseling services are usually limited to immediate temporary support and short-term follow-up through the use of peer counselors. The goal of counseling is the return of autonomous functioning and control, and prolonged dependency on the center is discouraged. Individual counseling is the rule; group models are reportedly less successful. Victim advocacy services include intervention with medical and law enforcement personnel when it is felt that the victim is receiving inappropriate or inadequate treatment, and continuing contact by telephone and in person throughout the prosecutory phase. Anonymous reporting is often arranged for those victims who choose not to report the rape or rape attempt to law enforcement agencies. Additional services may include transportation, babysitting, and a place to sleep either when the victim fears returning home or when her home is judged to be unsafe.

The aims of educational programs in the crisis centers are self-education; the dissemination of information on rape prevention and resistance, as well as what to do if rape occurs; and community and personal attitudinal changes.[7] There has been a focus on "demythologizing" the crime of rape, particularly with regard to the stereotypic assumptions about both the victim and the assailant. Public education programs have been conducted independently in cooperation with other groups or with existing medical and criminal justice institutions. Educational efforts are viewed as a necessary precursor to reforms of the law enforcement and health care systems. Reform goals have been initiated in cooperation with these institutions or by assuming a vocal, adversary

---

* A national directory of rape crisis centers is provided in *National Directory: Rape Prevention and Treatment Resources*, published by the National Center for the Prevention and Control of Rape, US Department of Health and Human Services, Rockville, MD, 1981.

position. Rape crisis centers have variously recommended or demanded an increase in women police officers, sensitivity to victims' needs, and clarification of hospital and police protocols. Many centers have collaborative relationships with both hospitals and law enforcement agencies so that the counselor remains with the victim throughout the required procedures. Center advocates attend rape trials and, on occasion, will "pack the court" as an additional method of public pressure to change courtroom behavior.

Despite the similarity of goals and services, each program has unique aspects which stem from the nature of the group itself as well as from the resources and attitudes of the community in which the center is located. Many centers remain alienated from professional institutions, but others work closely with existing medical and legal resources. Although most counseling is done by nonprofessional women, programs for training these women in the techniques of crisis intervention for rape victims have involved professionals in both medical and legal spheres. Despite the lack of psychological sophistication, counselors have been creative and innovative in providing support to victims and families.[7] It is likely that psychiatric consultative and backup services would be welcomed by many centers.

Institutional-based rape crisis programs should not be considered an improved alternative which replaces the community rape crisis centers. Community groups may tend to attract younger and/or feminist women, and more traditional and/or older women will use institutional services. It is anticipated that community programs will continue to be necessary to provide support and to encourage referrals to appropriate medical and law enforcement facilities. Community programs also provide a wide spectrum of services not easily provided by traditional institutions, such as a safe place to sleep when the victim is fearful of returning home after the rape, or a companion to guide her through the time-consuming and traumatic experiences of the criminal justice procedure should she decide to prosecute. Finally, community groups continue to provide leadership for educating the public, and this will be reflected ultimately in changes in attitude on the part of the victim as well as the juror.[7]

Often the concerns of lay groups derive from their perception of the attitudes of professionals. Notman and Nadelson[3] have stated, "Until recently many psychiatrists have felt that rape was not a psychiatric issue, and further that psychiatrists had little to offer the rape victim. They often shared the view that the victim 'asked for it.'" The victim was then seen as acting out her unconscious fantasies, and, therefore, she was not "really" a victim. Thus the rape victim had not been offered the sympathetic understanding usually extended to people in crisis. Rape falls into a group of emotionally charged issues in which prejudice prevents the objectivity that would be available if it were regarded as a traumatic experience. As noted, another manifestation of this prejudice has been the concern that a rape victim was making a false accusation, a concern that has not been supported by the evidence in the vast majority of cases.

Professionals have shared the mythology about the rape victim, who they perceive as a young, sexually attractive woman in some way exposing herself to the danger that could be avoided in the ordinary course of living. Or they may believe that, after having initially agreed upon sexual intercourse, she is accusing her partner of rape in order to save herself from criticism. Holding these views fulfills several functions. It protects individuals who hold them from anxiety about their own vulnerability, and it states that "it can't happen here." This defensive position is further expressed by the focus on the sexual aspect of rape. If it is sexual, then the victim and the rapist could be seen as seeking sexual gratification together. The professional then can be protected from feelings of guilt or responsibility.

In our recent experience, concomitant with the development of a rape crisis program, changes have occurred in the attitudes of participating professionals with an increasing awareness of the crisis nature of the experience and an increased empathy for the individual victim.

The potential role of the psychiatrist or mental health professional is multifaceted, with clinical, administrative, teaching, supervisory, and research aspects. The role of the mental health professional with regard to the legal system is not entirely clear. As Hilberman notes, however, "It is not the function of the clinician to decide whether the victim has 'really' been raped. Rape is a legal and not a medical term. The fact that the victim perceives herself as having been violated remains the significant event."[7]

In the immediate aftermath of the rape, issues of personal safety and control emerge as primary concerns. The victim has just had an experience in which her very existence may have been threatened, with total loss of control of what was done to her. Her immediate needs are for a sense of physical safety as well as for assistance in assuming some control over what has happened to her and what will happen to her in her dealings with both individuals and institutions. The presence of an empathic and supportive individual—who may be a counselor, clinician, or friend—will enhance her sense of safety. She should not be left alone. She should be encouraged to talk and to ventilate her feelings with reassurance and validation of her responses. Whether this occurs in the police station, the physician's office, or the hospital emergency room, the issues are the same. In order to be effective, the counselor must have available information about medical and legal procedures so that the victim can be informed. Decisions about procedure, including reporting to the hospital or law enforcement agencies, must be made by the victim. Although the counselor may have some opinions about what she ought to do, coercion has no place in the management of the rape victim.[7]

Burgess and Holmstrom[32] summarize the assumptions they make in counseling victims. Their context is a short-term, issue-oriented crisis model with the goal of restoring the victim to her previous level of functioning as quickly as possible. Because the crisis disrupts the victim's lifestyle in four areas—physical, emotional, social, and sexual—all of these issues are appropriate areas of scrutiny. The victim is assumed to be normal, that is, an individual who was managing her life adequately prior to the crisis. The rape is viewed as a crisis situation, and previous problems unassociated with the rape are not considered priority issues for discussion. When other issues of concern are identified which would require the use of a different approach, appropriate referrals are suggested to the victims.

An analysis of rape crisis requests[8] suggests that there are four major categories of need, namely, for police intervention, medical intervention, psychological intervention, and emotional control (especially with victims who present in an incoherent state). There is an additional group who may not perceive that anyone can be of help to them; these people present with ambivalence, if not hostility, about any intervention.

The following sections, as summarized by Hilberman,[7] are appropriate areas for counseling intervention in the immediate phase.

The Assault

Considered here will be the circumstances and setting of the rape; the victim's conversation with the assailant; physical and verbal threats; details of behavior; amount and kind of resistance; the use of alcohol or drugs by either victim or assailant; and the victim's emotional and sexual reactions. The counselor's ability to learn about the details of the assault will clarify which of these concerns are most problematic. The focus may be on the rape as a first sexual encounter, or on intense guilt for not putting up a fiercer struggle. The victim's coping strategy before and during the assault will become an issue after the assault.

Medical Concerns

Medical concerns include the quality of the victim's treatment in the hospital; interactions with medical and nursing staff; extent and type of physical injury; the possibilities of pregnancy and venereal disease; and the pelvic examination. The pelvic examination is a frequent focus for the victim's anger. Because many victims experience the pelvic examination as another rape, adequate preparation is important. Victims are often fearful that their bodies are irrevocably damaged.

Law Enforcement

Questions directly related to law enforcement include the following: Does the victim plan to report the rape? If she has reported, how was she treated? What kinds of questions was she asked? Was she encouraged in, or dissuaded from, the pressing of charges against the assailant? Part of the counseling process is to help the victim vent her feelings about her treatment, as well as to validate her feelings.

Prosecution

The key prosecutory questions can be combined as follows: Does the victim plan to press charges, cooperate with the police investigation, and appear in court, and how does she feel about this? This is often an issue of high priority for the victim, who must make this decision at a time when it is difficult to think clearly about anything. Concrete information is usually helpful. For example, many victims think they are breaking the law by not reporting and prosecuting. The victim's rationale for not wishing to prosecute may be quite realistic, given the treatment of victims by the courts; or they may reflect her fears that she did indeed precipitate the rape. The counselor's role is to help the victim clarify for herself how she feels about these issues and to support the victim's decision, whatever it may be.

Social Support System

In terms of the social support system, the issues may be stated in three basic questions: Who are the important people in the victim's life? Whom does she plan to tell about the rape? What responses does she anticipate? How the rape may affect or change her relationship with significant others is invariably an issue in the immediate crisis period. An evaluation of the personal support available will determine in part the extent to which continued counseling becomes necessary; that is, the availability of a strong social support network will diminish the need for ongoing counseling intervention. In contrast to most personal crises, in which the counselor or therapist reinforces the importance of sharing the crisis with those who are significant in the person's life, no firm guidelines exist about communicating the event of the rape because of the real possibility that the revelation may disrupt the relationship. Thus a husband may perceive the rape as a deception by his wife, and the parents of an adolescent may project their own sense of guilt and become angry with the victim. At times, the counselor may have an important role to play in counseling the family. Family and friends must be sensitized to the meaning of the rape so that they are able to give honest support to the victim. Where there are preexisting conflicts in relationships, the rape may aggravate the situation. In cases in which the victim chooses not to tell close friends or family members, guilt or distancing may occur, for which the victim will need counseling assistance.

Physical Safety

If she lives alone, or was raped at home, the victim will likely be fearful of returning home. Moreover, the assailant (who most often has not been apprehended) may have threatened to return, or the victim may be fearful of this even when a threat has not been made. A temporary resolution may involve identifying a friend with whom the victim can stay as well as available options for the future if necessary.

Preparation for Victim Responses

As previously described, there is a wide spectrum of immediate responses to rape. A victim may not wish to talk, or she may show little overt emotional response. In any case, it is important for the counselor to prepare the victim for the range of reactions likely to occur, so that the victim becomes sensitized to her own feelings and has some awareness that the inevitable disruptions in lifestyle are normal. Mild sedation for sleep is usually indicated as well. Knowledge that the victim can call upon the counselor throughout this period provides additional reassurance that she will not be left in isolation. Although the counselor's role with the victim in the later reorganization phase cannot be defined specifically because of the complexity of victim needs and responses, it is important to keep in mind the issues we have raised.

MEDICOLEGAL CONSIDERATIONS

The physician treating the rape victim has several tasks, including immediate care of physical injuries, prevention of venereal disease, prevention of pregnancy, proper medicolegal examination with documentation by evidence collection for law enforcement purposes, and prevention or alleviation of permanent psychological damage. These tasks are extremely complex because there are very different systems operating and producing conflicting demands.

The *Report of the District of Columbia Task Force on Rape* describes many of the problems that had prevailed in hospital treatment of victims.[8] The task force suggested that doctors resist seeing rape victims because they want to avoid court appearances. They also suggested that some doctors minimize or neglect signs of trauma in an attempt to avoid being called in to testify. This may be related to the lack of training in the treatment of the physical and emotional trauma resulting from the rape or in the methods of evidence collection. Hospital policies vary widely. In some institutions, examinations are performed by gynecologists, but at others the lowest-ranking physician (without training in gynecology) sees the victim. Medical treatment is often inadequate and psychological treatment usually nonexistent. Victims have been known to wait for long periods of time to receive medical attention that is often perfunctory and impersonal. Issues concerning pregnancy and venereal disease may not be considered adequately. There may be no formal procedure for collection of evidence, and even when such procedure exists, it may not be followed. Many hospital policies require that parents give consent before a minor is treated; some automatically call the police whether a victim wishes to report or not. Some victims choose to forego treatment rather than have parents or police know of the rape. The problem of confidentiality in the doctor-patient relationship must be considered if testimony will be required of the physician or of the counselor working with the physician.

There are a number of formal reports and guidelines that have made recommendations for improving hospital services to rape victims.[33-37] The following major recommendations and considerations have been summarized by Hilberman.

1. At least one medical facility in any given community should have a formal program for the comprehensive treatment of rape victims, with such services available on a 24-hour basis. Those hospital or clinic facilities which do not have comprehensive programs should have a set of guidelines for treating rape victims.
2. Law enforcement agencies and the public should be made aware of the existence of comprehensive hospital services for rape victims.
3. Because treatment of the rape victim involves an interface between medical and legal issues, programs designed by medical facilities should operate within the context of their community and in cooperation with citizens' groups, law enforcement, and prosecutory agencies.
4. Treatment of the rape victim should be given high priority, second only to life-threatening illnesses or accidents, and should not be contingent on cooperation with the criminal justice system.
5. Adequate care of the victim is facilitated by a team treatment model. The team should include a support person, a nurse, a physician, and appropriate consultants, including a mental health professional. The support person should serve as an advocate/counselor/guide for the victim throughout the hospital process and should have familiarity with both crisis intervention techniques and criminal justice procedures. The nurse, usually a member of the regular emergency room staff, should coordinate the total treatment plan, assessing needs and explaining procedures. There are varying opinions about whether the physician should be a gynecologist, family practitioner, or specialist

in trauma. Because the physician's medicolegal role makes it highly probable that the victim will perceive him/her as an investigator rather than as an ally, counseling responsibilities are best handled by other team members. The role of the psychiatrist or other mental health professional as a consultant has been discussed earlier. Finally, although it is desirable to be able to offer the victim a choice regarding the sex of the team personnel, sensitivity and experience may be more important determinants of a successful intervention.

6. All hospital personnel who will have contact with the victim should be educated to the special problems of rape victims. The training program should include crisis intervention theory and practice, sensitization to the physical and emotional trauma of rape, and medicolegal issues. It is desirable that training efforts be accomplished in collaboration with citizens' groups and local criminal justice agencies.

7. Hospitals should have clear procedural guidelines for victim care and evidence collection with a specific and unambiguous description of the role and function of each member of the rape-crisis team. The medicolegal examination can be facilitated by prepackaged "rape kits," which contain all the information and equipment necessary for examination and evidence collection.

8. Crisis intervention should be immediately available to all victims, their families, and significant other persons at the time of initial contact with the hospital.

9. The victim should be fully informed and consent obtained for all treatment procedures performed in the emergency room and afterward, with special emphasis on those steps taken to prevent pregnancy and venereal disease. The victim may be experiencing considerable confusion at the time of the hospital visit, and written information furnished to her at the hospital serves as reassurance that the appropriate preventive measures were taken. Otherwise, the patient may be uncertain about what further protection she may need after release from the hospital.

10. Follow-up treatment may be complicated by the profound denial which often follows in the immediate aftermath of the rape. The victim may attempt to "forget" the assault and may not keep subsequent appointments. For this reason, it becomes especially important to provide all available services during the initial crisis contact; this may be the only intervention for a given victim. Follow-up efforts may be more successful if they involve contact with the original treatment team members rather than with new institutions and personnel. Thus the team physician should arrange to see the victim, with the support person maintaining continuing contact. When formal mental health referrals are indicated, the need for such services must be explained so that the victim does not assume that because she was raped, she must be mentally ill. All follow-up treatment plans must be contingent on the patient's informed choice, and all referral services should be suggested on the basis of their sensitivity to rape-crisis issues as well as on their general professional capabilities.

11. The issue of financial responsibility for the rape victim's medicolegal examination has been the object of considerable attention. Although some states have statutes providing for financial compensation to

victims of violent crimes, only recently have rape victims been considered appropriate beneficiaries of such laws. Inasmuch as the victim is expected to go through the ordeal of reporting to hospital and law enforcement personnel and then to face the trauma of the trial, it seems inappropriate that she also should be expected to absorb the cost of the state's evidence. Payment for hospital services rendered should not be the responsibility of the victim but should come from public funds.

12. Although interagency collaboration is necessary to provide comprehensive services, all efforts should be made to protect the confidentiality of the victim. During the course of the examination, information about the victim may surface that is relevant to medical treatment but irrelevant and potentially damaging in court (for example, pre-existing venereal disease or contraceptive usage in a single woman). Team members must use caution in what is entered into the woman's medical record, and guidelines should be established to protect her confidentiality.

13. Although medical treatment cannot be made contingent on reporting to police, it is desirable for law enforcement agencies to know about the incidence of rape. An anonymous or "blind" report system might be instituted in which the location and modus operandi of the assailant are described but the name of the victim withheld.

There are at present a growing number of hospital-based rape crisis programs that have incorporated these recommendations. Each program has unique features based on the nature of the area served, but the availability of community resources, state laws, and the local criminal justice procedures have strikingly common characteristics in all these programs. Clear and unambiguous guidelines can be the basis for establishing and maintaining an effective and sensitive rape crisis intervention program in any community.

REFERENCES

1. *American Heritage Dictonary.* Houghton Mifflin, Boston, 1982, p 1026.

2. EVARD, J: *Rape: The medical, social and legal implications.* Am J Obstet Gynecol 111:197-199, 1971.

3. NOTMAN, MT, NADELSON, CC: *The rape victim: Psychodynamic considerations.* Am J Psychiatry 133:4, 1976.

4. *Uniform Crime Reports for the United States.* Federal Bureau of Investigation, Washington, DC, 1982.

5. RUSSELL, D, HOWELL, N: *The prevalence of rape in the United States revisited.* Signs, Summer 1983, pp 688-695.

6. BURGESS, AW, HOLMSTROM, LL: *Rape trauma syndrome.* Am J Psychiatry 131:981-986, 1974.

7. HILBERMAN, E: *The Rape Victim.* American Psychiatric Association, Garamond/Pridemark Press, Baltimore, 1976.

8. *Report of the District of Columbia Task Force on Rape.* Subcommittee of District of Columbia City Council, July 1973.

9. AMIR, M: *Patterns of Forcible Rape.* University of Chicago Press, Chicago, 1971.

10. RAPKIN, J: *The epidemiology of forcible rape.* Am J Orthopsychiatry 49(4):634-647, October 1979.

11. HAYMAN, C, LANZA, C: *Sexual assault on women and girls.* Am J Obstet Gynecol 103(3):480-486, 1971.

12. GIACINTI, TA, TJADEN, C: *The Crime of Rape in Denver.* Denver Anti-Crime Council, 1973.

13. BROWNMILLER, S: *Against Our Will.* Simon & Schuster, New York, 1975.

14. Beth Israel Hospital Rape Crisis Intervention Project, Boston, 1983.

15. WEIS, K, BORGES, SS: *Victimology and rape: The case of the legitimate victim.* Issues in Criminology 8(2):71-115, 1973.

16. JANOFF-BULMAN, R: *Characterological versus behavioral self-blame: Inquiries in depression and rape.* J Pers Soc Psychol 37(10):1798-1809, 1979.

17. *Rape and its victims: A report for citizens, health facilities and criminal justice agencies.* In *The Police Response: A Handbook.* Center for Women Policy Studies, Washington, DC, 1975. (Copies available from Law Enforcement Assistance Administration, Washington, DC.)

18. HIBEY, RA: *The trial of a rape case: An advocate's analysis of corroboration, consent, and character.* In SCHULTZ, LG (ED): *Rape Victimology.* Charles C Thomas, Springfield, IL, 1975.

19. WOOD, PL: *The victim in a forcible rape case: A feminist view.* In SCHULTZ, LG (ED): *Rape Victimology.* Charles C Thomas, Springfield, IL, 1975.

20. BARD, M, ELLISON, K: *Crisis intervention and investigation of forcible rape.* The Police Chief, May 1974.

21. HOLMSTROM, LL, BURGESS, AW: *Sexual behavior of assailants during reported rapes.* Arch Sex Behav 9(5):427-439, 1980.

22. GATES, MJ: *The rape victim on trial.* Paper presented at Special Session on Rape, American Psychiatric Association, Anaheim, CA, 1975.

23. *Report of the task force to study the treatment of the victims of sexual assualt.* Task Force of the County Council of Prince George's County, MD, March 1973.

24. *House of Delegates redefines death, rape and undoes the Houston amendments.* American Bar Association Journal 61:463-473, 1975.

25. LOH, WD: *Q: What has reform of rape legislation wrought? A: Truth in criminal labeling.* Journal of Social Issues 37(4):28-52, 1981.

26. TYHURST, JS: *Individual reactions to community disaster: The habitual history of psychiatric phenomena.* Am J Psychiatry 107:764-69, 1951; LENDENMANN, E: *Symptomatology and management of acute grief.* Am J Psychiatry 101:141-146, 1944.

27. GLOVER, E: *Notes on the psychological effects of war conditions on the civilian population. Part I: The Munich crisis.* Int J Psychoanal 22:132-146, 1941; GLOVER, E: *Notes on the psychological effects of war conditions on the civilian population. Part III: The blitz.* Int J Psychoanal 23:17-37, 1942; SCHMIDEBERG, M: *Some observations on individual reactions to air raids.* Int J Psychoanal 23:146-176, 1942; RADO, S: *Pathodynamics and treatment of traumatic war neurosis (traumatophobia).* Psychosom Med 4:362-369, 1942.

28. DEUTSCH, H: *Some psychoanalytic observations in surgery.* Psychosom Med 4:105-115, 1942.

29. JANIS, IL: *Psychological Stress.* John Wiley & Sons, New York, 1958.

30. WEISS, RJ, PAYSON, HE: *Gross stress reaction I.* In FREEDMAN, AM AND KAPLAN, HJ (EDS): *Comprehensive Textbook of Psychiatry.* Williams & Wilkins, Baltimore, 1967.

31. SUTHERLAND, S, SCHERL, D: *Patterns of response among victims of rape.* Am J Orthopsychiatry 40(3):503-511, 1970.

32. BURGESS, AW, HOLMSTROM, LL: *The rape victim in the emergency ward.* Am J Nurs 73(10):1740-1745, 1973; BURGESS, AW, HOLMSTROM, LL: *Rape: Victims of Crisis.* Robert J Brady, Bowie, MD, 1974.

33. KATZ, S, MAZUR, MA: *Understanding the Rape Victim.* John Wiley & Sons, New York, 1971.

34. McCombie, SL (ed): *The Rape Crisis Intervention Handbook.* Plenum Press, New York, 1980.

35. Schmidt, P: *Rape crisis centers.* Ms 14-18, September 1973.

36. Wasserman, M: *Rape: Breaking the silence.* The Progressive 19-23, November 1973.

37. National Center for the Prevention and Control of Rape: *National Directory: Rape Prevention and Treatment Resources.* US Department of Health and Human Services, NIMH, Rockville, MD, 1981.

CHAPTER 16
MALE GENITAL EXHIBITIONISM

Park Elliott Dietz, M.D., M.P.H., Ph.D.
Daniel J. Cox, Ph.D.
Stephen Wegener, Ph.D.

Exposure of the male body for the purpose of shocking women was described as early as the fourth century B.C. by Theophrastus.[1] The first clinical description of exhibitionism was provided in 1877 by Laséque,[2] who noted that exhibitionists usually expose from a distance, make no attempt at sexual intercourse with their victims, and often return to the same place at the same time of day. Indecent exposure accounts for one third of all recorded sexual offenses in Canada,[3] the United States,[4] and England and Wales.[5] Detected recidivism rates vary from 17 percent to 41 percent, depending on the duration of the study.[3,6,7] Exhibitionism is the second most common sexual deviation encountered at mental health facilities in England.[7] The prevalence of exhibitionism is unknown because mental health facilities typically see exhibitionists only after they have been convicted and because only 15 percent to 25 percent of exposures are reported to the police.[6,8,9]

The mental health and criminal justice systems have different concerns and definitions regarding those who expose themselves. Although mental health focuses on the diagnosis and treatment of the individual, criminal law is designed to deter and to punish offensive actions. This chapter begins by considering clinical and legal definitions of exhibitionism and genital exposure, then explores the varied theoretical models of exhibitionism, the assessment and treatment approaches characteristic of each model, and the criminal sanctions and dispositions for those convicted of unlawful exposure.

Women have been reported to engage in genital exhibitionism,[10,12] but these cases are extremely rare.[13] They do not appear in the criminal courts and do not follow the typical compulsive male modus operandi. Consequently they will not be dealt with in the remainder of the chapter.

DEFINITIONS AND DESCRIPTION

Clinical Definitions

Mohr and colleagues defined exhibitionism as "the expressed impulse to expose the male genital organ to an unsuspecting female as a final sexual gratification."[3] Today the most widely accepted definition of exhibitionism is "repetitive acts of exposing the genitals to an unsuspecting stranger for the purpose of achieving sexual excitement with no attempt at further sexual activity with the stranger."[14] This definition excludes appropriate exposure (for example, precoital sex play), accidental exposure (for example, public urination), and exposure owing to other pre-existing disorders (for example, epilepsy, psychosis). In order to distinguish the mental disorder from its criminal expression and to take account of the fact that exhibitionists may have designs on their victims beyond exposure, we propose a new definition: Exhibitionism is a sexual deviation (paraphilia) characterized by a persistent or recurring desire to expose the genitals to an unsuspecting stranger for the purpose of achieving sexual excitement.

Legal Definitions

Two centuries ago "open and notorious lewdness" was recognized by the secular courts of law but construed as an offense "against religion and morality." This offense was committed "by frequenting houses of ill fame" or "by some grossly scandalous and public indecency," the latter of which was punishable by fine and imprisonment.[15] At common law, exposure to more than one person was necessary to constitute a crime. British cases of the mid-nineteenth century illustrate this point. It was not an offense for a man to expose himself to a 12-year-old girl in a public churchyard[16] or to a barmaid alone in a public bar,[17] but it was an offense for a man to expose himself to three women passengers on an omnibus.[18] Although certain other offenses "against religion and morality" are extinct or endangered (namely, drunkenness, adultery, fornication, and the having of bastard children), the progeny of prohibitions against lewdness are a vigorous breed.

In England, indecent exposure is currently an offense under Section 4 of the Vagrancy Act, 1824, when an individual "wilfully, openly, lewdly and obscenely expos[es] his person with intent to insult any female" and under Section 28 of the Town Police Clauses Act, 1847, when an individual "wilfully and indecently exposes his person."[5] Note that under the latter, proof of intent to insult or to shock a female is not necessary for conviction.[19]

In the United States, criminal statutes under which exhibitionists could be prosecuted include those relating to "lewd and obscene conduct," "open lewdness," "public lewdness," "public indecency," "indecent exposure," and "exposure of the sexual organs." Many of these statutes are worded so as to encompass a range of behaviors far broader than the furtive displays to strangers and children characteristic of exhibitionists. Public urination, nude sunbathing, "streaking," and commercial sex shows—none of which is related to the clinical entity of exhibitionism—are encompassed by many of these statutes. As noted later in this chapter, exhibitionists have sometimes been adjudicated as "sexual psychopaths" or "sexually dangerous persons" under sexual psychopath laws.

Constitutional challenges to indecency and lewdness laws have included claims that they are overly vague (a Fourteenth Amendment challenge) and that they breach the defendant's First Amendment right of free speech and association. Elements of these crimes that have been the basis of appeals include the definition of "public place," the definition of "private parts" or "genitals," the number of observers or witnesses necessary, the nature and degree of intent that must be proved, and the effect of the victim's consent.[20]

The New York public lewdness statute[21] illustrates a few of these issues. Derived in part from the Penal Law of 1909, the current New York statute states:

> A person is guilty of public lewdness when he intentionally exposes the private or intimate parts of his body in a lewd manner or commits any other lewd act (a) in a public place, or (b) in private premises under circumstances in which he may readily be observed from either a public place or from other private premises, and with intent that he be so observed.

When originally enacted in 1965, this statute did not include items (a) and (b) and thus seemed to require that the conduct occur in a public place. The addition of items (a) and (b) in a 1968 amendment clarifies that the offense is committed by one who, though himself in a private place, exposes himself to others who are in a public place, such as pedestrians passing his window. Nudity in a public place is insufficient to establish public lewdness;[22] there must be a showing of lewd conduct from which it can be inferred that the defendant intended to act in a lewd manner.[23,24]

New York recognizes no crime of indecent exposure. A statute[25] that prohibited "exposure of a female" was repealed in 1983 and re-enacted as a statute prohibiting "exposure of a person":[26]

> A person is guilty of exposure if he appears in a public place in such a manner that the private or intimate parts of his body are unclothed or exposed. For purposes of this section, the private or intimate parts of a female person shall include that portion of the breast which is below the top of the areola. This section shall not apply to any person entertaining or performing in a play, exhibition, show or entertainment.

Obviously this statute encompasses a great deal more than the exposures characteristic of exhibitionists.

Many states have adopted language similar to that in the Model Penal Code[27] in revising their criminal codes. The Model Penal Code provides for two offenses under which exhibitionistic acts would most likely be charged. The more specific of them is Section 213.5, defining **indecent exposure:**

> A person commits a misdemeanor if, for the purpose of arousing or gratifying sexual desire of himself or of any person other than his spouse, he exposes his genitals under circumstances in which he knows his conduct is likely to cause affront or alarm.

Less specific is Section 251.1, defining **open lewdness:**

> A person commits a petty misdemeanor if he does any lewd act which he knows is likely to be observed by others who would be affronted or alarmed.

Both of these Model Penal Code definitions succeed in avoiding the requirements that the offense occur in a public place or in the presence of others, each of which has to be proved under the common law definition and under some statutes. Much of the commentary and appellate litigation concerning these offenses deals with these elements of the older formulations, for example, whether a trespasser on private property is in a public place or whether the presence-of-others requirement is fulfilled when the observer and the exposed party are located in separate buildings. Although it avoids these problems, each Model Code definition retains its share of ambiguity. For example, on what basis are triers of fact to infer that a defendant had a "sexual" (erotic) purpose in order to return a conviction of indecent exposure? What is the standard to be applied in determining whether an act was "lewd" for the purpose of returning a conviction of open lewdness?

Pennsylvania has enacted indecent exposure[28] and open lewdness[29] statutes nearly identical to the Model Penal Code. Effective since 1973, these statutes have been clarified through rulings by Pennsylania courts. (Note, however, that courts in other jurisdictions could reach contrary conclusions.) A superior court held that neither the indecent exposure act nor the open lewdness act requires proof of intent to affront or to alarm the general public.[30] Proof that the defendant's conduct was sexually motivated was absent when the defendant faced a wall in an alley, extracted his penis, and subsequently shook it in view of a 7-year-old-girl.[31] Under the Pennsylvania open lewdness statute, it has been held that deliberate or malicious intent on the part of the defendant is not required as an element of the offense, as long as the lewdness is open and notorious.[32] Masturbation while seated in a motor vehicle in a public place constituted open lewdness,[33] but exposure of a portion of the genitals through a hole in the defendant's bathing trunks was not open lewdness absent evidence of any act marking his conduct as open and notorious or indicating that he was aware of the hole in his trunks.[32]

Offenders and Victims

On the basis of arrest records, it appears that exposure incidents occur most frequently in the spring (April through June), during daylight hours, and in public outdoor spaces. It happens less frequently during the winter (December through February), in the evening hours, and in private enclosed spaces.[34]

The age of onset of exhibitionistic behavior shows a bimodal distribution, peaking in the age ranges of 11 to 15 years old and 21 to 24 years old. The most frequent age at arrest, however, is in the mid-20s.[3] In one study a third of exhibitionists were from father-absent families.[3] Among exhibitionists age 21 years or over, 52 percent to 79 percent had been married at some time.[3,5,35] Although it has been observed that exhibitionists have childless marriages more frequently than members of the general population,[36] this may be an artifact of the young average age at apprehension.[3]

Efforts to describe the "typical" exhibitionist with psychological tests[37-39] or psychodynamic concepts,[40-42] though intellectually appealing, have not been shown to be useful in predicting recidivism or in selecting effective treatment. Arrested exhibitionists are not necessarily representative of all exhibitionists, and studies based on arrested men must be interpreted with this problem in mind.

SEXUALLY RELATED OFFENSES

An alternative to reviewing legal and mental health records is to survey a large sample of individuals about their victimization experiences.[9] A shortcoming of this approach is that it detects acts of indecent exposure by men who are not clinically diagnosable exhibitionists. Among college women sampled from the United States and Hong Kong, 57 percent and 56 percent, respectively, knew other women who had been victims of indecent exposure, and 33 percent and 35 percent had themselves been victims. Most of the victims reported being over age 10 years when first victimized, and their most distressing exposure incidents had been perpetrated by strangers (64 percent and 98 percent in the United States and Hong Kong, respectively). Although generally this is not reported to be a traumatic experience, 18 percent of each sample reported it to be "severely" or "very severely" distressing. Interestingly, there were very few differences between the reports of women from these two culturally divergent samples.[9]

This chapter focuses on the evaluation and disposition of the paraphiliac exhibitionist, for whom exposure is the preferred or exclusive means of achieving sexual gratification. Consequently, the following discussion of causes and treatment is not applicable to all individuals guilty of indecent exposure or open lewdness. Those whose actions are attributable solely to intoxication, brain damage, or schizophrenia, for example, would not be treatable with the techniques described here.

CAUSAL AND THERAPEUTIC THEORETICAL MODELS

This section briefly reviews the contemporary conceptualizations of exhibitionism according to psychodynamic, behavioral, and biological models. These various etiological models are not mutually exclusive but are expounded independently in order to highlight their unique features. Although treatments have been developed that are consonant with each model, it should be noted that effective treatments do not necessarily address underlying causes.

Psychodynamic Model

Freud viewed exhibitionism as normal childhood behavior. In adults, however, such activity is seen as indicating a fixation at an earlier period of development owing to a traumatic event. Psychoanalytic theory suggests that one such fixating, traumatic event may be the experience of castration anxiety which occurs during the oedipal stage of development.[43] The act of genital exposure and the victim's response serve to reassure the exhibitionist that he has in fact not been castrated, thereby decreasing his unconscious anxiety. The anxiety-reducing nature of the act enables the individual to continue to repress the oedipal urges and conflict.[44] More recent work by Gebhard et al[36] conceptualizes exhibitionism in a similar vein, finding that "some exhibition is largely an affirmation of masculinity, a cry of 'Look, here is proof I am a man!'"

Psychodynamic theorists suggest that what triggers the exhibitionism is not need for sexual contact, but rejection; a need to assert oneself in the social hierarchy; or failure in a male role activity. These events increase anxiety arising from repressed, underlying conflicts. This anxiety is displaced and acted out in a symbolic form—in this case, genital exhibition.

Exhibitionism is generally viewed as a neurotic condition. However, some authors, notably Allen,[45] consider exhibitionism to be a perversion with the fixation taking place at an early pre-verbal developmental stage. In either case, there is little direct empirical support for these theories beyond case reports. These case-treatment studies typically have involved psychoanalytic investigation of a single subject with the therapist reporting direct and interpretive observations and speculations.

The therapeutic model generated by psychodynamic theory centers around the uncovering of repressed psychic contents. Insight into the neurotic symptom (the exhibitionistic behavior) is believed to liberate the psychic energy associated with the repressed material, enabling the individual to strengthen his ego. Theoretically there is an accompanying reduction in anxiety and guilt, leading to a decrease in exposures.

Behavioral Model

Behavioral theorists conceptualize exhibitionism as a constellation of behaviors, each of which has been acquired according to the laws of learning. These behaviors are learned from the individual's interactions with his environment. Many theorists suggest that such learning can occur as the result of a single experience, a phenomenon known as single-trial learning. Roper[46] states the position as follows:

> Exhibitionism can also be looked upon as a maladaptive behavior according to principles of behavior therapy, using classical concepts of Hull and Pavlov. The aberrant form of sexual gratification can be seen to be the result of a fortuitous combination of environmental circumstances reacting upon personality factors which at the time are vulnerable. The subsequent gratification of the act causes reinforcement so that the pattern becomes consolidated.

As is the case with psychodynamic theory, there are single-subject investigations to support this theory.[46] However, other case studies[47] as well as clinical experience do not support this notion of single-trial learning.

McGuire, Carlisle, and Young[48] have proposed a more complex learning pattern. The initial deviant act, whether actual or fantasized, intended or accidental, serves as fantasy material for use during masturbation. These fantasies are repeatedly and powerfully reinforced by the subsequent orgasms. Thus, the "response strength" of exhibitionistic fantasies increases with each masturbatory act, and this behavior is then displayed in real-life situations.

This emphasis on internal (fantasy) events as influential in the learning process has been supported in a study conducted by Evans.[49] He investigated the masturbatory fantasies of 52 sexual deviants, including 10 exhibitionists, and found that 79 percent reported deviant fantasies. In a treatment study, Evans[49] reported that exhibitionists with deviant sexual fantasies required six times as many aversive conditioning sessions (median = 24 sessions) as did those with "normal" fantasies to achieve no exhibitionistic acts or urges. Evans[50] compared a group of successfully treated exhibitionists with treatment failures in aversive shock therapy. The treatment failures differed from those successfully treated on measures that would relate to response strength, for example, length of time since the onset of exhibitionistic behavior, frequency of behavior, and use of deviant fantasies during masturbation. The two groups did not differ on measures of demographic variables or of appropriate heterosexual activity. Rooth and Marks[51] also found an inverse relationship between treatment outcome and deviant fantasy activity. Ancillary supportive evidence comes from reports[52,53] indicating that exhibitionists who are successfully treated have a reduction of deviant fantasies as well as of deviant behavior.

Although covert rehearsal of exhibitionistic fantasies appears to play a role in the development and maintenance of overt deviant behavior, it is not well documented how the initial fantasy stimulus arises. McGuire and colleagues[48] state that early sexual experiences provide fantasy material. Working from a social learning perspective, Brownell[54] posits that older adults may serve as models for the child's view of sexual behavior. This point poses a thorny theoretical problem for behavioral etiological theories of exhibitionism.

Cox and Daitzman[55] combine theories proposed by others[46,48] in suggesting that "fortuitous conditions" lead to in vivo or imagined genital exposure which is reinforced immediately or which provides material for subsequent masturbatory activity. The reinforcing event may be in the form of orgasm, anxiety reduction, sense of power importance, or imagined sexual prowess secondary to the victim's shock. This model adheres to the essential behavioral paradigm wherein a behavior that is followed by a reinforcing event is strengthened and has a higher probability of recurring. Behavioral theories for the development and maintenance of exhibitionism are supported by the available empirical evidence and provide a more parsimonious explanation than psychodynamic formulations.

The therapeutic model generated by behavior theory uses learning principles to interrupt the learned chain of behaviors comprising the exhibitionistic act. A model describing the chain of behaviors (Fig. 16-1) has been proposed by Cox and Xavier.[56] In this model an external triggering stimulus is interpreted in a negative manner by the exhibitionist, leading to an emotionally aroused state. The individual, as a result of past learning experience, responds to this state by fantasizing exposure and the pleasurable (reinforcing) consequences of that act. This fantasy increases arousal, both psychologically and physiologically, and is followed by efforts to seek and to locate a victim. Fantasized rehearsals of the pending exposure and the immediate consequences often directly precede actual exposure. The exhibitionistic act is usually reinforced by heightened sexual arousal, subsequent orgasm, anxiety reduction, and a sense of potency. The nature of the triggering stimulus, the content of the fantasized rehearsal, and the type of likely consequences vary according to the exhibitionist's past history. Cox and Xavier[56] postulate that increased sexual arousal is accompanied by a reduction of critical judgment and self-control as the chain of events progresses. Behavioral interventions may be used at a number of critical decision points (see Figure 16-1) in the chain of events. These interventions are aimed at developing alternative coping strategies, reducing anxiety, and changing the perceived consequences of the exhibitionistic act.

Biological Theories

The history of biological theories of crime and of sexual deviation is replete with dogma, hope, and disproof. Enlargement of the prostate was once thought to cause exhibitionism, but this theory has been abandoned.[34] Each of the other biological abnormalities that has been suggested as a cause of exhibitionism has

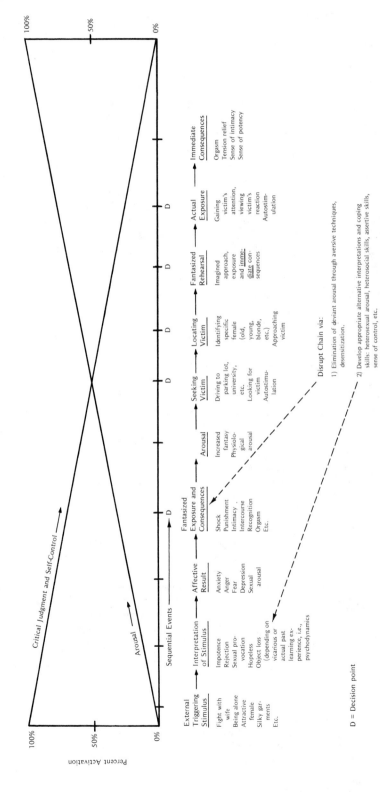

FIGURE 16-1 Shown here is a model of immediate sequential events leading to male genital exposure.

SEXUALLY RELATED OFFENSES

also been suggested as a cause of other criminal and sexual conduct. Abnormalities of brain function (temporal lobe electrical activity, limbic system dysfunction, cortical loss in dementia, and the long-abandoned concept of "degeneracy"), endocrine hormone production (particularly plasma testosterone) and heredity (notably the 47,XYY and 47,XXY chromosomal abnormalities and the "hereditary taint" hypothesis) have been proposed as explanations for exhibitionism. Each also has been proposed as an explanation for many other types of crime and sexual deviance (see the review by Shah and Roth[57]). None of these abnormalities has been shown to be characteristic of any significant proportion of exhibitionists. Nonetheless, as noted below, pharmacologic manipulation of hormone levels has proved useful in the treatment of exhibitionism and other paraphilias whether or not any biological abnormality has been detected in the individual being treated.

Sex offenders who receive comprehensive genetic, neurological, and endocrine evaluations always have appeared to have a higher incidence of abnormalities in these systems than has been assumed for men in general (see Krafft-Ebing[58] for a century-old collection of cases that suggests this phenomenon; and see Berlin and Coyle[59] for a smaller, recent collection for whom radically improved assessment technologies were available). This finding may, of course, be entirely a reflection of sampling and referral bias, or it may represent a true difference between these populations. Only truly random or representative samples of sex offenders subjected to careful evaluation will provide data that can differentiate these alternatives when compared with data from appropriate comparison groups. Although the incidence and role of biological abnormalities remain uncertain, the fact that biological systems are important determinants of many aspects of erotic behavior is indisputable. Thus, biological abnormalities are not prerequisite to biological treatment.

ASSESSMENT AND TREATMENT

This section devotes disproportionate attention to pharmacological treatment. This is not because we regard pharmacological treatment as more important or more effective. Rather, it is because there is no specific psychodynamic treatment for exhibitionism or other paraphilias, because behavioral treatments have been reviewed more exhaustively elsewhere[55,60,61] (also see chapter 13 in this volume), and because there is no other literature that specifically reviews pharmacological treatment of exhibitionism.

Psychodynamic Approach

Psychodynamically oriented writings have not reported specific pretreatment assessment procedures beyond the use of clinical interviews or formal psychoanalytic technique. Emphasis typically is placed on assessing general psychological functioning rather than on specific variables related to exhibitionistic behavior. Case reports[46,62] describing psychodynamically oriented treatment have suggested several variables that have been found to be associated with poor treatment outcome: neurologic damage, sociopathy, lack of alternative sexual outlets, psychosis, and denial of exhibitionistic behavior. These reports indicate that being legally remanded to treatment neither precludes nor guarantees a positive outcome.

Psychodynamically oriented therapy has been evaluated only in single or multiple case studies,[62-68] nearly all of which report positive treatment outcomes for small numbers of patients. Among the psychodynamic approaches that have been used are psychoanalysis, insight-oriented individual psychotherapy, group therapy, and hypnotherapy. However, psychodynamically oriented treatment is often lengthy. Mathis and Cullens[69] conducted insight-oriented group therapy in an outpatient setting; they treated 45 exhibitionists, of whom 13 terminated prematurely and 15 were still in treatment after 3 years.

Behavioral Approach

Outcome studies of behaviorally oriented treatment have identified a number of variables that may affect treatment. Evans[49,50] has emphasized the importance of investigating the individual's sexual fantasy life. Of particular importance is the type of masturbatory fantasy (especially whether the favorite fantasies are conventional or are about exposing), the frequency of masturbatory activity, and any deviant fantasy during sexual intercourse. It would appear that other measures of response strength, such as duration of the exhibiting behavior and rate of such acts per week for the previous 6 months, also need to be evaluated.

Brownell[54] recommends assessment of heterosexual fears and skills. Research has indicated that many individuals with sexual perversions have aversions to heterosexual practices.[70] Although this may not be the case with all exhibitionists, further investigation is warranted. Other reports[54,71] have indicated that inadequate or inappropriate heterosexual behavior could play an important role in maintenance of deviant behavior. In a similar vein, Cox and Xavier[56] have suggested assessment of alternative coping strategies for handling anxiety.

Specific treatment approaches often require specific assessment procedures. If hypnotherapy is to be considered, level of hypnotizability should be assessed before treatment is initiated.[46] Treatment of exhibitionists with either covert sensitization, assisted covert sensitization, or systematic desensitization requires the exhibitionist to "imagine scenes" as part of treatment. The individual's ability to imagine vividly lifelike events is critical and must therefore be evaluated.

Behavior therapies that have been documented to be successful in controlled studies generally involve the use of aversive stimuli. Aversive shock therapy (AST) involves the application of painful electric shock while fantasizing, viewing slides, or listening to audiotapes of exposure situations. AST is a well-documented treatment with exhibitionists who do not masturbate to fantasies of exposure.[49-51,53] Alternative approaches are recommended when the individual reports such deviant masturbation fantasies.

Covert sensitization uses imagined aversive events (nausea, vomiting, arrest, being seen in the act by one's family) coupled with imagined exhibitionistic behavior. Avoidance learning is also employed. In this technique imagined avoidance of exposure is paired with positive images and relief. The procedure for covert sensitization is well described, but the results, though positive, are not as well supported owing to the smaller number of individuals treated.[55,72]

Maletzky[52] developed assisted covert sensitization, in which the imagined aversive event paired with the imagined exposure is intensified by presenting a foul-smelling odor. In a summary of his work to date, Maletzky[73] reported on

155 patients treated with this technique, 62 of whom also received some other form of treatment. All the patients were followed for at least 1 year, and 135 had no reported exposures and no arrests for exposure. A few exhibitionists required booster sessions when exhibitionistic urges and fantasies returned following a particularly provocative stimulus.

Shame aversion therapy[74] requires the exhibitionist to expose himself to a mixed sex audience while the audience asks questions regarding his thoughts, feelings, and actions. In a similar procedure (aversive behavioral rehearsal) Wickramasekera[75] had exhibitionists rehearse their deviant activity while verbalizing their feelings to prevent dissociation. Reports of these interventions indicate uniformly positive outcomes, and the treatment is impressive for its brevity (typically one to five sessions) and for its minimal reliance on the individual's imagination or on elaborate equipment. However, because this can be an extremely unpleasant experience for the patient, many exhibitionists may refuse this procedure.

Although no controlled comparisons have been made, behavioral approaches using aversive stimuli as one component seem to be more effective, at least within a short time frame (12 to 18 months), than other behavioral approaches.[55] Clinical practice typically demands a multifaceted treatment to exhibitionism. Indeed, it is noteworthy that fewer than half the behavioral studies reviewed used solely aversive techniques. Hackett[76] advocates such a mulitfaceted approach, employing in vivo aversive conditioning and providing training in assertiveness and social skills.

The model proposed by Cox and Xavier[56] (see Figure 16-1) indicates where in the chain of behaviors comprising the exhibitionistic act various types of intervention may be applied. The techniques selected, from those with documented efficacy, will depend on characteristics of patients, therapists, and treatment settings. Based on the available literature, successful behavioral treatment employs an aversive conditioning element. Adjunctive psychotherapy, social skills training, or marital therapy may be necessary to deal with other deficits or particular stressors that precipitate the deviant acts.

Biological Approach

The best procedure for the physiological evaluation of male sexual arousal is direct measurement of penile tumescence under baseline and stimulus conditions. This is accomplished in a laboratory using a device designed to measure penis circumference or volume and to provide a continuous record of these measurements. Exhibitionists show increased penile blood volume responses (PBVRs) to their preferred stimuli.[53] Phallometry, as this technique is known, can be used to distinguish reliably between heterosexual arousal and exhibitionism.[77] In his review of psychophysiological assessment in sexual functioning, Geer[78] finds that PBVRs do an acceptable job of discriminating among individuals with different sexual object preferences. However, a number of difficulties have also been reported with these assessments. Bancroft[79] notes that PBVRs do not necessarily reflect behavior and that such responses can be elicited by fantasy alone. Moreover, approximately 35 percent of exhibitionists do not demonstrate penile erection during exposure, and a few men can voluntarily inhibit a penile response during evaluation sessions.[51,80,81] Thus, PBVRs should be used cautiously to assess and to predict exhibitionistic behavior.

Phallometric assessment of erotic responsiveness is currently available in only a limited number of research and clinical settings. The large number of phallometric studies has been comprehensively reviewed by Langevin.[61] Detailed information on the instrumentation and use of a phallometric laboratory is also available.[82,83]

No biological assessment procedure is essential on a routine basis. In the absence of other clinical indications, physical examination, electroencephalography, brain-imaging techniques, and hormone assays each have rather limited usefulness in the area of our concern; they also result in a certain number of false-positive findings. The exhibitionist under consideration for the drug treatments described below should certainly have a physical examination (with special attention to signs of tardive dyskinesia if any neuroleptic—that is, antipsychotic—drug is being considered and to ophthalmologic examination if thioridazine—a particular neuroleptic drug—is being considered); assays of serum testosterone, luteinizing hormone, and follicle-stimulating hormone; and liver function tests. If drug treatment is undertaken, these blood tests should be repeated periodically.

No pharmacologic treatment is approved by the United States Food and Drug Administration (FDA) specifically for the treatment of exhibitionism. This lack of endorsement does not bar licensed and qualified physicians from prescribing or administering particular drugs for the treatment of exhibitionism. The decision to use a drug for an unapproved purpose must, however, be based on informed and reasonable professional judgment; it should also reflect a careful balancing of benefits against risks. Appropriate informed consent by the patient is ethically and legally necessary. (For commentary on relevant US law, see Kessler,[84] McEniry and Willig,[85] and Shapiro.[86])

Two classes of drugs have been used in the treatment of paraphiliac sex offenders, including exhibitionists, in recent years: neuroleptics and antiandrogens. However, none of the drugs in either class has received FDA approval for this particular use. In Europe and Canada these drugs have largely replaced the use of estrogens, surgical castration, and neurosurgical procedures in the treatment of paraphiliac sex offenders.

NEUROLEPTIC MEDICATIONS

Antipsychotic medications have been used to treat concurrent psychotic illnesses among sex offenders and, based on their inhibitory effect on the pituitary-gonadal system, have sometimes been used to treat paraphiliac sex offenders who do not have a concurrent psychosis.

Given the risk of tardive dyskinesia with long-term administration of neuroleptics, one would probably not prescribe them for an exhibitionist with no other indication for such a drug. Other things being equal, however, thioridazine might be regarded as the preferred neuroleptic for schizophrenic patients (or others requiring neuroleptics) who are also exhibitionists.

Benperidol

This neuroleptic medication is chemically related to haloperidol, but it is not available in the United States. Both uncontrolled[87] and controlled[88,89] studies have suggested promising behavioral effects, though the effects on the relevant hormones are much weaker than those of antiandrogens.[88]

Thioridazine

Of all the widely used neuroleptic drugs, thioridazine has the most pronounced inhibitory effect on the pituitary-gonadal system, resulting in the greatest lowering of testosterone and luteinizing hormone (LH)[90] and a higher incidence of difficulties in developing and maintaining an erection.[91]

Kamm[92] reported a lessening of sexual preoccupation with thioridazine, but not with other neuroleptics, in a 19-year-old woman who had a diagnosis of organic brain syndrome and who frequently exposed herself to men. Thioridazine is occasionally mentioned[93] as having "been suggested" for the treatment of exhibitionism and other paraphilias and is sometimes discussed among clinicians as a treatment possibility in such cases. Thioridazine has been used to decrease the likelihood of exposure among high-risk patients in the early weeks of behavioral treatments.[73] No controlled clinical trials with exhibitionists have been reported.

ANTIANDROGENS

Antiandrogens are substances that significantly reduce the physiological effects of androgens (male sex hormones), particularly testosterone. Thus, the term "antiandrogen" refers to a class of substances defined by their biological effects rather than by their chemistry. By convention, the term is used to refer to drugs chemically related to hormones. Naturally occurring hormones, a few of which have antiandrogenic effects, are not conventionally referred to as antiandrogens.

Antiandrogens are used in conjunction with other behavioral or psychotherapeutic treatments. The medication affects the patient's deviant behavior only while an effective level of the drug is maintained. Thus, other treatments are essential to achieve the desired long-term changes in deviant behavior. Two antiandrogens—medroxyprogesterone acetate and cyproterone acetate—have promise for the treatment of exhibitionism and other paraphilias.

Medroxyprogesterone Acetate

None of the clinical trials of medroxyprogesterone acetate reported to date is based on an experimental design that meets current standards for clinical drug trials. The standard technique for evaluating drug effectiveness is the randomized clinical trial,[94] in which patients are randomly allocated to two or more treatment groups. Randomized designs allow an experimental drug to be compared with placebo (a biologically inert substance) or with a standard treatment. Ideally, neither the patient nor those evaluating his response to treatment know which treatment group he is in. Techniques have been developed for obtaining patients' consent to participate in experiments while preserving randomization and blind conditions.[95,96] When both patient and evaluator are "blind" to the treatment the patient is receiving, the study design is referred to as a "double-blind trial." Randomized double-blind trials have not been conducted with medroxyprogesterone acetate.

Approved by the FDA for use in treating certain gynecologic diseases and marketed as a contraceptive in at least 76 countries,[97] medroxyprogesterone acetate is approved by the FDA neither as a contraceptive nor for the treatment of sexual deviations. The drug is a synthetic steroid manufactured by the Upjohn Company in an oral form (Provera) and in a long-acting injectable form

(Depo-Provera). It decreases testicular production of testosterone and usually prevents compensatory increases in luteinizing and follicle-stimulating hormones.[59,98,99] Administered to adult males in long-acting injections at a dose of 200 to 500 mg every 7 to 10 days, it produces reductions in plasma testosterone, erotic imagery, frequency of erections, and frequency of erotic activity. All these effects are reversible when treatment is stopped. The 100 mg per ml concentration is less painful than the 400 mg per ml concentration; no more than 250 mg should be injected at a single site.[98,100] The dosage for each patient requires adjustment to a level that achieves the desired clinical effects (reduced sexual drive or libido) without causing total impotence. It has been claimed that a few patients undergo a "psychic realignment" to more socially acceptable erotic imagery as a concomitant of counseling during their medication-induced "vacation from sex drive,"[101] but most patients who discontinue medication relapse.[100]

Weight gain, mild lethargy, and hypertension are commonly reported with medroxyprogesterone acetate, but the effect that causes greatest concern is decreased sperm production which, although initially reversible, might result in infertility in light of reports of progressive testicular atrophy during prolonged treatment. A number of other side effects have been reported among the legions of women who have taken the drug, but their frequency in men is unknown.

Medroxyprogesterone acetate was first used in the treatment of a sex offender in 1966.[101-103] One of the first patients treated was an exhibitionist with an extensive police record who was exposing himself as often as 10 times daily; he rapidly stopped exposing himself, although some obsessive sexual ideation continued after 7 months of treatment.[103] Another man with a history of shoplifting and exposing himself in a department store stopped doing both during treatment but relapsed when he dropped out of treatment for three weeks.[101] Other exhibitionists are included among those for whom successful treatment has been reported, but the reporting of aggregate data and the fact that some cases are reported in more than one of the papers from Johns Hopkins[59,98-104] preclude an accurate count of the number of exhibitionists treated or calculation of their success ratio. The report by Berlin and Meinecke[98] tabulates data on four heterosexual exhibitionists with pretreatment rates of exposure (by self-report and institutional records) ranging from twice weekly to five times daily. During medroxyprogesterone acetate treatment spanning 10 to 27 months, there were no known episodes of exposure; three dropped out of treatment, and each of them relapsed. In the same series, a homosexual pedophile exhibitionist who probably engaged in several incidents per year had no known incidents during 3 years, 9 months of treatment.

Cyproterone Acetate

This medication is not available in the United States. Cyproterone acetate's endocrinologic effects were first reported on the basis of animal tests.[105] The drug competes with testosterone at peripheral target organ sites, blocks hypothalamic androgen receptors, and has a nonspecific progestogenic effect by which LH secretion is inhibited, resulting in a decrease in serum testosterone. Treatment of men at a dose of 50 to 250 mg orally per day produces rapid reduction in libido and potency and arrest of sperm production. When treatment is stopped, libido, potency, and sperm production recover rapidly.

Double-blind comparisons between cyproterone acetate and either placebo or other drugs have shown that cyproterone acetate results in reductions of serum testosterone and luteinizing hormone,[88] reported erotic arousal and activity,[106] and measured erotic arousal to favorite stimuli.[107] Testicular biopsies have shown minimal testicular damage.[108] Other undesired effects have been reported, including slight gynecomastia (increased breast tissue)[109] and loss of energy.[110] No irreversible adverse effects have been reported.

Documentation of successful treatment of exhibitionists with cyproterone acetate is limited to case reports[111] and to reports based on the treatment of groups of sex offenders or groups of men with paraphilias for whom only aggregate data are presented.[112] Davies[109] reported that a small (but unspecified) number of men with a history of repeated indecent exposure committed no known offenses during 6 months to 3 years of treatment with cyproterone acetate. In a review of seven studies from six countries, Ortmann[113] reported a remarkable decrease in detected recidivism rates among mixed groups of sex offenders treated with cyproterone acetate.

CRIMINAL SANCTIONS AND DISPOSITIONS

The clinical material in this chapter has concerned the paraphiliac exhibitionist, whose mental disorder is evident primarily by his repeated exposure. In considering criminal sanctions and dispositions, it is essential to recognize that men who are not exhibitionists also expose themselves. Dietz[114] has distinguished between preferential sex offenders (such as exhibitionists) and situational sex offenders (such as the nonexhibitionist who exposes himself as a prank or while under severe marital stress, intoxicated, or psychotic). The preferential exposer has a diagnosable mental disorder (exhibitionism) that may be treated with the methods described above. The situational exposer may or may not have a treatable disorder (such as alcoholism or organic brain syndrome). To the extent that sentencing is individualized or rehabilitation sought, this distinction becomes critical.

By all accounts, the vast majority of indecent exposure and open lewdness offenders receive noncustodial sentences, though laws in every state provide for periods of incarceration for these and cognate offenses. In this section we consider the statutory penalties for these offenses, the operation of sexual psychopath statutes, the insanity defense for exhibitionists, and mechanisms for providing treatment to exhibitionists who have been convicted for unlawful exposure.

Statutory Penalties

Prior to the Model Penal Code,* statutes dealing with "indecent exposure," "public lewdness," "lewd and lascivious behavior," and other variations on this theme most often classified the offense as a misdemeanor carrying a maximum

---

* The factual material in this and the following paragraph derives from the encyclopedic commentaries on the Model Penal Code prepared by Professors Peter Low and John Calvin Jeffries, Jr.[115]

term of 3 months, 6 months, or 1 year. A few statutes provided for imprisonment for as long as 10 years. The narrower provisions of the Model Code limit the offense of indecent exposure to displays intended to arouse or to gratify erotic desire, while retaining a broader offense of open lewdness that encompasses displays lacking such erotic intent. Exposure by an exhibitionist would usually constitute indecent exposure, but exposure by a prankster would usually constitute open lewdness.

In the Model Code, indecent exposure is graded as a misdemeanor, ordinarily carrying a maximum term of 1 year; open lewdness is graded as a petty misdemeanor, ordinarily carrying a maximum term of 30 days imprisonment. Statutes revised in light of the Model Code carry maximum penalties of 10 days to 2 years for indecent exposure and of 6 months to 1 year for open lewdness. Although the drafters of the Model Code provided harsher penalties for indecent exposure than for open lewdness, Pennsylvania is the only state that took this approach among the 16 states that revised their statutes dealing with both offenses between 1962 and 1980. Two states (Arizona and Wisconsin) enacted revisions that provide for harsher penalties for open lewdness than for indecent exposure, and the remaining 13 states provide for equal sanctions.

Sexual Psychopath Statutes

As of this writing, fewer than 19 states and the District of Columbia have special statutory provisions under which certain persons charged with or convicted of sex offenses (in some states limited to particular offenses) may be adjudicated as "sexually dangerous," "sexual psychopaths," or similarly worded provisions. The precise triggering conditions, commitment criteria, and procedures for commitment and discharge vary among jurisdictions.[116,117] Repeal of these statutes has been recommended by the Group for the Advancement of Psychiatry[118] and by the American Bar Association.[117] The process of repeal is underway in the state legislatures: Seven states repealed such statutes between 1978 and 1980.[119] Since then additional states have either repealed or modified their statutes.[117]

Many of the remaining sexual psychopath statutes allow for anyone convicted of a sex offense to be considered for possible disposition as a sexual psychopath. A few (for example, Massachusetts and Washington) even specify indecent exposure or lewdness as one of the predicate sex offenses (see Favole's statutory compendium[120]). In the two cases in which it has had occasion to consider the issue, the United States Supreme Court has recognized the necessity of due process hearings in the commitment of persons as sexual psychopaths.[121,122]

One of the key factual issues to be addressed at such hearings is whether the individual poses a danger to others. In the case of persons whose sole sex offense has been an exposure, the inquiry should begin with a determination as to whether the individual is a preferential sex offender. If he is not, that is, if his exposure was situational, sexual psychopath proceedings against him should be abandoned. If he is a preferential sex offender, the issue of the type of danger he poses becomes critical. Some exhibitionists have other paraphilias as well (for example, pedophilia or sexual sadism) and may pose a risk of physical harm to others on this basis. Ordinarily, however, the only risk posed by an exhibitionist is that of repeated exposures.

The probability that an untreated exhibitionist will expose himself in the future is extremely high; whether this should be construed as "dangerous" is a separate and debatable issue. Based on his review of case law, Dix[116] concludes that "[g]enerally it seems clear that most statutory criteria do not require physical harm." The California Court of Appeals in 1964 upheld the finding that an exhibitionist who exposed himself to young girls was within the meaning of a mentally disordered sex offender statute requiring that the defendant be shown to be a "menace to the health or safety of others."[123]

In the District of Columbia, 16 of 31 persons committed to St. Elizabeths Hospital as sexual psychopaths from July 1, 1961, through October 30, 1968, had committed an exposure offense.[124] In reviewing a challenge to one such commitment, the District of Columbia Circuit Court of Appeals[125] noted:

> The unanimous testimony of all the expert witnesses that serious psychological harm would result from public exposure only to unusually sensitive adult women and small children leads us to conclude that the future sexual misconduct of the appellant, if any, is not sufficiently likely to cause the sort of harm required by the statute to justify further commitment.

The dangerousness of exhibitionists was further explored by the same court the following year,[126] but the waters were left even more muddy when Chief Judge Bazelon construed the **type** of harm anticipated to be an element of both the **likelihood** of harm and the **magnitude** of harm inquiries.

The Insanity Defense

Some of the most patently unjust outcomes have occurred when exhibitionists charged with indecent exposure have been found not guilty by reason of insanity. One such man was "confined in St. Elizabeths Hospital for more than 4 years" even though the "criminal penalty for conviction of that charge was a 90-day-to-one-year prison term." Moreover, the appellate court found that that "appellant's testimony casts doubt on whether he is receiving any treatment."[127]

An insanity defense would rarely be in the interests of one charged with indecent exposure or lewdness. A defendant facing the prospect of indefinite commitment as a sexual psychopath would be one of the few for whom an insanity acquittal might be preferable, particularly in jurisdictions in which insanity acquittees are accorded better treatment than sexual psychopaths. If the defendant suffers from a psychotic disorder, an insanity defense might be viable in jurisdictions with either a M'Naghten or an American Law Institute (ALI) test of insanity (see chapter 8). If the defendant's sole mental disorder is exhibitionism, a defense of insanity would have to be based on the volitional prong of ALI or on an irresistible impulse test. Although a few commentators have implied that exhibitionists and other paraphiliac offenders have an impaired ability to control their conduct,[59,98,128] others have suggested that paraphiliac persons, though unable to control their cravings, are as able as anyone else to control their conduct (that is, whether, how, and when they act on their cravings).[114]

Providing Treatment to the Convicted Exhibitionist

The proportion of men convicted of unlawful exposure who also commit a violent offense or sexually molest children is higher than that for men in the general population, but the vast majority of exhibitionists are never convicted of other offenses against persons.[129,130] Partly in recognition of this fact, exhibitionists are often placed on probation.

If the sentencing court wishes to insure that the exhibitionist will receive treatment, it is necessary to require treatment as a condition of probation and to provide some mechanism by which the court will be notified if the probationer does not participate in the treatment. Exhibitionists, like other sexual offenders, often have little desire to abandon their deviant behavior, which they find gratifying apart from the occasional legal complications. Many participate in treatment only to prevent imprisonment and drop out at the first opportunity.

We regard behavior therapy with an aversive component as the treatment of choice for exhibitionism, and we consider antiandrogens plus psychotherapy to be suitable as a supplement or alternative to behavior therapy. We do not, however, believe that courts should prescribe treatment. Rather, courts should use their influence with the legislature and with mental health care providers to encourage the development of appropriate treatment programs for prisoners, probationers, and parolees. In our view, the decision as to whether the potential benefits of a particular treatment outweigh its risks should be left to the patient when the only risk of harm to others is a likelihood of exposure incidents.

A few commentators (for example, Halleck[131]) have questioned whether an offender can provide competent, informed, and truly voluntary consent to antiandrogen treatment while facing the alternative of incarceration or the threat of incarceration. In the case of exhibitionists, we think this can be handled by making treatment a condition of probation but leaving the choice of treatment to the patient and his therapist.

REFERENCES

1. CHRISTOFFEL, H: *Male genital exhibitionism.* In LORAND, S AND BALINT, M: *Perversions: Psychodynamics and Therapy.* Gramercy, New York, 1956, pp 243-264.

2. LASÉQUE, EC: *Les exhibitionnistes.* Union Méd (Paris), Series 3:23:709, 1877.

3. MOHR, JW, TURNER, RE, JERRY, MB: *Pedophilia and Exhibitionism: A Handbook.* University of Toronto Press, Toronto, 1964.

4. SMUKLER, AJ AND SCHIEBEL, D: *Personality characteristics of exhibitionists.* Dis Nerv Sys 36:600, 1975.

5. CAMBRIDGE DEPARTMENT OF CRIMINAL SCIENCE: *Sexual Offences.* Macmillan, London, 1957.

6. FRISBIE, LV: *Recidivism among treated sex offenders: A study of 1921 male discharges from a California state hospital.* Department of Mental Hygiene, Research Division, Sacramento, 1963.

7. BANCROFT, H: *Behavioral treatment of sexual deviations.* In LEITENBERG, H (ED): *Handbook of Behavior Modification and Behavior Therapy.* Prentice-Hall, New York, 1976.

8. GITTLESON, NL, EACOTT, SE, MEHTA, BM: *Victims of indecent exposure.* Br J Psychiat 132:61, 1978.

9. COX, DJ, TSANG, K, LEE, A: *A cross-cultural comparison of the incidence and nature of male exhibitionism among female college students.* Victimology 7:231, 1982.

10. HERMANN, K AND SCHRODER, GE: *Un cas d'exhibitionisme chez une femme.* Acta Psychiatr Neurol Scand 10:547, 1935.

11. ZAVITZIANOS, G: *Fetishism and exhibitionism in the female and their relationship to psychopathy and kleptomania.* Int J Psychoanal 52:297, 1971.

12. HOLLENDER, MH, BROWN, CW, ROBACK, HB: *Genital exhibitionism in women.* Am J Psychiatry 134:436, 1977.

13. SCHNEIDER, RD: *Exhibitionism: An exclusively male deviation?* Int J Offender Ther Comp Criminol 26:173, 1982.

14. AMERICAN PSYCHIATRIC ASSOCIATION: *Diagnostic and Statistical Manual of Mental Disorders,* ed 3. American Psychiatric Association, Washington, DC, 1980, p 272.

15. BLACKSTONE, W: *Commentaries on the Laws of England, Vol. 4.* Clarendon Press, Oxford, 1769, p 64.

16. Reg. v. Watson, 2 Cox Cr. Cases 376 (Q.B. 1847).

17. Reg. v Webb, 1 Den. 345, 169 Eng. Rep. 271 (Q.B. 1848).

18. Reg. v. Holmes, 6 Cox Cr. Cases 216 (C.C.A. 1852).

19. POWER, DJ: *Sexual deviation and crime.* Med Sci Law 16:111, 1976.

20. SMITH, SR: *Legal stand toward exhibitionism.* In COX, DJ AND DAITZMAN, RJ (EDS): *Exhibitionism: Description, Assessment, and Treatment.* Garland Press, New York, 1980, pp 11-38.

21. N.Y. Penal Law § 245.00 (McKinney 1980).

22. People v. Gilbert, 72 Misc. 2d 75, 338 N.Y.S. 2d 457 (1972).

23. People v. Hardy, 77 Misc. 2d 1092, 357 N.Y.S. 2d 970 (1974).

24. People v. Ventrice, 96 Misc. 2d 282, 408 N.Y.S. 2d 990 (1978).

25. N.Y. Penal Law § 245.01 (McKinney 1980).

26. N.Y. Penal Law § 245.01 (McKinney Supp. 1983).

27. AMERICAN LAW INSTITUTE: *Model Penal Code: Proposed Official Draft* (changes and editorial corrections in May 4, 1962). American Law Institute, Philadelphia, 1962.

28. 18 Pa. Cons. Stat. Ann. § 3127 (Purdon 1983).

29. 18 Pa. Cons. Stat. Ann. § 5901 (Purdon 1983).

30. Com. v. Back, 389 A.2d 141, 255 Pa. Super. 603 (1978).

31. Com. v. Rodriguez, 442 A.2d 803, 296 Pa. Super. 349 (1982).

32. Com. v. Botzum, 302 A.2d 381, 225 Pa. Super. 268 (1973).

33. Com. v. Gonzales, 396 A.2d 428, 261 Pa. Super. 339 (1978).

34. MACDONALD, JM: *Indecent Exposure.* Charles C Thomas, Springfield, IL, 1973.

35. ARIEFF, AJ AND ROTMAN, DB: *One hundred cases of indecent exposure.* J Nerv Ment Dis 96:523, 1942.

36. GEBHARD, PH, GAGNON, JH, POMEROY, WB, CHRISTENSON, CV: *Sex Offenders: An Analysis of Types.* Harper & Row, New York, 1965.

37. McCREARY, C: *Personality profiles of persons convicted of indecent exposure.* J Clin Psychol 31:260, 1975.

38. RADAR, CM: *MMPI profile types of exposers, rapists, and assaulters in a court services population.* J Consult Clin Psychol 45:61, 1977.

39. SINGER, BA: *Defensiveness in exhibitionists.* J Personality Assessment 43:526, 1979.

40. GLASSER, M: *The role of the superego in exhibitionism.* Int J Psychoanal Psychother 7:333, 1978.

41. ROSEN, I: *Exhibitionism, scopophilia and voyeurism.* In ROSEN, I (ED): *Sexual Deviation,* ed 2. Oxford University Press, Oxford, 1979, pp 139-194.

42. FORGAC, GE AND MICHAELS, EJ: *Personality characteristics of two types of male exhibitionists.* J Abnorm Psychology 91:287, 1982.

43. GREENACRE, P: *Perversions: General considerations regarding their genetic and dynamic background.* Psychoanalytic Study Child 23:47, 1968.

44. FENICHEL, O: *The Psychoanalytic Theory of Neurosis.* Norton, New York, 1945.

45. ALLEN, DW: *A psychoanalytic view. In* Cox, DJ AND DAITZMAN, RJ (EDS): *Exhibitionism: Description, Assessment, and Treatment.* Garland Press, New York, 1980, pp 59-82.

46. ROPER, P: *The use of hypnosis in the treatment of exhibitionism.* Canad Med Assn J 94:72, 1966.

47. GOLDBERG, A: *A fresh look at perverse behavior.* Int J Psychoanal 56:335, 1975.

48. McGUIRE, RJ, CARLISLE, JM, YOUNG, BG: *Sexual deviations as conditioned behaviour: A hypothesis.* Behav Res Ther 2:185, 1965.

49. EVANS, DR: *Masturbatory fantasy and sexual deviations.* Behav Res Ther 6:17, 1968.

50. EVANS, DR: *Subjective variables and treatment effects in aversion therapy.* Behav Res Ther 8:147, 1970.

51. ROOTH, FG AND MARKS, IM: *Persistent exhibitionism: Short-term response to aversion, self-regulation, and relaxation treatments.* Arch Sex Behav 3:227, 1974.

52. MALETZKY, BM: *"Assisted" covert sensitization in the treatment of exhibitionism.* J Consul Clin Psychol 42:34, 1974.

53. ABEL, GG, LEVIS, DJ, CLANCY, J: *Aversion therapy applied to taped sequences of deviant behavior in exhibitionism and other sexual deviations: A preliminary report.* J Behav Ther Exp Psychiatry 1:59, 1970.

54. BROWNELL, KD: *Multifaceted behavior therapy. In* Cox, DJ AND DAITZMAN, RJ (EDS): *Exhibitionism: Description, Assessment, and Treatment.* Garland Press, New York, 1980, pp 151-186.

55. COX, DJ AND DAITZMAN, RJ: *Behavioral theory, research, and treatment of male exhibitionism.* Prog Behav Modification 7:63, 1979.

56. COX, DJ AND XAVIER, NS: Behavioral treatment of male exhibitionism: A review. Unpublished material, 1978.

57. SHAH, SA AND ROTH, LH: *Biological and psychophysiological factors in criminality. In* GLASER, D (ED): *Handbook of Criminology.* Rand McNally, Chicago, 1974, pp 101-173.

58. KRAFFT-EBING, R von (WEDECK, HE, TRANS): *Psychopathia Sexualis: A Medico-Forensic Study.* GP Putnam's Sons, New York, 1965.

59. BERLIN, FS AND COYLE, GS: *Sexual deviation syndromes.* Johns Hopkins Med J 149:119, 1981.

60. COX, DJ AND DAITZMAN, RJ (EDS): *Exhibitionism: Description, Assessment, and Treatment.* Garland Press, New York, 1980.

61. LANGEVIN, R: *Sexual Strands: Understanding and Treating Sexual Anomalies in Men.* Lawrence Erlbaum Associates, Hillsdale, NJ, 1983.

62. WITZIG, JS: *The group treatment of male exhibitionists.* Am J Psychiatry 125:179, 1968.

63. RICKLES, NK: *Exhibitionism.* JB Lippincott, Philadelphia, 1950.

64. MUTTER, CB: I. *A hypnotherapeutic approach to exhibitionism: Outpatient therapeutic strategy.* J Forensic Sci 26:129, 1981.

65. ZECHNICH, R: *Exhibitionism: Genesis, dynamics and treatment.* Psychiatr Q 45:70, 1971.

66. BOSS, M (ABELL, LL, TRANS): *Meaning and Content of Sexual Perversions: A Dasein-analytic Approach to the Psychopathology of the Phenomenon of Love.* Grune & Stratton, New York, 1949, pp 71-79.

67. LONDON, LS AND CAPRIO, FS: *Sexual Deviations.* Linacre Press, Washington, DC, 1950, pp 295-360.

68. SPERLING, M: *The analysis of an exhibitionist.* Int J Psychoanal 28:32, 1947.

69. MATHIS, JL AND CULLENS, M: *Enforced group treatment of exhibitionists.* In MASSERMAN JH (ED): *Current Psychiatric Therapies, Vol II-1971.* Grune & Stratton, New York, 1971, pp 139-145.

70. RAMSEY, RW AND VAN VELZEN, V: *Behavior therapy for sexual perversions.* Behav Res Ther 6:17, 1968.

71. ANNON, JS: *The extension of learning principles to the analysis and treatment of sexual problems.* Dissertation Abstr Int 32(6-B):3627, 1971.

72. BROWNELL, KD, HAYNES, SC, BARLOW, DH: *Patterns of appropriate and deviant sexual arousal: The behavioral treatment of multiple sexual deviations.* J Cons Clin Psychol 45:1144, 1977.

73. MALETZKY, BM: *Assisted covert sensitization.* In COX, DJ AND DAITZMAN, RJ (EDS): *Exhibitionism: Description, Assessment, and Treatment.* Garland Press, New York, 1980, pp 187-251.

74. SERBER, M: *Shame aversion therapy.* J Behav Ther Exp Psychiatry 1:213, 1970.

75. WICKRAMASEKERA, I: *A technique for controlling a certain type of sexual exhibitionism.* Psychotherapy: Theory, Res and Prac 9:207, 1972.

76. HACKETT, TP: *The psychotherapy of exhibitionists in a court clinic setting.* Sem Psychiatry 3:297, 1971.

77. LANGEVIN, R, PAITICH, D, RAMSAY, G, ANDERSON, C, KAMRAD, J, POPE, S, GELLER, G, PEARL, L, NEWMAN, S: *Experimental studies of the etiology of genital exhibitionism.* Arch Sex Behav 8:307, 1979.

78. GEER, JH: *Sexual functioning: Some data and speculations on psychophysiological assessment.* In CONE, JD AND HAWKINS, RP (EDS): *Behavioral Assessment.* Brunner/Mazel, New York, 1977, pp 196-209.

79. BANCROFT, J: *Deviant Sexual Behaviour: Modification and Assessment.* Clarendon Press, Oxford, 1974.

80. LAWS, DR AND RUBIN, HH: *Instructional control of an autonomic sexual response.* J Appl Behav Analysis 2:93, 1969.

81. ROSEN, RC: *Genital blood flow measurement: Feedback applications in sexual therapy.* J Sex Marital Ther 2:184, 1976.

82. EARLS, CM AND MARSHALL, WL: *The current state of technology in the laboratory assessment of sexual arousal patterns.* In GREER, JG AND STUART, IR (EDS): *The Sexual Aggressor: Current Perspectives on Treatment.* Van Nostrand Reinhold, New York, 1983, pp 336-362.

83. LAWS, DR AND OSBORN, CA: *How to build and operate a behavioral laboratory to evaluate and treat sexual deviance.* In GREER, JG AND STUART, IR (EDS): *The Sexual Aggressor: Current Perspectives on Treatment.* Van Nostrand Reinhold, New York, 1983, pp 293-335.

84. KESSLER, DA: *Regulating the prescribing of human drugs for nonapproved uses under the Food, Drug, and Cosmetic Act.* Harvard Journal of Legislation 15:693, 1978.

85. MCENIRY, MA AND WILLIG, SH: *The Federal Food, Drug, and Cosmetic Act and the medical practitioner.* Food Drug Cosm Law J 29:548, 1974.

86. SHAPIRO, SA: *Limiting physician freedom to prescribe a drug for any purpose: The need for FDA regulation.* Northwestern University Law Review 73:801, 1978.

87. FIELD, LH: *Benperidol in the treatment of sexual offenders.* Med Sci Law 13:195, 1973.

88. MURRAY, MAF, BANCROFT, JHJ, ANDERSON, DC, TENNENT, TG, CARR, PJ: *Endocrine changes in male sexual deviants after treatment with anti-androgens, oestrogens or tranquilizers.* J Endocrin 67:179, 1975.

89. TENNENT, TG, BANCROFT, JHJ, CASS, J: *The control of deviant sexual behavior by drugs: A double blind controlled study of benperidol, chlorpromazine, and placebo.* Arch Sexual Behav 3:261, 1974.

90. Brown, WA, Laughren, TP, Williams, B: *Differential effects of neuroleptic agents on the pituitary-gonadal axis in men.* Arch Gen Psychiatry 38:1270, 1981.

91. Kotin, J, Wilbert, DE, Verburg D, Soldinger, SM: *Thioridazine and sexual dysfunction.* Am J Psychiatry 133:82, 1976.

92. Kamm, I: *Control of sexual hyperactivity with thioridazine.* Am J Psychiatry 121:922, 1965.

93. Bastani, JB: *Treatment of genital exhibitionism.* Compr Psychiatry 17:769, 1976.

94. Byar, DP, Simon, RM, Friedewald, WT, et al: *Randomized clinical trials: Perspectives on some recent ideas.* New Engl J Med 295:74, 1976.

95. Zellen, M: *A new design for randomized clinical trials.* New Engl J Med 300:1242, 1979.

96. Schafer, A: *The ethics of the randomized clinical trial.* New Engl J Med 307:719, 1982.

97. Rosenfield, A, Maine, D, Rochat, R, Shelton, J, Hatcher, RA: *The Food and Drug Administration and medroxyprogesterone acetate: What are the issues?* JAMA 249:2922, 1983.

98. Berlin, FS and Meinecke, CF: *Treatment of sex offenders with antiandrogenic medication: Conceptualization, review of treatment modalities, and preliminary findings.* Am J Psychiatry 138:601, 1981.

99. Meyer, WJ III, Walker, PA, Wiedeking, C, Money, J, Kowarski, AA, Migeon, CJ, Borgaonkar, DS: *Pituitary function in adult males receiving medroxyprogesterone acetate.* Fertil Steril 28:1072, 1977.

100. Berlin, FS: *Sex offenders: A biomedical perspective and a status report on biomedical treatment.* In Greer, JG and Stuart, IR (eds): *The Sexual Aggressor: Current Perspectives on Treatment.* Van Nostrand Reinhold, New York, 1983, pp 83-123.

101. Money, J, Wiedeking, C, Walker, P, Migeon, C, Meyer, W, Borgaonkar, D: *47,XYY and 46,XY males with antisocial and/or sex-offending behavior: Antiandrogen therapy plus counseling.* Psychoneuroendocrin 1:165, 1975.

102. Money, J: *Discussion of Chapter 9.* In Michael, RP (ed): *Endocrinology and Human Behaviour.* Oxford University Press, London, 1968, p 169.

103. Money, J: *Use of an androgen-depleting hormone in the treatment of male sex offenders.* J Sex Res 6:165, 1970.

104. Blumer, D and Migeon, C: *Hormone and hormonal agents in the treatment of aggression.* J Nerv Ment Dis 160:127, 1975.

105. Hamada, H, Neumann, F, Junkmann, K: *Intrauterine antimasculine Beeinflussing von Rattenfeten ein stark gestagen wirksames Steroid.* Acta Endocrin 44:380, 1963.

106. Cooper, AJ: *A placebo-controlled trial of the antiandrogen cyproterone acetate in deviant hypersexuality.* Compr Psychiatry 22:458, 1981.

107. Bancroft, J, Tennent, G, Loucas, K, Cass, J: *The control of deviant sexual behaviour by drugs: I. Behavioural changes following oestrogens and anti-androgens.* Br J Psychiatry 125:310, 1974.

108. Laschet, U and Laschet, L: *Psychopharmacology of sex offenders with cyproterone acetate.* Pharmakopsychiatrie Neuro-Psychopharmakologie 4:99, 1971.

109. Davies, TS: *Cyproterone acetate for male hypersexuality.* J Int Med Res 2:159, 1974.

110. Cooper, AJ, Ismail, AAA, Phanjoo, AL, Love, DL: *Antiandrogen (cyproterone acetate) therapy in deviant hypersexuality.* Br J Psychiatry 120:59, 1972.

111. Van Moffaert, M: *Social reintegration of sexual delinquents by a combination of psychotherapy and anti-androgen treatment.* Acta Psychiatr Scan 53:29, 1976.

112. Schumann, HJ von: *Die Resozialisierung von sexuell abnormen Patienten durch kombinierte Antiandrogen-Applikation und Psychotherapie.* Psychother Psychosom 20:321, 1972.

113. Ortmann, J: *The treatment of sexual offenders: Castration and antihormone therapy.* Int J Law Psychiatry 3:443, 1980.

114. DIETZ, PE: *Sex offenses: Behavioral aspects.* In KADISH, SH (ED): *Encyclopedia of Crime and Justice,* vol 4. Free Press, New York, 1983, pp 1485-1493.

115. AMERICAN LAW INSTITUTE: *Model Penal Code and Commentaries (Official Draft and Revised Comments): Part II: Definition of Specific Crimes.* American Law Institute, Philadelphia, 1980.

116. DIX, G: *Special dispositional alternatives for abnormal offenders: Developments in the law.* In MONAHAN, J AND STEADMAN, HJ (EDS): *Mentally Disordered Offenders: Perspectives from Law and Social Science.* Plenum Press, New York, 1983, pp 133-190.

117. AMERICAN BAR ASSOCIATION: *Proposed Criminal Justice Mental Health Standards.* ABA, Chicago, IL, 1984.

118. COMMITTEE ON PSYCHIATRY AND LAW: *Psychiatry and Sex Psychopath Legislation: The 30s to the 80s.* Group for the Advancement of Psychiatry, New York, 1977.

119. MONAHAN, J AND DAVIS, SK: *Mentally disordered sex offenders.* In MONAHAN, J AND STEADMAN, HJ (EDS): *Mentally Disordered Offenders: Perspectives from Law and Social Science.* Plenum Press, New York, 1983, pp 191-204.

120. FAVOLE, RJ: *Mental disability in the American criminal process: A four issue survey.* In MONAHAN, J AND STEADMAN, HJ (EDS): *Mentally Disordered Offenders: Perspectives from Law and Social Science.* Plenum Press, New York, 1983, pp 247-295.

121. Specht v. Patterson, 386 U.S. 605 (1967).

122. Humphrey v. Cady, 405 U.S. 504 (1972).

123. People v. Stoddard, 227 Cal. App. 2d 40, 38 Cal. Reptr. 407 (1964).

124. Letter from Dr. Dorothy S. Dobbs, St. Elizabeths Hospital, November 15, 1968, cited in Millard v. Harris, 406 F.2d 964, 982 (D.C. Cir. 1968) (Wright, J., concurring).

125. Millard v. Harris, 406 F.2d 964 (D.C. Cir. 1968).

126. Cross v. Harris, 418 F.2d 1095 (D.C. Cir. 1969).

127. Darnell v. Cameron, 348 F.2d 64 (D.C. Cir. 1965).

128. RILEY, MR: *Exhibitionism: A psycho-legal perspective.* San Diego Law Review 16:853, 1979.

129. ROOTH, G: *Exhibitionism, sexual violence and paedophilia.* Br J Psychiatry 122:705, 1973.

130. BERAH, EF AND MYERS, RG: *The offense records of a sample of convicted exhibitionists.* Bull Am Acad Psychiatry Law 11:365, 1983.

131. HALLECK, SL: *The ethics of antiandrogen therapy.* Am J Psychiatry 138:642, 1981.

PART 5
LEGAL IMPLICATIONS OF PERSONALITY DISORDERS

This section examines diagnostic categories of mentally disturbed persons presenting special problems for the legal and correctional systems. The reaction of some mental health evaluators is to assume that a large portion of the persons encountered in these diagnostic groups are not criminally responsible, are often unfit for criminal trial, and quite uniformly do not respond to any kind of therapeutic intervention. This is because patients with personality disorders and disorders of impulse control appear undeterred by punishment and seem compelled to repeat their criminal behavior in self-destructive fashion.

If these views were presented as forensic clinical judgments, such evaluations could remove large numbers of charged offenders from accountability to the legal system of the country and from access to specialized treatment and care related to their behavior. The common law system does not, and never has, supported such sweeping positions. Offenders in each of these categories should be examined individually, based on their own characteristics and the legal requirements for the crimes with which they are charged. Some offenders in these categories can respond favorably to the specialized treatment described in this chapter. The trend of American criminal law, however, as indicated earlier in chapter 8 by Dr. Shah, is conservative; the scope of the insanity defense is currently being limited, not expanded. Serious mental disturbance of a nature generally beyond that examined in this chapter is being required as a threshold to any application of the defense, and the "volitional arm" of the traditional responsibility test is looked upon with considerable disfavor and is being repealed in many jurisdictions.

In the first chapter in this section, Dr. Simon Dinitz, a sociologist, takes a very broad view of developments in this field. He examines the definitional-diagnostic problems of the antisocial personality concept and the latest attempts at clarification by the American Psychiatric Association. Dr. Dinitz finds little new in the description of the disorder in the third edition of the *Diagnostic and*

Statistical Manual of Mental Disorders (DSM III), except for its greater emphasis on early adolescent onset of the behavior pattern. The thrust of the diagnosis is upon continuous and chronic antisocial behavior that persists into adult life and becomes evident prior to the age of 15. Dr. Dinitz agrees with the manual's estimate of 3 percent of males and 1 percent of females in the American population fitting this definition. Much more controversial are the estimates of antisocial personality offenders in American prisons. Figures are offered from surveys of prevalence ranging from 20 percent to upward of 80 percent in correctional facilities.

The author provides detailed descriptions of the multivariant factors considered in diagnosing antisocial personality under the many clinical diagnostic concepts in the field. He also offers the observation that the dominant criminological-sociological research efforts of this country have not focused adequately upon biological factors despite the rather obvious indicators in this direction. Dr. Dinitz welcomes in his concluding remarks a return to this field of medically and biologically oriented forensic science specialists, a view supported by the editors in the interest of multidisciplinary research in this field.

The other chapter in this part was clearly stimulated by the publication of *DSM III.* Its subject is disorders of impulse control, particularly those involving antisocial or criminal behavior, as dealt with in the American Psychiatric Association's new manual. The authors Dr. Monopolis and Dr. Lion, have had considerable clinical experience with many of these disorders.

The authors concentrate attention on a central problem in the manual's treatment of the subject: the description of a "failure to resist" the impulses covered in the category. Is this concept the same as inability or incapacity to resist? Does it mean that the behavior is not premeditated? The authors also question the universality of the experience of relief or pleasure on completion of the action. From clinical experience, the authors point to evidence of rage or guilt reactions after outbursts of explosive rage rather than of either relief or pleasure. A detailed description is provided of the clinical features of each entity, a discussion of its etiology, and a review of accepted therapeutic measures applicable to each entity. Particularly sparkling are the pithy comments of the clinician authors in the discussions of etiology and treatment of these disorders.

There is an analysis of the use of these impulse categories as defenses on insanity grounds in criminal cases. Research data are admittedly quite scarce. The legal utility of the disorders as defenses seems remote when one considers the authors' description of the limitations of the diagnoses: that they should be applied only in the absence of other psychopathology. For example, they suggest that kleptomania should not be diagnosed when the patient is stealing as part of a general criminal career or when the conduct arises out of schizophrenic delusional disorder.

The newest of the entities, pathological gambling, has been seen in the trial courts only in a few instances. Insanity defenses were successful in two cases, and there were "hung jury" mistrials in two others. Appellate courts have begun to reject such verdicts, however, especially when the pathological gambling is accompanied by other criminal conduct, often in an effort to recoup gambling losses and when the plea of criminal irresponsibility is argued to cover the entire range of the person's criminal behavior. It is still too early after publication of *DSM III* to assess its impact on clinical testimony and legal applications in regard to these categories of impulse disorder. The chapter by

Drs. Monopolis and Lion should be an important contribution to the determination of these issues. The chapter's close adherence to the categories of *DSM III* and the authors' specific clinical commentaries on treatment methodologies in each category should help considerably in the everyday, practical application of the new manual in forensic mental health programs across the United States.

CHAPTER 17
THE ANTISOCIAL PERSONALITY
Simon Dinitz, Ph.D.

Antisocial personality is a clinical disorder whose course, mechanism, and etiology remain unknown.[1] Genetic, physiologic, interactional, and sociocultural etiologies have been advanced to explain this intractable behavioral disorder which is not recognized as a form of mental illness by present legal standards. From M'Naghten to the American Law Institute Model Penal Code, the sociopath has been considered to be fully responsible for his or her conduct. In this, as in other spheres, the law and psychiatry are at odds. Thus, in 1952, the *Diagnostic and Statistical Manual of Mental Disorders** of the American Psychiatric Association *(APA)* described antisocial sociopaths as

> chronically anti-social individuals who are always in trouble, profiting neither from experience nor punishment and maintaining no real loyalty to any person, group, or code. They are frequently callous and hedonistic, showing marked emotional immaturity with lack of sense of responsibility, lack of judgment, and an ability to rationalize their behavior so that it appears warranted, reasonable and justified.

The second (1968) edition of the manual and the 1969 APA glossary contain no mention at all of such traditional and now obsolete terms as sociopathy and psychopathy. This most recent change in classification replaces sociopathy with antisocial personality, the latter described as follows:

> This term is reserved for individuals who are basically unsocialized and whose behavior pattern brings them repeatedly into conflict with society.

---

* American Psychiatric Association: *Diagnostic and Statistical Manual of Mental Disorders;* ed. 1, 1952; ed. 2, 1968; ed 3, ed. 3, 1980. APA, Washington, DC.

They are incapable of significant loyalty to individuals, groups, or social values. They are grossly selfish, calloused, irresponsible, impulsive, and unable to feel guilt or to learn from experience. Frustration tolerance is low. They tend to blame others or offer plausible rationalizations for their behavior. . . .

In the 1980 edition of the *Diagnostic and Statistical Manual of Mental Disorders (DSM III)* of the American Psychiatric Association, the essential attributes of an antisocial personality disorder are described in these terms:

> a history of continuous and chronic antisocial behavior in which the rights of others are violated, persistence into adult life of a pattern of antisocial behavior that began before the age of 15 and failure to sustain good job performance (when applicable) over a period of several years.

After listing a variety of specific behavioral precursors in childhood such as lying, stealing, fighting, and resisting authority, the *DSM III* notes that most of the unlovely and illegal conduct of the antisocial personality tends to diminish after age 30, especially sexual promiscuity, criminality, and vagrancy. In addition to the major antisocial attributes, associated features of this personality disorder include signs of personal distress, complaints of tension, intolerance to boredom, depression, interpersonal difficulties which persist into late adult life, and impaired capacity for rewarding relationships with family and friends. This disorder, continues the *DSM III* exposition, "is often extremely incapacitating . . ., more commonly penal than medical."

DSM III estimates that the prevalence of this disorder in men is 3 percent and in women, 1 percent; that the onset in male persons is already evident in early childhood and in girls about the time of the onset of puberty. *DSM III* notes that there is considerable familial aggregation of this disorder. The more impoverished and disorganized the household, the greater the prevalence.

In truth, *DSM III* confuses more than clarifies—hardly surprising in so amorphous a disorder. Particularly disturbing are the criteria (symptoms) specified to confirm this disorder. Of the 12 criteria (behaviors) listed prior to age 15, only three are needed to qualify for inclusion. All but a few of these 12 would apply to most lower-class boys and to many in better economic circumstances as well: truancy, school suspension, delinquent conduct resulting in some sort of official action, running away from home at least twice, persistent lying, repeated sexual intercourse of a casual nature, alcohol or substance abuse, theft, vandalism, poor school performance (below expectations), chronic violations of home and school rules, and initiation of fights.

At the adult level, four of nine symptoms are considered adequate for this diagnostic label: poor work performance, irresponsible parenting, chronic illegal behavior, inability to maintain enduring attachment to a sexual partner, irritability and acting out, fiscal irresponsibility, failure to plan ahead, disregard for the truth, and recklessness.

From this analysis it is evident that no additional specificity is added in *DSM III*, compared with the earlier diagnostic criteria, except for the focus on the adolescent behavioral concomitants of this disorder.

Previously and less specifically referred to as psychopathy,* constitutional psychopathic state, and psychopathic personality, sociopathy has been attributed to genetic, biologic, interpersonal, and cultural causes.[2]

Clinical evidence indicates that the antisocial personality constitutes from 1 to 3 percent of all adults of both sexes.[3] Even if this estimate is somewhat overdrawn numerically, sociopathy is an economically and socially expensive mental disorder. Furthermore, this chronic and disabling disease, which is probably characterized by a shortened life span,[4] was earlier estimated to affect approximately 20 percent of the adult correctional population in the United States.† On the other hand, more recent studies of released male felons from prisons have diagnosed nearly 80 percent as displaying antisocial personality.[5] (See chapter 19 for further discussion of the antisocial personality in prison populations.)

Whatever the precise etiology—the extraordinary disruption of the modern family, the increased geographic mobility, the "eclipse" of community, the elaboration of the female-headed household as a major type—the increased social disorganization occasioned by urbanization seems to have exacerbated the problem. The sociopath creates problems for the urban community; the urban community negatively influences the sociopath. The spiral effect is to be seen in *Children Who Hate,*[6] the "core" members of gangs,[7] and the changing composition of inmate populations. Experienced corrections people are more than ever disturbed by this trend and freely confess that they are unable to deal successfully with these highly disruptive inmates.

Despite the size of the sociopathic population and the belief of many clinicians that sociopathy is probably an irreversible personality disorder, little headway has been made in effective treatment techniques. In general, most correctional officers feel that no effective therapy exists and, even worse, that antisocial sociopaths are not amenable to treatment.[8] If sociopathy could be studied, its epidemiology delineated, and its social and biomedical characteristics elucidated, some of the defeatism which now characterizes the corrections system might be alleviated.

EARLY FORMULATIONS

The contemporary conception of the antisocial personality which forms the theoretical basis of present conceptions of the nature of sociopathy has evolved from formulations that have been advanced by numerous investigators, most of whom have derived their theories and insights from clinical experience.

---

* Psychopathic personality was the generic term used to refer to a large group of disorders that were regarded by many physicians and clinicians as diverse in nature and as having too little in common to justify subsuming them under the general term. Furthermore, practitioners seldom used the term except to refer, not to the more heterogenous group, but to one, and only one, of the disorders—psychopathy.

† Cleckley, H., *The Mask of Sanity* (CV Mosby, St.Louis, 1950), appendix A. Bernard Glueck investigated 608 Sing Sing inmates, 18.9 percent of whom were found to be sociopaths (quoted in S. Maughs: *A concept of psychopathy and psychopathic personality: Its evolution and historical development.* Journal of Criminal Psychopathology 2:480, 1941).

Pinel is credited with first describing this phenomenon in modern terms.[9] His classification and description of manie sans delire (mania without delusions), although mixing a variety of disorders, dealt with this previously unexplained phenomenon. His tripartite classification (impulsive insanity and moral idiocy, hypomania, and melancholia activa), broadened the conception of mental illness and led others to question the prevailing notion of the time that the intellect is always involved in mental illness.

The American psychiatrist Benjamin Rush expressed similar ideas as early as 1812, speaking of moral alienation, defective organization of moral faculties, and deranged will. While postulating a special moral sense, in accordance with faculty psychology, Rush—like Pinel—recognized that mental illness may involve other than intellectual faculties.

These formulations influenced the English physician J. C. Prichard. His comprehensive descriptions of sociopathy (under the titles of moral insanity and moral imbecility) drew attention to states characterized by an affective and feeling disorder, rather than by understanding and intellect. Although his description of nonintellectual "insanity" was a bold step in the classification of mental diseases, he grouped all disorders on the basis of symptomatology and consequently included disorders other than sociopathy.

Garofalo,[10] one of the major founders of positive criminology, attempted to evade the issue of moral insanity by suggesting that biological factors might be present:

> Should [such moral anomalies as the sociopath] be regarded as a new nosologic form—the moral insanity of the English writers? The existence of this form of alienation is questionable, to say the least. In spite of utmost efforts to discover traces of insanity, one is often obliged to admit that the individual under examination possesses an intelligence which leaves nothing to be desired, that he exhibits no nosologic symptom, unless it be the absence of a moral sense, and that, to quote a French physician, whatever be the subject's unity of mind, "the psychic keyboard has only one false note and only one."

Garofalo further noted that these children are born with "ferocious instincts." For these criminals with imprudence, lack of insight, and moral insensibility, who exhibit complete indifference to shame, he substituted the term "constitutional inferiority" for "moral insanity."

Lombroso,[11] the father of modern criminology and a forensic psychiatrist, embraced the conception of the chronically antisocial individual as a moral imbecile, noting that he was guiltless, highly aggressive, impulsive, boastful, and particularly insensitive to social criticism and physical pain. Lombroso wanted such persons placed in asylums:

> At first sight this proposition seems absurd . . . . But proper attention has not been paid to the fact that it is just such . . . cases, intermediate between reason and insanity, in which, therefore, the criminal asylums are most useful and of most service in guaranteeing the public safety.[12]

Partridge is credited with the introduction of the term sociopath, suggesting that persons with this disorder should be considered defective as a consequence of improper socialization.[13] Utilizing psychoanalytic theory, Partridge located the sociopathic person's maladjustment in the developmental process. A study of 50 sociopathic persons revealed, Partridge contended, that the sociopathic person fails to progress through the stages of normal child development and retains adjustment techniques common to early childhood. He described this disorder as a permanently fixed concentration on oral needs. His studies led him to conclude that

> [The sociopathic] personality is a persistent behavior pattern or tendency in which there is usually excessive demand . . . which when there is a failure of direct or immediate satisfaction, is reacted to by a tendency to develop characteristic ways of dominating situations; by emotional displays we call tantrums, by sulks; by running away . . . .[11]

Thompson[15] offers a somewhat similar conception. To him, sociopathy is a personality deviation characterized by an inability to adjust adequately and consistently to social standards. Thompson maintained that this deviation stems from a basic mental defect that renders the sufferer incapable of developing an adequate sense of time, particularly with regard to self. Lack of guilt, insufficient judgment, impulsiveness, and inability to profit from experience are secondary symptoms which result from this basic defect.

Henderson[16] used the term psychopathic state to refer to the antisocial sociopathic person and included three groups under this rubric: the predominantly aggressive, the predominantly passive or inadequate, and the predominantly creative. The latter state suggests the genius as a variant of the sociopathic personality.* In essence, Henderson described the sociopathic person as unstable, explosive, and egocentric. Psychic immaturity is the prime feature of the condition:

> He cannot accept things as they are; he is unable to fit into the life of the herd, but tends to lead an independent, individualistic type of existence with no thought or feeling for his family, his friends, or his country. He is blunted emotionally . . . for a time he may prove charming . . . . For some inscrutable reason he fails to grow up, he remains at the level of a primitive savage with a distaste for reasoning and an "impermeability to experience" . . . . The judicial, deciding, selecting process described as intelligence, and the energizing, emotivating, driving powers called character, are not working in harmony.[17]

Cleckley[18] has provided the most inclusive and thorough conceptualization of the antisocial sociopathic personality, maintaining that the latter is a distinguishable, deeply rooted clinical entity. The disorder adversely affects interper-

---

* Kozol, a more recent contributor, also related genius and sociopathy and stated that the same dynamics operate in both. The level of assault differs—the genius creates, whereas the sociopathic person makes attacks for "kicks;" yet both are characterized by identical factors, Kozol maintained. There is dissociation between basic impulse patterns and the development of social pseudoconformity. Sociopathic persons learn to conform for their own benefit; however, this educative process appears unrelated to the primitive impulse structure. This separation accounts for the lack of internal control and the primitiveness of goals which characterizes them (Maughs, op cit, p 484).

sonal relations and is demonstrated best when the sociopathic person confronts problems of living.

The antisocial sociopathic personality, according to Cleckley,[19] is characterized by the following:

1. Superficial charm and good intelligence
2. Absence of delusions and other signs of irrational thinking
3. Absence of nervousness and other psychoneurotic manifestations
4. Unreliability
5. Untruthfulness and insincerity
6. Lack of remorse or shame
7. Inadequately motivated antisocial behavior
8. Poor judgment and failure to learn by experience
9. Pathologic egocentricity and incapacity for love
10. General poverty of major affective relations
11. Specific loss of insight
12. Unresponsiveness in interpersonal behavior
13. Fantastic and uninviting behavior, with drink and sometimes without
14. Suicide rarely carried out
15. Sex life impersonal, trivial, and poorly integrated
16. Failure to follow any life plan

More precisely, Cleckley described the sociopathic person who is likely to end up in prison as easy to talk with, friendly, and frequently of superior intelligence. Outer perceptual reality is not distorted; social values may be accepted verbally, and excellent logical reasoning prevails. The sociopathic individual with great verbal facility foresees consequences of action and criticizes former mistakes. These excellent rational powers, so apparent verbally as well as in hypothetical situations, do not carry over into behavior. Despite the rationality, the sociopathic person shows poor judgment in behavior and has a perplexing ability for creating situations in which no rational person would participate. Furthermore, this person suffers from specific loss of insight. The sociopathic person neither knows how others feel in relation to him or her nor appreciates subjectively the values and major emotional concerns others have for him or her. There is a total absence of appraisal of self as a real and moving experience. The sociopathic person has all the qualities by which insight is gained, and awareness of major facts, all the words of understanding; yet these facts neither enter into the person's evaluations nor prompt the person to change his or her behavior. The discrepancy between his or her favorable orientation and ability to reason and his or her behavior is enigmatic.

This baffling paradox is clearly revealed in the sociopathic person's inadequately motivated antisocial behavior, the failure to develop a life plan, and the person's untruthfulness. As part of the antisocial conduct, he or she commits crimes for small stakes and under great risks. Yet there is no evidence of a compulsive or neurotic component. This person does not formulate long-term goals but seems to be motivated to fail in life. The sociopathic person cannot be trusted in personal accounts of the past, statements of present intentions, or promises for the future. This person lies, seemingly without purpose, and, with ready sincerity, manipulates truth to gain personal immediate ends.

The sociopathic person's untruthfulness is coupled with personal unreliability and irresponsibility. He or she is irresponsible, now matter how binding the obligation, in trivial as well as serious matters. Although the antisocial sociopathic individual intermittently reveals convincing and conforming loyalty, predicting when he or she will or will not be responsible appears to be impossible. It does not seem to be related to mood, objective stress, or amount at stake for oneself or for others. Furthermore, this person feels no shame or remorse; the antisocial sociopathic person usually projects blame on others, and the blaming of oneself is hollow, casual, and instrumental. This person is seemingly incapable of object love and is generally unresponsive in interpersonal behavior. Although he or she may be attentive to small courtesies, perhaps even obliging and generous, he or she cannot show consistent, ordinary responsiveness to kindness and trust. This person is not usually motivated by altruistic concern, although he or she may superficially claim to be; nor can he or she express genuine human emotions. In brief, the sociopathic person is impoverished in affective reactions.

Cleckley suggests that the sociopathic person has no deep commitment either to persons or to ideas. He or she often overindulges in sexual behavior, alcohol, drugs, and other "thrill-producing" substances. Sexual behavior is random, provoked frequently by whimlike impulses of little intensity and is free of emotional involvement.

Cleckley adopted the term "semantic disorder" or "semantic psychosis" to refer to the clinical entity characterized above. The sociopathic personality mimics the human personality and wears a "mask of sanity." He or she is unaware of and lacks the ability to become cognizant of what the most important life experiences mean to others. Major emotional accompaniments or affective competencies are missing. This person's response to life is dissociated, and components of normal experience are not integrated into a wholly human reaction.

In a major break with current wisdom and empirical research, the late Samuel Yochelson,[20] a psychiatrist, and his colleague, Stanton Samenow, a psychologist, propose the widely disputed thesis that the antisocial personality disorder is in reality a cognitive disorder or, more simply, a lifestyle built on distortions in thinking. According to Yochelson and Samenow, this imprinted "criminal personality" features an early onset—5 or 6 years of age—and a patterned mode of coping with reality that is amoral in character. The antisocial personality is not the product of the environment but rather of a "series of choices that he makes starting at a very early age."

The Yochelson-Samenow thesis is based on clinical investigation of 240 cases at St Elizabeths Hospital in which over 50 specific thinking distortions were noted. The most important concerns the self-defeating utilization of a high energy level geared to the pursuit of excitement. The antisocial personality cycles from a near manic activity level (nonutilitarian) to fatigue and boredom and back again in this quest.

This disorder, despite appearances to the contrary, is characterized by pathological fears in the subject. These subclinical fears are widespread, persistent, and intense. They include a persistent preoccupation with death and injury, illness and pain, and an even more intense dread of social and ego vulnerability (being "put down"). The antisocial personality cannot cope with these threats and in guarding against them becomes even more ego vulnerable.

Perhaps the most unique quality of this disorder is what the authors refer to as the zero state. (I am a zero, a nothing.) In this **unchangeable** ego state, the subject has the lowest self-esteem and believes that others share this definition of the subject with him or her—a conception reminiscent of Cooley's "looking-glass self." In this disorder the subject was "born to lose."

Because of these deficits and fears and needs, the antisocial personality suffers chronic anger, which he or she attempts to relieve through manipulation and intimidation of all others. Pride, manliness, and overt displays of machismo are part of the behavioral picture as well.

Equally central clinically is the **power thrust** seen in hobbies (for example, motorcycles), work (money making), appearance (fashionable), speech (tailored to the occasion), and sex (conquest). Key adjectives used by Yochelson and Samenow in describing this cognitive disorder are exploitation, manipulation, destruction, surface sentimentality, overt respectability, rigidity, imperviousness, and a good many others—all negative.

Such persons think concretely (unable to deal with abstractions except superficially); are inconsistent (not even a consistency in their inconsistency); emphasize their uniqueness and superiority; strive for perfection in dress, speech, and presentation; and are loners (lack of trust), irresponsible, and unable to take the role of the other. All in all, over 50 such chronic and implacable thinking distortions motivate the subjects' behaviors and dictate their choices.

Yochelson and Samenow portray the antisocial personality as competent and responsible. His or her choices are deliberate and optimize his or her unquenchable need for power, exploitation, and excitement. Treatment intervention demands that this personality be continually confronted with the thinking distortions and prevented from manipulating the therapist and the situation. The presenting personality must be stripped and, with the responsible involvement of the patient, painstakingly remolded. The prognosis in this encounter is poor because the subject is fated (heredity and organicity as destiny) to remain a social pariah with considerable potential for doing harm to others.

In many ways, the "semantic disorder" of Cleckley is replaced by the terms cognitive disorder or thinking distortions in this understandably controversial description by Yochelson and Samenow of the "criminal personality." Nevertheless, in taking a "nature over nurture" position, Yochelson and Samenow's writing is a throwback to the pioneers of the Italian positivist school and, in particular, to Garofalo and his thesis of the "natural" criminal and children born with "ferocious instincts."

In contrast, Gough,[21] in a social psychological treatment of sociopathy, contends that the sociological theory of role playing as described in the work of the symbolic interactionists, such as Harry Stack Sullivan in psychiatry, provides a synthesis of known facts of sociopathy and formulated deductive hypotheses for empirical testing. The antisocial personality, according to Gough, is pathologically deficient in role-taking ability. This deficiency is characterized by an inability to view the self as an object and to identify with another's point of view. Inasmuch as other aspects of sociopathy are associated with this deficiency, Gough concluded that the causes of sociopathy must be sought in the causes of inadequacy in role-playing ability.

ETIOLOGIC PERSPECTIVES

Defective Role Taking

Apart from clinical studies, the antisocial sociopath has been relatively neglected as a subject of research. There have been very few social psychological studies.

Following Gough, Baker[22] investigated skill in taking the role of the other and hypothesized that in a group of male prisoners, antisocial sociopathic personalities would be less able than nonsociopathic personalities* to empathize with their cellmates, all of whom had shared a cell with these cellmates for at least 4 weeks. Each subject and his cellmate filled out four adjective checklists: for self (A); for cellmate (B); prediction of self-checks for cellmate (C); and subject's guesses as to how he appears to his cellmate (D). Predictions made by each subject on checklists C and D were compared with the cellmate's actual choices on checklists A and B, thus providing two measures of empathy, including the percentage of correct predictions on checklist C and the percentage of correct predictions on checklist D. The first indicates ability to perceive qualities or traits others use in assessing one's self. Although the samples are small (21 sociopathic persons and 13 nonsociopathic persons), the differences in C and D percentages are statistically significant; sociopathic persons are less able to empathize with others.

Arguing that antisocial sociopathic people cannot take the time to put themselves in the role of the other before they act† and therefore are poor tension binders, Albrecht and Sarbin[23] hypothesized that such persons would be most responsive to annoying stimuli. Administering a 172-item annoyance questionnaire to 60 male subjects (20 diagnosed as sociopaths, 27 diagnosed as neurotics, and 13 without psychiatric diagnosis), they found significant differences between groups on total mean scores, with sociopaths having the highest, normals intermediate, and neurotics lowest mean annoyance scale scores.

McCord and McCord offer one of the more recent formulations of the sociopath and specify guiltlessness and lovelessness as the core characteristics of the antisocial sociopathic personality.

> The [antisocial personality] is an asocial, aggressive, highly impulsive person, who feels little or no guilt and is unable to form lasting bonds of affection with other human beings.[24]

These characteristics, it would appear, are considered basic to the antisocial sociopath syndrome; they are consistently employed in almost all contemporary uses of the concept.

The McCords attempted to evaluate the contributions of milieu therapy on young, aggressive, sociopathic boys at the Wiltwyck School in New York, wherein both individual and group therapy were combined in a warm, permissive environment. After painstaking study, the authors concluded that milieu therapy causes radical alterations in personality of the subjects. However, such an environment is easily manipulated by sociopathic personalities; if the subjects had been followed after release, much of the optimism concerning successful treatment might have been dispelled by observing the behavior of sociopathic boys in a nonaccepting environment.

Sociological and Psychiatric Variables

In the most thorough sociological and psychiatric study of the antisocial personality to date, Robins[25] directed a 10-year research project representing a 30-year longitudinal study of the adult status of 524 child-guidance clinic patients

---

* Subjects were assigned to categories on the basis of MMPI profiles.
† This point is basic to Gough's role-taking theory of sociopathy, following Mead (Mead, GH: *Mind, Self and Society.* University of Chicago Press, Chicago, 1934).

at the St. Louis Municipal Psychiatric Clinic. This patient group was made up predominantly of male offspring of American-born Protestant parents of low socioeconomic status; blacks were excluded from the investigation. Ninety percent of the subjects were located, 82 percent were interviewed, and 98 percent were successfully traced through adult records. On the basis of interview and record information, and for each of the 19 areas of the subject's life in which he might have failed to conform to societal norms,[26] specific criteria for sociopathic behavior were established.* These criteria allowed two psychiatrists to agree as to whether 80 percent of the subjects were well or ill† and to make reasonably specific diagnoses for 71 percent of the subjects. Robins does not indicate the degree to which the remaining 29 percent, who could not be specifically diagnosed, differed from those who were successfully diagnosed. (This latter point introduces possible unknown biases.)

The 94 sociopathic personality subjects from St. Louis were compared with four other specific diagnostic groups that occurred frequently enough to permit statistical comparisons (anxiety neurosis, hysteria, schizophrenia, and alcoholism) and with a group of 100 control subjects from the same city, matched on race, area of residence, sex, age, and intelligence quotient.

This important research was concerned basically with three areas of delineation: distinctive symptoms of the sociopathic personality; a portrait of adult sociopathic personality; and childhood behavior predictive of later diagnosis. The findings in these three areas were complex, were subject to differences in interpretation, and were not analyzed or presented in a wholly satisfactory fashion.

As for symptoms, persons diagnosed as sociopathic personalities in the St. Louis study had more symptoms than any other diagnostic group; the three most common symptoms being financial dependency, poor work history, and multiple arrests. Four symptoms distinguished the sociopathic personality group at a statistically significant level from the other four groups: poor marital history, impulsiveness, vagrancy, and the use of aliases. The presence of one or more of the latter symptoms turned out to be among the best indicators of later sociopathic personality diagnosis.

The portrait of the St. Louis patient diagnosed as a sociopathic personality as an adult is contaminated by the use of 19 symptom areas to diagnose subjects; the very criteria used for diagnosis were later treated as characteristics of the sociopathic personality. However, four noncircular aspects of sociopathy are also presented: social adjustment, health, psychiatric symptoms, and treatment.

In general, persons diagnosed as sociopathic personalities in the St. Louis study had a disproportionately high death rate, more than twice the national rate; felt themselves to be sicker than other groups; were extremely mobile;

---

* The median number of areas in which subjects given the diagnosis of antisocial sociopathic personality met the various criteria for failure to conform to societal norms was first reported to be 11. In the next paragraph it was reported that 13 of the 19 symptoms occurred in at least half the subjects diagnosed as antisocial sociopathic personalities. Five pages later it was noted that 69 percent of the sociopathic group had at least nine of these 19 symptoms.

† The psychiatrists were aware that the topic of interest was antisocial sociopathic personality; a relatively high proportion (15.6 percent) of the subjects were diagnosed sociopathic. It may well have been that "blind" evaluators would not have found such a high proportion to be sociopathic.

more often lived in the core city; were currently more often unemployed; had experienced long periods of unemployment; usually held a low-ranking blue-collar job; rarely held a job for long; functioned longer in jobs in which they had little supervision; earned less when employed; were downwardly mobile in occupation; had low educational attainment; experienced little upward mobility from their fathers; were more frequently recipients of aid from public agencies; had the lowest percentage with established credit ratings; were more often divorced than any other group, and less often currently living with spouse; tended to marry spouses with serious behavior problems; married somewhat younger than either patient or control groups; were slightly more often childless; were parents to children who were already showing marked emotional problems, few of whom graduated from high school; had the lowest rates of induction into the armed forces; were extreme medical and disciplinary problems in the service; and had aborted terms of military service.

The St. Louis patients also had unusually high proportions of nontraffic arrests, being arrested at least once for a major crime; had more convictions when arrested than all other subjects; were less likely to "burn out" in criminal behavior over time; evinced high rates of problem drinking; and were either currently experimenting with drugs (5 percent) or were or had been addicted to drugs (10 percent).

The sociopathic personalities in the St. Louis study were also more often isolated from relatives and neighbors; belonged to very few formal organizations; had many neurotic and somatic symptoms; had rarely sought psychiatric care; had been frequently hospitalized in mental hospitals (21 percent); and had been more often previously diagnosed as sociopathic when hospitalized.

The above characteristics have been closely linked with lower social class status by sociologists, especially Matza,[27] Kahl,[28] and Komarovsky.[29] Social class may well be intervening to produce these marked differences and traits, although Robins made a concerted but somewhat ineffectual and unconvincing effort to contraindicate social class as an explanatory variable.

Robins' treatment of social class as a variable is at best less than ideal. Her study group is somewhat vaguely broken into "blue collar" and "white collar" on the basis of father's occupation; 24 percent of the former and 13 percent of the latter were found to be sociopathic. This represents a ratio of almost 2:1. It may be that sociopathy is concentrated in the lower class, owing to the relative breakdown in socialization or to the sociopathic person's having drifted downward. Another possible alternative is that psychiatrists see such antisocial behavior of the lower class as sociopathy, exhibiting middle-class perspective as professional judgment. Perhaps all three may be operating, although Robins argues against the latter. However, the argument would have been stronger if she had presented the average number of symptoms necessary for diagnosis as sociopathic for the lower and middle classes separately.

Finally, as for childhood behavior predicting sociopathy, Robins suggested that these symptoms would include aggression or theft for a boy; many episodes of diverse antisocial behavior, at least one of which could bring the child before a juvenile court; antisocial involvement with strangers and organizations as well as with parents and teachers; gratuitous lying; a history of truancy, staying out late, and refusing to obey parents; little guilt over behavior; irresponsibility concerning both being where one was supposed to be and taking care of money; interest in sexual behavior and experimenting with homosexual behavior; bed wetting; and poor grooming. Only self-exposure and vandalism, among the antisocial symptoms, were innocuous. Girls resembled boys in the antisocial symptoms, except that they exhibited sexual misbehavior more frequently and prominently and experienced the onset of difficulties more visible at a later age.

Robins noted that antisocial behavior by the fathers of the patients is predictive of antisocial behavior for patients, particularly paternal desertion, arrest, excessive drinking, failure to support the family, and chronic unemployment. However, as for the effects of the family setting on sociopathic personality per se, Robins noted only that parental rejection does not appear to lead to sociopathy, and early separation from an antisocial father does not appear to prevent the development of sociopathy in the child. In the latter case, this may be due to the lessened ability of the mother alone to exercise control over the child.

In conclusion, Robins suggested that a more precise study of the sociopathic personality could be made from a longitudinal study of consecutive births, thus minimizing the selectivity inherent in subjects volunteering or being forced to seek attention at mental health or child-guidance clinics. Such would be a difficult but potentially rewarding enterprise.

BIOLOGICAL SUBSTRATES OF SOCIOPATHY

Despite the long-standing interest, particularly on the part of European criminologists, in the biologic substrates of chronically antisocial behavior, few modern American criminologists have considered it relevant to examine these aspects of criminal conduct. There are, of course, a variety of justifications for this neglect. For one thing, academic criminology in the United States is located in departments of sociology rather than in schools of law or medicine, as has been traditional in Europe and Latin America. Given their training and orientation, few sociologists are versed in, or sympathetic to, a biologic perspective. Instead, American criminology has been distinguished by its strong sociocultural emphasis and its view of criminal behavior as essentially learned and adaptive conduct. Another and perhaps even more important reason for this neglect of biologic investigation has been the sorry history of the biological perspective in the last hundred years. The extravagant claims, meager empirical evidence, naivete, gross inadequacy, and stated or implied concepts of racial and ethnic inferiority in the work of the constitutionalists, the morphologists, the European traditionalists, and the early endocrinologists deservedly discredited the biological framework in the study of crime. Finally, American psychiatrists, at least those interested in criminology, have long been wedded to a psychodynamic orientation in which the focus is on the psychogenic and familial bases of intrapsychic and interpersonal pathologies rather than the psychophysiologic. Given this intellectual climate and disreputable history of biological theorizing, it is little wonder that even the very few important empirical observations of a biologic nature have been generally overlooked by criminologists.

Nevertheless, recent, though limited, studies of the antisocial sociopathic personality have been conducted by physiological psychologists, biologists, and physicians, most of whom have focused on the physiologic responses of the sociopathic person as distinguished from other inmates. It was in 1949 that Funkenstein and associates[30] parenthetically mentioned the cardiovascular lability of chronically antisocial individuals. Funkenstein, a psychiatrist, and his colleagues reported on 15 sociopathic persons (13 men and 2 women) selected from a group of court referrals to the Boston Psychopathic Hospital. They characterized these subjects, ranging in age from 21 to 39 (mean = 25), as hostile recidivists. All had committed crimes of violence and exhibited no clinical signs of anxiety, although they often claimed to be "nervous." Even though none of these subjects volunteered any complaint of subjective discomfort, after an injection of 50 mg of epinephrine, 13 of the 15 sustained a systolic blood pressure rise of 75 mm Hg as compared with only 19 of the 85 psychotic and neurotic patients and five of the 15 controls.

In 1955, the psychologist Lykken[31] reported on the performance of 19 "primary" sociopathic felons (12 of whom were men) on eight assorted psychological tests. On the two tests measuring autonomic function, the "primary" sociopathic personalities produced a diminished galvanic skin response (GSR) to lying and a diminished conditionability of the GSR as compared with the noninstitutionalized controls. The first difference, the GSR to lying, approached the 0.05 level of significance. These differences were statistically different when the "primary" sociopathic persons were compared with a group of 19 incarcerated "neurotic" sociopathic personalities (that is, the inmates who were labeled sociopathic by the prison staff but who did not meet Cleckley's clinical criteria).

In 1964, the social psychologists Schacter and Latane[32] reported that 15 imprisoned sociopathic men showed greater increase in pulse rate following an epinephrine injection than did 15 inmate control subjects. (Whether the controls of Schacter and Latane more closely related to Lykken's "neurotic" sociopathic subjects or to his controls is a moot point.)

In 1965, the psychologist Lippert[33] compared 21 "sociopathic" delinquents with 21 nonsociopathic delinquents and found that their patterns of spontaneous GSR frequency were characterized by (1) lower resting levels, (2) lesser increases during experimental manipulation, (3) decreases below resting levels following experimental manipulation, and (4) increased adaptation to repeated stimuli.

In 1968, Hare,[34] like Lippert, found that 21 primary psychopathic subjects had higher skin resistance and less variability at rest than 12 nonpsychopathic controls. Furthermore, the psychopathic subjects' GSR, cardiovascular, and orienting responses to mild stimuli, such as the solution of arithmetic problems, were less than in the controls.

Hakerem[35] observed an exaggerated pupillary response in a group of patients who were later identified as "psychopaths." This parenthetical observation was neither pursued nor published.

In the most recent and elegant assessment of the status of research in sociopathy, Hare[36] underscores the assumption, now increasingly postulated, of a physiologic basis for this disorder. Substantial emphasis has been placed on some prominent biologic correlates of sociopathy, outlined below.

1. The electroencephalogram (EEG) patterns of some antisocial personalities resemble those of children. This has led some investigators to the hypothesis of delayed maturation of some cortical neuronal mechanism.[37] These abnormal EEGs, often found in their parents as well, are characterized by a predominantly slow wave pattern, a pattern found in states of hypoarousal.
2. In some antisocial personalities, Hare argues that limbic system dysfunction, as evidenced in an abnormal slow wave EEG, seems to be involved.

3. From this evidence, one may conclude that psychopathy may depend on a decreased state of cortical excitability and on an attenuation of sensory input.[38]

4. Moreover, some sociopaths display not only these symptoms of hypoarousal, but those of sensory deprivation as well. For example, consistently observed is the paradoxical increase in aggressivity and other emotionality in certain sociopaths treated with drugs, such as barbiturates, neuroleptics, and ethanol—substances which usually aggravate states of sensory deprivation and promote passivity.[39]

5. Certain antisocial personalities demonstrate a pathologic need for stimulation and appear to be at a low end of an arousal continuum.[40] One would expect from these observations that some sociopathic persons would avoid the use of depressants. Indeed, Robins[41] found this to be the case. However, Hill[42] found depressants to improve the behavior of aggressive sociopathic personalities.

6. Some antisocial personalities exhibit stereotyped behavior.[43] In view of poor space-time integration and the stereotypical behavior, there is a likelihood that basal ganglia dysfunction may be involved.

7. There are definite sexual differences in the median age of the onset of antisocial personality, and symptoms may not be entirely socioculturally determined. Whereas in boys symptoms occur at 7 years of age, they are less severe in girls and occur later, at age 13. There may be a sex-related difference in certain kinds of sociopathy together with a possible biological explanation, as indicated in the research by Robins.

8. Sociopathic or antisocial personality types improve as a function of age, supporting the concept of delayed maturation. However, only a certain type of sociopathic personality will improve, and others will continue to demonstrate symptoms for life unless otherwise modified.

9. On the basis of the assumption that sociopathic behavior is somehow a consequence of hypoarousal, MacCulloch and Feldman[44] suggested that stimulants such as amphetamine might have utility in the treatment of sociopathic persons. However, Hare[45] rightly adds social processing to this chemotherapy as a potential means of rehabilitation.

HETEROGENEITY OF SOCIOPATHY

It is clear that much of the recent research in sociopathy suggests a highly probable biological etiology, yet often there has been little statistical validation of this hypothesis within and between studies from different laboratories. Possible explanations of this lack of validation may lie in the operational definitions of sociopathy and the selection of different sociopathic types for experimentation purposes.

After attempting to replicate the pioneering work of Schacter and Latane, in which a unique biologic response was described in sociopathic individuals, it became clear to us that even the rigorous selection procedures used by them had failed to provide us with a homogeneous group; marked variability in biologic and other measures made interpretation meaningless. We soon concluded that much of this variation, also noted by others, could be explained on the basis of at least two subgroups, as described below.

Our own multidisciplinary investigation, begun in 1965 at the Ohio Penitentiary and involving 19 "primary" sociopathic personalities (10 mixed and 14 nonsociopathic personalities, as defined by clinical, psychometric, and criminal history criteria), revealed that the "primary" sociopathic individuals were not homogeneous with regard to such sociocultural variables as previous antisocial history, family characteristics, psychological profiles, and attitudes. As a result, using the Lykken Scale scores as the criterion, the "primary" sociopathic subjects were divided into two types—"hostile" and "simple." These types were clearly and significantly different from each other on nearly all the sociocultural and psychological measures. Most importantly, only the "simple" (reasonably nonaggressive) sociopathic persons demonstrated the cardiac lability to epinephrine previously ascribed to sociopathic persons in general.[46] The exaggerated autonomic responses of simple sociopathic persons demonstrate that their characteristic overt behavior is paralleled by a characteristic physiologic behavior.

It is possible, based on research at various Ohio prisons, that a logical case can be made for both abnormal autonomic and abnormal social behaviors in the simple sociopathic persons, resulting from a single, simple, structural biological defect. The most parsimonious lesion consistent with the available physiologic data is simply a diminished function (partial or total) of the catecholamine-secreting nerve endings, including those involved with sensory receptors. Such a sympathetic denervation would produce a denervation sensitivity long familiar to psychologists. Such a supersensitivity—of whatever origin—is testable by current technology. This hypothesis in no way precludes extension of the defect to monoaminergic interneurons modulating both sensory input and motor output at higher levels of nervous system integration.

It is reasonable to assume that a defect already observed for three disparate effectors—heart, skin, and pupil—is general among catecholamine-secreting neurons. Inasmuch as other evidence, both physiologic and anatomic,[47] indicates that the sympathetic nervous system modulates sensory input at several levels—including interoceptors and exteroceptors themselves—one result of such a general sympathetic nervous system defect would be a reduction and distortion of incoming stimuli in the simple sociopathic person. In point of fact, both Schoenherr[48] and Herr[49] have already demonstrated an elevated threshold for electric shock in sociopathic prisoners. Such diminution and distortion of sensory data on a chronic basis must markedly modify conditioned responses to emotion-laden stimuli, thereby distorting the attitudes and values erected during the formative years.

It is conceivable and desirable that lesions such as those mentioned could be reversed or at least compensated by medical means. Such medical treatment would probably suffice as a preventive measure when applied prior to the onset of the disease. However, in those in whom detection is delayed until the syndrome has developed, the defect will have influenced behavior already; years of faulty programming would continue to determine behavior even after any original biologic basis had been removed or compensated. Hence, even a medical solution to the sociopathic person's problem would be insufficient. If our assumptions are correct, therapeutic intervention, of necessity, will have to include resocialization.

The issue is far from being resolved. We are still very much in ignorance of the course, mechanisms, and etiology of the behavior pattern and mental status currently called antisocial personality. Despite increased pharmacologic treatment of those designated as sociopathic personalities, the chronically antisocial individual is likely to tax our ingenuity and patience in the foreseeable future to perhaps an even greater extent than in the past. In conclusion, there is considerable room for pessimism, notwithstanding the return of the medical and biologically oriented specialists to the field.

REFERENCES

1. KAELBLING, R AND PATTERSON, R: *Eclectic Psychiatry.* Charles C Thomas, Springfield, IL, 1966, p 371.

2. An excellent summary of these attributions may be found in CLECKLEY, H: *Psychopathic States.* In ARIETI, S (ED): *American Handbook of Psychiatry.* Basic Books, New York, 1962, pp 567-588. See also NOYES, A AND KOLB, I: *Modern Clinical Psychiatry.* WB Saunders, Philadelphia, 1963, pp 460-464; ROBINS, E: *Personality disorders. II. Sociopathic types: Antisocial disorders and sexual deviations.* In FREEMAN, A AND KAPLAN, H (EDS): *Comprehensive Textbook of Psychiatry.* Williams & Wilkins, Baltimore, 1967, pp 955-956; and MCCORD, W AND MCCORD J: *Psychopathy and Delinquency.* Grune & Stratton, New York, 1956, pp 47-81.

3. GREGORY, I: *Psychiatry.* WB Saunders, Philadelphia, 1961, pp 52-67.

4. ROBINS, L: *Deviant Children Grown Up.* Williams & Wilkins, Baltimore, 1966, pp 90-92.

5. GUZE, SB: *Criminality and Psychiatric Disorders.* Oxford University Press, New York, 1975. See also MONAHAN, J AND STEADMAN, HJ: *Crime and mental disorder: An epidemiological approach.* In TONRY, M AND MORRIS, N (EDS): *Crime and Justice.* University of Chicago Press, Chicago, 1983.

6. REDL, F AND WINEMAN, D: *Children Who Hate.* The Free Press, Glencoe, IL, 1951.

7. YABLONSKY, L: *The Violent Gang.* Macmillan, New York, 1962.

8. ROBINS, op cit, p 2; FREEDMAN AND KAPLAN, op cit, p 958; NOYES AND KOLB, op cit, pp 464-465; CLECKLEY, op cit, pp 585-587; MCCARTHY, DJ AND CORRIN, KM: *Medical Treatment of Mental Diseases.* JB Lippincott, Philadelphia, 1955, pp 415-418.

9. MAUGHS, S: *A concept of psychotherapy and psychopathic personality: Its evolution and historical development.* Journal of Criminal Psychopathology 2:465-499, 1941.

10. GAROFALO, R: *Criminology.* Little, Brown & Co, Boston, 1914, p 80.

11. LOMBROSO, C: *Crime: Its Causes and Remedies.* Little, Brown & Co, Boston, 1911, pp 365-366.

12. Ibid, p 423.

13. MAUGHS, op cit, p 487.

14. Quoted in HENDERSON, PK: *Psychopathic States.* WW Norton, New York, 1939, p 27.

15. THOMPSON, GN: *Psychopathy.* Archives of Criminal Psychodynamics 4(2):736-749, 1961.

16. HENDERSON, op cit.

17. HENDERSON, op cit, pp 128-129.

18. CLECKLEY, H: *The Mask of Sanity,* ed 4. CV Mosby, St Louis, 1964.

19. Ibid, pp 363-400.

20. YOCHELSON, S AND SAMENOW, S: *The Criminal Personality.* J Aronson, New York, 1976 (2 vols).

21. GOUGH, H: *A sociological theory of psychopathy.* Am J Sociol 53:359-366, 1948.

22. BAKER, B: Accuracy of Social Perceptions of Psychopathic and Non-Psychopathic

Prison Inmates. Unpublished manuscript, 1954, summarized in SARBIN, TR: *Role theory*. In LINDZEY, C (ED): *Handbook of Social Psychology*. Addison-Wesley, Reading, MA, 1954, p 246.

23. ALBRECHT, R AND SARBIN, TR: Contributions to Role-Taking Theory: Annoyability as a Function of the Self. Unpublished manuscript, 1954, cited in LINDZEY, op cit, p 246.

24. MCCORD AND MCCORD, op cit, p 2.

25. ROBINS, op cit, pp 90-92.

26. Ibid, p 80.

27. MATZA, D: *Poverty and Disrepute*. In MERTON, RK AND NISBET, R (EDS): *Contemporary Social Problems*. Harcourt, Brace & World, New York, 1966, pp 619-669.

28. KAHL, J. *The American Class Structure*. Rinehart & Company, New York, 1957, pp 205-215.

29. KOMAROVSKY, M: *Blue-Collar Marriage*. Random House, New York, 1964.

30. FUNKENSTEIN, DH, GREENBLATT, M, SOLOMON, HC: *Psychophysiological study of mentally ill patients*. Am J Psychiatry 106:359-366, 1949.

31. LYKKEN, DT: *A study of anxiety in the sociopathic personality*. Ph.D. dissertation, University of Minnesota, University Microfilms, Ann Arbor, 1955, No 55-944.

32. SCHACTER, S AND LATANE, B: *Crime, cognition and the autonomic nervous system*. In LEVINE, D (ED): *Nebraska Symposium of Motivation*. University of Nebraska Press, Lincoln, 1964, pp 271-274.

33. LIPPERT, WW: *The electrodermal system of the sociopath*. Ph.D. dissertation, University of Cincinnati, University Microfilms, Ann Arbor, 1965, No 65-12921.

34. HARE, RD: *Psychopathy, autonomic functioning, and the orienting response*. J Abnorm Psychol 73 (Suppl): 1-24, 1968.

35. Personal communication, September 1968.

36. HARE, RD: *Psychopathy*. John Wiley & Sons, New York, 1970, p 33.

37. KILOH, L AND OSSELTON, JW: *Clinical Electroencephalography*. Butterworth, Washington, 1966; LINDSLEY, DB: *The ontogeny of pleasure: Neural and behavioral development*. In HEATH, RG (ED): *The Role of Pleasure in Behavior*. Harper & Row, New York, 1964, pp 3-22; SCHEIBEL, ME AND SCHEIBEL, AB: *Some neural substrates of postnatal development*. In HOFFMAN, M AND HOFFMAN, L (EDS): *Review of Child Development Research*, Vol 1. Russell Sage Foundation, New York, 1954, pp 481-519.

38. HARE, op cit, p 36; LINDNER, LA, GOLDMAN, H, DINITZ, S, ALLEN, HE: *Antisocial personality type with cardiac lability*. Arch Gen Psychiatry 23:260-267, 1970.

39. Cleckley, H, op cit.

40. QUAY, HC: *Psychopathic personality and pathological stimulation seeking*. Am J Psychiatry 122:180-183, 1965; PETRIE, A: *Individuality in Pain and Suffering*. University of Chicago Press, Chicago, 1967; EYSENCK, HJ: *The Biological Basis of Personality*. Charles C Thomas, Springfield, IL, 1967.

41. ROBINS, LN: *Deviant Children Grow Up*. Williams & Wilkins, Baltimore, 1966.

42. HILL, D: *Amphetamine in psychopathic states*. Br J Addiction 44:50-54, 1947.

43. HARE, op cit, p 89.

44. MACCULLOCH, MJ AND FELDMAN, MP: Personality Structure and Its Relation to Success in the Treatment of Homosexuals by Anticipatory Avoidance Conditioning. Unpublished manuscript; HARE, op cit, p 117.

45. HARE, op cit, p118.

46. ALLEN, HE: *Bio-Social Correlates of Two Types of Antisocial Sociopaths*. Ph.D. dissertation, Ohio State University, University Microfilms, Ann Arbor, 1969, No 70-13971; ALLEN, HE, LINDNER, LA, HOLDMAN, H, DINITIZ, S: *The social and bio-medical correlates of sociopathy*. Criminologica 6:68-75, 1969; ALLEN, HE, LINDNER, LA, GOLD-

MAN, H, DINITZ, S: *Hostile and simple sociopaths: An empirical typology.* Criminology 9:27-47, 1971; GOLDMAN, H, LINDNER, L, DINITZ, S, ALLEN, H: *The simple sociopath: Physiologic and sociologic characteristics.* Biol Psychiatry 3:77-83, 1971; LINDNER, LA, GOLDMAN, H, DINITZ, S, ALLEN, H: *Antisocial personality type with cardiac lability.* Arch Gen Psychiatry 23:260-267, 1970; GOLDMAN, H: *Diseases of arousal.* Quaderni di Criminologia Clinica 2:175-194, 1973.

47. BULBRING, E: *Biophysical changes produced by adrenaline and noradrenaline.* In VANE, JR, VOLSTENHOLME, GEW, O'CONNER, M (EDS): *Adrenergic Mechanisms.* Little, Brown & Co, Boston, 1961, pp 275-287; BURN, JH: *The relation of adrenaline to acetylcholine in the nervous system.* Physiol Rev 25:377-394, 1945; CHERNETSKI, KE: *Sympathetic enhancement of peripheral sensory input in the frog.* J Neurophysiol 27:493-515, 1964; ELDRED, E, SCHNITZLEIN, HN, BUCHWALD, J: *Response of muscle spindles to stimulation of the sympathetic trunk.* Exp Neurol 2:187-195, 1960; LOWENSTEIN, WR AND ALTIMIRANO-ORREGO, R: *Enhancement of activity in a paciniam corpuscle by sympathomimetic agents.* Nature 178:1292-1293, 1956; BEIDLER, LM: *Mechanisms of gustatory and olfactory receptor stimulation.* In ROSENBLITH, WA (ED): *Sensory Communication.* John Wiley & Sons and MIT Press, New York and Cambridge, MA, 1961, pp 294-307; RODRIGUEZ-PEREZ, AP: *On the existence of accessory unmyelinated fibers in the Meissner's corpuscles of the pulp of the human toe.* Dermatologica 129:468-474, 1964.

48. SCHOENHERR, J: *Avoidance of noxious stimulation in psychopathic personality.* Ph.D. dissertation, UCLA; University Microfilms, Ann Arbor, 1965, No 64-8334.

49. HARE, RD: *Detection threshold for electric shock in psychopaths.* J Abnorm Psychol 73:268-272, 1968.

CHAPTER 18

DISORDERS OF IMPULSE CONTROL: EXPLOSIVE DISORDERS, PATHOLOGICAL GAMBLING, PYROMANIA, AND KLEPTOMANIA

Spyros J. Monopolis, M.D.
John R. Lion, M.D.

The disorders of impulse control are a group of clinical syndromes described in the third edition of the American Psychiatric Association's *Diagnostic and Statistical Manual of Mental Disorders (DSM III)*.[1] There are five categories of these disorders: the intermittent explosive disorder, the isolated explosive disorder, pyromania, kleptomania, and pathologic gambling. A sixth category, the atypical impulse control disorder, is also listed but reserved for conditions that clearly do not fall into the above; these "atypical" categories exist in many of the affective and thought disorder conditions described within the manual and allow for the diagnosis of unusual syndromes that may ultimately shape more specific clinical entities. This chapter will review briefly each of the existing clinical syndromes and comment on their diagnostic features and utility.

GENERAL COMMENTS

At the onset, it should be noted that the disorders of impulse control are a heterogeneous group of entities, quite different from each other and linked only by the common characteristics of (a) a failure to resist an impulse, drive, or temptation that gives rise to the act, (b) psychological tension that rises until the act is committed, and (c) some sense of relief or release upon completion of the act or a sense of gratification or pleasure during the act or thereafter. These characteristics are listed in the manual as inherent features of the impulse disorders, yet they pose certain problems for the practitioner, clinician, or forensic expert. For example, "failure to resist an impulse" is a controversial concept. Does this mean that the behavior is unpremeditated? Temper outbursts usually seem unpremeditated; but pyromania, shoplifting, and pathologic gambling involve degrees of willful planning and foresight. Thus the basic tenet of these disorders representing a capitulation to an impulse or a temptation is problematic. The matter of there being an increased sense of tension before the impulsive act and an experience of pleasure or "release" during or after the commission of the act is also somewhat questionable. From the clinical standpoint, tension and release do not invariably occur. For example, persons exhibiting explosive temper outbursts may experience tension prior to their violence, but pleasure is rarely present during the act itself or thereafter; rage or guilt are common emotions as sequelae.

TERMINOLOGICAL DIFFICULTIES

On reviewing the disorders of impulse control, one is immediately struck with the different heritage of terms and the varying data bases surrounding the entities. The intermittent explosive disorder, for example, represents a transplant of the old "explosive personality" described in the second edition of the *Diagnostic and Statistical Manual (DSM II)*. The explosive personality was a rather sturdy entity most clinicians agreed upon.[2] Yet the characterologic terms posed contradictions for members of the American Psychiatric Association Task Force on Nomenclature who focused on observable behavior. An explosive personality was not always explosive; in fact, over a period of time it was rarely so. Virtually all explosive personalities interviewed by clinicians were "nonexplosive" at the time of their office visit (this is not to say that they were free of other characterologic traits). Therefore, how could one call this person explosive? Paranoid personalities, in contrast, seem to be more consistently paranoid, and schizoid individuals seem to be usually aloof. Obviously representing a rather statistical view of psychopathological base rates, such was the reasoning behind the deliberations resulting in the latest *Diagnostic and Statistical Manual;* the net result was to take the explosiveness of the explosive personality and redefine the latter as a disorder of impulse control. The term was also neurologized, so to speak, and made a limbic system disturbance. This reflected experience some task force members and consultants had with this disorder and with the study of aggression.

In juxtaposition to the intermittent explosive disorder, pathological gambling was introduced as an entirely fresh entity. Historically, there existed a literature on the topic of gambling, but it was predominantly found in case reports psychoanalytic in nature. A much larger and more scientific literature exists on the subjects of episodic dyscontrol,[3] violence and aggression,[4-6] and brain dysfunction,[7-8] all of which helped shape the entity of the intermittent explosive disorder.

Pyromania and kleptomania had more traditional roots in the history of psychiatry, again mainly the focus of psychoanalytic interest. Because the two entities reflected observable behavior that had underpinnings of psychological dysfunction, they were itemized as disorders of impulse control.

Some entities among the impulse disorders seem more sensible than others in terms of reflecting clinical practice. Pyromaniac patients are not uncommonly seen in general psychiatric or forensic institutions, but kleptomaniacs are uncommon. Patients with the intermittent explosive disorder are often perceived as having behavior disturbances more appropriately the domain of the criminal justice system than the province of clinical psychiatry.

Pathological gambling, however, is probably the most questionable construct, at least in theory, when offered as a defense of insanity. To some extent, the entity is similar to the term pathologic intoxication in *DSM II*, now called idiosyncratic alcohol intoxication in *DSM III*. Here, the prefix "pathologic" denoted a qualitatively different form of behavior characterized not by simple drunkenness but by a form of intoxication liberated by minimal alcohol intake and involving central nervous system manifestations.

Most critics skeptical of the term pathological gambling ask, "What, then, is normal gambling?" The question is not easy to answer from the viewpoint of clinical medicine; it would appear that pathological gambling is simply a losing form of gambling, representative of bad luck coupled with a driven compulsiveness that can be observed. Suffice it to say that the fate of this term for any future manual is unclear.

The disorders of impulse control are not the only entities to suffer from inconsistencies in diagnostic rigor. Some personality disorders are just as variable. For example, the avoidant personality is described almost poetically in *DSM III* as a disorder "in which there is a hypersensitivity to potential rejection, humiliation, or shame; an unwillingness to enter into relationships unless given unusually strong guarantees of uncritical acceptance; social withdrawal in spite of a desire for affection and acceptance; and low self-esteem." In sharp contrast, the antisocial personality has numerous qualifying parameters such as "truancy (positive if it amounted to at least five days per year for at least two years, not including the last year of school)" or "inability to sustain consistent work behavior as indicated by . . . too frequent job changes (e.g., three or more jobs in five years not accounted for by nature of job or economic or seasonal fluctuation)."

The lesson to be learned here is that the criteria for some diagnoses in the manual are very hard, some quite soft. The same is obviously true with the disorders of impulse control. As will be seen from the diagnostic criteria for all the disorders of impulse control, other major psychopathology has to be excluded; affective, thought, behavior, and personality disorders should **not** be the basis for the specific impulse disorder. In other words, a patient's kleptomaniac activities should not be due to a schizophrenic disorder in which he or she may be delusional and hence steal articles of some delusionally symbolic worth. Kleptomania should not be due to antisocial propensities in which stealing is part of a criminal's life, and the intermittent explosive disorder should not be due to a conduct disturbance, such as an attention deficit disorder in which there is generalized impulsivity. In clinical practice, however, these distinctions are difficult to make, and the forensic expert may indeed see a patient who engages in kleptomaniac activities and who has a history of schizophrenia but who is not actively psychotic at the time of the commission of the kleptomaniac act. The same is true of pyromania; mental retardation may coexist, or the patient may have schizoid traits. The differential diagnosis may thus be problematic. Psychological testing may be useful to detect or to substantiate an underlying thought disorder, organicity, or other major psychopathology.

INSANITY DEFENSE ISSUES

Little objective data exist on the matter of how often the disorders of impulse control are used as the basis for an insanity defense. Ratner and Shapiro[9] have indicated the successful use on a few occasions of episodic behavior disorders[3] as legal exculpation for violent crime. The term episodic behavior disorder is, however, not synonymous with any particular disorder of impulse control but is an all-inclusive description of a wide range of behaviors that include affective, thought, and behavior disturbances. These are all paroxysmal in nature, thought to be epileptoid in etiology. Pyromania and kleptomania are rather distinctive clinical entities, and both have been used as the basis for insanity pleas, though precise statistics are not available with respect to frequency of such use. Pathological gambling is so subtly different from "nonpathologic" gambling that one might wonder about its viability for an insanity defense. Yet McGarry[10] indicates that the term has served as a basis for insanity pleas at trial court level in three states and in two federal jurisdictions. Furthermore, the plea has led to insanity acquittals in two states and a hung jury in two others. Although McGarry is tolerant of the clinical entity of pathological gambling, he feels it illogical to assume that the lack of volitional control over the isolated act of gambling is the same as the lack of such control over the criminal acts carried out in the service of the impulse to gamble. McGarry is thus critical of the exculpatory use of the term and forecasts that such use will ultimately not be sustained by the appellate courts of this country.

INTERMITTENT EXPLOSIVE DISORDER

Clinical Features

This condition refers to patients who have sudden and paroxysmally recurring outbursts of impulsive violence. The outbursts come on without clear warning and remit quickly; in common parlance, the term "temper" would be used to describe the rage attacks. Patients who demonstrate the intermittent explosive disorder overrespond to stimuli and react to some social situations with all-or-none behavior. They have difficulties with the modulation of anger and become physically aggressive toward persons or property. Between the outbursts of rage, they often appear calm, peaceful, and even reflective. The diagnostic criteria of the illness are excerpted below from the current *Diagnostic and Statistical Manual*.[1]

Diagnosis

    A. Several discrete episodes of loss of control of aggressive impulses resulting in serious assault or destruction of property.
    B. Behavior that is grossly out of proportion to any precipitating psychosocial stressor.
    C. Absence of signs of generalized impulsivity or aggressiveness between episodes.
    D. Not due to Schizophrenia, Antisocial Personality Disorder, or Conduct Disorder.

Etiology, Pathogenesis, Dynamics

The above features are purely descriptive. As previously mentioned, there is little statistical or systematic empirical basis for this disorder, and the qualifying parameters are clinical descriptions. Men are more likely to demonstrate this disorder than are women. The complications of the illness seem rather obvious and include penal incarceration and hospitalization. The disorder commonly makes its appearance in the second or third decade of life. No clinical course is outlined in *DSM III*.

The neurological flavoring of the diagnosis has already been alluded to with regard to the biology of aggression. In this matter of temper, some clinical data have suggested that organic factors play a role in some expressions of aggression in man, especially paroxysmal outbursts in intermittent explosive disorders. Thus in *DSM III*, certain neurologic features are described as important. These include historical antecedents to temper outbursts, such as head injuries or hyperactivity, or predisposing factors such as perinatal trauma and encephalitis. Evidence of organic brain dysfunction or actual seizure states manifested by alterations in consciousness, confusion, or memory deficits are relevant. Inasmuch as epilepsy is often accompanied by subjective symptoms like changes in taste or smell, followed by drowsiness or amnesia, these symptoms are also mentioned in the manual. Laboratory tests may be of value in the diagnosis of the intermittent explosive disorder. A sleep electroencephalogram (EEG) may reveal paroxysmal discharges or a spike focus indicative of brain dysfunction. Neurologic examination for "soft signs" and psychological tests for organicity may detect underlying cortical dysfunction that plays a role in the patient's aggressive outbursts. In summary, the etiology of the intermittent explosive disorder is seen as partially organic and its pathogenesis reflective of central nervous system dysfunction.

Many conditions mimic this disorder. The differential diagnosis thus includes the antisocial personality, dissociative disorders, psychotic disorders, attention deficit disorder, and an organic brain syndrome.

Despite little knowledge about this disorder, its inclusion in *DSM III* is extremely important and acknowledges that aggression may be a subject for study by clinicians. Psychiatrists have long been reluctant to study violent patients and have relegated them to the disciplines of criminology and sociology. Thus it may facilitate the understanding of aggression to include the intermittent explosive disorder among conventional mental disease entities.

The only existing literature on the intermittent explosive disorder pertains to the matter of precision of diagnosis, using official nomenclature. Monopolis and Lion[11] have studied 20 cases of the disorder among 830 admissions to a general psychiatric unit over a 2-year period (an incidence of 2.4 percent). Cases of intermittent explosive disorder were found to be diagnosed principally in reference to the basic diagnostic criteria cited in this chapter. With the exception of the EEG, few clinicians used neurologic indices for identifying their cases, despite the manual's emphasis of these organic factors as associated features of the disorder.

A number of authors have studied what is tantamount to the intermittent explosive disorder without calling it by that name. Monroe[3] has devoted a portion of his monograph on episodic behavior disorders to a description of patients who have recurring repetitive outbursts of temper or atypical mood or thought disorders reflective of limbic system dysfunction. Bach-y-Rita and coworkers[12] have described patients with recurring outbursts of rage and drawn attention to recurring clinical features of these individuals.

Treatment

Unlike case reports for the treatment of kleptomania or pathologic gambling, little literature exists for the specific treatment of the intermittent explosive disorder. But there is a vast literature pertaining to the treatment of aggressive individuals, many of whom do not have a crisply defined intermittent explosive disorder yet suffer from aggressive tempers. Treatment for the specific intermittent explosive disorder relies upon drugs and psychotherapy. In regard to drugs, a variety of pharmacologic agents have been used, most with the rationale that outbursts of temper reflect an epileptoid disorder, hence the drug of choice is an anticonvulsant.[13] Most recently, carbamazepine has been used as an agent to control limbic system kindling and temper.[14] Lion[15] has described the basic strategy underlying the psychotherapeutic treatment of impulsive aggression and indicates that there are two strategies in the treatment of such patients. First, these patients need to be aware of anger as it builds up so that they can identify it as early as possible and verbalize their feelings. Impulsive patients generally have an impoverished affective awareness and tend to translate the premonitory mood associated with physical violence into some kind of adverse behavior such as drinking, often to quench the incipient rage. The drinking, in turn, exacerbates the violence. Second, Lion emphasizes the need to teach people to fantasize the outcome of a violent act. Cognitive appreciation for the sequelae of an aggressive outburst is an essential prerequisite for violence-prone patients' control of their impulsivity. These patients tend to act first and think afterward and need to be retrained to reflect on the consequences of their violence. Pschodynamic factors are also important because patients with violent tempers are sensitive to conflicts over sexuality, body size, or territoriality.

Patients manifesting the intermittent explosive disorder often become convicted of criminal assault. Many see little need for any kind of psychiatric treatment and perceive their temper outbursts as simply a part of their personality. Court-mandated therapy is thus a useful means of propelling them into a treatment program which may ultimately attenuate their violent propensities. Lion and coworkers[16] have described outpatient group psychotherapy as a useful modality of treatment for these patients.

ISOLATED EXPLOSIVE DISORDER

Clinical Features

This disorder will be mentioned only briefly because it is so rare. The disorder refers to a single outburst of rage, an outburst of catastrophic proportions but one which cannot be classified as psychotic. The diagnosis would seem to be a difficult one to make, though anecdotally many clinicians recall hearing of patients who have "gone amok" and committed a heinously violent act such as a mass murder. The condition has been described by Menninger[17] in his accounts of the "third order of dyscontrol" and, earlier, by Wertham,[18] who used the expression "catathymic crisis." Both authors refer to a single and isolated assaultive or destructive rage which may build up over a period of time within the individual and then erupt into overt behavior. Megargee[19] has described the "overcontrolled" personality who is very rigid and guarded and who is prone to an unmodulated and explosive outburst of rage. Formal literature on the forensic aspects of the isolated explosive disorder is lacking.

The diagnostic criteria for this condition are excerpted below from *DSM III*[1]:

Diagnosis

A. A single, discrete episode in which failure to resist an impulse led to a single, violent, externally directed act that had a catastrophic impact on others.

B. The degree of aggressivity expressed during the episode was grossly out of proportion to any precipitating psychosocial stressor.

C. Before the episode there were no signs of generalized impulsivity or aggressiveness.

D. Not due to Schizophrenia, Antisocial Personality Disorder, or Conduct Disorder.

Etiology, Pathogenesis, Dynamics

Little is known or has been described regarding the above factors in this disease process. Although the violent act is often bizarre or senseless and typically involves victims unknown to the assailant, isolated accounts of this disorder often reveal that the perpetrator was under great emotional stress. He may have translated an intolerable intrapsychic crisis into an isolated behavioral act which represented the ultimate discharge of murderous rage without evidence or development of a psychosis. These accounts, however, are speculations after the fact; the isolated explosive disorder has not been sufficiently studied to validate any recurring dynamics or etiological factors. As such, its appearance in *DSM III* could be regarded as tentative.

Treatment

No specific therapy is identified for the disorder; because the outburst of violence occurs just once, treatment obviously would be dictated by the specifics of the individual case, and hospitalization would seem to be in order to reach appropriate clinical understanding.

PYROMANIA

Clinical Features

This condition refers to patients who feel compelled to set fires repeatedly and for no monetary or overtly retributive gain. The fire setting is a highly symbolic act in the mind of the fire setter and, unlike arson, is a seemingly purposeless act that is carried out impulsively. There appear to be no clearly associated psychiatric disturbances in these patients. The diagnostic criteria of the illness are excerpted below from *DSM III*.[1]

Diagnosis

A. Recurrent failure to resist impulses to set fires.

B. Increasing sense of tension before setting the fire.

C. An experience of either intense pleasure, gratification, or release at the time of committing the act.

D. Lack of motivation, such as monetary gain or sociopolitical ideology, for setting fires.

E. Not due to an Organic Mental Disorder, Schizophrenia, Antisocial Personality Disorder, or Conduct Disorder.

Etiology, Pathogenesis, Dynamics

A large and descriptive literature exists on pyromania, mostly psychoanalytic in nature, highly theoretical, and based on isolated case reports. Freud[20] linked fire setting to enuresis and later saw the act as a masturbatory equivalent, and Fenichel[21] more explicitly identified pyromania with urethral eroticism. Other early writers, like Stekel,[22] described what they felt to be an association between fire setting and sadism or homosexuality. Later investigators who interviewed children fire setters commented more globally on the extensive family pathology present in the cases they saw and reported that fire setting often occurred after the child witnessed parental infidelity or sexual intercourse between parents.[23,24] Yarnell[25] found that latency age children (ages 6 to 12 years) who set fires had fantasies about burning a family member who had either withheld love from them or was a rival for the love of the parents. They set fires in or close to their home. Associated behavior problems among this group of children included running away, truancy, stealing, aggression, and learning disabilities. Enuresis was frequently present.

Incidence and prevalence statistics vary widely in different published series. The term "fire setting" is often used interchangeably with "pyromania," thus confusing the data. In a heterogeneous series of 1145 fire setters seen in a variety of clinical settings by Lewis and Yarnell,[26] these authors found that two thirds of the individuals were men over the age of 16, and only 13 percent were girls or women. The peak incidence was at the age of 17. Monkemoeller[27] reported that 37 percent of his series of fire setters were females. Vandersall and Wiener[28] reported that among 660 children seen in an outpatient clinic, 2.1 percent were fire setters; whether these children set fires for revenge or money or were pyromaniacs is unknown. In looking at Lewis and Yarnell's data,[26] it appears that about 40 percent of their series represented true pyromaniacs.

Much attention has been given to the clinical triad of enuresis, pyromania, and cruelty to animals as indicative of future criminal violence; however, more recent empirical data[29] has shown this triad to have no predictive value.

Neurological impairment accompanied by poor academic achievement and borderline intellectual functioning has been described among fire setters as a whole.[30] Kuhnley and coworkers[31] reported a high frequency of attention deficit disorder among fire setting children. Vandersall and Wiener[28] noticed that school failure was common, and Yarnell[25] and Lewis and Yarnell[26] remarked that fire setters may have below normal intelligence.

Pyromaniac patients have been observed by some clinicians to be regularly present at neighborhood fires and find particular fascination with fire-fighting apparatus. They may become involved in setting off false alarms. In Lewis and Yarnell's[26] series of firesetters, 5 percent were reported to have set the fire merely to extinguish it themselves or to watch it extinguished, hence drawing attention to the often-cited association between firemen and pyromaniacs. In fact, no data exist regarding the representation of firemen among either general fire setters or true pyromaniacs. Sexual satisfaction or masturbation or orgasm during the watching or setting of fires is rarely present.

A number of behaviors mimic true pyromania and thus need to be considered in the differential diagnosis. These would include normal play behavior by children, conduct disorders, antisocial personality, and criminal arson.

Treatment

Pyromaniac people as a group are usually resistant to treatment because of their poor motivation, denial, lack of insight, and resistance to assuming responsibility for their actions. They are also very passive, and it is difficult in therapeutic work to confirm the psychodynamics that are presumed to underlie the etiology of the behavior. The use of intensive individual psychotherapy has been reported by Macht and Mack;[32] however, no follow-up data have been reported.

Psychiatric hospitalization may provide the needed protective environment to treat underlying psychopathology and may help the patient cope with destructive urges. According to published accounts of case reports, outpatient treatment and probation supervision for long periods are necessary in order to prevent recurrences of the pyromaniac activity.[32-35]

KLEPTOMANIA

Clinical Features

This condition refers to individuals who experience an impulse to steal objects that they neither need nor wish to keep or to sell. Although kleptomaniacs break the law in the commission of their acts, they are not antisocial. The object stolen is often one of symbolic significance to the patient. Kleptomaniacs usually act alone and without accomplices. They steal objects such as books, undergarments, or even food, although they carry money with them. Some kleptomaniac patients are reported to return the stolen item secretly or to dispose of it, but most evidently keep such items. As in the case of pyromania, no consistent psychiatric disorders are associated with this group of patients. The diagnostic criteria of the illness are excerpted below from *DSM III*.[1]

Diagnosis

A. Recurrent failure to resist impulses to steal objects that are not for immediate use or their monetary value.
B. Increasing sense of tension before committing the act.
C. An experience of either pleasure or release at the time of committing the theft.

D. Stealing is done without long-term planning and assistance from, or collaboration with, others.

E. Not due to Conduct Disorder or Antisocial Personality Disorder.

Etiology, Pathogenesis, Dynamics

Kleptomania, like pyromania, has been primarily the focus of psychoanalytic writers who have studied isolated causes and reported on psychodynamic considerations. Thus Wimmer[36] talked of the role of hunger and orgasm among the kleptomaniac patients, and Abrahamson[37] classified the disease as a neurotic entity, similar to nymphomania or pyromania. Anna Freud[38] considered stealing as rooted in the early "oneness" between mother and child.

Winer and Pollock[39] have described the repetitive course of kleptomania, pointing out that the urge to steal waxes and wanes within an individual and may be a function of his or her internal conflicts. Other workers[40, 41] have described autonomic sensations that accompany the shoplifting episodes such an anxiety, perspiration, or dyspnea, although it would seem that such symptoms are quite nonspecific and common to any endeavor that has legal consequences for the individual concerned. Remorse or guilt following an episode of kleptomania has been described, but this would also seem to suffer from the same criticisms as above.

The terms "kleptomania" and "shoplifting" have been used synonomously (but erroneously) as though the two were the same entities. Thus it is difficult to discern in the published literature which statistics apply to true kleptomaniac patients and which to criminal shoplifters. Arieff and Bowie[42] indicated that in a 5-year period, 77 percent of shoplifting cases studied in a psychiatric hospital had a psychiatric diagnosis (psychoneurosis, mental deficiency, psychosis, or organic disorder). Meyers[40] emphasized the marked disturbance in the sexual lives of shoplifters, as well as the presence of somatic symptoms and signs such as headache, respiratory symptoms, or gastrointestinal disturbances. In a 5-year study of female shoplifters brought to court, Gibbens, Palmer, and Prince[43] found that about 15 percent had a history of previous inpatient mental treatment. Schizophrenia, depression, manic-depressive illness, psychotherapy, and alcoholism were the most common diagnoses. Meyers[40] observed that the majority of male shoplifters were single and that female offenders were married. Men stole books much more frequently than did women.

The main condition that plays a role in the differential diagnosis is a criminal stealing in which there is obvious gain and clear planning. Conduct disorders and the antisocial personality must also be considered in the differential diagnosis.

Treatment

Unfortunately, the available literature on kleptomania usually consists of single case reports or small series of cases.[44-47] No systematic studies have been undertaken. On the basis of clinical knowledge about the tendency for kleptomaniacs to repeat the act, some form of court-mandated psychiatric treatment would seem warranted.

PATHOLOGICAL GAMBLING

Clinical Features

This condition refers to compulsive involvement in gambling with concomitant deterioration in personal and social functioning. The gambler gives up all else in life and concentrates mainly on winning or gaining restitution of debts incurred through gambling. Pathological gamblers are unable to stop their activities but spiral ever downward to the point of confrontation by legal authorities. The diagnostic criteria of the illness are excerpted below from *DSM III*.[1]

Diagnosis

    A. The individual is chronically and progressively unable to resist impulses to gamble.

    B. Gambling compromises, disrupts, or damages family, personal, and vocational pursuits, as indicated by at least three of the following:

        1. arrest for forgery, fraud, embezzlement, or income tax evasion due to attempts to obtain money for gambling.
        2. default on debts or other financial responsibilities.
        3. disrupted family or spouse relationship due to gambling.
        4. borrowing of money from illegal sources (loan sharks).
        5. inability to account for loss of money or to produce evidence of winning money, if this is claimed.
        6. loss of work due to absenteeism in order to pursue gambling activity.
        7. necessity for another person to provide money to relieve a desperate financial situation.

    C. The gambling is not due to Antisocial Personality Disorder.

Etiology, Pathogenesis, Dynamics

Most of the older literature pertaining to gambling comes from psychoanalytic writers. Very small series or isolated case reports form the bulk of these descriptions. Freud[48] viewed gambling as a repetition of the childhood compulsion to masturbate, and Bergler[49] commented on the gambler's unconscious desire to lose. Other writers have talked in general terms about the unconscious determinants of winning or losing or the need to appease others or to be appeased by luck.

    Writing about current views of gambling, Custer[50] based his experience on a Veterans Administration service for compulsive gamblers. He felt that only a minority of the treated population were neurotic. However, precise figures on this aspect of diagnosis are lacking. Moran[51] described neurotic, impulsive, and psychopathic gamblers in a survey of 50 pathological gamblers referred for psychiatric treatment.

Pathological gambling is more common among men than among women.[1] Pathological gambling and alcoholism are more common in the fathers of men and in the mothers of women with the disorder than in the general population.[1] Custer[52] estimates that there are several million "compulsive" gamblers in the United States. No other data are available for the specific disorder of pathological gambling; the demographics of gambling in general have been studied, one source being a 1975 survey done at the University of Michigan, cited by Custer,[50] and another cited by Moran.[53]

The stages of the development of the pathological gambler have been described by Dupouy and Chatagnon[54] as consisting of initiation, habituation, suffering, and impairment. The authors discuss the fact that most gamblers are introduced to this activity by friends or relatives. Petty gambling usually starts in early adolescence. Serious gambling begins around age 17. According to Custer,[52] there appear to be three phases in the development of pathological gambling: (1) *Winning phase*—the gambler wins at the beginning of his career. (2) *Losing phase*—eventually he or she experiences failures. In order to make up for the losses, the gambler starts betting amounts of money that deplete personal resources and he or she becomes increasingly indebted to others. Excuses and lying are frequent. Work attendance and productivity are diminished. Family relationships deteriorate. The pressure of lenders increases. (3) *Desperation phase*—over time, occupational, family, social aspects of the gambler's life deteriorate further. Eventually the inability to pay excessive debts leads to illegal activities, such as forgery, embezzlement, income tax evasion, fraud, or robbery. It may take from 1 to 20 years to reach this stage of desperation, but the average is 5 years.

According to Lesieur,[55] as options diminish, the compulsive gambler becomes entrapped in an extremely powerful and panic-ridden state that leads with certainty to personal downfall.

Forensic experts may have difficulty distinguishing pathological gambling from "nonpathological" gambling. In the former, the patient usually has no antisocial history and has a good work history until such time as the gambling takes hold. Predatory or psychopathic traits are absent, and the patient usually is conscientious in all other areas of life. Other differential diagnoses include malingering and conduct disorder. Some patients develop a true euphoria as they gamble and do not eat or sleep; in time, the full-blown clinical picture of mania is seen. Thus affective disorders, such as manic-depressive disorder, are in the differential diagnosis.

Treatment

A host of techniques has been used with pathological gamblers, including psychoanalysis,[49] group therapy,[56] and isolated case reports of behavior modification paradigms.[57, 58] The program developed by Custer consists of inpatient treatment with outpatient follow-up. Hospitalization lasts 3 to 4 weeks and consists of various psychosocial treatment modalities.[50, 52]

Pathological gambling is a chronic and incapacitating psychosocial disorder that requires long-term intervention. Modeled after other addiction treatments, Gamblers Anonymous (GA) was founded in Los Angeles in 1957. It is a self-help organization of pathological gamblers helping each other with abstinence.[59] Pokorny[60] found that spouses played a crucial role in the illness of pathological gambling and affected the outcome of therapy. Gam-Anon and Gam-a-Teen provide gamblers' spouses and children opportunity for therapy.

Once identified as a pathologic gambler, the individual patient requires some form of court supervision in order to remain in treatment.

REFERENCES

1. *Diagnostic and Statistical Manual of Mental Disorders,* ed 3. American Psychiatric Association, Washington, DC, 1980.
2. LION, JR (ED): *Personality Disorders: Diagnosis and Management (revised for DSM III),* ed 2. Williams & Wilkins, Baltimore, 1981.
3. MONROE, RR: *Episodic Behavior Disorders: A Psychodynamic and Neurophysiologic Analysis.* Harvard University Press, Cambridge, MA, 1970.
4. AMERICAN PSYCHIATRIC ASSOCIATION: *Clinical Aspects of the Violent Individual, Task Force Report #8.* American Psychiatric Association, Washington, DC, July 1974.
5. LION, JR: *Evaluation and Management of the Violent Patient.* Charles C Thomas, Springfield, IL, 1972.
6. LION, JR AND PENNA, M: *The study of human aggression.* In WHALEN, R (ED): *The Neuropsychology of Aggression.* Plenum Press, New York, 1974, pp 165-184.
7. MARK, VH AND ERVIN, FR: *Violence and the Brain.* Harper & Row, New York, 1970.
8. SWEET, WH, ERVIN, FR, MARK, VH: *The relationship of violent behavior to focal cerebral disease.* In GARATTINI, S AND SIGGS, EG (EDS): *Aggressive Behavior.* John Wiley & Sons, New York, 1969, pp 336-352.
9. RATNER, R AND SHAPIRO, D: *The episodic dyscontrol syndrome and criminal responsibility.* Bull Am Acad Psychiatry Law 7:422-432, 1979.
10. MCGARRY, AL: *Pathological gambling: A new insanity defense.* Bull Am Acad Psychiatry Law 11:301-308, 1983.
11. MONOPOLIS, S AND LION, JR: *Problems in the diagnosis of intermittent explosive disorder.* Am J Psychiatry 140:1200-1202, 1983.
12. BACH-Y-RITA, G, LION, JR, CLIMENT, C, ET AL: *Episodic dyscontrol: A study of 130 violent patients.* Am J Psychiatry 127:1473, 1971.
13. MONROE, RR: *Anticonvulsants in the treatment of aggression.* J Nerv Ment Dis 160:119-126, 1974.
14. TUNKS, ER AND DERMER, SW: *Carbamazepine in the dyscontrol syndrome associated with limbic system dysfunction.* J Nerv Ment Dis 164:56-63, 1977.
15. LION, JR: *The role of depression in the treatment of aggressive personality disorders.* Am J Psychiatry 129:347-349, 1972.
16. LION, JR, CHRISTOPHER, R, MADDEN, DJ: *A group approach with violent outpatients.* Int J Group Psychother 27:67-74, 1977.
17. MENNINGER, K: *The Vital Balance.* Viking Press, New York, 1963.
18. WERTHAM, F: *The Show of Violence.* Doubleday, New York, 1949.
19. MEGARGEE, EI: *Undercontrolled and overcontrolled personality types in extreme antisocial aggression.* Psychological Monographs: General and Applied 80(3): Whole No. 611, 1966, pp 1-29.
20. FREUD, S: *Civilization and its discontents.* In STARCHEY, J (ED): *The Complete Psychological Works of Sigmund Freud,* vol 21. Hogarth Press, London, 1961, p 59.
21. FENICHEL, O: *The Psychoanalytic Theory of Neurosis.* WW Norton, New York, 1945, pp 371-372.
22. STEKEL, W: *Peculiarities of Behavior.* Liveright, New York, 1924, pp 124-181.

23. SIMMEL, E: *Incendiarism*. In EISSLER, K (ED):*Searchlights on Delinquency.* International University Press, New York, 1949, pp 90-101.

24. KAUFMAN, I, HEIMS, LW, REISER, DE: *A re-evalution of the psychodynamics of firesetting.* Am J Orthopsychiatry 31:123-136, 1961.

25. YARNELL, H: *Firesetting in children.* Am J Orthopsychiatry 10:272-286, 1940.

26. LEWIS, NDC AND YARNELL, H: *Pathological Firesetting.* Nervous and Mental Diseases Monograph #82:8-26, 1951.

27. MONKEMOELLER, X: *Zur Psychopathologie des Brandstifters.* Hans Gross Archiv Kriminal-Authropologie Kriminalistik 48:193, 1912.

28. VANDERSALL, TA AND WIENER, JM: *Children who set fires.* Arch Gen Psychiatry 22:63-71, 1970.

29. JUSTICE, B, JUSTICE, R, KRAFT, IA: *Early warning signs of violence: Is a triad enough?* Am J Psychiatry 131: 457-459, 1974.

30. MAVROMATIS, M AND LION, JR: *A primer in pyromania.* Diseases of the Nervous System 38:954-955, 1977.

31. KUHNLEY, EJ, HENDREN, RL, QUINLAN, DM: *Firesetting by children.* J Am Acad Child Psychiat 21:560-563, 1982.

32. MACHT LB AND MACK, JE: *The firesetter syndrome.* Psychiatry 31:277-288, 1968.

33. STEWART, MA AND CULVER, KW: *Children who set fires: The clinical picture and a follow-up.* Br J Psychiatry 140:357-363, 1982.

34. KOSON, DF AND DVOSKIN, J: *Arson: A diagnostic study.* Bull Am Acad Psychiatry Law 10:39-49, 1982.

35. FINE, S AND LOUIE, D: *Juvenile firesetters: Do the agencies help?* Am J Psychiatry 136:433-435, 1979.

36. WIMMER, A: *De la kleptomanie.* Ann Med Psychol 79:1-12, 1921.

37. ABRAHAMSON, D: *The Psychology of Crime.* Columbia University Press, New York, 1960.

38. FREUD, A: *Normality and Pathology in Childhood.* International University Press, New York, 1965.

39. WINER, JA AND POLLOCK, GH: *Disorders of impulse control.* In KAPLAN, HI, FREEDMAN, AM, SADOCK, BJ (EDS): *Comprehensive Textbook of Psychiatry/III.* Williams & Wilkins, Baltimore, 1980, pp 1817-1829.

40. MEYERS, TJ: *A contribution to the psychopathology of shoplifting.* J Forensic Sci 15:295-310, 1970.

41. DUPOUY, R: *La kleptomanie.* Journal de Psychologie Normale et Pathologique 2:404-426, 1905.

42. ARIEFF, AJ AND BOWIE, CG: *Some psychiatric aspects of shoplifting.* Journal of Clinical Psychopathology 8:565-576, 1967.

43. GIBBENS, TCN, PALMER, C, PRINCE, J: *Mental health aspects of shoplifting.* Br Med J 3:612-615, 1971.

44. ZAVITSIANOS, G: *The kleptomaniacs and female criminality.* In SCHLESINGER, LB AND REVITCH, E (EDS): *Sexual Dynamics of Anti-Social Behavior.* Charles C Thomas, Springfield, IL, 1983, pp 132-158.

45. SOCARIDES, CW: *Pathological stealing as a reparative move of the ego.* Psychoanal Rev 41:246-252, 1954.

46. ALLEN, A: *Stealing as a defense.* Psychoanal Q 34:572-583, 1955.

47. MARZAGAO, LR: *Systemic desensitization treatment of kleptomania.* J Behav Ther Exp Psychiatry 3:327-328, 1972.

48. FREUD, S: *Dostoevsky and parricide.* In STARCHEY, J (ED): *The Complete Psychological Works of Sigmund Freud,* vol 21. Hogarth Press, London, 1961, pp 177-194.

49. BERGLER, E: *The Psychology of Gambling.* Harrison, London, 1958.

50. CUSTER, RL: *Gambling and addiction.* In CRAIG, RJ AND BAKER, SL (EDS): *Drug Dependent Patients.* Charles C Thomas, Springfield, IL, 1982, pp 367-381.

51. MORAN, E: *Varieties of pathological gambling.* Br J Psychiatry 116:593-597, 1970.

52. CUSTER, RL: *An overview of compulsive gambling.* Carrier Foundation Letter 59, February 1980, Carrier Foundation, Belle Mead, NJ.

53. MORAN, E: *An assessment of the report of the royal commission on gambling 1976-1978.* Br J Addict 74:3-9, 1979.

54. DUPOUY, R AND CHATAGNON, P: *Le joueur. Esquisse psychologique.* Ann Med Psychol 87:102-112, 1929.

55. LESIEUR, HR: *The Chase Career of the Compulsive Gambler.* Anchor Press/Doubleday, New York, 1977.

56. BOYD, WH AND BOLEN, DW: *The compulsive gambler and spouse in group psychotherapy.* Int J Group Psychother 20:77-90, 1970.

57. GREENBERG, D AND RANKIN, H: *Compulsive gamblers in treatment.* Br J Psychiatry 140:364-366, 1982.

58. BANNISTER, G, JR: *Cognitive and behavior therapy in a case of compulsive gambling.* Cognitive Therapy Research 1:223-227, 1977.

59. SCODEL, A: *Inspirational group therapy: A study of Gamblers Anonymous.* Am J Psychother 18:115-125, 1964.

60. POKORNY, MR: *Compulsive gambling and the family.* Br J Med Psychol 45:355-364, 1972.

PART 6
ROLE OF MENTAL HEALTH PROFESSIONALS IN THE COURTS AND PRISONS

This last part returns to themes developed in earlier sections and chapters of this text. Each chapter is comprehensive in approach. Two of the chapters, the first and second contributions, deal with entire fields of forensic application: One concerns mental health services in the correctional system; the other concerns mental health professional roles in various types of civil law litigation.

The contribution by Loren Roth on correctional psychiatry was first prepared for the earlier volume and updated for this book. It is a modern exegesis on the contribution of therapeutic techniques to correctional objectives. In the opinion of the editors it is one of the most ambitious and definitive writings on this subject by a single author in this field. Dr. Roth lays down principles for effective therapeutic programs in the prisons. He asserts that the services must be designed to duplicate the best standards of psychiatric practice in any location. Correctional psychiatry cannot hope to succeed, even in modestly set objectives, if it is willing to accept second-class or even third-class status. Furthermore, it must assert its operational independence from correctional authorities in the interest of accomplishing its therapeutic aims with criminal offenders.

The author admits that mental health programs in the prisons have often failed in the past; but rather than curtail or abandon the effort, he urges expanded efforts in correctional psychiatry and medical care. Coercive treatment of antisocial behavior is described as ineffective and unacceptable in the current philosophy of the field; therapeutic techniques of proven value are stressed with emphasis on crisis intervention and longer-term treatment for seriously mentally ill offenders. Among the inmate population, between 15 percent and 20 percent exhibit pathology of serious enough proportions to warrant therapeutic attention and intervention. Dr. Roth describes various patient groups found in the prisons and methods used to provide treatment. He also indicates a role for the mental health professional in dealing with violence in the prisons, not only in evaluation and treatment for violent mentally ill inmates, but in studying epidemiological and environmental factors in prison that contribute to institutional disruption and violence.

Dr. Roth is not an advocate of full-time, salaried, career forensic psychiatrists and psychologists in the prisons. His support for therapeutic and operational autonomy and for programs closely related to mental health goals outside the correctional framework argues vigorously against a career-dependent, lifetime commitment by individual professionals to a single security unit. He suggests shorter career assignments and part-time opportunities for prison-based professional personnel as well as close affiliation with university departments, residency training, and the range of resources of schools of public health wherever they are available and convenient for prison involvement for practice, training, and research. The vistas for improved therapeutic and consultative roles for mental health professions in the correctional system presented in this chapter should rekindle the interest of even the most disenchanted among our readers. We can only hope that Dr. Roth's followers will grow and multiply in the years ahead.

In the chapter on participation in civil law litigation, Herbert Modlin of the Menninger Foundation—one of the pioneers in the development of the specialty of forensic psychiatry and of quality residency training in the field, as well—has prepared a review of the several areas of civil law in which mental health evaluation and testimony may be helpful to attorneys and the courts. He offers sage advice briefly and concisely, based upon over 30 years of experience as a trial witness.

The author points out that there is much more involvement for mental health professionals in civil litigation than in the more publicized criminal justice system. He enumerates the wide range of civil cases in which mental health testimony is currently utilized. In the following pages, the author illustrates the problems in each area and the legal standards required for testimony on the various legal questions involved.

The last two chapters in part 6 concentrate upon mental health professional involvement in court matters on both the civil and criminal sides as consultants, evaluators, and, ultimately, as courtroom expert witnesses. Both are fresh contributions to this new volume.

Much has been written on psychiatric expert testimony; the literature on the psychologist as an expert in the courts is much less in volume and quality. In the past, this was due in large part to the legal restriction imposed upon psychological experts in regard to the scope of their testimony. The restrictions were highly unrealistic and repressive. They never did represent the true character of either the scientific or the clinical skills of the field. Currently, these limitations have been totally removed in virtually all American jurisdictions. The psychologist expert is currently evaluated in court—a threshold issue of admissibility to be determined in the discretion of the trial judge—on his or her personal expert qualifications and experience concerning the matters at issue in the particular case—not on the basis of a preconceived, inaccurate model of the psychologist of the past.

Psychologist Wallace Kennedy of Florida State University writes from obvious experience in all phases of trial litigation. He reviews the general requirements for recognition as an expert, with stress on the doctoral degree; licensure; board certification, if relevant to the case; and practical experience in the field. He advises young psychologists to offer their services first in the municipal courts of smaller communities in order to build their skills and composure in a more congenial atmosphere in which the participants are willing to tolerate, to teach, and to welcome the novel witness. Only after this should they venture into the busier, more impersonal, highly competitive urban courthouses and, perhaps last of all, into the tightly run, elitist federal district courts of the jurisdiction. This is good advice, but it is often difficult to follow, because the lawyers who select the experts may have greater and more urgent needs for psychological consultation and expert testimony in the crowded urban circuits. As soon as a psychologist of talent and weighty credentials indicates a willingness and aptitude for law and the courts, the invitations to participate in the more exciting and compelling cases in the city jurisdictions and in the federal courts (constitutional rights cases, interstate issues, and so forth) may begin to tempt even the less experienced court neophyte.

The author has organized his presentation into three primary parts: the content areas of expert testimony in psychology; the characteristics of an effective expert witness; and the common errors or pitfalls that psychologist experts can be prone to in the cold exposure of the combative courthouse. In each of these areas, Dr. Kennedy's suggestions in regard to courtroom effectiveness build well upon the foundation provided by Thomas Grisso in his chapter on psychological assessment. As Dr. Kennedy points out, scientifically unchallengeable testimony can be rendered useless to the fact-finder in the court by flawed presentation: inaudible mumbling; incoherent and disorderly coverage of the data; over-sophisticated, jargon-loaded description without adequate explanation. Nearly all of what Dr. Kennedy suggests in these pages is easily adaptable to the testimonial needs of other mental health professionals in psychiatry, social work, and nursing, and, in fact, to most other areas of expertise in court.

The last chapter of this part and the final chapter of the text was prepared by two of the editors, Dr. Curran and Dr. McGarry. It reviews psychiatric roles in the courtroom in a variety of capacities—as educator; investigator; clinical evaluator; interpreter; trial strategy adviser; venue and jury selection adviser; drama coach and critic; rewrite editor; and personal emotional or therapeutic support for the parties, certain witnesses, or the trial counsel themselves, who may experience stress during litigation.

The chapter examines basic professional qualifications for the specialty of forensic psychiatry and compares these standards with the usual practices of American trial court judges in ruling upon admissibility of expert psychiatric testimony.

Considerable attention is given in the chapter to preparation of reports which become the basis of later courtroom testimony. The authors deal with issues of pretrial preparation and consultation with the trial attorney who has utilized the expertise of the forensic specialist.

The chapter also reviews the recommendations in the American Bar Association's report on standards for mental health aspects of criminal justice, particularly those relating to admissibility and scope of psychiatric and psychological testimony.

In an overall way, this last chapter illustrates, as do several other chapters in the book, the need of forensic specialists to be aware of the legal rules applicable to their roles in the American judicial system. The effective forensic evaluator must be aware of these rules **before appearing** in court as well as while engaging in presenting testimony.

This last point brings us full circle in our text: The opening chapter by editors Saleem Shah and Louis McGarry was devoted to an examination of professional qualifications, including legal training and the development of forensic skills of assessment and treatment. The last chapter stresses these same matters from a consultative-testimonial point of view. It is our hope as editors that our readers, both those who are currently in training and those who are already engaged in forensic practice, will find these contributions from the opening pages to these last chapters useful and instructive in their work, now and in the future.

CHAPTER 19
CORRECTIONAL PSYCHIATRY
Loren H. Roth, M.D., M.P.H.

Psychiatry practiced in prisons must at all times strive to duplicate the best of psychiatric practice in other settings and must share its goals.[1] In the past, few psychiatrists could assert that their accomplishments have been effective or well received in American prisons and jails.[2-8] Nevertheless, this discussion will indicate that more, rather than less, genuine psychiatric and medical services are needed in the penal system if any success is to be achieved. I also propose the thesis that correctional psychiatry cannot simultaneously be the handmaiden of the penal bureaucracy and also serve its own traditional therapeutic aims.[9] Furthermore, an effective program of correctional psychiatry will hardly be even a possibility until psychiatrists and those who look to psychiatry for guidance and service in prisons recognize that the majority of inmates, both violent and nonviolent, are not mentally ill.[10-12]

With notable exceptions, few psychiatrists are enthusiastic about the likelihood of coercive cure for antisocial behavior.[13] An effective and useful prison psychiatry program must be committed firmly and must be knowledgeable about the special aspects of health services delivery within a prison environment; it must be inmate-oriented rather than society-oriented in its goals; and it consciously must avoid preoccupation with whether inmates recidivate, either owing to the direct effects of the psychiatrist or in agreement with the psychiatrist's clinical or intuitive "prediction" of their fates.

The purpose of this chapter will be to acquaint the psychiatrist with the special information necessary to achieve these aims so that the practitioner entering this environment may maintain professional skills, interest, and empathy for the prisoner patients rather than retreat from the institutional scene in haste, depression, and anger.

DEFINITION OF THE FIELD

Historical Review

The construction of prisons was a Quaker-inspired reform movement of the late 18th and early 19th centuries.[14] Prisons were intended to allow the offender to reflect on his or her crimes and to repent in order that he or she might regain freedom. Rather than promoting reform, the deleterious effects of certain prison practices on the physical and mental health of inmates were soon noted.

> In the early years of the Auburn Prison, administrators tried an experiment to test the efficiency of the Pennsylvania system. They selected eighty of the most hardened convicts and placed them in solitary confinement and enforced idleness from Christmas 1821 through Christmas 1823. So many of these men succumbed to sickness and insanity that the experiment was scrapped in 1823.[15]

A somewhat similar report came from William Farr in England. Farr, considered one of the fathers of epidemiology, noted that "prisoners rarely labour under any serious disease at the time of their committal." However, although "eight inmates were executed [in] 1837 . . . the average annual number of deaths due to imprisonment was 51."[16] The inhumanity of the prison system was thus apparent at an early point. The subsequent conceptual problem for psychiatry has been whether, in modesty, it might assist in rendering a too frequently inhumane system of punishment and incapacitation (albeit labeled reform) to become generally more humane, more solicitous of the person, or alternatively, whether psychiatry would do better to advocate a more scientific penology, one oriented more toward treating illness and correcting individual deficiencies in order to decrease inmate recidivism.

Halleck[3] and Fitzpatrick[17] have summarized the contributions of 19th- and 20th-century psychiatry and psychoanalysis to corrections and criminology. These sources delineate the main figures, their theories regarding criminality, the psychological evaluation of offenders, and the provision of mental health services. The details will not be repeated here. Suffice it to note that of the 100 milestones given by Halleck in the history of American psychiatry and the criminal (1800 to 1960), many seeming advances have proved themselves as much problems as solutions[18,19] (for example, the creation of special institutions for the "criminally insane," or sexual psychopathic legislation which mandated medical rather than penological treatment for sex offenders).[20]

In the 19th century, physicians led the way in encouraging the examination of the criminal offender as an individual. Psychiatry "attempted to discover scientific explanations for the behavior of criminals rather than relegating them completely to moral condemnation or to pessimistic theories of social inevitability."[3] Although the biological approach of the late 19th and early 20th centuries was naive at best and calamitous at worst (for example, sterilization of criminals during the early 20th century), medical and psychiatric interest in the biology of antisocial and aggressive behaviors has continued to be strong until the present day (see studies of the neurophysiology, endocrinology, and genetics of aggressive and violent behavior).[21,22] Nevertheless, a serious question can be raised today as to whether the general subject matter of the biology of crime lies at all within the province of correctional psychiatry. Unitary theories linking one or another biological entity to criminal behavior have had a characteristic and disappointing history, namely, early enthusiasm and later rejection as more scientific data become available. This dictum, for example, seems to apply to the findings and discussions over the last 15 years regarding the contribution of the XYY chromosomal variant to aggressive behavior.[23] Furthermore, many psychiatrists have taken the position that to the extent that biological interventions for offenders involve great risk to them, and to the extent that there is some question about the "voluntariness" of the inmates' request for such intervention, these modalities should be made available to offenders only during periods of freedom and when they are no longer under legal control.[24]

During the early 20th century, psychiatrists working in both court clinics and prisons devoted considerable effort to examining inmates in order to determine how many were mentally ill. Throughout the 1920s and 1930s, the psychiatrist who worked with the criminal held a relatively esteemed position.[3] From the 1930s until the 1960s, however, the amount of psychiatric services provided to prisoners failed to keep pace with the prison population. Over many decades, numerous surveys have revealed a paucity of psychiatrists actively involved in prisons and jails.[3,25-29] In 1976, the United States Bureau of Prisons employed 14 full-time psychiatrists for some 27,000 inmates. Six additional positions were unfilled. During the 1970s, the Alabama penal system employed virtually no mental health professional employees or consultants for its 3800 inmates.[29] Within the psychiatric profession the prestige of correctional psychiatry declined. Psychoanalytic theories of criminality gained prominence during the 1940s[3,17] but failed to furnish a practical rationale for the treatment of the offender. The 1950s were characterized by the growth of special medical-penological programs for the handling of the recalcitrant offenders (for example, the opening by the State of Maryland in 1955 of the Patuxent Institution for the treatment of "defective delinquents").[13] Small groups of interested psychiatrists met together and began to publish specialized journals devoted to offender treatment; for example, the Association for Psychiatric Treatment of Offenders (APTO), which publishes the *International Journal of Offender Therapy and Comparative Criminology*, formerly the *Journal of Offender Therapy*. Other specialty journals in the area of correctional psychiatry, past and present, include the *Journal of Criminal Psychopathology*, *The Prison Journal*, *Corrective and Social Psychiatry*, and the *Journal of Behavior Technology Methods and Therapy* (formerly *Corrective Psychiatry and Journal of Social Therapy*).

It is probable, however, that neither the formulation of specific psychiatric theories of offender pathology and treatment nor the provision of conventional or special mental health services to the prisoner population has been the most influential contribution of correctional psychiatry (and the other behavioral and helping sciences). Throughout the 1940s and 1950s—but especially in the 1960s—the discipline helped promote a view of corrections and the prison system that re-emphasized its potential for habilitation and also made the contribution that individualized rather than mass handling of offenders would more likely promote their "rehabilitation." During the 1940s and the 1950s, the Federal Bureau of Prisons gradually emerged as the national pacesetter in corrections, introducing new concepts such as "diagnosis," "classification," and the use of professional personnel such as psychiatrists and psychologists to help rehabilitate inmates.[14] The innovations of the Federal Bureau of Prisons were incorporated into many state systems. A wide variety of programs, albeit piecemeal but educational and vocational in nature, were also introduced in prisons with hope not only that inmates would be less idle but also that through the inmate's participation in such programs he or she would be rehabilitated. Although Karl Menninger's advice, given in 1927, that psychiatric reports should influence all sentencing, release, and transfer of inmates was never operationalized,[3] the dictum that "the object so sublime" is to "make the punishment fit the crime" was replaced (at least in rhetoric if not in fact) by a correctional notion that "the object so sublime" is to "make the punishment fit the criminal." Under such a conception, psychiatrists during the 1960s and 1970s became involved in a wide variety of correctional roles, including evaluation of offenders for purposes of sentencing and classification, in-prison treatment of offenders, preparole assessment, and program development and training of other correctional workers. A few psychiatrists were even destined to function as "wardens" within specialized settings.[4,30-35]

A representative statement was made in 1971 concerning one generally accepted role for psychiatry and corrections: "In the quest of individualized treatment psychiatry becomes a valuable ally to the law in its efforts to identify and diagnose those offenders who can benefit from something more than simply punitive incapacitation."[31] This quotation is by no means an isolated one. There has been a tendency for many psychiatrists interested in law and corrections to formulate a medical type approach with respect to the offender. Benjamin Karpman observed in 1949 that "[we] have no more reason to punish them for behavior over which they have no control than [we have] to punish an individual for breathing through his mouth because of large adenoids."[36] Sheldon Glueck predicted, "There will be no prisons—only hospitals."[37] Arthur Zitrin noted that "modern psychoanalytic concepts will not make very much of a distinction between those who are evil and those who are sick. I think they're all sick in different kinds of ways. That's my point, and I think the prescription for the different kinds of sicknesses is what the psychiatrist can help with."[38] Of course, psychiatrists are not the only ones to have struggled with these issues:

> It is time to admit that the sick and the wicked are not scientifically distinguishable: time to scrub this distinction out of our laws and to do away with the consequential rigid classification of custodial institutions into the medical and the penal; and time to replace the once-for-all sentencing decision by a more flexible system under which the treatment of offenders, whether medical or nonmedical, is continuously adjusted to the results achieved.[39]

The language and logic of medicine, although most likely appropriate for only a small number of offenders, were in the midst of being extended to great numbers of them.

The Present Scene

Both corrections and psychiatry have changed since 1971. Even if there was no consensus as to who was responsible for the mass violence and deaths at Attica Prison, there was general agreement that rehabilitation of inmates would never be achieved within the usual milieu of the large and closed institution.

Following the Attica tragedy, correctional philosophies diverged. One school maintained, despite past rhetoric and seeming failures,[40,41] that the truth was that the corrections model "has never been tried."[42-44] This school hoped that individual handling; the correct matching of the offender with the proper treatment modality; and the development of smaller, more personalized, community-based institutions would promote offender rehabilitation.

Convinced that institutions have harmed more than helped their inmates, other national groups in the early 1970s called for increased community handling of offenders and for a moratorium on the construction of new jails and prisons. It was argued that only the dangerous offender should be confined.[45,46] Finally, prominent critics of corrections, convinced that in fairness and in fact rehabilitation cannot be the primary justification for incarceration, called for an end to hypocrisy.[47] Prisons serve multiple functions, including punishment, incapacitation of offenders, and deterrence to other offenders. It is unlikely that these objectives will ever be subservient to that of "rehabilitation." In part, the point of these critics has been that the tools of individual offender rehabilitation—namely, the disparate sentence, the contingent parole,[48] and the indeterminate sentence[49]—not only are unfair but also compound rather than ameliorate the destructiveness of the prison experience.

The new trends of corrections thus emphasize both a decrease in discretionary handling of offenders and an improvement in the prison milieu, more as a matter of human decency and in order to do the "least harm" rather than to "treat the inmate." Rehabilitation is hoped for but not necessarily expected. Participation by inmates in programs of self-improvement is to be encouraged but is to be voluntary and optional; the inmate's release is not to be contingent on such participation.[50,51] As noted by Norval Morris, the rehabilitative model of corrections "suffers fundamentally from a belief that psychological change can be coerced."[47] But whether the new corrections of the 1980s will be only an excuse for continuing neglect of inmates and for more severe and more lengthy, rather than more certain, punishments remains to be seen. If anything, the prison and jail milieu as it exists today is as bad as, or worse than, the milieu of the previous decade.

If the corrections approach is now at a point of some consternation both with itself and its clients, what can be said of psychiatry? In truth, there is also a ferment undermining some of the traditional concerns of correctional psychiatry. It is questioned whether the terms "psychopathy" and "sociopathy" do not conceal more than they convey[52,53] and whether psychiatry has not in the past clearly oversold itself as a predictor of both dangerousness and recidivism.[54,55] As with others in corrections, psychiatrists have become more modest concerning their ability both to intervene successfully and to predict the future behavior of antisocial persons. If psychiatrists traditionally have criticized the operation of prisons and jails, a similar questioning by corrections of the proper role of psychiatry is not now out of place.

Future Directions: Psychiatry and the Normal Offender

As might be anticipated from the previous discussion, this author advocates no pivotal role for psychiatry in the long-term direct treatment and handling of the "normal offender." The psychiatrist's track record here is unproved, and his or her skills are not unique. Without the incentive of release, it remains to be seen whether inmates will voluntarily seek such treatments as group psychotherapy, still the mainstay of correctional psychiatric treatment.[56,57] When release is an incentive, the ensuing consequence is often "game playing" by the inmate and role diffusion for the psychiatrist. These reservations regarding the role of psychiatry vis-à-vis the direct treatment of the normal inmate, however, by no means belittle the role the psychiatrist can and should play in crisis intervention for even the "normal" incarcerated inmate, nor do they limit the importance that psychiatry ought to attach to promoting "normalization" of the prison environment, helping decrease wherever possible its harshness, and helping increase its opportunity for individual growth.

Future Directions: Psychiatry and the Mentally Ill Offender

Here there is a problem of definitions. Only a small percentage of inmates suffer from well-defined severe psychiatric disorders (that is, the psychoses). Furthermore, a recent comprehensive review of the relationship between criminal behavior and mental illness suggests that the former is rarely produced by the latter.[10] The clearly mentally ill offender is wanted by no one—not the prison, the prison hospital, the hospital prison, nor the state mental hospital. The disruptive, aggressive, but nonpsychotic prisoner becomes administratively defined as "mentally ill" in order to facilitate recurring geographical cures. The trained psychiatrist is seldom available to treat or to help manage either of these groups. Considering the small number of psychiatrists who have actually been available in the past to prison and jail systems (and in all likelihood will be available in the future), psychiatry would do well if it could attempt to meet the genuine mental health needs of these persons, let alone attend to the problems of "normal" offenders.

In summary, future correctional psychiatry would do well to be more modest in its aims. At least for the foreseeable future, prisons and jails are here to stay, and seems unlikely that "rehabilitation" will ever constitute the primary function of these institutions. Curious and motivated psychiatrists now have an opportunity to offer their services voluntarily to those inmates who genuinely seek them. In addition they can play a helpful role in providing consultation to the prison community. In my view it is in the area of direct services to the mentally ill inmate and in crisis intervention, however, that the psychiatrist's future role in corrections most clearly lies.

THE INMATE EXPERIENCE

Overcrowding exacerbates the stresses of institutional life and compounds the endemic problems of prisons and jails, including poor living conditions, lack of meaningful work, interinmate violence, sexual exploitation, and weakening of the inmate's usual affectional ties. Unfortunately, however, the prison population of the United States now constitutes an all-time high of about 431,829 inmates.[58] Depending upon their crimes, most of these inmates will serve from 2 to 5 years behind bars. In addition, approximately 210,000 persons are daily residents in local jails.[59]

With rare exceptions, these offenders are seldom provided custody in surroundings that approximate the "free world." In numerous states during the 1970s and 1980s, prison and jail conditions have been declared in violation of constitutional guarantees respecting both the physical and psychological needs of their inmates.[60-65] In 1982, 29 states were operating their corrections systems under some kind of federal court order or sanction.[62] Consider, for example, the recent litigation in Alabama in which sweeping court orders have mandated widespread reform in all areas of prison life, the implementation of such reform to be monitored by a court-appointed human rights committee:

> The living conditions in Alabama prisons constitute cruel and unusual punishment. Specifically, lack of sanitation throughout the institutions—in living areas, infirmaries, and food service—presents an imminent danger to the health of each and every inmate. Prisoners suffer from further physical deterioration because there are no opportunities for exercise and recreation. Treatment for prisoners with physical or emotional problems is totally inadequate.[66]

Moreover, the jail milieu is usually worse, not better, than the customary prison setting.[60,61]

Of importance to the correctional psychiatrist then is that he or she gain some acquaintance with the prison or jail setting, the manner in which incarceration provokes stress for the inmate, and the ways in which the inmate characteristically adapts to this stress. Extremely useful sources of information—not frequently enough consulted by either correctional officials or correctional psychiatrists—are the inmates' own accounts of the prison or jail experience.[67,68]

The Jail Experience

Save for the clearly inadequate inmate relieved to be back in custody, to be jailed is to be uncertain, frightened, or angry:

> "Why did I do it?" "If only I hadn't done that." "Why did I get into this mess?" . . . Regret and remorse probably reach the greatest intensity in the first few days when the impact of the disjointed experience is the greatest, but this type of reflection on the offender's past continues throughout the presentencing phase.[67]

Only about 10 percent of jail inmates are charged with felony offenses. Nationally, on a given day, about 42 percent of jail inmates have been convicted and are serving brief sentences, usually of less than 1 year.[61] The remainder of jailees await arraignment, trial, or transfer. A significant portion of jailees have alcoholic or drug problems.[60] Problems of substance withdrawal are frequent. Increasingly, the chronically mentally ill, no longer able to be treated in state mental institutions or anywhere else, are jailed for minor misbehavior.[68-70] In some jurisdictions other mentally ill persons may be temporarily held, awaiting eventual transfer to mental institutions.[60] "Many jail inmates are really disguised health and welfare cases that require some other mode of help or treatment."[61,70] The petty offender and the jail repeater know that their stay will be a short, if nonproductive, one. The offender charged with a more serious crime faces the uncertainty of bail, plea bargaining, and eventual sentence or return to prison. Usually there is nothing to do to cope with this uncertainy, only idle time to be spent.

The hours are spent crowded with other prisoners in narrow aisles in front of the cells or in small day rooms. [The offender] plays cards, dominoes, reads, and sleeps.

It should not be surprising then that the jail experience, albeit briefer, is frequently as stressful as, or even more stressful than, longer-term imprisonment. Suicide, self-mutilation, displaced violence toward other inmates in the form of sexual and other types of violent outbursts, panic and/or social withdrawal are the potential outcomes of such stress. These are the outcomes that the correctional psychiatrist hopes to help avert.[71,72]

The Prison Experience

Generalization is dangerous when attempting to characterize the impact of somewhat disparate institutions upon disparate persons for variable lengths of time. For example, in spite of oppressive surroundings and punitive handling, occasionally an inmate finds both courage and individuality within the self and grows, seeks opportunity, or otherwise matures in prison, even when such growth may not always lead to a happy conclusion. For others, habituated by many years of dependency and regimentation or otherwise psychologically so disposed, "free-world" skills atrophy, and the prison becomes their only home.[73]

Neither of the above adaptations to prison is perhaps as frequent as the inmate's tendency to learn "to do time"; to make accommodations with both the inmate subculture and the prison staff to live as comfortably as possible in prison and to secure release at the earliest possible time. Nonconformity with prison norms and even rebellion are, of course, also seen. This became a particular problem in the 1970s as the prisons were clogged with younger, more dangerous, and more repetitively violent inmates[74]—inmates not so inclined to accept the solidarity aspects of the old-time "convict code" and to join the inmate subculture. Perhaps the fairest summary statement, though, is that most inmates want only that their time go as smoothly and as quickly as possible.

Relatively few well-designed studies have systematically assessed the impact of the prison experience upon inmate psychology or performance.[68,73-77] There are, however, many sensitive accounts of prison life and the psychology of incarceration.[2,4,68,78] Of direct relevance to correctional psychiatry are the following themes and features of ordinary prison life.

AUTHORITY AND CONTROL

A powerful dynamic in prison settings that affects the equilibrium of both inmates and staff revolves around authority relationships. In the closed prison society, this issue of control profoundly affects multiple behaviors of the dyads and triads of prison life: individual inmates or inmate groups vis-à-vis each other, inmates versus custodial staff, and either or both of these groups versus "treatment staff." For example, homosexual contacts in prison, though at times a reflection of otherwise unachievable intimacy or a matter of simple sexual release per se, even more frequently reflect issues of control (that is, who is to have status and power among the inmate group). It will be rather quickly established whether the new inmate will be labeled a "punk" and exploited or instead will fight back. In fact, the aggressor or active partner who engages in homosexual acts in prison often does not regard himself as homosexual. To take another example, prison practices that possibly promote better mental health of inmates (for example, privacy of visits, absence of strip searches, freedom for inmates to form friendships at varying levels of the prison community) seemingly cannot be instituted or maintained because of custodial concerns that "operational control" of the prison be at all times maintained. Other themes relating to control may confront the psychiatrist more directly when he wishes to institute treatment of a clearly mentally ill inmate (for example, rumor among the inmate population), or the inmate himself may question the rationale for the treatment. Meanwhile, the psychiatrist knows that if he fails to help the prisoner and to modulate the inmate's erratic behavior, the prison system has at its disposal, and will employ, alternative means of control which the psychiatrist may abhor, such as isolation or segregation. Throughout incarceration, then, the inmate fears and resists further control or restriction, the custodial staff fears its absence, and the psychiatrist or other treatment staff easily becomes caught in the same dilemma.

THE TEMPORAL PROFILE OF INCARCERATION

In order to understand the stress for the inmate of the prison experience and the inmate's subsequent coping behavior, it is useful, if somewhat arbitrary, to divide the prison experience into temporal phases: early, middle, and late (prerelease).

The early phase of incarceration bears some similarity to reception into jail. There is further wrenching of the inmate's community ties as contacts with wives, families, or girl friends diminish. An initial data-gathering phase, "classification," may ensue during which the offender is in limbo regarding what is to be expected of him during his prison stay and what will be his prerogatives within the prison.[79] For some inmates the length of their sentence hangs heavy, and there is accompanying denial of their probable future and much fantasy concerning early release. The inmate may pursue continued legal activity. Meanwhile, adjustments must begin to be made with fellow inmates as the new inmate's reputation is established with his peers. Epidemiologic studies give some testimony to the relative difficulties of adjustment during this early period of incarceration. For example, suicides in prison, neither so frequent nor as great a risk as in jails, are more apt to occur during the early period of incarceration,[80] as are episodes of inmate violence against one another or against prison staff.[81] In another study, the proportion of inmates appearing at sick call was found to be highest during the first year of imprisonment.[82] In various ways during this initial period, the inmate must learn to do his time "a day at a time," otherwise he may be "broken" by the prison.

The temporal profile of incarceration is U-shaped, the middle phase of imprisonment representing a period of somewhat greater psychological stability, albeit frequently at the expense of inmate autonomy, and with some accompanying deadening of routine. The time spent in prison is seldom constructive. The inmate's identification with the prison subculture and his preoccupation with its diversion and currency (gambling, cigarettes, contraband drugs, and liquor) impede any constructive psychological change within him and make him susceptible to the pressures of the other inmates. Disappointing news from home, missed visits, periods of time spent in isolation-segregation secondary to minor misbehavior, victimization secondary to quarrels with other inmates, and dashed parole hopes may provoke breakdowns, occurring in different groups of inmates with varying frequencies.

> Indeterminate sentences also may contribute to denial by encouraging false hopes. For inmates having such sentences there is a formalized, unwritten minimum time which must be served which varies with the nature of the offense. Inmates, who are not made aware of this or cannot accept it, may very early become intensely involved in institution programs and then react to a denial at their first parole hearing with depression, anger, or abandonment of behavior that would ultimately lead to release.[4]

Coping with anger is particularly difficult as the inmate attempts to build a record of institutional adjustment that will not preclude release. Though this observation is somewhat dated, and the trend in correction over the last decade has been toward fixed sentencing and more structured release decision making,[83,84] the sentiment expressed is nevertheless still highly relevant. Inmates are seldom honestly apprised by correctional officials of their realistic chances for release, and accepting the time to be served is a psychological hurdle contributing to bitterness and resentment of inmates concerning their prison handling. To control his impulses, or for purposes of self-protection, the inmate may himself seek segregation status or isolation from other inmates. Although during the earliest phase of incarceration the occasional inmate may express the view that he is getting what he deserves or that he "got off light," as the time passes, the ongoing punishment and deprivation seem to most inmates progressively more unjust and excessive. Numerous commentators have, of course, criticized the excessive lengths of American prison sentences, sentences that, if anything, may increase rather than decrease in length throughout this decade.

The final phase of incarceration, that of prerelease, is again a period of relative disequilibrium for the inmate. Similar to the experiences of others in the "free world" (for example, the terminal phases of a military or even a school career), the inmate is "short term." "Being short" may be a period of weeks, months, or even years for the inmate who is serving a very lengthy sentence. "Being short" is essentially a psychological perception that the prison stay is going to end. There are new realities to be faced upon release, realities that the inmate is ill-equipped to meet. These burdens are also compounded by the inmate's firsthand knowledge of societal opportunity structures, such as the nonavailability of jobs upon release. During this late phase there may be frequent visits to the prison hospital, requests for sleeping medication, irritability, and excessive caution taken by the inmate so that his ongoing behavior will not otherwise jeopardize the expected release. However, other men will engage in behaviors that delay release (for example, the inmate who runs away from a minimum-security setting shortly prior to expected discharge). Prison staff speculate that the inmate "knew he wouldn't make it anyway," and so he sabotaged his release. Because release will occur, clearly any psychological growth that the inmate might achieve during the prerelease period is relevant to adjustment outside the prison. The release period seems therefore a particularly relevant one in terms of crisis intervention.

PSYCHIATRIC PROBLEMS OF PRISONERS

A range of psychiatric pathologies, both traditional and somewhat special, may be exhibited by prisoners. Surveys that have quantified the number of inmates who are mentally ill, or the percentage of all offenders who are mentally ill (whatever their legal status), have reached varying conclusions, depending upon the definitions used, the methods employed, and the nature of the population surveyed.[10,11] Other offenders who are clearly disturbed may be diverted or transferred from regular prisons or jails into special facilities for mentally ill offenders. These offenders include those being evaluated for competency to stand trial, those found incompetent, those found not guilty by reason of insanity, those who were mentally ill at the time of sentencing, and those who became mentally ill while serving prison terms.[85] Steadman and his associates[86] found that 20,143 mentally disordered offenders were admitted in 1978 to state and federal facilities. Of the 256 facilities to which these offenders were admitted, the vast majority (224, 88%) were smaller, secondary facilities, for example, forensic units within state hospitals or inpatient mental health units within state prisons. Twelve percent of the facilities (32) were larger, primary facilities. Whether they are run by corrections or mental health professionals, such facilities are typically identified as hospitals for the "criminally insane." Such diversion from prison or jail may reflect as much the vagaries of legal and administrative processing as the mental state of the inmate per se.

There is increasing judicial and administrative criticism of the nature of treatment actually provided to mentally ill offenders in the traditional "hybrid institutions," mixed medical-penal fortress type settings, as well as judicial recognition that due process protections must be afforded mentally ill inmates prior to transfer to a hospital setting.[87, 88] Examples of such criticism in the recent past concerned the care and handling afforded mentally ill inmates at the Matteawan State Hospital for the Criminally Insane in New York[89] and the improvements recommended for Lima State Hospital, a special security mental facility in Ohio.[90] Consequently, improved psychiatric services will need to be made available for inmates, including those who are seriously mentally ill, within the traditional prison environment or within special psychiatric units to be established within prisons. Such a development has taken place within some states. New York, for example, has established a few "satellite units" within its prisons for short-term mental health treatment and special housing for the mentally ill. A similar direction is now planned for Pennsylvania.

The experienced correctional psychiatrist is never surprised to encounter mentally sound inmates detained within special facilities for the mentally ill and psychiatrically untreated inmates within prisons and jails. Labels are highly misleading when attempting to understand the careers of mentally ill offenders.

THE MENTALLY ILL PRISONER

It may be stated that at various times approximately 15 percent to 20 percent of prison inmates manifest sufficient psychiatric pathology to warrant therapeutic attention or intervention.[10, 11, 31, 35] A 1976 court-ordered reclassification of Alabama prisoners arrived at a figure of 20 percent who badly needed psychological help. The number of prisoners manifesting psychoses or otherwise severe psychiatric disturbances is, however, considerably less than 20 percent, probably on the order of 5 percent or less of the total prison population.[10, 11, 35] Other surveys have revealed an even smaller percentage of offenders who are severely mentally ill (those diagnosed schizophrenic).[91] The work of the St. Louis group led by Dr. Samuel B. Guze is perhaps the best known in this area because of its systematic approach and precise diagnostic formulations. Only 1 percent of released male felons were diagnosed as schizophrenic. A high percentage of male felons (78%) were, however, diagnosed as sociopathic or exhibiting an "antisocial personality," a behavioral disorder defined by the St. Louis group as including a history of police trouble in addition to other variable features (a history of excessive fighting, school delinquency, poor job record, wanderlust, and so forth). Guze's survey revealed that 43 percent of the sample manifested definite alcoholic problems, and 11 percent of the felons had questionable alcoholic problems; 85 percent of those interviewed were diagnosed as either sociopathic, alcoholic, or drug dependent. National surveys have also recently demonstrated extensive drug and alcohol problems among prisoners.[92] Other estimates of the proportion of prison inmates manifesting "personality disorders" have arrived at a far smaller proportion of diagnosable disorders.[93] Bach-y-Rita has reviewed the problems of trying to establish such diagnoses in prisons. The physician may fail to appreciate both the cultural and the institutional determinants of the inmate's prison behavior and psychology. The diagnosis of personality disorder is also variably made by attending to behavioral criteria, psychological criteria, or to a combination of these. Guze's work illustrates the conceptual and definitional problems for correctional psychiatry. Although antisocial personality is both a social and a personal tragedy, equating correctional psychiatry with the treatment and management of personality disorders overwhelms and bankrupts meager psychiatric resources.

Some brief observations should be offered concerning the management of personality disorders in prison because these are the "disorders" most likely to be encountered. Traditionally, individuals with personality disorders manifest rather fixed or long-standing character traits or behaviors that may trouble others as much as, or more than, these traits or behaviors trouble the person himself. A number of personality disorders may be found among prison inmates, including passive-aggressive personality disorders, antisocial personality disorders (sociopathy-psychopathy), and explosive personality disorders. A central problem in prison for these men is one of behavioral inhibition, the prevention or modification by the closed prison environment of the inmate's traditional methods of coping (for example, taking immediate physical action, self-medication, or flight). Vaillant[94] has nicely summarized this issue. In the closed prison setting where flight is impossible and where behavior is under stricter control, anxiety and depression may be both feared and experienced, even by those inmates who are seemingly "sociopathic." Such is not always counterproductive. During crises the task for the correctional psychiatrist is to communicate to the inmate, "I am sorry that you are feeling bad, but I think that you can manage the feeling."[94] The inmate's request for medication, for some "time out" in the prison hospital, or for a facilitated change from his present living quarters to other quarters in order to avoid either perpetrating or being the victim of violence should be neither immediately acceded to nor rejected out of hand as "manipulative." Rather, more information should be gathered by the psychiatrist while he makes simultaneous efforts to reassure the inmate concerning his own competence and potential to manage both his feelings and his behavior. Although occasionally one of the above interventions may be appropriate, the overriding goal is to help the inmate confront, understand, and handle the frustrations of the prison experience without necessarily having to act upon them. For example, aiding the impulsive inmate to experience, but also to tolerate, "depression" or anxiety may prevent rather than encourage other potential outcomes of prison frustrations for inmates with personality problems (resulting in violence, time spent in isolation-segregation, self-mutilation, drug abuse, reactive psychoses).[95]

In-prison management or treatment of inmates with personality disorders should be distinguished from attempts at "rehabilitation." With regard to rehabilitation, there is some consensus: individual psychotherapy is not likely to increase substantially future law-abiding behavior. This is particularly true when the inmate is young and has an extensive criminal record.[96] Group therapy, peer pressure (milieu) approaches,[56, 94] or behavioral approaches seem more promising here.[97] A panel on research on rehabilitative techniques (working under the aegis of the National Research Council) has recently summarized what is new and promising in the arena of offender rehabilitation. This report[98] provides a number of important suggestions for improving the scientific evaluation of such rehabilitative efforts.

Whatever the modality of treatment used for the personality-disordered inmate, scrupulous honesty, consistency of approach, limit-setting when necessary, and a "here and now" orientation are required. It is important for the correctional psychiatrist not to maintain a pejorative attitude toward these men and their treatment; neither, however, is excessive sympathy or "excuse making" valued or useful for the inmate. If genuine respect for the inmate is communicated, there may be an opportunity for the individual inmate and the psychiatrist to form a working alliance.[10] This is particularly feasible when the inmate himself comes to realize that his behaviors, past and present, are dysfunctional. He may welcome some help in changing these behaviors, especially when the psychiatrist has already demonstrated his "wares" through aiding in the resolution of some in-prison minimum crisis.

Other Psychiatric and Psychological Profiles

Inadequacy, rather than stereotypic "meanness" or "badness," is a clinically more impressive finding in many prison or jail inmates. The statistical unlikelihood that incarceration will follow most offending behavior ensures that offenders either less adept at crime commission or otherwise socially least able to defend themselves against the law are the ones who will be incarcerated. For example, because serving time is in some respects more statistically normative for blacks than for whites, black prisoners often impress the psychiatrist as more "normal," more "put together," than white prisoners. Women prisoners, who make up less than 5 percent of all inmates, may appear even more deviant, when compared with the stereotype or ideals of womanhood, than do male prisoners when they are compared with other men. Whether one considers male or female inmates, however, the vast majority of them are minimally educated, originate from lower socioeconomic strata, and have experienced frequent parental and otherwise severe social deprivation.[91, 99, 100] For men (in addition to the aforementioned diagnoses of antisocial personality, alcoholism, and drug dependency), schizophrenia, mental retardation, and perhaps epilepsy may be overrepresented in prison and jail populations.[11, 35, 91, 101, 102]

From an epidemiologic perspective these last three diagnoses are probably not directly related to crime prevalence or causation but may represent demographic influences and the effect of differential handling of offenders (less competent offenders more likely may be sent to, and spend longer times in, institutions). For women offenders the remaining psychiatric diagnosis likely to be encountered is hysteria.[91] Some discussion is therefore appropriate concerning prison and jail treatment for the most difficult of these psychiatric and psychological problems—the psychoses (frequently of schizophrenic type) and mental retardation.

JAIL PSYCHOSES

Psychotic jail inmates frequently fail to obtain needed medical help. One problem is the aforementioned lack of medical personnel available to evaluate, to diagnose, and to treat these conditions adequately.[26] In addition to the functional psychoses, attention must be given in jails to an adequate differential diagnosis, including both substance abuse and substance withdrawal (typically amphetamines, sedative-hypnotics, opiates, or alcohol), other metabolic and organic conditions, head trauma, postconvulsive states, and reactive psychoses secondary to incarceration. In theory the treatment of these conditions should be similar to treatment in other locales, but numerous bureaucratic, political, and administrative considerations seemingly overwhelm a decent medical approach.

The jail that contains an adequate medical or mental health component is the exception.[70] Although implementation of national standards (professional approaches) for providing jail and/or prison medicine has begun,[72, 103–105] that effort is sometimes more a matter of rhetoric than reality. Over the last decade, the American Medical Association has successfully implemented a program of jail health care accreditation, and 400 of the nation's jails participated. However, seven times as many facilities were not reached.[103] The psychotic inmate must be detected and then treated in some continuing fashion. All too frequently known psychotic inmates are transferred from jails to hospital settings for a brief stay; inadequately or too briefly treated; returned to the jails, frequently not on medication or without instructions as to the manner of continuing necessary care; and thus, again untreated in jail, the cycle is repeated. If transfer to a hospital is possible, because of legal considerations it cannot be expedited. The psychotic inmate may never be detected or evaluated because of the absence of trained jail personnel, the attitudes of jail personnel toward inmates, or the nonavailability of physicians. Although there is no magic solution to these problems, they should be confronted, and certain recommendations can be made.

Jail personnel need to be trained in the recognition of psychotic conditions and given the best current explanations for their emergence. This is best accomplished through the traditional "case approach" rather than didactically. Daily or twice-daily physician contact with newly admitted, disturbed inmates is recommended. "Voluntary" transfer to a hospital setting may be advisable and possible for a few inmates and is required in cases of alcohol or sedative-hypnotic withdrawal. Although mental hospital treatment may need to be mandated for a few inmates, a surprisingly large number of psychoses may be successfully managed in the jail itself, if adequate facilities and manpower are provided. Ideally, the jail should include a separate section or infirmary, adequately staffed on a 24-hour basis, for the care and management of such clearly ill inmates. Isolation and "strip cells" are not necessary and only confound the treatment. Well-publicized court cases have forced creation of special jail mental health units in some jurisdictions, particularly in overcrowded city and county jails in urban areas.[106]

Ensuring adequate detection, treatment, and continual follow-up of jail inmates within the jail, as opposed to transfer (although not desirable in all cases), is practically the only way that institutional Ping-Pong can be avoided with no one taking genuine medical responsibility for the inmate. Providing this type of jail health care should be the responsibility of a civilian health care organization or community department of health, rather than the jail per se, though the care is provided in the jail. "Contracting out" to local hospitals, clinics, or medical partnerships to provide treatment is one mechanism to ensure that the inmate is afforded treatment equal to that which he might receive if he were not in jail.

PRISON PSYCHOSES

The psychotic inmate in the general prison population may be feared and victimized, and there is tremendous pressure on the prison psychiatrist to "dispose" of this inmate in some manner. In one study of federal prisoners, it was found through record review that 4 percent of inmates had apparently suffered a first psychosis while incarcerated.[11] Again a differential diagnosis should be pursued, and the automatic response should be neither "schizophrenic" nor "transfer."

The successful management of prison psychoses may often be accomplished by voluntary transfer within the prison to a hospital section, to an infirmary, or even to "outpatient" care within the prison, though prison officials may resist or sabotage such handling. Providing medication in prison poses certain problems. Its administration must be closely and medically supervised and not left to the discretion of the correctional staff. Abuse of the major tranquilizers by inmates is generally not a problem. Antipsychotic drugs simply do not make the nonpsychotic inmate "feel good." Unlike the antianxiety agents (for example, Valium) or the sedative-hypnotic drugs (barbiturates or Doriden), antipsychotic drugs are not useful prison currency. More problematic here is inmate refusal of treatment, a right increasingly recognized and one that should be accorded, at least in the absence of clear-cut and imminent danger to self or others.[107] Psychotic inmates are not the main perpetrators of prison violence. In the absence of previous history of physical aggression, many so-called paranoid and even frankly delusional inmates may nevertheless avoid overt difficulties, even though they are at risk of being "gotten" first by other inmates who misinterpret their behavior or who are afraid of them. If involuntary treatment is necessary, the increasing trend is to follow procedures providing the equivalent civil protections prior to, and accompanying, such involuntary treatment.[87, 88, 107, 108]

In *Vitek v. Jones*,[87] the United States Supreme Court ruled that prior to transfer from prison to a mental hospital setting, refusing inmates must be provided with due process protections, including representation and a hearing before a neutral decision maker. Case law in this area is rapidly changing. The prudent course is also to provide similar protections for inmates transferred for involuntary treatment to in-prison mental health units, whether they are operated by mental health or corrections professionals.[109] Various court cases have raised the specter that treatment of institutionalized offenders with antipsychotic drugs (or the use of certain behavioral techniques) may constitute more of a management or "control" device than a medical one per se.[88, 107, 110] The individual practitioner must look to his or her heart and training, ensuring that his or her approach is in fact a professional one, that appropriate medical orders and examinations have been provided, and that an individual treatment plan has been formulated. He or she is also advised to consult the most recent case of statutory law in the jurisdiction regarding in-prison treatment. Psychopharmacology, although generally required and helpful in the management of psychotic conditions, should not be automatic or administered without simultaneous attempts at supportive counseling and efforts to understand and to modify any intercurrent stresses contributing to the inmate's presenting picture.

Mention should be made here of segregation and the impact of isolation (sensory deprivation) upon all inmates, including "normal" individuals and those suffering personality problems or the more severe varieties of mental illness. Surprisingly, there is poor documentation of a systematic sort concerning the impact of segregation, though numerous case reports and clinical accounts do testify to the negative impact of the segregation experience on some inmates.[2, 93] A visit to any set of segregation cells reveals great commotion, banging on pipes, and mirrors extended through bars, permitting one man to communicate with another. In the absence of communication and sometimes even despite it, deterioration may occur. Agitation, lethargy, withdrawal, and self-mutilation in order to "experience" something or for purposes of attention getting may occur.[93] Hallucinatory or delusive experiences emerge or are exacerbated. For example, a study of the seclusion experience at a psychiatric hospital showed a possible increase in patient hallucinatory experiences consequent to seclusion as well as patient delusional and affective responses of fear, terror, anger, and resentment.[111]

The correctional psychiatrist should institute a daily "rounding" to check on the conditions of those inmates who may have been placed in segregation. Although ethical and professional conflicts emerge, especially when the psychiatrist contemplates transfer of the disturbed inmate to a setting other than segregation, these uncertainties must be faced. The psychiatrist should ask himself, "How would I treat this inmate in a conventional hospital setting?" and then attempt to come as near this ideal as possible. The problem is that the psychiatrist may be seen as attempting to lessen the punishment without having the final authority to modify a system of management or control which he or she may deplore. Isolation-segregation cells are "prisons within prisons" and raise a similar debate concerning the functions of correctional psychiatry, as does the prison itself. In the face of clear-cut psychoses, psychiatrists cannot fail to treat or at least to offer the opportunity for treatment to the disturbed inmate. As a quid pro quo for his or her willingness to treat and to examine inmates in segregation, the psychiatrist should simultaneously attempt to alter the basic prison handling of these men and women.

MENTAL RETARDATION

Mentally retarded inmates, constituting perhaps 10 percent of all inmates (with some variation in this overall percentage from one jurisdiction to another), are seldom served by meaningful prison programs or by prison personnel devoted to their special needs.[112, 113]

Mentally retarded inmates are more easily and more frequently victimized by other inmates. They are impaired in social intelligence as well as intellectual functioning. They have more difficulty understanding institutional rules and regulations and more frequently violate them with subsequent punishment.[112] Prisons lack the special programs necessary for habilitation of the retarded. These problems have underscored the continuing question, Should not these mentally retarded offenders be handled differently, preferably from the onset of their legal involvement? For example, the illegal behavior of the retarded could be reviewed by an Exceptional Offender's Court,[114] and more attention could be devoted to determining whether or not retarded offenders are competent to stand trial.[115] The retarded offender's disposition could more frequently be that of community supervision, or supervision in a special institutional setting, rather than that of a prison.[112] These remedies are attractive, but until now such suggestions have come against hard reality, namely, the nonavailability of adequate alternative programs to implement these ideas. This is particularly true with regard to special institutions. There is little benefit for the mentally retarded offender, especially for the nondangerous offender, in being lumped together with sexual psychopaths;[20] severely mentally ill offenders; or, as many would argue, even "defective delinquents," as was the case at the Patuxent Institution. The needs of the retarded are different, and it is pointless for such persons to spend years languishing in "special institutions" awaiting nonexistent treatment. For now, the best that can be said is that the correctional psychiatrist needs to be aware of the existence and the special vulnerabilities of this group of offenders and to know that the stresses of incarceration may fall particularly hard upon them. On the more positive side, much of the pessimism of the past concerning the habilitation of the retarded is lessening. For many, though not all, retarded offenders, and in accord with the principle of "normalization,"[116] the routines and reinforcements of the normal prison setting may be even more therapeutic than other poorly conceived special treatment programs. For other offenders, more structured programs of a behavioral or operant sort might be warranted.[101] As noted by Rowan,[112] what is truly needed for the retarded offender, and what is now missing, is a "wide range of alternative" approaches to meet the varying needs of all such inmates.

Prison Violence

To recall the words of Rap Brown, violence within prisons and jails is now as "American as cherry pie."[74, 117] Although inmates seldom injure prison or jail staff, they are hurting and even killing one another with increasing frequency. In 1970, an inmate in California ran one chance in a hundred of suffering serious injury during the year; by 1974, his chances of injury had increased fourfold.[118] From mid-1974 to mid-1976, a period of a little more than two years, there were eight homicides at the federal penitentiary at Lewisburg, Pennsylvania.[74]

The great majority of episodes of interinmate violence are neither random nor inexplicable. The Federal Board of Inquiry, studying the homicides at Lewisburg, noted that "in most of the homicides the victims were assaulted for some specific reason. They apparently were not killed indiscriminantly but in retaliation for something they had done."[74] This "something" frequently related to homosexual entanglements. Both assailants and victims had long prior records. Other studies or reviews have come to similar conclusions. Interinmate violence is associated with homosexuality, racial and political tensions, hustling (inmate squabbles concerning cigarettes, drugs, or contraband), enforcement of debts, paybacks to informers, and paybacks or exchanges between members of rival prison gangs or cliques. These situational precipitants to violence need not, of course, always culminate in violence. Rather, such precipitants interact with inmate behavioral predispositions, inmate psychology, and inmate psychopathology. As Toch[118] has observed, although the relationship is not one-to-one, there is some association between the likelihood of an inmate committing a violent act in prison and his having a previous history of violence while on the street. In California, for example, Mexican-American inmates are proportionately overrepresented among prison aggressors, perhaps a reflection of the special concern of this group with demonstrating *machismo,* or "manliness." Similar to street violence, prison violence is generally committed by the younger inmates.[119] These facts highlight the irony of continuing debates concerning corrections and rehabilitation. Limiting the prison to "dangerous" offenders, or decreasing discretionary handling of dangerous offenders to make their automatic incarceration the result, makes the prison all the more volatile and destructive to its residents.

Studies of prison violence point to other factors now likely contributing to increases in interinmate violence, namely, the progressive overcrowding of prisons and jails.[63, 120] Violent prisoners have been shown to be hypersensitive to physical encroachment,[121] and other researchers have demonstrated a positive correlation between disruptive behavior of inmates and the average number of square feet of living space available to the inmate.[122] Separation of aggressive or rapist inmates from one another appears to promote a reduction of group violence.[123] These studies suggest that despite the concerns of the critics, if prison violence is to be reduced, either additional, smaller, and more personalized prisons must be built or, alternatively, inmate sentences must be reduced in duration to decrease present overcrowding.

The relationship between prison violence and inmate psychopathology or mental illness has not, however, been as adequately studied. Probably no more than between 10 percent and 15 percent of inmates who are seriously violent or disruptive in prisons suffer from the psychoses, and even these figures are high estimates.[81, 123] Bach-y-Rita and Veno have described a group of 62 men, habitually violent both within and without prisons. One group of men was notable for the extent of their associated self-mutilation and scarring; this group warranted a diagnosis of explosive personality or impulsive character disorder. These men described episodes of intolerable anxiety, restlessness, and depression. Another subgroup (13 of 62 men) were quiet and withdrawn and had subtle delusional systems not apparent to an unskilled examiner.[124] In another survey, Uhlig[123] reviewed the records of 365 mentally disturbed and disruptive New England offenders, most of whom were apparently violent or aggressive in prison. Of these, 41.9 percent were diagnosed as severe character or personality disorders, 11.5 percent were identified as having a functional psychosis, and the remainder were apparently undiagnosed. It was found that 41.6 percent of the men had spent previous periods in state mental hospitals (beyond time for evaluation), though at the time of the survey almost all of them were back in the prisons. Uhlig's study demonstrated that an adequate approach to these men remains to be developed; neither the traditional mental hospital nor the prison has been able to offer very much.

Achieving significant reductions in interinmate violence will require changes in the prison milieu and penological practices[78] over which the correctional psychiatrist may have little control. This matter has recently been reviewed by Roth.[125] Correctional psychiatrists should help jail and prison administrators take an epidemiological, or environmental, look at episodes of prison violence. The location, timing, and precipitants of these episodes may suggest structural or staffing changes that will reduce their frequency. Data that indicate that fights occur in disproportionate numbers when inmates quarrel over access to an insufficient number of telephones suggests a need for more telephones, not necessarily more psychotherapy or more segregation.[125]

Some violence in the prison is, however, adaptive and necessary and should be extinguished only with caution (for example, the inmate in danger of being raped must learn to fight back, or, alternatively, he may need to spend a great deal of time in self-sought segregation). Nevertheless, the psychiatrist has a role to play in violence prevention in the prison.

The mentally ill violent inmate deserves psychiatric evaluation in addition to, if not instead of, repetitive handling in the prison segregation unit. Correctional officers may fail to detect psychosis which may be treatable via conventional means. With the cooperation of the inmate, a complete medical workup should be performed, including attention to situational precipitants of violence, inmate psychology, and psychobiological and neurological factors that may be associated with violence.[21] Crisis intervention may prove useful for inmates who, with support, will communicate a wish to be less violent and who view their violent outbursts as distasteful or upsetting rather than as absolutely necessary for survival in the prison. Psychological interventions addressed to issues of dependency or passivity, hurt masculine pride or helplessness, or the need for retaliation will usually hit home.[126, 127] Finally, although no medication is as yet specific for violence, the pharmacopoeia for aggression is expanding.[128, 129] Assuming the request of the inmate, medication trials directed at decreasing violent outbursts may be considered for selected inmates whose response to prison provocation seems excessive, even given the nature of the prison milieu. Lithium carbonate treatment seems particularly promising.[129, 130]

Suicides in Prisons and Jails

Preventing all suicides or attempted suicides in prisons and jails is a task beyond the capabilities of the correctional psychiatrist. Nevertheless, more studies are being performed in this area,[68, 77, 80, 131-133] and a few guidelines may be given. The risk of completed suicide is far greater in jails or in holding areas at the time of initial confinement or pretrial than later on during a prison term. In fact, considering the deprivations associated with the typical prison experience, the psychiatrist may wonder why even more men do not take their lives in prison. A number of profiles have been given for jail inmates who are at risk for completed suicide, including (1) the young, impulsive inmate charged with a violent crime who is hypersensitive to confinement and makes a lethal attempt within the first day or week of incarceration; (2) the slightly older inmate who is hopeless and clinically depressed, who may have a past psychiatric history, and who threatens suicide and is reacting to a loss of supports from outside the jail;[134] (3) the good-citizen type charged with a first offense who is shamed by arrest; and finally (4) the more chronic offender who has lost his moorings to the world and cannot face doing any more time.[135] Successful suicides in jail are frequently drug or alcohol users or those charged with these offenses.[134, 136] A recent study by the National Center on Institutions and alternatives of 344 jail suicides developed the following profile of a typical jail suicide: a 22-year-old single white male charged with public intoxication; with no history of mental illness, prior suicide attempts, or arrests. Less than 3 hours after incarceration, the victim hanged himself with material from his bed.[133] Whether within jails or prisons, hanging is the most frequent method of successful self-destruction, though other methods may be attempted, including cutting, overdosage, and ingestion of poisons or cleaning materials. To be distinguished from the above are more manipulative suicide attempts, such as cuttings or nonlethal swallowings (as of glass or razor blades), which are generally accomplished by younger inmates with previous histories of violence and/or self-mutilation. In addition to manipulation, some cutters do so for purposes of tension reduction, to serve as a defense against depersonalization. These latter profiles, though in some sense more benign, do not ensure that the inmate will not go on to completed suicide.

Suicides within prisons have not been well studied. Toch[68] presents some useful psychological autopsies of men who took their lives in prison; for example, the seemingly gentle inmate, nine years in prison, who becomes progressively fearful of other inmates; who is drawn into fights; who eventually clashes with correctional staff for the first time; and who then, within a few months, electrocutes himself in a segregation unit.[68] As noted by Sloane,[132] "anomic (suicide) attempts develop after a period of months or years of imprisonment as gradual feelings of helplessness and hopelessness envelop the individual who finds himself powerless to change his situation." Although severe depressions are unusual in prison settings, loss of loved ones and abandonment by formerly involved friends, lovers, or spouses may provoke clinical depressions with some potential for completed suicide in prison.

Toch has summarized in great detail the social psychology of nonlethal inmate self-injury in jails and prisons, a valuable work which should be consulted. It is instructive to note that the demography of self-injury differs between jails and prisons. In jails the men at greatest risk for self-injury are the older, the married, the drug user, the violent, and the white or Latin. In prison the men at greatest risk for self-injury are the young, the single, the nonuser of drugs, the violent, and the white or Latin. For women inmates the risk factors include youth, drug use, violence, and Latin background. Demographic differences parallel psychological ones. For example, Latin inmates are particularly vulnerable to abandonment by relatives, and women inmates tend to have the greater problem with loneliness.

Management of the suicidal inmate and prevention of jail or prison suicides pose problems similar to those noted in the area of prison violence. Truly ameliorative efforts require improvement of the jail or prison milieu;[125, 132] for example, in the jail, increasing the frequency and improving the quality of exchanges between prisoners and their families in order to decrease the shock of incarceration. As another example, suicide may seem an attractive possibility to a not-so-powerful inmate, both shamed and angered by a homosexual rape.[137] Preventing the suicide would require preventing the rape, which might require providing all inmates with their own cells, providing increased opportunities for family visits or furloughs,[138] and altering the prison or jail environment to a less challenging one to the "manhood" of inmates likely to commit rape. On the more modest individual level, certain actions can be recommended. Correctional psychiatrists and other correctional workers, particularly jail personnel, should be acquainted with the high-risk profiles mentioned above. The risks are, of course, only comparative and not absolute. Firm predictions cannot be made. However, correctional officers can be trained to pick up danger signals in certain men in order that they be placed under surveillance. An adequate history must, of course, be obtained when the inmate is admitted to jail, and correctional staff must be acquainted with clinical profiles of depression. The use of isolation cells or the typical padded cell is not recommended for the suicidal inmate. Such sensory deprivation merely compounds the problem. Inmates at risk of suicide or threatening suicide should instead be transferred to a specially staffed portion of the jail or prison unit where around-the-clock surveillance is possible.[106] In jails, most successful suicides occur at night or early in the morning, and coverage throughout these hours is necessary. In addition to this general approach, attention also should be given to the general medical problems of the inmate, particularly that adequate facilities and techniques for drug detoxification (methadone treatments) are available. A decrease in both violence and suicide in jails consequent to an adequate program of detoxification has been reported.[139] Many depressed inmates will respond to conventional treatments for depression. Severe cases will probably require transfer to a mental hospital.

A difficult problem is the inmate with a history of self-cuttings who again threatens to kill himself or who has made a minor gesture, either in the jail or in the prison. A psychological or "investigative" approach should be pursued. It is well to begin by asking the inmate what it is he is trying to achieve or to communicate. With adequate exploration, some purposes may be judged to be manipulative and may need to be refused.[80]

Difficult Characters

The correctional psychiatrist may be asked to evaluate or to treat prison or jail inmates whose behavior is both puzzling and annoying to the prison workers, such as the inmate manifesting brief, confusional episodes; the inmate who is hyperactive or who has "down" periods; the inmate whose talk makes no sense; and the inmate who feels perpetually abused and who is in continuous conflict with prison workers concerning his handling and his rights. Differential diagnosis should be pursued in these instances, giving careful attention in puzzling cases to the possibility of institutional drug or alcohol abuse, glue or solvent sniffing, or other uses of prison contraband.[140] A high proportion of prison inmates have, of course, been drug or alcohol abusers.[92, 102, 141] In selected institutions the proportions run as high as 40 percent to 60 percent. "Turning on" with drugs or alcohol is one of the few prison diversions; drugs and alcohol are nearly always available in prisons, and overdoses may culminate in death. Treatment of these substance-abusing inmates may be quite difficult because inmate denial of abuse is the norm, and the "pleasures" of abuse are great. Urine drug screens may need to be run as well as other routine laboratory work (for example, testing of hepatic enzymes for liver damage). The thrust of the psychological treatment should be to achieve some consensus with the inmate that substance abuse is dysfunctional for him or her[142] and that more meaningful activities for the inmate may yet be found or created in the prison or jail.

The Ganser syndrome requires brief mention as an entity especially associated with forensic psychiatry and prisons. This is a disorder occupying an intermediate position between disease and malingering, psychosis and neurosis.[143] In this rare condition, the patient, frequently an inmate, gives clearly wrong or nonsensical answers to questions. The nature of the answers given, however, suggests that the patient understands the questions. A hysterical mechanism is presumably involved, but "organic" etiology should be excluded. Benefits may accrue to the inmate by virtue of his being believed to be mentally ill or "insane." The Ganser syndrome is short-lived. The treatment should be watchful waiting, monitoring of the realistic pressures that are upon the inmate, and confronting him with the consequences of his behavior—at least until it is possible to determine whether this is an instance of malingering or genuine psychosis.[144]

Regarding inmates who are in continuous conflict with prison staff (or with the prison medical department) concerning their rights or handling, the watchword is "be wary." This type of inmate is a repetitive visitor to the prison sick call and the correctional psychiatrist's station and will complain to anyone who will listen, including the chaplain, the caseworker, and the warden. Many of these men have every reason to complain, and their complaints should be remedied. For others, such complaints may be more defensive. One set of complaints is replaced by another in a never-ending psychological rejection of the prison experience. Paradoxically, "curing" these men, ridding them of their complaints, may make them worse, even precipitating a prison psychosis. The main way these inmates relate to others within the prison is through complaints.

Mentally Abnormal Offenders

Achieving the goals of fair, just, and effective handling for the mentally abnormal offender seems utopian.[88, 145-148] An entire monograph or two—not a portion of a chapter—would be required to discuss fully the problems posed, including the historically confused response to these offenders characteristic of both legal and mental health professionals. The lumping appellations "mentally abnormal offender" or "mentally disordered offender" have not helped; these terms are hardly an improvement over the terms "criminally insane" or "insane criminals."

For the present purposes, the following prisoners may be defined as "mentally abnormal offenders": offenders undergoing observation for their competency to stand trial or for criminal responsibility;[149-151] offenders deemed incompetent to stand trial; offenders found not guilty by reason of insanity (a small proportion of all mentally abnormal offenders);[88] certain sexual offenders;[20] sentenced offenders who are or who become mentally ill;[109, 152] "defective delinquents,"[13, 88, 112] repetitive or dangerous criminals judged in need of special psychological handling,[146] and other offenders such as those who may now, in several states, be found guilty but mentally ill. Many of these special-category prisoner-patients are the subject of other chapters of this text and will not be discussed here.

These disparate types of offenders are, because of putative mental illness and putative dangerousness, frequently evaluated or treated in maximum-security or other inpatient settings. These may be penal or medical in name.

Whatever they are called, in most cases such settings often resemble prisons more than hospitals, as the following quotations graphically reveal:

> The story is the same everywhere. The mentally ill offender is confined in a grim storehouse. Treatment is grossly inadequate. There is virtually no therapy.[147]

> These hospitals . . . suffer . . . the traditional ailment of hospitals for criminally insane and dangerous mentally retarded patients. Geographic and professional isolation, staff difficulties, preoccupation with security measures and uncertain but probably overcautious release policies are among those usually mentioned in this context.[153]

Over the last two decades leading mental health law cases[87, 90, 154-158] have addressed the rights of these offenders. Litigation has involved procedures for their hospitalization and release and their right to treatment and their right to refuse treatment. Variable progress has been reported in some jurisdictions concerning the care of these persons.[159] The correctional psychiatrist's relationship to these offender-patients is complicated. By virtue of written reports or testimony given to the court about the offender's mental state or dangerousness, the correctional psychiatrist may hold the key to the offender's release or commitment. The treater (de facto if not de jure) may also be the keeper. Although this dilemma may be avoided (and should be avoided) partly by the provision of independent forensic examination related to release and recovery, such is not always possible.[160] Moreover, and unfortunately, the psychiatrist and the court may not be acquainted with the legal criteria upon which judgments are to be made concerning these offenders and by which the relevance of psychiatric evidence is established. Finally, both the legal criteria and the medical data may be distorted or ignored by all parties in order to accomplish a disposition for the offender. The mentally ill jail inmate, a "minor offender," may be transferred to the maximum-security hospital ostensibly under the suspicion of incompetency to stand trial but actually to obtain treatment not otherwise available. The violent offender may be diverted temporarily from his probable fate into a status of incompetency to stand trial that suits the strategic needs of either the prosecution or the defense.[161] The violent but not mentally ill inmate may be defined as mentally ill in order to rid the prison of him. The patient declared not guilty by reason of insanity, who is not mentally ill but nevertheless judged "dangerous," may be retained for further treatment as mentally ill. Though a valid societal goal, balancing the needs of society with the needs of the offender-patient encourages psychiatric and judicial hypocrisy, both knowingly and unknowingly.

Correctional psychiatrists working with mentally abnormal offenders must, therefore, always be proactive. This includes their acquiring an understanding of the laws and the legal concepts involved, in addition to exhibiting a willingness to challenge these laws and their operation when such jeopardize the treatment of offender-patients.[162] Without a proactive stance, the psychiatrist working with mentally abnormal offenders becomes mainly "dispositional grease," allowing a nonrational system to escape scrutiny.

Mentally ill offenders should not be treated involuntarily without their having been afforded the civil protections of due process hearings similar to those available to the nonincarcerated.[88, 109] An important trend relates to the regionalization of forensic facilities, to the disbanding of conglomerate statewide maximum-security prison hospitals or hospital prisons, and to their replacement—as much as possible—with smaller hospitals or satellite clinics located within wings of conventional state hospitals or prisons.[88, 89, 145, 146, 159, 163]

The dangerousness of mentally ill offenders has been overestimated in the past. This is another illustration of the fallacy of lumping together mentally abnormal offenders in maximum security hospitals on the basis of alleged, though unproven, common characteristics. The care of mentally ill offenders in the future will occur to a greater extent in traditional institutions (conventional prisons or hospitals) rather than in "hybrids" (in between special security institutions). These "third alternatives" pose intractable administrative problems and have manifested a very poor track record.

In the past, prisoners who have become mentally ill in prison or jails have not been permitted to seek care voluntarily in hospitals. Such care had to be mandated. Furthermore, the prisoner typically lost certain benefits while in hospital (loss of good time or denial of parole eligibility). These practices are being criticized as unfair to prisoners and a denial of their right to medical care.[88, 159] With the development of smaller, less onerous treatment alternatives for the mentally ill inmate, such practices ought to be modified.

Finally, the question arises concerning responsibility for the delivery of mental health care to mentally ill offenders. Who should be responsible: the prison or jail which hires its own personnel, or a department of mental health or other equivalent medical organization? The latter is practically the only way to ensure that the medical needs of the offenders are not completely subsumed to those of custody. Prison hospitals run by doctors are, nonetheless, prisons. A compromise (one that cannot always be achieved and that is not perfect for every inmate) is that the inmate be treated within a hospital that is within a prison.[145, 163] The prison hospital should have some autonomy operating under the aegis of medical, rather than penal, administration. This is the least hypocritical solution to a difficult problem. Mentally ill offenders are, nevertheless, offenders. Their handling thus involves consideration of social factors which go considerably beyond medical factors. As with prisoners with other types of health problems, the offender's access to high-quality mental health care should be similar to that of patients who are not incarcerated.[160] Developing quality medical facilities within jails and prisons, adequately staffed and medically administered, is one way out of this dilemma and is far preferable to the proliferation of special-security hospitals.

Dangerous Psychopaths

Psychopathic offenders are the most controversial of inmates. This chapter cannot resolve the issue of whether psychopathy is a mental disorder.[52, 53, 146] The British, in particular, have been plagued by uncertainties as to how to manage and to conceptualize the handling of these offenders. As a practical matter, in the United States, psychopathy is most often not treated as a mental disorder. At any rate, neither British nor American psychopathy is with any degree of reliability "medically treatable."[146] The term itself is objectionable and pejorative. Psychiatrists more optimistic about the possibility of psychiatric intervention point out:

> Psychopathy is an administrative term comparing patients whose only common feature is their persistently difficult behavior and in whom three causative areas can be found, often in complex combination: (1) extremes of personality types . . .; (2) extreme mishandling in childhood . . .; and (3) formes frustes of organic brain damage . . . and psychosis . . . . To make generalizations for psychopaths any more than one does for schizophrenia, alcoholism or nephritis, may be proved wrong in the long run.[164]

The above citation is relevant to whether any of these men (who may be extremely difficult to manage in prison) should be placed in special prisons or special prison units having medical input, or whether such offenders should be handled in regular prisons. This issue most clearly confronts the "behavior control" issue, because the great majority of these men are not classically mentally ill and they may also resist such special handling. In Britain it has been recommended that psychopathic offenders be treated in prisons rather than in hospitals, not in prison hospitals or in "special" hospitals, but in "training units" established in prisons and featuring regimens of intensive work and social activities.[146] Psychiatrists, though, are to head the unit "because of the long association of the medical profession with the treatment of personality disorders."[146] It is important that admission to the units be voluntary.

In the United States, this debate has been manifested in several contexts. In order to maximize resources and to defuse the regular prisons, consideration has been given to whether regional penal facilities should be established which would receive and treat "special offenders" (for example, "special offenders" resident in New England prisons).[124] These "special offenders" are not too precisely defined. As a common feature they seem to be not only violent and/or mentally ill, but also troublesome to the prison authorities. Although the problem addressed is no doubt real, this proposal and other recommendations for special prisoners have been reviewed with skepticism by a few.[124, 165]

Better known nationally have been other controversies concerning programs of behavior modification for "troublesome" or violent prisoners. For example, the Special Treatment and Rehabilitative Training (START) program of the Federal Bureau of Prisons consisted of the involuntary transfer of inmates to living conditions involving considerable deprivation (isolation cells) with subsequent progressive amenities provided to the offender commensurate with progress.[88, 166] START was "stopped" by the Federal Bureau of Prisons consequent to litigation and to the controversy engendered. A federal district court ruled that transfer to the START program involved "a major change in the conditions of confinement" and that the inmate "is entitled, at a minimum, to the type of hearing required by the Supreme Court in *Wolff v. McDonnell*."[167]

What is the correctional psychiatrist to make of this? A previous section of this chapter has suggested that psychiatric management and treatment of many violent prisoners might be helpful to the prisoners and indirectly to potential victims; such help, if voluntarily requested by inmates, should be encouraged. Morris has provided a useful description of a voluntary prison treatment program for violent offenders, noting also that such a program cannot be directed solely or even primarily toward institutional troublemakers. [168] Morris's ideas have recently been implemented in a portion of the Butner Federal Correctional Institute in North Carolina. Students of corrections eagerly await the outcome from this model prison.

Coercion and isolation must not be euphemistically labeled "treatment." What is treatment from the perspective of society may constitute yet another form of punishment to the offender. Given the past failures of psychiatric approaches in this area, and considering the ethical dilemmas, correctional psychiatric participation in the treatment of "dangerous psychopaths" is not recommended unless (1) such treatment is self-sought by the inmate, and (2) the inmate's decision either to enter into or to continue in the treatment bears no direct relationship to subsequent release from prison.

THE ROLE OF THE CORRECTIONAL PSYCHIATRIST

This chapter has articulated a point of view not always highlighted in discussions of prison and jail work; namely, that the primary purpose of correctional psychiatry is to make available to inmates on a voluntary basis those medical and psychological opportunities that would or should be available to them in the outside community. Treatment should be addressed to the mental disorder per se, to the prison-induced mental instability, or to the behavioral disorder as this is defined by the inmate. Furthermore, it is advocated that release generally not be dependent upon the psychiatrist's estimate of "cure," either of mental disorder or of criminality. This position is the middle ground between the unacceptable opposites of the "crime of treatment" and the "crime of no treatment."[8] Society defines the punishment; the inmate defines the subsequent treatment and requests it.

Experts in correctional psychiatry, however, conceptualize the role of the correctional psychiatrist differently.[56, 168-172] A brief review will illustrate both the strengths and the problems of other correctional roles, in addition to the clinical role, that the correctional psychiatrist may play.

The Psychiatrist as Agent of Change

Some believe that the psychiatric interventions with inmates discussed above are relatively fruitless and that the correctional psychiatrist can function more broadly as a consultant to, and a shaper of, the institutional milieu (for example, by promoting decarceration; the abolition of large, inhumane prisons; training or sensitizing correctional officers to be less punitive or more psychologically minded; advocating reforms to decrease the deprivations of incarceration; and advocating use of prison furloughs, conjugal visits, and so forth.) As Suarez put it, "Psychiatry would do better to spend its time treating the institution itself rather than the individual inmates within it."[171] Considering the small number of correctional psychiatrists available, it is only through directing attention to the overall milieu that the psychiatrist can influence the treatment of more than a few inmates.[125,169] This consultative approach, which may involve "taking the warden home to dinner," properly aims at making the prison environment more human and constructive.

Often, however, this consultative approach does not stop at this point. It may be traditionally argued that "the wall that exists between custody and treatment must go,"[169] or that psychiatry should help "the staff members change their focus toward rehabilitation and away from infantalizing custody."[171] This is the point of departure between the present author and other commentators. Although prisons must become more humane (and making a full range of services and opportunities, including psychiatric services, available to inmates is a step in this direction), American penology has repetitively confirmed that prisons and jails will never be primarily treatment-oriented rather than punishment-oriented institutions. Correctional officers confronted by problems to inmate violence and recidivism; correctional administrators confronted with a poverty of resources; treatment staff confronted by the limitations of closed or semiclosed institutions; and all others, including inmates, know that these institutions do not and cannot exist primarily for purposes of treatment. To assert that this is possible is to defy the logic of the word prison. Furthermore, the psychological reality of the inmate is that

> Deprivation of freedom is punishment and no amount of semantics will make it otherwise. Inmates know and feel this and staff should admit it. There are no more bitter inmates that those who are sentenced for "rehabilitation" and who find only a long period of isolation and sometimes repression behind the walls.[173]

Paradoxically, the ability of psychiatrists to influence the milieu and to communicate with inmate-patients is notable only when they are willing to admit that treatment is not the sole or even the major purpose of incarceration. Above all, the correctional psychiatrist must always play it straight: "The lesson perhaps is that in prison one may be a more effective therapist if he does not claim to be one."[172]

Thus, although consultation to the milieu can be very much encouraged as a role complementary to that of individual inmate treatment, the correctional psychiatrist should not believe that even with changes in the milieu, prisons or jails will become genuine treatment-type institutions. Furthermore, because of external constraints, more often the milieu does not change, or milieu changes which are instituted are not maintained. The psychiatric consultant, despairing of providing any type of treatment in such a milieu, leaves the prison or jail, and once more mentally ill inmates are left with no access to traditional services. This is the danger of preoccupation with consultation to the milieu as the sole or major role for the correctional psychiatrist.

Rehabilitation

This chapter has not presented a very optimistic view concerning rehabilitation of inmates.[174] Rehabilitation is the payoff that law and society hope for from correctional psychiatry, a payoff that traditionally has been associated with psychiatric participation in sentencing, in institutional classification procedures, in preparole assessment, and in other diagnostic activities.[31, 35, 36] Again, it is beyond the scope of this chapter to explore these areas in any depth or to review the voluminous and somewhat discouraging literature on rehabilitation. From the perspective of the present author, it is quite unwise to condition the provision of psychiatric services to inmates on the premise that such will be rehabilitative or will decrease recidivism. First, with few exceptions,[96] there is no evidence for such a claim. One would not want to take the position that the value of fixing a fractured leg in prison is dependent upon whether or not the inmate steals again. Furthermore, forcing characterologic change (necessary in a few inmates for purposes of "rehabilitation") in the absence of clear-cut mental illness, dangerousness, mental incompetence, and treatability would constitute very questionable behavior for psychiatrists.[175] The paradox is that behavioral interventions that truly "work" in correcting offenders (assuming such interventions are not genuinely accepted by inmates) may be either unethical, illegal, or both. Finally, orienting the provision of psychiatric services in prison to reducing recidivism, given the present state of knowledge, exposes the correctional psychiatrist and inmates to a series of embittering encounters—encounters that jeopardize legitimate institutional treatment endeavors. The correctional officers jibe the psychiatrist—"He's back again, Doc; I thought you treated him already"—while the correctional psychiatrist knows, or should know, that psychological, social, and situational factors that contribute to inmate recidivism easily overpower psychological changes seemingly accomplished during incarceration. Despite the data, there are always new enthusiasts for rehabilitation, new nostrums proposed for old problems.[176]

Sentencing, Classification, and Parole

A few comments are relevant concerning sentencing, classification, and psychiatric activities relevant to parole. These activities, which may be of some use to the inmate but which even more frequently are of use to the institution, must immediately be distinguished from activities falling under the mantle of the doctor-patient relationship. Confidentially is absent, the information is shared with others, and it cannot be predicted whether the information gathered will help or hurt the inmate, at least from the inmate's perspective. All this must be explained to the inmate from the outset. Maintaining the confidentiality of even conventional treatment efforts may be very difficult in prison. The inmate must be apprised of the extent of confidentiality of communications. When inmates threaten violence or discuss escape, the psychiatrist is placed in a tenuous position. The correctional bureaucracy presses for information that the psychiatrist possesses and that constitutes a threat to the institution. The resolution of this dilemma relates to informed consent. Coincident with treatment—individual treatment, group treatment, crisis intervention—the psychiatrist should be forthright regarding information that, if it was known to him or her, he or she would feel necessary to act upon.[177] The psychiatrist must also know that no records, kept anywhere in the prison, are immune from scrutiny. If it is to be "confidential," it must be kept in the head. Generally, the correctional psychiatrist who participates in institutional decision making concerning an inmate should not be doing the treatment.

> Mental health professionals who participate in administrative decision-making processes, such as, but not limited to parole and furlough relating to a prisoner, should be other than those mental health professionals providing direct therapeutic services to that prisoner. *(Standards of the American Public Health Association)*[160]

Sentencing and classification issues may be considered jointly. Regarding sentencing evaluations, it is noted:

We devote our evaluation to understanding what is happening with the individual, how the offense fits in this context, and what the individual needs in terms of therapy and rehabilitation, including some specific discussion of these needs and the agencies that might meet them.[171]

Psychiatric evaluations for purposes of sentencing may help avert prison sentences for some offenders. In the federal prison system, offenders may be sent to institutions for brief periods of observation prior to final sentencing. The assumptions concerning the utility of psychiatric participation in sentencing are as follows: first, that differential programming or treatment is available and that its pursuit will make a difference; and second, that the court will be influenced by the psychiatrist's recommendation. One of the few empirical studies of this latter issue discovered this not to be the case. Psychiatric reports did not generally affect the type of sentence given.[178] If this is to be a useful activity for the correctional psychiatrist, psychiatrists must request and should receive feedback concerning the utility of reports, whether they are followed, and whether they make a difference. As in the area of classification, the most worthwhile psychiatric contributions involve identifying clear-cut mental illness and maintaining sensitivity to mental retardation and other factors that might contribute to institutional victimization in the event that the offender is incarcerated. The dynamics of the offender's behavior, and not merely conclusions, should be given. It is highly doubtful whether a psychiatrist's diagnosis of "personality disorder with a need for a structured setting" is very enlightening to a court.

The classification controversy may be briefly summarized. Classification is a type of diagnostic workup or evaluation from multiple perspectives, which occurs prior to or shortly after incarceration. There are no psychiatric classification systems in widespread use today. A few such psychiatric systems have been described.[44, 79] An effort by Yarvis, dividing 25 incarcerated offenders into three groups, is illustrative. One group is essentially psychiatric in nature, neurotic offenders with minor histories of criminality. The second is a social deviance group, offenders with lengthy criminal histories. The last group of offenders manifested a clear-cut psychiatric illness as well as recurrent criminality.[179]

The critical question regarding classification is, why do it? Ideally the goal is classification in some form of "treatment" (matching offender types and needs with individual programs designed to meet these needs). In practice, most classification systems are utilized for purposes of institutional management, such as evaluating risk (Can the offender be in the community rather than in the institution?) or the inmate's need for a security level within an institution, or deciding what part of the institution's resources it is worthwhile or efficient to devote to the inmate.[79] Compromising most classification efforts is the lack of adequate back-up programs that might accomplish the goals of classification. The correctional psychiatrist involved in classification often experiences this effort, like other institutional "diagnosis," as a haphazardous, nontheoretical attempt.[180] In practice, the choices involve such matters as assignment to one cellblock or another, whether or not the inmate will be recommended to obtain a high school equivalency education, and what type of security is required for visits. As in other types of consultative work, the psychiatrist's dilemma is whether to recommend what he or she believes is necessary but which may not be available, or simply to choose on the basis of what the prison has to offer. Psychiatrists make their chief contribution, however, in adequately diagnosing mental illness, mental retardation, and neurological illness, and in clinically identifying other conventional medical entities which may require attention. Additionally, the inmate may discuss fears of victimization in the prison environment or sexual anxieties which, with the inmate's consent, may be communicated to other correctional workers for purposes of prevention.

Chapter 6 reviews the prediction of dangerousness, which is the variable of greatest interest to the parole authority. The trend in corrections is toward decreased discretionary handling with regard to parole.[83] Many states have ended indeterminate sentencing. The critical questions concerning psychiatric participation in parole relate to the uncertain status of the psychiatrist's expertise in these matters and to the propriety of psychiatric participation in this phase of corrections. To know that youth and a previous history of violent episodes, or a history of alcohol abuse, bespeak a poor prognosis is useful, but a psychiatrist is not needed to point this out, because information is contained in the record. A psychiatrist can profitably comment on whether the inmate is presently mentally ill if the inmate is known to have been so previously and if this remains a question. The psychiatrist can review the stresses previously or presently operative on the inmate and can explain their relationship to the inmate's behavior and give some pointers concerning danger signals or situational variables that should be considered following release.[181] Transitional mental health care can be recommended.

The assumption here is that such reports will not be presented or written by correctional psychiatrists whose roles in the prison have been in the treatment area. This is a difficult point. As the treating psychiatrist grows to know an inmate, he or she may be of the opinion that the inmate has shown psychological growth and that further incarceration would not be helpful, or that the inmate is no longer dangerous. The temptation is to want to present this material to the parole board, especially if the inmate requests or allows it.[9, 160, 172]

Unfortunately, such psychiatric behavior eventually confounds the prison treatment efforts. A further problem is that the inmates's release, as a realistic matter, may not depend to a great extent on the psychiatric report. Like other inmate reports from educational or vocational counselors, or Alcoholics Anonymous supervisors, these reports become excuses not to release the inmate but, instead, to recommend more treatment or improvement. The punishment and the treatment are again confounded. Because of these complexities, it is again stressed that it is best for the treating psychiatrist to separate his or her work from that of the evaluating psychiatrist. Agreement on this matter should be reached by negotiation and discussion between the treating psychiatrist and the inmate at the outset of any treatment effort. Moreover, it is important for the evaluating psychiatrist to explain to the inmate that the purpose of a diagnostic or preparole interview is to help the parole board reach its decision. What inmates most want from prison is to get out. This is completely understandable, but it must be taken into account as the psychiatrist assesses the value of his or her own participation in release decision making.

The Preservation of Therapeutic Identity

Numerous factors in the prison and jail conspire to degrade the correctional psychiatrist's identity. A few readers might argue that the skepticism evinced in this chapter concerning prison "treatment" (rehabilitation as the rationale for correctional psychiatric services) does exactly this. Such a conclusion would be a misreading of this chapter. The point has been to argue for the provision of standard medical services for inmates, whether or not these are rehabilitative. Prisoners require access to psychiatric services not because they are prisoners or because such services will necessarily reduce crime but because prisoners are people. For this matter, a similar point of view could be expressed concerning other human service programs in prisons and jails (for example, providing adequate programs of educational or vocational training for inmates). Given the fact of imprisonment, using prison opportunities should be a matter of choice for the inmate—a choice, however, that he or she must be able to make. It is in this sense that psychiatry as well as other human services can contribute to a humanizing of the prison environment; a lessening, though not an abrogation, of punishment.

Whatever the role of the correctional psychiatrist may be, there are many strains placed upon it.[6, 172] For example, doing crisis intervention (dealing with problems of prison violence, suicide, drug taking, or other disequilibriums), as well as treating the acutely mentally ill, exposes the correctional psychiatrist to the charge that he or she is mainly an institutional "pacifier" or "tranquilizer"— not a very appealing role. It has been said by experienced therapists that "to be limited to such a role, however useful it might be, is in fact a prostitution of . . . basic orientation as a therapist."[169] The role of "troubleshooter," if accomplished with empathy, may profit inmates as well as the institution. Such a role, however, if delivered with cynicism or disregard for longer-term gains that the offender might make by coping with the crisis, makes the correctional psychiatrist nothing but a "cop doctor"; a doctor interested mainly in the control of inmates for the purposes of others. This custodial role must be condemned strongly.[6] Psychiatrists must therefore continually reassess and re-evaluate their approach to in-prison problems, reviewing both the frustrations and the satisfactions that such problem-solving has engendered, asking themselves whose agent they are, or whose agent they have become.

Other sources of ambiguity concerning the correctional psychiatrist's role are the attitudes of the inmates and the correctional officers. The prisoners, mentally ill and not mentally ill alike, "may hold no special reverence for psychiatrists or physicians, who are considered just some more authority figures with whom to contend."[172] Although the physician may consider himself "a helping person in the medical and mental health tradition, inmates [are] naturally disbelieving."[172] Inmate skepticism concerning the value of psychiatry is sometimes reinforced by the correctional officers, even when psychiatric intervention may be appropriate: "Why do you want to mess around with those shrinks?" "If you don't watch what you say, you'll end up on the funny farm for good." "You're not crazy, what do you need those shrinks for?"[182] The majority of inmates are not mentally ill, nor do they wish to be so labeled or so handled.[172] Halleck was one of the first to write of "the criminal's problems with psychiatry."[57] The inmate is loath to give up a "bad" role, which has adaptive as well as destructive components, and instead to adopt a "sick" role.

The resolution of these problems is not simple. The correctional psychiatrist must maintain a straightforward approach in dealing with both inmates and correctional officers. The "sick" metaphor, though only a metaphor, is too powerful and has too many connotations to be usefully applied to most inmates. Even when treating those inmates who are mentally ill, the correctional psychiatrist does better to focus on inmate behaviors or feelings that are presently dysfunctional or painful, and on which some agreement can be reached with the inmate that the treatment is for his or her sake rather than for others. Word spreads quickly in prison or jail about "who is on whose side." If the correctional psychiatrist is honest and consistent in dealings with inmates, help will be sought, even if the inmate does not view his or her own behavior as sick or crazy.

Correctional officers sometimes ridicule psychiatric treatment because they view it as often ineffective and because they view the psychiatrist as hopelessly naive; as someone, for example, who does not realize how dangerous the inmates really are and who fails to grasp the idea that inmates can "never be trusted." Correctional workers "often look upon the clinician as a menacing figure who wishes to unleash recklessly all the uncontrolled impulses of the criminal."[169] Correctional officers may resent the opportunities for treatment or for other types of training that may be afforded to inmates "who have done bad things"—the kinds of treatments or opportunities that many correctional officers themselves have never had. These attitudes will not disappear entirely, nor is remedying them entirely within the correctional psychiatrist's purview. If, however, the correctional psychiatrist maintains his or her "cool" and attempts to understand the problems that beset the officers as well as the inmates, then communication is facilitated.[183] Correctional officers are generally neither cruel or inhuman. In the main they are persons with limited future options, persons struggling hard to do a difficult and sometimes dangerous job. The continuing confrontation of the correctional officers with the failures, yet never with the successes, of the prison or jail system culminates too frequently in anger or apathy. As the correctional psychiatrist experiences the prison or jail environment, he or she begins to appreciate the problems of the correctional officers. Informal exchanges between psychiatrists and correctional officers may then obviate some of the difficulties. As is true of the psychiatrist, what the correctional officer (and admittedly also the inmate) really needs is time away from the prison.

One solution to these problems is clear-cut. Few psychiatrists should work full time in a prison or a jail for very long. Psychiatrists who maintain affiliations outside the prison or jail or who themselves are known to be "short-timers" may be better trusted by inmates than the career correctional psychiatrist. Working elsewhere while doing prison or jail work permits the correctional psychiatrist to maintain professional standards and other professional associations while providing time for reflection about what he or she is doing in the prison. Similarity of psychiatric practice is thereby encouraged, whatever the setting. The cross-fertilization between the community and the prison improves the quality of mental health work that may be performed by correctional psychiatrists and by other professionals under their supervision. The unwelcome outcome of full-time work in correctional psychiatry, similar to that experienced by the correctional officers (anger, apathy, or a custodial mentality), is thus avoided. As Halleck[2] points out, many correctional psychiatrists do very little work, a problem that is essentially similar to "institutionalization" of the inmates and the guards.

Related to the point that professionals can function best on a part-time basis in prisons and jails is the recommendation that medical units in prisons and jails be staffed and run autonomously from the prison administration. Ideally, university-based personnel, residents in psychiatry (with supervision), and public health and private psychiatrists who are members of a group or a hospital should provide part-time psychiatric coverage for prisons or jails. This concept, however, is often resisted by the prison administration, which has a vested interest in maintaining control over its personnel. To some degree, of course, the prison officials are correct—a naive psychiatrist can wreak havoc in an institution—but the point here is one of achieving the proper balance. The proper mix for a prison psychiatric unit might include both full-time and part-time professionals; the full-time professionals could serve as liaisons to the institution and the milieu and help teach the part-time personnel the institutional mores, and the part-time personnel could maintain community contacts and could stimulate an up-to-date professional attitude for the unit.

Why Work in a Prison?

If what has been presented so far seems dismal, there is another side. Why would a psychiatrist want to work in a prison or jail? This is an interesting question. At least judged by their behavior, most psychiatrists have answered this question in the negative, namely, they wouldn't. Nevertheless, many psychiatrists exposed initially through the military service, the public health service, or even through psychiatric residency experience get "bitten" by prisons and jails and eventually do at least some part-time work there. The psychiatrist who takes the time, who can be persuaded even to visit a prison or jail, requires no convincing that (1) the need for his or her service is great, (2) the milieu is simultaneously deplorable and yet of considerable intellectual interest, and (3) with a clever approach it simply must be the case that something better could be happening there. Grandiosity and messianic zeal are, of course, no long-term friends for correctional psychiatry; yet, given the indicting picture that prisons and jails present, it is not that difficult for the psychiatrist to be inspired to make some contribution. There are, of course, other motivations. Every correctional psychiatrist recalls many positive relationships established with inmates (and a few with correctional officers, too), even if the inmate has continued to be in difficulty or the outcome was not known. The recent comprehensive study by Gunn and coworkers[184] also suggests that the mental health of some prisoners can be improved during the period of imprisonment. A great deal can be learned in prisons and jails concerning social organization, individual and group adaptation to stress, problems of violent and antisocial behavior, and problems of health delivery and health planning for underserved groups. Prisons and jails are logical catch areas and in this sense can serve as testing grounds for concepts in social and community psychiatry. Curiosity and a willingness to provide service for an underserved population are well rewarded. For at least some psychiatrists it can honestly be said, "Try it, you'll like it—at least a little bit." Providing better service for patients, rather than preventing crime, is, however, the orientation most consistent with the psychiatrist's experience and expertise.

REFERENCES

1. CORMIER, BM: *The practice of psychiatry in the prison society.* Bull Am Acad Psychiatry Law 1:156-183, 1973.
2. HALLECK SL: *Psychiatry and the Dilemmas of Crime. A Study of Causes, Punishment and Treatment.* Harper & Row, New York, 1967.

3. HALLECK, SL: *American psychiatry and the criminal: A historical review.* Int J Psychiatry 6:185-208, 1968.

4. *A Handbook of Correctional Psychiatry,* vol. 1. U.S. Bureau of Prisons, Department of Justice, Washington, DC, 1968.

5. CORMIER, BM: *The Watcher and Watched.* Scribner Tundra Books, New York, 1976.

6. POWELSON, H AND BENDIX, R: *Psychiatry in Prison.* Psychiatry 14:73-86, 1951.

7. CUMMING, RG AND SOLOWAY, HJ: *The Incarcerated Psychiatrists.* Hosp Community Psychiatry 24:631-632, 1973.

8. *Psychiatry in prisons: Treatment or punishment? (Symposium).* Psychiatric Opinion 11(3), 1974.

9. SHESTACK, JJ: *Psychiatry and the dilemmas of dual loyalties.* American Bar Association Journal 60:1521-1524, 1974.

10. MONAHAN, J AND STEADMAN, HJ: *Crime and mental disorder: An epidemiological approach.* In TONRY, M AND MORRIS, N (EDS): *Crime and Justice: An Annual Review of Research,* vol 4. University of Chicago Press, Chicago, 1983, pp 145-189.

11. ROTH, LH AND ERVIN, F: *Psychiatric care of federal prisoners.* Am J Psychiatry 128:424-430, 1971.

12. MESNIKOFF, AM AND LAUTERBACH, CG: *The Association of violent dangerous behavior with psychiatric disorders: A review of the research literature.* The Journal of Psychiatry and Law 3:415-445, 1975.

13. RAPPEPORT, JR: *Enforced treatment—is it treatment?* Bull Am Acad Psychiatry Law 2:148-158, 1974.

14. ALLEN, HE AND SIMONSEN, CE: *Corrections in America: An Introduction.* Glencoe Press, Beverly Hills, CA, 1975, pp 18-66.

15. Ibid, pp 42, 43.

16. MACMAHON, B AND PUGH, TE: *Epidemiology Principles and Methods.* Little, Brown & Co, Boston, 1970, p 7.

17. FITZPATRICK, JJ: *Psychoanalysis and crime: A critical survey of salient trends in the literature.* Ann Am Acad Political Social Sci 423:67-74, 1976.

18. RUBIN, S: *Psychiatry and the prison: A negative report.* Int J Psychiatry 6:214-218, 1968.

19. RUSSELL, DH: *Dimensions of forensic psychiatry.* Int J Psychiatry 6:219-221, 1968.

20. GROUP FOR THE ADVANCEMENT OF PSYCHIATRY: *Psychiatry and Sex Psychopath Legislation, the 30's to the 80's* 9(98):831-956, 1977.

21. SHAH, SA AND ROTH, LH: *Biological and psychophysiological factors in criminality.* In GLASER, D (ED): *Handbook of Criminology.* Rand McNally, Chicago, 1974, pp 101-173.

22. MEDNICK, SA AND FINELLO, KM: *Biological factors and crime: Implications for forensic psychiatry.* Int J Law Psychiatry 6:1-15, 1983.

23. WITKIN, HA ET AL: *Criminality in XYY and XXY men.* Science 193:547-555, 1976.

24. ROTH, LH: *Voluntary castration.* Hastings Cent Rep 6(5):4,30, 1976.

25. *Lack of prison psychiatrists puts strain on psychologists.* Behavior Today 7(30), July 26, 1976, pp 2,3.

26. AMA CENTER FOR HEALTH SERVICES RESEARCH AND DEVELOPMENT: *Medical Care in US Jails.* American Medical Association, Chicago, 1973.

27. COMPTROLLER GENERAL OF THE UNITED STATES: *Report to the Congress. Prison Mental Health Care Can Be Improved by Better Management and More Effective Federal Aid.* General Accounting Office, Washington, DC, November 23, 1979.

28. CIBA FOUNDATION: *Medical Care of Prisoners and Detainees,* Symposium 16. Associated Scientific Publishers, Amsterdam, 1973.

29. Newman v. State of Alabama, 503 F.2d 1320, 1322-24 (5th Cir. 1974, cert. denied, 421 US 948, 1975).

30. LEVINSON, RB: *Treatment in correctional facilities.* In CARNAHAN, WA (ED): *Legal Prob-*

lems of Correctional, Mental Health and Juvenile Detention Facilities. Practicing Law Institute, New York, 1975, pp 551-557.

31. SMITH, CE: *Recognizing and sentencing the exceptional and dangerous offenders.* Federal Probation 35(4):3-12, 1971.

32. STANFORD, P: *A model, clockwork-orange prison.* New York Times Magazine, September 17, 1972, pp 71-84.

33. STÜRUP, GK: *Treating the "Untreatable"—Chronic Criminals at Hertstedvester.* The Johns Hopkins University Press, Baltimore, 1968.

34. GRODER, M: *An angry resignation.* Corrections 1(6):27-36, 1975.

35. KIM, LIC AND CLANON, TL: *Psychiatric services integrated into the California correction system.* International Journal of Offender Therapy 15:169-179, 1971.

36. KARPMAN, B, CITED BY ROBITSCHER, J: *Definition, description and dynamics of the mentally ill offender as seen from the law and psychiatry.* Address at Institute of the Mentally Ill Offender, Thomas Jefferson University, Philadelphia, 1970.

37. GLUECK, S, CITED IN RUSSELL, DH: *Dimensions of forensic psychiatry.* Int J Psychiatry 6:219-221, 1968.

38. ZITRIN, A: *Comments in NYU colloquium: President Nixon's proposal on the insanity defense.* J Psychiatry Law 1:297-334, 1973.

39. WOOTON, B: *The place of psychiatry and medical concepts in the treatment of offenders: A layman's view.* Canadian Psychiatric Association Journal 17:365-375, 1972.

40. BAILEY, WC: *Correctional outcome: An evaluation of 100 reports.* Journal of Criminal Law, Criminology, and Police Science 57:153-160, 1966.

41. MARTINSON, R: *What works? Questions and answers about prison reform.* The Public Interest, Spring 1974, pp 22-54.

42. QUAY, HC: *What corrections can correct and how.* Federal Probation 37(2):3-5, 1973.

43. MACDOUGALL, EC: *Corrections has not been tried.* Criminal Justice Review 1:63-76, 1976.

44. WARREN, MQ: *Classification of offenders as an aid to efficient management and effective treatment.* Journal of Criminal Law, Criminology, and Police Science 62:239-258, 1971.

45. NATIONAL COUNCIL ON CRIME AND DELINQUENCY: *The non-dangerous offender should not be imprisoned.* Crime Delinquency 21:315-322, 1975.

46. NATIONAL ADVISORY COMMISSION ON CRIMINAL JUSTICE STANDARDS AND GOALS: *Corrections.* US Government Printing Office, Washington, DC, 1983, pp 595-606.

47. SERRILL, MS: *Critics of corrections speak out.* Corrections 2:3, 1976.

48. Bronstein, AJ: *Rules for playing God.* Civil Liberties Review Summer 1975, pp 116-121.

49. DERSHOWITZ, A: *Let the punishment fit the crime.* New York Times Magazine, December 28, 1975, p 7.

50. LEVINSON, RB AND DEPPE, DA: *Optional programming: A model structure for the federal correctional institution at Butner.* Federal Probation 40(2):37-44, 1976.

51. FLYNN, EE: *Turning judges into robots.* Trial, March 1976, pp 17-23.

52. GUNN, J AND ROBERTSON, G: *Psychopathic personality: A conceptual problem.* Psychological Med 6:631-634, 1976.

53. LEWIS, A: *Psychopathic Personality: A Most Elusive Category.* Psychol Med 4:133-140, 1974.

54. *Clinical Aspects of the Violent Individual.* Task Force Report 8. American Psychiatric Association, Washington, DC, 1974.

55. VAN DER KVAST, S: *Can the psychiatrist foretell criminal behavior?* International Journal of Offender Therapy and Comparative Criminology 20(2):148-152, 1976.

56. HALLECK, SL: *Rehabilitation of criminal offenders—a reassessment of the concept.* Psychiatric Annals 4(3):61-85, 1974.

57. HALLECK, SL: *The criminal's problem with psychiatry.* Psychiatry 23:409-412, 1960.

58. *Prisoners at midyear 1983.* In *Bureau of Justice Statistics Bulletin.* US Department of Justice, Bureau of Justice Statistics, Washington, DC, October 1983.

59. *Jail inmates 1982.* In *Bureau of Justice Statistics Bulletin.* US Department of Justice, Bureau of Justice Statistics, Washington, DC, February 1983.

60. GOLDFARB, R: *Jails: The Ultimate Ghetto.* Anchor Books, New York, 1976.

61. MATTICK, HW: *The contemporary jails of the United States: An unknown and neglected area of justice.* In GLASER, D (ED): *Handbook of Criminology.* Rand McNally, Chicago, 1974, pp 777-848.

62. RAWLS, W, JR: *Crises and cutbacks stir fresh concerns on nation's prisons.* New York Times, January 5, 1982, p A-1.

63. Costello v. Wainwright, 397 F Supp 20 (MD Fla 1975), mod, 525 F2d 1239 (5th Cir 1976), 539 F 2d 547 (Sept. 27, 1976).

64. CLEMENTS, CB: *Psychological roles and issues in recent prison litigation.* In GUNN, J AND FARRINGTON, DP (EDS): *Abnormal Offenders, Delinquency, and the Criminal Justice System.* John Wiley & Sons, New York, 1982, pp 37-59.

65. PRIGMORE, CS AND CROW, RT: *Is the court remaking the American prison system? A brief overview of significant court decisions.* Federal Probation 40(2):3-10, 1976.

66. Pugh v. Locke: James v. Wallace, 406 F Supp 318, 329-330 (MD Ala 1976).

67. IRWIN, J: *The Felon.* Prentice-Hall, Englewood Cliffs, NJ, 1970.

68. TOCH, H: *Men in Crisis: Human Breakdowns in Prison.* Aldine, Chicago, 1975.

69. SWANK, GE AND WINER, D: *Occurrence of psychiatric disorder in a county jail population.* Am J Psychiatry 133:1331-1333, 1976.

70. LAMB, HR AND GRANT, RW: *The mentally ill in an urban county jail.* Arch Gen Psychiatry 39:17-22, January 1982.

71. PETRICH, J: *Psychiatric treatment in jail: An experiment in health-care delivery.* Hosp Community Psychiatry 27:413-415, 1976.

72. DUNN CS AND STEADMAN, HJ: (EDS): *Mental Health Services in Local Jails: Report of a Special National Workshop. Crime and Delinquency Issues: A Monograph.* US Department of Health and Human Services, Alcohol, Drug Abuse, and Mental Health Administration, Washington, DC, 1982.

73. *Inmate 66 years finds life in prison is what he prefers.* New York Times. August 19, 1976, p 30.

74. Board of Inquiry, United States Penitentiary, Lewisburg, PA, June 8-June 15, 1976. US Bureau of Prisons, Washington, DC, 1976.

75. BANISTER, PA, ET AL: *Psychological correlates of long-term imprisonment. I. Cognitive variables.* Br J Criminol 13:312-323, 1973.

76. HESKIN, KJ, ET AL: *Psychological correlates of long-term imprisonment. II. Personality variables.* Br J Criminol 13:323-330, 1973.

77. BUKSTEL, LH AND KILMANN, PR: *Psychological effects of imprisonment on confined individuals.* Psychol Bull 88:469-493, 1980.

78. JOHNSON, R AND TOCH, H (EDS): *The Pains of Imprisonment.* Sage Publications, Beverly Hills, CA, 1982.

79. NATIONAL ADVISORY COMMISSION ON CRIMINAL JUSTICE STANDARDS AND GOALS: *Classification of offenders.* In *Corrections.* US Government Printing Office, Washington, DC, 1973, pp 197-218.

80. RIEGER, W: *Suicide attempts in a federal prison.* Arch Gen Psychiatry 24:532-535, 1971.

81. ROTH, LH, ROLLIN, AM, ERVIN, FR: *Violent and nonviolent prisoners: A comparison.* Paper given at session on institutional violence. Annual meeting, American Psychiatric Association, Dallas, 1972.

82. TWADDLE, AC: *Utilization of medical services by a captive population: An analysis of sick call in a state prison.* J Health Soc Behav 17:236-248, 1976.

83. *Setting prison terms.* In Bureau of Justice Statistics Bulletin, US Department of Justice, Bureau of Justice Statistics, Washington, DC, August 1983.

84. SIGLER, MH: *Abolish Parole?* Federal Probation 39(2):42-48, 1975.

85. MONAHAN, J AND STEADMAN, HJ (EDS): *Mentally Disordered Offenders: Perspectives from Law and Social Science.* Plenum Press, New York, 1983.

86. STEADMAN, HJ, ET AL: *Mentally disordered offenders.* Law and Human Behavior 6:31-38, 1982.

87. Vitek v. Jones, 445 U.S. 480 (1980).

88. WEXLER, DB: *Criminal Commitments and Dangerous Mental Patients: Legal Issues of Confinement, Treatment, and Release, Crime and Delinquency Issues.* National Institute of Mental Health. DHEW No. (ADM) 76-331, Washington, DC, 1976.

89. *Matteawan State Hospital to Shut Down by April 1.* New York Times, August 2, 1976, p 51.

90. Davis v. Watkins, 384 F Supp 1196 (ND Ohio 1974).

91. GUZE, SB: *Criminality and Psychiatric Disorders.* Oxford University Press, New York, 1976.

92. *Prisoners and drugs.* In Bureau of Justice Statistics Bulletin, US Department of Justice, Bureau of Justice Statistics, Washington, DC, March 1983.

93. BACH-Y-RITA, G: *Personality disorders in prison.* In LION, JR (ED): *Personality Disorders, Diagnosis and Management.* Williams & Wilkins, Baltimore, 1974, pp 308-317.

94. VAILLANT, GE: *Sociopathy as a human process. A viewpoint.* Arch Gen Psychiatry 32:178-183, 1975.

95. BACH-Y-RITA, GE: *Habitual violence and self-mutilation.* Am J Psychiatry 131:1018-1020, 1974.

96. CARNEY, FJ: *Evaluation of psychotherapy in a maximum security prison.* Semin Psychiatry 3:363-375, 1971.

97. BRAUKMANN, CJ, ET AL: *Behavioral approaches to treatment in the crime and delinquency field.* Criminology 13:299-331, 1975.

98. MARTIN, SE, SECHREST, LB, REDNER, R (EDS): *New Directions in the Rehabilitation of Criminal Offenders.* National Academy Press, Washington, DC, 1981.

99. SUTKER, PB AND MOAN, CE: *A psychosocial description of penitentiary inmates.* Arch Gen Psychiatry 29:663-667, 1973.

100. KOLLER, KM AND CASTANOS, JN: *Family background in prison groups: A comparative study of parental deprivation.* Br J Psychiatry 117:371-380, 1970.

101. GIAGIARI, S: *The mentally retarded offender.* Crime Delinquency Lit 3:559-577, 1971.

102. ROFFMAN, RA AND FROLAND, C: *Drug and alcohol dependencies in prison: A review of the response.* Crime Delinquency Lit 22:359-366, 1976.

103. ANNO, J: *The role of organized medicine in correctional health care.* JAMA 247:2923-2925, 1982.

104. *Standards for Health Services in Prisons.* American Medical Association, Chicago, July 1979.

105. *Standards for Health Services in Jails.* American Medical Association, Chicago, July 1979.

106. Inmates of Allegheny County Jail v. Pierce, 612 F.2d 754 (3d Cir. 1979); opinion and order of DJ Cohill, April 17, 1980, on remand, 487 F. Supp. 638 (W.D. Pa. 1980).

107. WINICK, BJ: *Legal limitations on correctional therapy and research.* Minnesota Law Review 65:331-422, 1981.

108. SCHWITZGEBEL, RK: *Legal Aspects of the Enforced Treatment of Offenders. Crime and Delinquency Issues: A Monograph Series.* US Department of Health, Education, and Welfare, Alcohol, Drug Abuse, and Mental Health Administration, Washington, DC, 1979.

109. HARTSTONE, E, STEADMAN, HJ, MONAHAN, J: *Vitek and beyond: The empirical context of prison-to-hospital transfer.* Law and Contemporary Problems 45:125-136, 1982.

110. Nelson v. Heyne, 491 F 2d 352 (7th Cir., 1974) cert den 417 US 976 (1974).

111. WADESON, H AND CARPENTER, WT: *Impact of the seclusion room experience.* J Nerv Ment Dis 163:318-328, 1976.

112. ROWAN, BA: *Corrections.* In KINDRED, M, ET AL (EDS): *The Mentally Retarded Citizen and the Law.* The Free Press, New York, 1976, pp 650-675.

113. BROWN, BS AND COURTLESS, TF: *The mentally retarded in penal and correctional institutions.* Am J Psychiatry 124:1164-1169, 1968.

114. FOX, SJ: *The Reform Movement and Tactical Problems.* In KINDRED, M, ET AL (EDS): *The Mentally Retarded Citizen and the Law.* The Free Press, New York, 1976, pp 627-638.

115. U.S. v. Masthers, 539 F 2d 721, 1 MDLR 187, 1976.

116. WOLFENSBERGER, W: *The Principle of Normalization in Human Services.* National Institute on Mental Retardation. Leonard Crainford, Toronto, 1972.

117. COHEN, AK, COLE, GF, BAILEY, RG (EDS): *Prison Violence.* DC Heath, Lexington, MA, 1976.

118. TOCH, H: *Police, Prisons, and the Problem of Violence.* Crime and Delinquency Issues. NIMH, Center for Studies of Crime and Delinquency. DHEW Publication No. (ADM) 76-364, 1977.

119. Bennett, LA: *The study of violence in California prisons: A review with policy implications.* In COHEN, AK, COLE, GF, BAILEY, RG (EDS): *Prison Violence.* DC Heath, Lexington, MA, 1977, pp 149-168.

120. CLEMENTS, CB: *Crowded prisons: A review of psychological and environmental effects.* Law and Human Behavior 3:217-225, 1979.

121. KINZEL, AF: *Body-buffer zone in violent prisoners.* Am J Psychiatry 127:99-104, 1970.

122. MEGARGEE, EI: *Population density and disruptive behavior in a prison setting.* In COHEN, AK, COLE, GF, BAILEY, RG (EDS): *Prison Violence.* DC Heath, Lexington, MA, 1976, pp 135-144.

123. UHLIG, RH: *Hospitalization experience of mentally disturbed and disruptive, incarcerated offenders.* J Psychiatry Law 4:49-59, 1976.

124. BACH-Y-RITA, G, VENO, A: *Habitual: A profile of 62 men.* Am J Psychiatry 131:1015-1017, 1974.

125. ROTH, LH: *Treating violent behaviors in prisons, jails, and other special institutional settings.* In ROTH, LH (ED): *Clinical Treatment of the Violent Person. Crime and Delinquency Issues: A Monograph Series.* National Institute of Mental Health, Washington, DC, 1985. (in press).

126. WOODS, SM: *Violence: Psychotherapy of pseudohomosexual panic.* Arch Gen Psychiatry 27:255-258, 1972.

127. LION, JR: *Evaluation and Management of the Violent Patient.* Charles C Thomas, Springfield, IL, 1972.

128. *Drugs in the treatment of human aggression.* J Nerv Ment Dis 160:75-145, 1975.

129. TUPIN, JP: *Psychopharmacology and aggression.* In ROTH, LH (ED): *Clinical Treatment of the Violent Person. Crime and Delinquent Issues: A Monograph Series.* National Institute of Mental Health, Washington, DC, 1985 (in press).

130. SHEARD, MH, ET AL: *The effect of lithium on impulsive aggressive behavior in man.* Am J Psychiatry 133:1409-1413, 1976.

131. DANTO, BL (ED): *Jail House Blues, Studies of Suicidal Behavior in Jail and Prison.* Epic Publications, Orchard Lake, MI, 1973.

132. SLOANE, BC: *Suicide attempts in the District of Columbia prison system.* Omega 4:37-50, 1973.

133. *Study challenges common assumptions about jailhouse suicides.* Newsletter, American Academy of Psychiatry and the Law 8:51, September 1983.

134. Fawcett, J and Marrs, B: *Suicide at the country jail.* In Danto, BL (ed): *Jail House Blues.* Epic Publications, Orchard Lake, MI, 1973, pp 83-106.

135. Danto, BL: *The Suicidal Inmate.* In Danto, BL (ed): *Jail House Blues.* Epic Publications, Orchard Lake, MI, 1973, pp 17-26.

136. Heilig, SM: *Suicide in jails—a preliminary study in Los Angeles County.* In Danto, BL (ed): *Jail House Blues.* Epic Publications, Orchard Lake, MI, 1973, pp 47-55.

137. Sagarin, E: *Prison homosexuality and its effect on post-prison sexual behavior.* Psychiatry 39:245-257, 1976.

138. Serrill, MS: *Prison Furloughs in America.* Corrections 1(6):3-12, 53-56, 1975.

139. Dole, VP: *Detoxification of sick addicts in prison.* JAMA 220:366-369, 1972.

140. Guenther, AL: *Compensations in a total institution: The forms and functions of contraband.* Crime and Delinquency 21:243-254, 1975.

141. Roth, LH, Rosenberg, N, Levinson, RB: *Prison Adjustment of Alcoholic Felons.* Q J Studies Alcohol 32:382-392, 1971.

142. Ziegler, R, Costello, R, Horvat, G: *Innovative programming in a penitentiary setting: Report from a functional unit.* Federal Probation 40(2):44-49, 1976.

143. Lehmann, HE: *Unusual psychiatric disorders and atypical psychoses.* In Freedman, AM, Kaplan, HI, Sadock, BJ (eds): *Comprehensive Textbook of Psychiatry,* vol 2. Williams & Wilkins, Baltimore, 1975, pp 1724-1725.

144. Bellino, TT: *The Ganser syndrome: A contemporary forensic problem.* International Journal of Offender Therapy and Comparative Criminology 17:136-137, 1973.

145. Liss, R and Frances, A: *Court-mandated treatment: Dilemmas for hospital psychiatry.* Am J Psychiatry 132:924-927, 1975.

146. *Report of the Committee on Mentally Abnormal Offenders (Butler Report).* Her Majesty's Stationery Office, London, 1975.

147. Brooks, AD: *The mentally disabled offender.* In Brooks, AD (ed): *Law, Psychiatry and the Mental Health System.* Little, Brown & Co, Boston, 1974.

148. Shah, SA: *The Mentally Disordered Offender.* In Allen, RC, Ferster, EZ, Rubin, JG (eds): *Readings in Law and Psychiatry.* The Johns Hopkins University Press, Baltimore, 1975, pp 571-586.

149. McGarry, AL, et al: *Competency to stand trial and mental illness.* Crime and Delinquency Issues, NIMH, Center for Studies of Crime and Delinquency. DHEW Publication No. (HSM) 73:9105, Washington, DC, 1973.

150. Group for the Advancement of Psychiatry: *Misuse of Psychiatry in the Criminal Courts: Competency to Stand Trial,* vol 8. Report No. 89, February 1974.

151. Roesch, R and Golding, SL: *Competency to Stand Trial.* University of Illinois Press, Chicago, 1980.

152. Steadman, HJ and Cocozza, JJ: *Careers of the Criminally Insane: Excessive Social Control of Deviance.* DC Heath, Lexington, MA, 1974.

153. *Psychiatry and the dangerous offender.* Med J Aust 1:1-3, 1972.

154. Baxstrom v. Herold, 383 U.S. 107 (1966).

155. Nason v. Superintendent of Bridgewater State Hospital, 233 N.E.2d 908 (Mass 1968).

156. United States ex rel Schuster v. Herold, 410 F 2d 1071 (2nd Cir. 1969), cert. denied, 396 U.S. 847 (1969).

157. Jackson v. Indiana, 406 U.S. 713 (1972).

158. Jones v. U.S., 103 S.Ct. 3043 (1983).

159. Laben, JK and Spencer, JD: *Decentralization of forensic services.* Community Ment Health J 12:405-414, 1976.

160. Jails and Prisons Task Force: *Standards for Health Services in Correctional Institutions.* American Public Health Association, Washington, DC, 1976.

161. STEADMAN, HJ AND BRAFF, J: *Crimes of violence and incompetency diversion.* Journal of Criminal Law and Criminology 66:73-78, 1975.

162. MCGARRY, AL AND BENDT, RH: *Criminal vs. civil commitment of psychotic offenders: A seven-year follow-up.* Am J Psychiatry 125:1387-1394, 1969.

163. JABLON, NC, SADOFF, RL, HELLER, MS: *A unique forensic diagnostic hospital.* Am J Psychiatry 126:1663-1667, 1970.

164. SCOTT, PD: *The Butler committee's report. II. Psychiatric aspects.* Br J Criminol 16:177-178, 1976.

165. DESROCHES, F: *Regional psychiatric centers: A myopic view?* Canadian Journal of Criminology and Corrections 15:200-218, 1973.

166. HOLLAND, JG: *Behavior modification for prisoners, patients and other people as a prescription for the planned society.* Prison Journal 54(1):23-37, 1974.

167. Clonce v. Richardson, 379 F Supp 338, 348 (WD Mo, 1974).

168. MORRIS, N: *The Future of Imprisonment.* University of Chicago Press, Chicago, 1974.

169. PACHT, AR AND HALLECK, SL: *Development of mental health programs in correction.* Crime and Delinquency 12:1-8, 1966.

170. HELLER, MS: *The private reflections of a prison psychiatrist.* Prison Journal 54(2):15-33, 1974.

171. SUAREZ, JM: *Psychiatry and the criminal law system.* Am J Psychiatry 129:293-297, 1972.

172. KETAI, R: *Role conflicts of the prison psychiatrist.* Bull Am Acad Psychiatry Law 2:246-250, 1974.

173. ROTH, LH: *Treating the incarcerated offender.* Corrective Psychiatry Journal of Social Therapy 15(1):4-14, 1969.

174. SECHREST, L, WHITE, SO, BROWN, ED: *The Rehabilitation of Criminal Offenders: Problems and Prospects.* National Academy of Sciences, Washington, DC, 1979.

175. HALLECK, SL: *Legal and ethical aspects of behavior control.* Am J Psychiatry 131:381-385, 1975.

176. YOCHELSON, S AND SAMENOW, SE: *The Criminal Personality,* vol 1. Jason Aronson, New York, 1976, 1977.

177. ROTH, L AND MEISEL, A: *Dangerousness, confidentiality and the duty to warn.* Am J Psychiatry 134:508-511, 1977.

178. BOHMER, CER: *Bad or mad: The psychiatrist in the sentencing process.* J Psychiatry Law 4:23-48, 1976.

179. YARVIS, RM: *Psychiatric pathology and social deviance in 25 incarcerated offenders: An assessment.* Arch Gen Psychiatry 26:79-84, 1972.

180. SHOVNER, N: *"Experts" and diagnosis in correctional agencies.* Crime and Delinquency 20:347-358, 1974.

181. MONAHAN, J: *The Clinical Prediction of Violent Behavior. Crime and Delinquency Issues: A Monograph Series.* US Department of Health and Human Services, Alcohol, Drug Abuse, and Mental Health Administration, Washington, DC, 1981.

182. EDELMAN, SE AND FELTHOUS, AR: *Some methodological problems in studying violent offenders.* Bull Am Acad Psychiatry Law 4:67-72, 1976.

183. *A day on the job—in prison.* Corrections 2(6):6-12, 36-40, 44-48, 1976.

184. GUNN, J, ET AL: *Psychiatric Aspects of Imprisonment.* Academic Press, New York, 1978.

CHAPTER 20
CIVIL LAW AND PSYCHIATRIC TESTIMONY
Herbert C. Modlin, M.D.

Forensic mental health services have traditionally been associated mainly with criminal law applications: in the courtroom with the determination of litigants' sanity, and in prisons with prisoners' personal rehabilitation. However, only a small part of modern legal practice concerns criminal law. In the average three-year school curriculum, instruction in criminal law is given in a short, three-hour credit course for one semester. Most attorneys practice civil law; correspondingly, the collaboration of most practicing psychiatrists and psychologists with lawyers occurs in connection with legal problems focused on matters of civil law. Moreover, among mentally ill patients whose problems include involvement with the law, those problems are more likely to be civil than criminal, including personal injury suits, worker's compensation claims, divorce actions, child custody disputes, altercations with the Federal Internal Revenue Service, efforts to break or to preserve wills, issues concerning deeds and contracts, and professional malpractice claims.

PERSONAL INJURY SUITS

In the personal injury suits and malpractice claims that most commonly occupy potential, current, or former mental patients, the law of torts applies. The field of torts is complicated: "A really satisfactory definition of a tort has yet to be found."[1] A tort is a civil wrong (as opposed to a criminal wrong) perpetrated against one citizen by another. Tort refers to a transgression of legitimate rights such as invasion of privacy, defamation, misrepresentation, nuisance, negligence, trespass on real property, false imprisonment, assault and battery, and product liability.

In essence, the law imposed upon each of us is a civil duty to respect the person, name, reputation, property, privacy, and liberty of others. If we violate the rights of, or injure, another person regarding any of these, we may be liable to a tort claim for money damages. For a successful tort action to be pressed, X must prove that Y owed him a civic duty, that Y breached that duty, and that X suffered injury as a result.[2]

It has been estimated that about half of all the cases (not including divorce actions) on all the dockets of all the courts in the land are personal injury suits. In nearly all such claims, medical testimony is crucial; several physicians are ordinarily drawn into each case. Even when an attorney can prove liability, that a tort was committed, unless he or she can also establish through medical witnesses that the tort effected injury to the client, there is no basis for a successful law suit.

The functioning of psychiatrists in personal injury suits is usually in connection with the concept of traumatic neurosis. Although "traumatic neurosis" appears repeatedly in medical and legal literature, it is not an officially accepted diagnosis. It has never been listed in the *Diagnostic and Statistical Manual* published by the American Psychiatric Association, including the most recent, third, edition *(DSM III)*. The phrase has been applied in so many contexts and varying senses that its meaning is blurred and nearly useless.

In psychoanalytic literature, traumatic neurosis generally refers to a neurosis stemming from childhood experiences in which the immature ego is called upon to cope with untoward excitations or stresses.[3] The traumatic neuroses of war refer to a hodgepodge of reactions to a wide variety of precipitating agents.[4, 5] World War II spawned the tragic long-term "traumatic neuroses" engendered by concentration camp ordeals and the aftermath of atomic bombing.[6] In recent years the psychotraumatic effects of fires, tornadoes,[7] floods,[8] earthquakes,[9] sinking ships,[10] and other massive disasters have been studied and the term "traumatic neurosis" applied broadly. A companion phrase, "survivor syndrome," is becoming popular, as are delayed Viet Nam syndrome and rape trauma syndrome.

The clinical syndromes commonly seen postaccident are (1) posttraumatic stress disorder, in which free-floating anxiety may be experienced for months and sometimes for years; (2) conversion disorder, including anesthesia, paralyses, and torticollis; (3) somatiform disorder (psychophysiologic reactions), including chronic back pain, prolonged concussion syndrome, and cardiac neurosis; and (4) dependency reaction, an exacerbation of a characterologic passive-dependent reaction to stress. Depression, hypochondriasis, or dissociative reactions are rare.

POSTTRAUMATIC STRESS DISORDER

In 1976, Horowitz[11] suggested the overarching phrase "stress response syndrome" to encompass most of the clinical entities mentioned above. His work influenced the authors of *DSM III* to recognize a century of clinical observation and to devise a new diagnostic category, posttraumatic stress disorder. All the components of the syndrome are subjective complaints voiced by the victim or his or her family. Objective findings are minimal; thus diagnosis rests on accurate history taking. It is exceedingly important for physicians to interview patients' spouses and close family members because, characteristically, these patients are concrete, unimaginative, verbally unproductive, and inept observers of their own feelings and behaviors.[12] The symptoms of the syndrome are as follows:

1. **Anxiety.** Patients describe chronic, free-floating anxiety: "Something is about to happen." The accident to which they are reacting is past, but the persistent protective psychophysiologic set is anticipation of an imminent recurrence. The anxiety often becomes acute if the patient finds himself or herself again at the scene of the accident or in circumstances reminiscent of it. A phobic avoidance reaction may be the patient's most serious occupational disability. I have treated three structural steelworkers following falls which were not physically damaging; none of them went "back up" again. Following a frightening accident, a heavy construction equipment operator could not tolerate visiting construction sites, much less climbing into the cab of a vehicle. He is now working as a plant night watchman, earning a third of his former wages. An over-the-road trucker was involved in a head-on highway collision which overturned his cab. After 20 years of experience he had to give up driving. "Every time I get near a truck I get so nervous I can't open the cab door."

2. **Muscular tension.** Symptomatic complaints are restlessness, fatigability, insomnia, and a reiterated "I just can't seem to relax." The patient's spouse often vividly describes the patient's inability to sit still for long.

3. **Irritability.** When questioned, the patient will frequently acknowledge being a bit more difficult to live with, but here again the patient's spouse waxes eloquent about the patient's touchiness, flare-ups of anger, impatience, and loss of his or her former sense of humor. In over half the cases, the well-known "startle reaction" to sudden noises is an accompaniment. Radio, television, or conversation of well-meaning friends may cause an irritable lashing out or withdrawal. The patient's offspring, with some bewilderment and resentment, learn to avoid their explosive parent.

4. **Impaired concentration and memory.** Although these are common complaints, repeated psychological testing demonstrates no real memory loss at all. The patient's subjective sense of poor memory reflects self-preoccupied inattention to reality in the environment.

5. **Repetitive nightmares.** Frightening dreams directly or symbolically reproducing the experienced accident occur in about 75 percent of the cases and are pathognomonic of the syndrome. A spouse may report waking during the night to find the patient violently trembling and sitting bolt upright in bed.

6. **Sexual inhibition.** A notable lowering of sexual capacity is characteristic, sometimes to the point of complete impotence or frigidity. In working-class men this may be the most disturbing symptom of the syndrome, yet one that they can rarely talk about spontaneously.

7. **Social withdrawal.** Interpersonal involvement with relatives, friends, and neighbors is avoided. The patient discontinues regular church attendance, participation in recreational activities, movie going, and drops club memberships. By his behavior, he evidently is seeking "peace at any price."

A 52-year-old salesman was traveling in a midwestern town at dusk when his automobile stalled on some railroad tracks. In attempting to restart the car, he flooded the engine. As he waited a moment for the carburetor to drain, a slowly moving switch engine appeared and turned on its headlight. For 8 or 10 terrorized seconds the motorist helplessly gripped the steering wheel while the fiery-eyed monster bore down upon him. He received no physical injury from the impact, which nudged his car off the tracks, but he was so shaken that his legs buckled when he stepped from the car. When seen for psychiatric evaluation 8 months later, he complained of fearfulness, tension, restlessness, tearfulness, insomnia, repetitive nightmares, impaired concentration, irritability, and total sexual impotence. He had lost 20 pounds in weight and had been dismissed from his job. Almost anyone would be considerably shaken psychologically by such an experience but would recover in a few days or a week. For this particular man, the accident was disastrous.

Any of these symptoms may be part of other psychic illnesses, but together they constitute a specific handicapping reaction to the stress of an accident. Whenever three key symptoms—anxiety, startle reaction, and repetitive nightmares—are coexistent, a psychologically traumatic accident manifestly has occurred. In a few patients the syndrome may be complicated by a "spillover" of anxiety into the autonomic nervous system, resulting in familiar functional complaints such as palpitation, dyspnea, headache, dizziness, gastric distress, urinary frequency, and menstrual irregularity.

CONVERSION DISORDER (HYSTERICAL NEUROSIS)

The postaccident conversion reaction usually consists of symptoms referable to the body site of a physical impact. Suggestibility is a prominent feature.

> On a construction job a 10-pound sandbag fell from the third floor and struck a workman on the shoulder, knocking him to the ground. An hour later the victim, unable to work because of pain, was examined by the company physician who found no evidence of serious injury. After a week of physiotherapy he was deemed ready to return to the job, but he reported for work with a torticollis, his chin fixed over his left clavicle. Further examination revealed no physical basis for the distorted position, and psychiatric referral was accomplished. Hypnotic treatment relieved the disability, and the patient returned to work, although with some conscious anxiety.

> A 55-year-old carpenter, stepping back to admire a piece of work, fell into a hole 12 feet deep. Momentarily out of breath, he lay limply while fellow workers gathered around and warned him not to move "because something might be broken." He was raised by an improvised stretcher and transported to the nearest physician, whose cursory examination revealed considerable back pain and absent patellar reflexes. The physician unwisely mumbled something about "broken back," and the patient was sent by ambulance to a nearby hospital. Unfortunately, he shared a room with a patient with multiple sclerosis. When examined an hour after admission, he was hysterically paralyzed from the waist down.

The serious disability of such a patient is often traceable to therapeutic mismanagement. If time passes and the symptoms remain unalleviated, and if secondary gain of illness sets in—a limp, blindness, loss of voice, or torticollis becomes part of a chronic invalidism—remedial help is hard to apply.

SOMATIFORM DISORDER (PSYCHOPHYSIOLOGIC REACTION)

The well-known but poorly understood interweaving of psyche and soma is the postaccident condition least amenable to successful management. The persistent low back pain, the prolonged concussion syndrome, the cardiac neurosis—these are the most refractory problems.

A laborer lifts a heavy load, "something snaps," and pain develops quickly. Soft tissue injury is diagnosed and orthopedic treatment instituted. After 6 months the orthopedist, stating that the tissues should be well healed, can no longer attribute the persistent pain and disability to organic trauma. Eventually the patient may be persuaded to seek psychiatric evaluation, and the psychiatrist may be hard put to explain the disability convincingly on purely psychiatric grounds. The probable factor of secondary gain may loom large, but the primary mechanisms remain obscure.

DEPENDENCY REACTION

The exacerbation of a latent, passive-dependent solution to stress may appear in relatively pure culture or may complicate numerous other clinical syndromes. One common personality characteristic of these accident casualties might be labeled "inadequate." They often seem psychologically underdeveloped.

> A middle-aged plasterer working on a ceiling fell 8 feet to a terrazzo floor when his scaffold collapsed. He was badly frightened and suffered leg pain, but medical findings were essentially negative except for a linear hairline fracture of the right os calcis requiring no specific treatment. He sought psychiatric evaluation 2 years later because of persistent inability to work and chronic diffuse pain in both legs and hips, unconfirmed by physical findings. He lived with his widowed mother, who devoted much attention to his welfare. While on maneuvers during World War II, he twisted a knee and spent a year in Army hospitals. He was unable to work for an additional year after discharge from the service. In 1955, gastric symptoms were diagnosed as a preulcer state, and diet and medication were prescribed. A subsequent acute perforation of the stomach required only simple closure, but he could not work for 18 months.

This seemingly uncomplicated man struggled through life at a marginal level of adjustment. At a casual, uncritical glance, one might view him as an undistinguished but solid member of society—good to his mother, friendly to his peers, adequately performing his work. Closer inquiry revealed that he had a sixth-grade education, was pathetically awkward and fruitless in his approaches to women, and maintained continued psychological dependence on his mother and a steadily employed brother. Physicians, insurance companies, and the general public tend to find such a person irritating or contemptible. He may be called lazy, dishonest, or mercenary. To psychiatrists these are not sufficient explanations of his behavior, nor should they be. Human psychology is not that simple.

Any kind of accident, life-threatening or inconsequential, may trigger one of the psychopathologic reactions I have discussed. The unexpected, potentially dangerous near miss, in the absence of physical damage to the victim, usually triggers the anxiety reaction. The scaffold collapses, the steam pipe bursts, the crane tips over, the gasoline fumes flare into a flash fire. Such experiences undoubtedly would produce at least a degree of psychic disequilibrium even in "normal" persons.

Minor accidents—mild concussion, wrenched back, pratfall—usually produce a psychophysiologic reaction manifested by backache, recurrent headache, palpitation and dyspnea, leg weakness, and dizzy spells.

A young woman slipped and fell in a sitting position on a ramp in a department store. When examined by a psychiatrist a year later she was tense, hypersensitive, tearful, and unable to work because of diffuse lower-back pain unexplained by findings of repeated orthopedic examinations.

This type of valid postaccident disability is difficult for the average person to understand and to credit; one is prone to suspect malingering.

As a generality, there is a compensatory relationship between physical and psychic damage. The more extensive the tissue damage—fractures, lacerations, contusions, hemorrhage—the less likely a postaccident psychiatric disorder. Significant physical damage seems to bind or to neutralize the reactive anxiety or depression that the patient might reasonably be expected to exhibit; the person has something "real" to cope with instead of something intangible. The medical and nursing ministrations; bed rest; traction harness and plaster cast; visible evidence of "battle" injury to display; sedatives, analgesics, and narcotics; an acceptable, even required, temporary state of regressed invalidism; a legitimate, socially condoned period of convalescent inactivity—all these factors tend to inhibit the development of a complex of neurotic symptoms.

Conversely, a sudden, frightening accident causing little or no physical damage is more likely precipitant of psychiatric disorders. After the fact, the traumatized psyche is not put at rest between cool white sheets; the hyperirritable nervous system is not soothingly bandaged, poulticed, and fed intravenously; the invisible ego laceration is not legal tender for special considerations; and the victim's desire to retreat temporarily from everyday stresses is not socially approved. Incidentally, all these psychophysiologic treatments—immediate rest, sedation, isolation, enforced quiet, special attention under empathic medical authority—were encountered routinely by disturbed soldiers in Viet Nam with a resultant remarkably low incidence of psychiatric casualties. It is unfortunate that those hard-learned lessons of military psychiatry have not been more tellingly applied to counterpart civilian problems.

The course of the postaccident syndrome can be influenced by a variety of factors. Keiser devotes separate chapters of a book to the roles of physician, attorney, employer, insurance company, psychiatrist, family, and society.[13]

The havoc consequent to a severe stress depends upon the intrinsic strength of the target personality. The weaker the adaptive capacity of the psyche, the less insult is necessary to unbalance it. The more sudden and potentially dangerous the accident, the more likely it is to be psychologically unsettling, especially to an already teetering balance.

A young man involved in a head-on highway collision miraculously escaped physical injury. The girl riding with him was killed, and a passenger in the other car was seriously injured. His postaccident anxiety and depression are easy to understand; so severe a stress would be difficult for the most stable person to handle with unruffled poise.

It follows that observers using a common sense frame of reference are puzzled by, if not suspicious of, the considerable disability some persons manifest after seemingly minor or even trivial accidents. Their skepticism is based on the conviction that life consists only of what can be seen, that all people are approximately alike ("like me" is the usual point of comparison), and that a cause produces an event. Psychological science considers such thinking erroneous.

Individuals vary greatly in their personality strengths and weaknesses, and the capacity for flexible tolerance a victim brings with him to an accident must be duly weighed as one determinant of postaccident recovery from its psychological impact. "One man's meat is another man's poison." What to an observer appears a minor stress may constitute a major psychic assault to a given victim's uniquely vulnerable arrangement of internal resources and the particular set of external circumstances that happen at that time to be impinging upon him. Outsiders may well be unaware that the person is already near the breaking point from antecedent stresses of which the person himself or herself may not consciously be fully aware. The accident, then, can be a "last straw" phenomenon.

WORKER'S COMPENSATION CLAIMS

The broad intent of a state worker's compensation law is to provide subsistence in lieu of salary for an employee unable to work because of medical disability caused by a job-related incident. Additionally, the employee's medical expenses are paid. In cases of permanent disability, the weekly payments can be extended for a definite time period, usually 5 to 10 years.

Unlike tort law, worker's compensation law is not primarily concerned with proving fault or assessing penalty against a negligent other. If the employee is involved in a damaging accident or becomes ill because of the work environment, the employee is automatically compensated. All employers carry worker's compensation insurance; if there is a dispute, the contending parties are usually the employee and the insurance carrier.

In a representative case, a worker is injured. He is examined and treated by an orthopedist and in due course is declared able to return to work. The man objects because he is still tense, nervous, depressed, and suffering back pain. The insurance carrier, acting on the doctor's report, promptly stops weekly payments and refuses to honor further medical bills. The worker engages an attorney, usually through the union office, and the battle is joined. Enter the psychiatrist.

Persons suffering psychological decompensation from industrial accidents differ little clinically from psychologically injured victims of highway accidents. However, the incidence of psychophysiologic reactions in industrial cases is greater, and the factor of secondary gain more frequently complicates recovery. Industrial environments hold possibilities for a multitude of frightening accidents, some of them bizarre: a crane tips over; dynamite goes off prematurely; an operator's hair is caught in a whirring machine.

Worker's compensation laws cover most illnesses (called "industrial illnesses") identifiable with the employment situation, not just traumatic accidents. The proof of a causal link between the development of the illness or its exacerbation is often difficult. The issue of job stress that triggers psychiatric illness presents challenging evaluative problems to the psychiatrist; for example, the inherent chronic stress in the air traffic control officer's job, or the unrelieved pressure of a ceaselessly moving assembly line belt.

The dean of a graduate school resigned, and a senior professor was appointed acting dean. He assumed the new responsibilities and maintained his full teaching load. His double duty required much overtime work. One Sunday he suffered a severe coronary thrombosis in his office and, following complicated litigation, was held to have been a victim of job stress, entitled to full worker's compensation, including that for loss of future earnings. The psychiatrist's explanation of the compulsive, overconscientious professor's psychophysiologic mechanisms was helpful in winning his claim.

Evaluation of psychiatric disability in worker's compensation claims is frequently complicated by variables of the "system" encapsulating the employee—variables imposed by employer, insurance company, worker's compensation laws, doctors, the claimant's family, and patterns of the individual's culture.

At the beginning of the day's work, a welder stooped to get a welding rod and, on straightening up, cracked his head sharply against a steel beam. Briefly dazed, he fell to his knees. Half an hour later, complaining of severe headache and blurred vision, he told his foreman he needed to go to the emergency room of a hospital nearby. The foreman said, "Get out your toolbox or quit"—hardly an enlightened personnel policy. After another half hour he went to the hospital, was examined, and was sent home with medication and instructions to see his family doctor if he did not improve. The following morning his headache and neck pain were so severe that he could not lift his head from his pillow. The welder returned to the hospital and was admitted because of the neck problem, poor eye convergence, and a fleeting nystagmus. He was treated for brain concussion and cervical sprain and was discharged 10 days later to continue in treatment as an outpatient. At the end of 2 months he was pronounced sufficiently recovered for light work. In that postaccident period he experienced tension, restlessness, insomnia, sensitivity to noise, moodiness, and irritability. He snapped at his wife and railed at their children. His behavior proved a last straw for an already tottering marriage; his wife left with their children and sued for divorce. Through his union's assistance, he applied for worker's compensation and did receive two monthly checks. When the doctor reported him able to work, the checks were stopped without explanation. Thus within 3 months the patient had lost his job, his income, and his employability (because of incapacitating symptoms), as well as his wife, his offspring, and the ownership of his house. He was bewildered, demoralized, depressed, and nervous. He took his troubles to an attorney whose investigative procedure included sending him to be examined by an orthopedist, a neurologist, and a psychiatrist. Armed with appropriate medical information, the attorney got the compensation checks restarted and instituted suit against the former employer whose insurance carrier then arranged for the man to be examined by its company's orthopedist, neurosurgeon, and psychiatrist. So the months dragged on while the patient's bewilderment and self-preoccupation were intensified by diagnoses in the medical reports that ranged from malingering to brain damage to neurosis.

Although the liberal worker's compensation laws tend to encourage a dependency reaction, the possible monetary gain is of negligible psychological importance in most cases. Nearly all workmen receiving compensation lose financially, because the payments are less than they earn on the job.

Secondary Gain

The primary gain of psychiatric illness is inwardly directed. The patient's symptoms serve to maintain a degree of personality integration and balance, although at a level below good health. Secondary gain may be thought of as outwardly directed and is an attempt to achieve interpersonal balance or gratification.[14] As a consequence of the legitimate illness, the patient may realize relief from stress, pressure, and responsibility. The patient may have dependency needs met by a concerned and devoted spouse; he or she may acquire a morally condoned outlet for counteraggression toward an employer; or the patient may discover the seeming solution to concomitant life problems.

The 55-year-old construction worker may be able to avoid consciously acknowledging his slowly fading physical strength, his diminishing muscular agility, his increasing weariness at the end of the day, and his mildly waning sexual virility. He needs to believe that "I am as good a man as I ever was" and "experience is what counts on my job." He needs to maintain self-esteem, to deny how he is struggling to keep pace with the vigorous young apprentice working beside him. When this man suffers a sprained back, a bruised shoulder, a period of heat exhaustion in midsummer, or a brief coma from a minor blow to the head, his unconscious coping efforts are facilitated by a legitimate, face-saving way out of a troubling situation. Thus a protective, problem-solving invalidism may set in—it is a common psychological maneuver. In medicine it may complicate any illness—medical, surgical, obstetrical, or psychiatric—and it is not peculiar to postaccident reactions. In fact, the psychological mechanism of solving Problem A by succumbing to Problem B is a universal phenomenon of human behavior and is not peculiar to beneficiaries of medical or legal expertise.

> An oil well troubleshooter earned a comfortable living for his wife and three children through his skill in returning faltering wells to production; he frequently collected overtime pay because he and his small crew were on call day and night. The work was often hazardous, and several of his workmen were commonly out of work with injuries, but he accepted all job assignments and accomplished them with conscientious thoroughness, secure in the belief that he was immune to injury. At one difficult job on a freezing, snowy night, he slipped and fell twice from a truck, landing in a sitting position each time. He gave up and pulled his crew off the job for the first time in years. Although not seriously injured, incapacitating lower-back pain set in, became chronic, and he was "forced" to leave the oil wells for much less remunerative work as a salesman.

Many authors point to the inappropriateness of "gain" in secondary gain.[14-17] For such paradoxical gains the patient pays a high price and in the long run is always the loser. The "gain" is illusory and irrational and becomes part of the neurotic matrix of the disability. According to Slawson,[16] "because it affords dependent gratification, it can complicate recovery by triggering neurotic decompensation. Marked psychophysiologic regression may follow."

Monetary reward for illness may be an additional complication. "Compensation neurosis" is another piece of jargon in our working vocabulary. Its meaning is even more vague than "traumatic neurosis" because of the bias and emotion usually associated with it. It often takes on the character of an epithet. Here again, the reality of monetary gain is often an illusion, but the symbolism of money is part of our contemporary mythology. The dollar may represent emotional security, just compensation for suffering, a symbolic taking away of that which is precious from the aggressor; in short, a righteous retribution.[18]

Malingering

Malingering is the conscious, planned simulation of illness for the sake of gain. Individuals who simulate mental illness are uncommon, and those who do it successfully are rare. In contrast, patients who simulate health are common in clinical experience. In the personal injury problems in which we have been involved, time is on the clinician's side diagnostically. The symptoms have been present for months or years and have produced a consistent pattern of impaired functioning in most aspects of the patient's life.

The vast majority of patients who fail to improve from the effects of an industrial injury after a reasonable treatment effort are not malingering. Enelow[15] has classified these long-term nonrecoverers as (1) depressed patients; (2) hysterical personalities; (3) dependent, immature persons; (4) pseudo-self-sufficient persons; and (5) aging workers. A sixth category, sociopathic exploiters, contains most of the would-be malingerers.

Insurance company investigative and legal personnel surely see some claimants who are at least partly motivated by cupidity and who are prone to exaggerate complaints. Some claimants perceive the insurance company as skeptical, resistive, withholding, and even insulting, particularly where psychological disability is concerned. Commonly both tort and worker's compensation cases drag on for months or years, and the patient is caught up in the legal system which has only one method—the dollar—for compensating him or her for pain, suffering, disability, insecurity, fear, and economic loss. The patient is, in effect, required to maintain the illness in order to live in peace with his or her own conscience. If the person is no longer ill, then the claim is dishonest. Thus the patient continues to wear the neck collar, carry the cane, turn on the heat lamp, take the medication, and settle into a state of chronic invalidism. The clinical problem is to define which aspects of the symptom picture should be placed where on the continuum: primary illness, secondary gain, compensation, exaggeration, cupidity, or malingering.

SPECIAL MENTAL HEALTH LEGAL PROBLEMS

It is beyond the scope of this chapter to review the extensive literature and comprehensively present cases on a number of special clinical-legal problems that complicate the lives of patients and the attorneys on both sides of a dispute. A brief discussion of those special concerns follows.

Burns

Once the fright stemming from the fire and the acute pain of the burn have subsided, the severely burned patient faces a prolonged ordeal. A "traumatic neurosis" may ensue, with the typical nightmares prominent. Usually this phase is short and the patient's attention focuses on his or her unfamiliar body surface as the patient goes through debridement, baths, dressings, removal of dressings, aseptic isolation, skin grafting, infection, regrafting, and painful exercises for contractures. Regression is the rule, particularly in children.[19] Usually it is a reversible retreat, but often not entirely. Particularly if the reparative plastic surgery goes on, as it commonly does, for a matter of years, the process of return to "normalcy" is impeded. One patient has had 12 operations in 3 years, another 15 surgical procedures over a period of 4 years. Children are often less psychologically scarred than adults, who may have fluctuating depression and social withdrawal. After healing comes the adaptation to residual scarring, the stares of strangers, the partly disguised discomfort of relatives, refusal to eat in public, and a gnawing concern about the future of interpersonal relationships, particularly about sexual intimacy.[20]

Amputations

The phantom limb phenomenon has been well documented, but significant psychiatric sequelae are uncommon, because in most cases the limb disappears by telescoping into the amputation stump. A period of mourning for the lost member is common, occasionally intense enough to be called depression, but on the whole amputees are not particularly susceptible to disabling psychiatric illnesses.[21]

Scars

Cosmetic scarring is a problem with special implications for girls and young women on the basis of conventional social-sexual values. Complaining less than her concerned mother and lawyer, the scar victim is often protected by her own intact body image. She may experience the stares and questions of friends and strangers as odd, intrusive, and crude, because she rapidly learns not to see the scar in her mirror. The psychiatric consultant may have seen little definable psychological impairment, but the lawyer still presses for an opinion about the possible effects of the scar on the client's marital and occupational prospects.

Prolonged Pain

Much of the postaccident pain that psychiatrists hear described by patients is psychogenic, although an organic insult may have initiated it.[22] Occasionally there is a patient who has endured organic pain over a long period: persistent phantom limb pain, only partially relieved tic douloureux, or inoperable spinal oot irritation. A common result is a chronic, partially incapacitating personality change with tension, irritability, explosions of temper, loss of humor, impatience, fatigue, and self-preoccupation.

Children

The extent of postaccident disability in a child is primarily dependent upon the family's attitudes.[23, 24] If the mother repeatedly wails, "My baby is ruined," a child may well come to believe it. If the child receives special attention and privileges and is excused from domestic chores and responsibility for erratic behavior, he or she may adapt with alacrity, and his or her development will be impeded. Given a wholesome home environment, the power of the natural growth process, the merciful capacity to forget, and the need for peer companionship, it is unlikely that untoward psychic sequelae will permanently affect the child.

Sexual Molestation, Including Rape

Recent cases of note have included a young woman who was abducted from a dark and deserted plant parking lot, a woman of 62 who was attacked by a soldier on a military base, a girl of 6 who was molested by a utility meter reader, and the 15-year-old daughter of a hospitalized patient, who was seduced by a male social worker. Civil suit was entered in all these cases against the company, the government, or the hospital; claiming negligence, breach of civil duty, and damage. The current literature regarding such offenses is voluminous, and a "rape syndrome" has been described. Long-term effects of rape are measurably influenced by the quality of supportive understanding from intimates of the victim. Often her most important "therapeutic" aid is afforded by her husband. (For further extensive discussion, see chapter 15, "The Rape Victim and the Rape Experience.")

Problems of Causality

The law seeks certainty. Did the accident cause the plaintiff's present disability? If there were several "causes," what percentage of the disability was due to the accident? The worker's compensation commissioner and trial judge must resolve the dispute—"the buck stops there." The psychiatric witness will be pressed by both attorneys to be as definite as possible and may well feel pressured and beleaguered. If he or she can ethically say only "maybe," "in part," or "yes and no," he or she should resist dissuasion. The legalists have to do the best they can with the imprecise testimony.

The law is of some help, if the psychiatrists can accept it. The law states that if the accident caused the disability, activated a latent condition, or aggravated a pre-existing condition, the person at fault is liable. The tort offender takes the victim as he or she finds the victim. The employer takes the employee as he or she finds the employee. In other words, factors of predisposition are legally irrelevant. In practice, the opposing attorney tries to present all possible predisposing factors to influence the jury, in spite of the letter of the law.

The law also recognizes the "chain of events theory," with the accident forming the first "link." The case of the welder is illustrative: The original blow on the head, with legitimate organic and psychiatric disability, became compounded by the losses attendant to the accident (his wife, his home, and so forth). The law finds it impossible to sort out and to assign percentages of blame in so complex a series of misfortunes besetting a life, and so do I. In this case the state compensation assigned full responsibility to the welder's employer.

A typical "chain of events" begins with a back injury from lifting a heavy load and continues with pain, disability, loss of income, medical examination, differing medical opinions, myelogram, surgical disk removal, continued pain, nervousness, tension, insomnia, discouragement, silent concern over impotence, spinal fusion, continued disability, depression, lawsuit—and permanent invalidism.

Percentage of Disability

Particularly in worker's compensation cases, the doctor is expected to grade the client-patient's disability according to a table of percentages. The orthopedic surgeon is comfortable in estimating 50 percent impairment of a hand, 25 percent impairment of the body as a whole; the mental health practitioner is expected to offer similar estimates. In worker's compensation cases only occupational disability is relevant. A useful guide is the rating system devised by an expert committee of the American Medical Association.[25] It is a guide, and the psychiatrist may deviate from it, but adherence to it does enable the clinician to maintain a consistency in communicating his or her findings and conclusions. Lawyers frequently remind me of a reality: The client has his or her day in court, and that is it. The client cannot sue again 5 to 10 years later for lingering impairment from the original injury. Thus the attorney presses for an evaluation of the long-term mental effects of the accident: the persistent pain, the scar, the burn disfigurement, the sexual insult, and the occupational limitation. The attorney's questions are appropriate; so are vague answers. Psychiatrists are handicapped by a dearth of adequate follow-up studies in these fields and usually must reply according to clinical impressions. There is no doubt of the need for more reliable empirical research in the worker's compensation field.

Legal Competency

Mental competency or capacity is defined variously: competency to stand criminal trial, the related issue of mental responsibility at the time of commission of an offense, competency to manage one's affairs, and competency to make a will or to enter into a contract. I shall describe briefly the requirements for the latter three areas of competency: those in the civil law field. Other chapters of this text examine the criminal law requirements. (See particularly chapters 7 and 8.)

Testimentary Capacity

Elderly persons occasionally alter their wills in a seemingly capricious fashion, and suits to "break" a will are not uncommon. In a recent case, a woman of 84 bequeathed her sizable estate equally to two nephews. One of them visited her regularly; the other ignored her. In a codicil she left the negligent nephew $1000 and the attentive one the rest of her property.

In will contests there is no patient for the psychiatrist to examine. His or her professional opinion must be based on material the attorney presents as well as on information garnered from personal interviews of persons with knowledge about the testator on the day of the signing of the will or codicil. In court, the attorney will ordinarily propound a hypothetical question: "Doctor, assume that an 84-year-old woman with two nephews . . ." It is appropriate for the psychiatrist to assist in preparing the hypothetical question to include the data that substantiate his or her opinion; for example, the old woman's developing cataracts; her reduced social contacts; her periods of confusion and disorientation at night; and her bitter, sometimes irrational, views and remarks about the nephew in disfavor.

The law offers a guiding definition of competency to make a will. Did the testator, at the time he or she executed his or her will (1) understand the objects of his or her natural bounty and (2) the nature and extent of his or her property? Those are the issues to be examined in court. As indicated by the preponderance of evidence gained, the expert witness responds to the questions. If he or she answers "no," he or she should add "by reason of mental illness." The expert witness will then be asked to expand and to explain. A full review of relevant findings should then be presented to the court.

Contractual Capacity

The ruling legal questions here are (1) did the party to the contract understand the legal instrument he or she signed, and (2) did he or she understand the probable consequences of his or her act? A recently widowed man, hoping to regain social contacts, signed a contract for $1700 worth of lessons at a dance studio. After two lessons he realized the error of his decision and sued for contract release on the plea of his disabling depression and faulty judgment. A discouraged, aging farmer sold his property, then became more depressed when he found himself homeless and unemployed. He sued for return of his property on the basis of incapacitating depression and mental inability to anticipate the consequences of his action. Each of these cases presents difficult issues for mental health evaluation and requires thorough examination of the patient, the patient's motivations, and the full circumstances of the events in question.

Competency to Manage One's Affairs

The usual outcome of a mental competency issue in court is appointment of a guardian, conservator, or power of attorney for the impaired subject. The plea for a guardian is regularly entered by someone other than the subject, and legal dispute may arise.

An elderly woman, living with one of three nieces, began showering her and her family with gifts. The other two nieces became concerned and moved to have a guardian appointed. A man disturbed by his 65-year-old mother's liaison with a traveling salesman and her generous gifts of money to him petitioned the court to have a guardian appointed for his mother. Both women contested guardianship, and jury trials resulted.

The primary clinical problem in all civil law competency cases is estimation of judgment. There may be evidence of minor defects in recent memory and occasional behavioral errors, such as writing a check on the wrong bank or forgetting to pay a bill, but lack of evidence of significant personality deterioration and resultant defects in business and social judgment. A full psychological test battery yields reliable evidence of the defendant's competency (see the description of psychological assessments in chapter 5). My inclination, and that of the law, is to support the subject's freedom to manage his or her own affairs whenever feasible.

Medical Malpractice Cases

In light of the current malpractice problems, it seems incumbent on the medical and mental health professions to better past performances in the art of self-policing, to break with the traditional "conspiracy of silence," and to expose whatever incompetence of colleagues is known. Although many malpractice suits are petty, ill-advised, or opportunistic, some are undeniably legitimate.

Within the past two years, 12 litigants have been referred to the Department of Psychiatry and Law at the Menninger Foundation for professional evaluation of their claims that they suffered psychic injury from the negligence of medical practitioners. Three suits were brought against surgeons, two against obstetricians, and seven against psychiatrists, psychiatric hospitals, or mental health centers. In all such cases, two crucial questions must be settled: Did medical personnel services deviate significantly from a generally accepted standard of care, and did the quality of care received cause psychic suffering to the litigious patient?

Four of the psychiatric suits involved patients' suicides; and, again, there is no patient to question. The alternative evaluative procedure is a "psychological autopsy" which includes interviewing those with pertinent evidence to give, perusal of records, and preparation of a hypothetical question. The particular burden for the defense is how one substantiates and documents a professional standard of care and demonstrates that if the proper standard had been adhered to, suicide might have been prevented.

As an expert witness in medical malpractice suits, a psychiatrist is primarily a consultant to the legal firm, evaluating the evidence, pointing to the strengths and weaknesses regarding medical facts and ethics in the lawyer's brief, and suggesting further inquiry. The psychiatrist is not a legal investigator; it is the attorney's task to find and to present the evidence.

CONCLUSION

A survey of 100 consecutive civil law litigation patients referred to the Menninger Foundation reveals that all were referred by attorneys who were alerted to their clients' need of psychiatric attention by the tenor of reports submitted to them from orthopedists, neurosurgeons, and other physicians. The attorneys would assert that "the patient is very nervous," or "there is a psychosomatic complication," or "there is a functional overlay," or a similar verbal avoidance of the term "psychiatric."

In such referrals the psychiatrist may feel a dual responsibility to the attorney and to the patient. The psychiatrist functions as an agent of the lawyer in that the psychiatrist's clinical report becomes part of the lawyer's legal evidence; the consulting role is in a sense concretized by fee arrangement. Lawyers are aware that mental-health professionals do not accept a contingency fee, and if the client is unable to pay, it is desirable that the lawyer understand that he or she is responsible for the charges.

The written report to the attorney should be complete. It should inform the attorney as to what the expert witness can and cannot disclose if he or she is called into court to testify. A further advantage of a complete report is that it frequently negates the need for a court appearance. Armed with an authoritative report, the attorney may be able to negotiate a settlement and to avoid a trial. In 1980, we evaluated 15 traumatic neurosis cases and went to court only four times.

The report to the attorney will be shared with the opposing lawyer, the worker's compensation commissioner, the judge, and even with the client. Therefore it is necessary to have the patient understand that material he or she wishes not to be divulged will be kept confidential, if possible. This material may include the patient's illegitimate birth, an abortion, or marijuana smoking that has no bearing on matters relevant in the civil suit. Moreover, certain of the psychiatrist's speculations or educated hunches about the patient are better conveyed to the attorney orally, if at all, rather than in writing. Such imprudently dropped phrases as "latent homosexuality," "seductive hysterical character," or "sadistic fantasies" can be pursued in court by an astute cross-examining attorney to the point that their author regrets the conjectural excursion from clinical exactness.

REFERENCES

1. PROSSER, WH: *Handbook of the Law of Torts*, ed 3. West Publishing, St Paul, 1964.
2. BLACK, HC: *Black's Law Dictionary*. West Publishing, St Paul, 1951.
3. FURST, S (ED): *Psychic Trauma*. Basic Books, New York, 1967.
4. KARDINER, A: *The Traumatic Neuroses of War*. National Research Council, Washington, DC, 1941.
5. GRINKER, R AND SPIEGEL, J: *Men Under Stress*. Blakiston, Philadelphia, 1945.
6. KRYSTAL, H (ED): *Massive Psychic Trauma*. International Universities Press, New York, 1969.
7. TAYLOR, J, ZERCHER, L, KEY, W: *Tornado*. University of Washington Press, Seattle, 1970.
8. *Disaster at Buffalo Creek*. Am J Psychiatry 133:295-316, 1976.
9. WOLFENSTEIN, M: *Disaster*. The Free Press, Glencoe, IL, 1957.
10. LEOPOLD, RL AND DILLON, H: *Psychoanatomy of a disaster*. Am J Psychiatry 119:913-921, 1963.
11. HOROWITZ, M: *Stress Response Syndrome*. Jason Aronson, New York, 1976.
12. MODLIN, HC: *The postaccident anxiety syndrome: Psychosocial aspects*. Am J Psychiatry 123:1008-1012, 1967.

13. KEISER, L: *The Traumatic Neurosis.* JB Lippincott, Philadelphia, 1968.

14. LAUGHLIN, H: *The Neuroses.* Butterworth, Washington, DC, 1967.

15. ENELOW, A: *Malingering and delayed recovery from injury.* In LEEDY, J (ED): *Compensation in Psychiatric Disability and Rehabilitation.* Charles C Thomas, Springfield, IL, 1971.

16. SLAWSON, P: *Compensable psychiatric disability and the problem of secondary gain.* In LEEDY, J (ED): *Compensation in Psychiatric Disability and Rehabilitation.* Charles C Thomas, Springfield, IL, 1971.

17. MODLIN, HC: *Accidents and traumatic neurosis.* In FRANKEL, CJ (ED): *Lawyers Medical Cyclopedia.* Allen Smith, Indianapolis, 1973.

18. KNIGHT, J: *Money attitudes in rehabilitation.* In LEEDY, J (ED): *Compensation in Psychiatric Disability and Rehabilitation.* Charles C Thomas, Springfield, IL, 1971.

19. GOLDSTON, R: *The burning and the healing of children.* Psychiatry 35:57, 1972.

20. JORGENSEN, J AND BROPHY, J: *Psychiatric Treatment Modalities in Burn Patients.* Grune & Stratton, New York, 1975.

21. PARKS, C: *Psycho-social transitions: Comparison between reactions to loss of a limb and loss of a spouse.* Br J Psychiatry 127:204-210, 1975.

22. SHANFIELD, S AND KILLINGSWORTH, R: *The psychiatric aspects of pain.* Psychiatric Annals 7:24-35, 1977.

23. MACGREGOR, F, ET AL: *Facial Deformity and Plastic Surgery: A Psychosocial Study.* Charles C Thomas, Springfield, IL, 1953.

24. WATSON, EJ AND JOHNSON, A: *The emotional significance of acquired physical disfigurement in children.* Am J Orthopsychiatry 28:85-97, 1958.

25. COMMITTEE ON RATING OF MENTAL AND PHYSICAL IMPAIRMENT: *Mental illness.* JAMA 198:1284-1293, 1966.

CHAPTER 21
THE PSYCHOLOGIST AS EXPERT WITNESS
Wallace A. Kennedy, Ph.D., ABPP

Other than as a plaintiff, defendant, or jury member, a psychologist may serve three roles in the courtroom: as a common witness, as an expert witness, or as a tableside consultant.

Common witnesses serve as sensors of the trial courts, called upon to report observations of their senses. A common witness is permitted to provide the courts with personal recall: what was heard, seen, smelled, tasted, or felt through the skin. In addition, the common witness can give common interpretations to these sensations. These interpretations can be challenged or objected to, of course, but for the most part they are recognized by the law as essential to the proceedings, because the courts recognize a dependency upon witnesses who have personal experience with the issue at hand.

These raw sensory data and their common interpretation are at times too ambiguous, too complex, perhaps too misleading for the jury to use as they stand. At this point, the psychologist as expert witness can provide inferences and interpretations that are not permitted common witnesses. An **expert witness** draws inferences and offers scientific conclusions based on professional observations, inferences, and scientific findings, such as the person in question is retarded, illiterate, senile, brain-impaired, psychotic, and so forth. From the inferences the expert witness psychologist predicts such things as long-range dependency, employability, mental competence, emotional lability, and post-trauma academic ability.

A common witness can report that the 7-year-old plaintiff has changed since the accident: she is more active; she has tantrums; she can't remember what she has been told; she gets off the track in conversations; she no longer likes to read; and for the first time, she is having trouble with mathematics. The issue, however, is not that she has changed but how serious is the change? What will this mean to her lifestyle? Will it affect her livelihood? Will it be permanent? Does it relate to the head injury suffered in the accident or to any other event related to the automobile accident?

Children, always changing, go through stages; they continually grow out of one set of behaviors into another. But the jury has to make its decision now. It has to predict the future. And ultimately, it has to do this on its own.

Even so, the inferences and interpretations of the psychological expert witness provide a stalwart basis to support the jury's opinion. The psychological expert witness can take the isolated sensory inputs of the common witnesses, along with accumulated professional data, and lead the jury to an understanding of the cause and effect under consideration. Through a professional interpretation of carefully defined results from specific, appropriate professional assessment instruments and from professional experience with similar cases, the expert witness can lead the jury to understand that the particular behavior pattern evident in this 7-year-old child is to be expected from a seizure-producing, closed-head injury and anoxia. It is permanent, largely unremediable. It will lead to a 30 percent loss in function, which means the difference between college success and failure, between professional and clerking vocational potential, between good and poor interpersonal relationships. Given this professional interpretation, along with an expert probability statement about any competing cause, the jury can decide whether this represents a monetary loss to the child and, if so, how much this loss is worth over a lifetime. On the latter economic issues, of course, the jury will receive other expert testimony.

THE MAKING OF AN EXPERT WITNESS

The answer is simple to the question, What makes a witness expert? A witness becomes an expert when the trial judge rules the person as such. The fact that a psychologist has been ruled not to be an expert can lead to a mistrial when reviewed by a higher court. But the statement still holds: The psychologist is now an expert because a higher court judge ruled so.

Happiness in being an expert witness is patience, detachment, and high ego strength. A psychologist on the stand can be fought over by batteries of lawyers for two days, only to be banished from the courtroom, having been judicially determined not be an "expert." In my opinion, this abuse is tempered best by a quietly ticking meter that pays the psychologist portal to portal while all this warfare goes on around him.

Psychology as a profession has been accepted as a field of expertise at all levels of the court system, but the expert status of any individual psychologist depends upon six personal resumé factors: (1) education, training, licensure, and specialty board certification; (2) experience; (3) scholarship; (4) aptitude in the courtroom; (5) reputation; and (6) history as an expert witness. Each of the latter five should be nourished constantly by the psychologist who proposes to function as an expert witness. The stronger the psychologist is in each of these areas, the more likely is his or her acceptance by the courts and the more credible is his or her assistance to the jury.

Education, Training, Licensure, and Certification

Except in the more rural local courts and in limited matters, the doctorate is the entry degree for an expert psychological witness. The more credible this degree, the more likely the seating as expert. Accredited psychology doctorate programs; accredited clinical, counseling, or school internships; state licensure and advanced level of professional accreditation by national boards (e.g., a diplomate in clinical psychology from the American Board of Professional Psychology and a diplomate in forensic psychology from the American Board of Forensic Psychology) all improve the acceptability of the expert.

Predoctoral and postdoctoral training in the area of expert witnessing is important. Bootstrap training in biofeedback, neuropsychology, and learning disability—no matter how good—is difficult to sell to judge and jury and is no substitute for clearly defined course work, supervised undergraduate and postgraduate training, and national boards examination. Coming into court as a jack-of-all-trades may do in a rural county court, but in a federal district court specialization in education, training, and licensure is the sine qua non. And, because of the medical tradition of national boards separating experts from practitioners, in court, the diplomate in psychology makes a significant difference in credentials, because it is based upon an evaluation of one's advanced level of professional competence and functioning in specialized areas (e.g., clinical, industrial, or school psychology).

Experience

One of the few areas in professional practice in which seniority and experience almost universally are rewarded is in the courtroom as an expert witness. Of course, everyone has to start somewhere; graduate students, subpoenaed in their second year of training, have testified regarding psychological matters. But for the most part, expert testimony should not be based on first experience from a few cases of the condition under litigation. Remember, being an expert witness is for the most part voluntary; there should be no hesitation in admitting that there are areas in which one is not an expert.

However, if, in fact, a psychologist desires to become an expert in a particular area, then beginning in a narrow area is proper and appropriate. The average clinician, for example, might see only one sexually abused child in five years. But a year's tour of duty on a child abuse team at Children's Hospital in Boston might easily produce 200 such cases. In round numbers, juries like to hear something more than "a dozen" in answer to the question, "How many such cases have you seen?"

It is hoped that an inexperienced young psychologist will not be called upon to examine a presidential assassin, a terrorist, or a person who has set himself afire in the town square. But if he or she is, lack of experience can be admitted readily: The psychologist becomes the one-eyed man in the country of the blind, having seen at least one when no one else has seen any.

Scholarship

If a psychologist wishes to become an expert in the courtroom, papers delivered before learned societies, articles published in leading journals, even workshops and speeches carefully prepared and delivered before recognized groups, add immensely to expert status. These are not simply window-dressing, because by scholarship a psychologist not only appears a better witness but also has more to offer. Following a scholarly trail of an issue over the years not only produces a convincing resumé but also produces high-level professional growth that improves confidence on the witness stand as well as the ability to withstand pressure on the question of certainty.

Aptitude in the Courtroom

In addition to professional education, experience, and scholarship, there is the matter of aptitude for the courtroom. Serving as an expert witness involves appearing to be professionally expert; the psychologist's performance in the courtroom is critical to that image.

Many psychologists, for a variety of reasons, come unglued in the courtroom. They turn red, or red and white in blotches, or ashen; they sweat profusely; they stammer and mumble; they cannot find their place in a reference document and cannot read a simple page placed in front of them; they forget their own names. Or, worse, they become pedantic, dogmatic, and certain. Other psychologists are stimulated by the courtroom drama, think clearly, remain calm and unruffled, and by their poise and demeanor add to the impression of confident, professional competence.

Many strategies can improve skill in the courtroom, but obviously experience, practice, preparation, desensitization, and a well-organized file in hand all help. Speech and drama coaching, participation in Toastmasters and moot courts are helpful. Even so, a few psychologists have a particular knack or talent for this performance. The best advice seems to be that the psychologist should either work very hard at becoming an expert expert witness or should let it entirely alone. No good comes to the individual or to the profession when an unprepared, inexperienced, unskilled, and untalented psychologist occasionally attempts to pose as a forensic psychology expert.

Reputation

As a psychologist matures professionally, a reputation is established for performing certain tasks well, or not well, including being an authority on some matters. Reputation is sometimes established on the basis of job title or description, sometimes by role in the community, and, of course, sometimes by performances in court. Consistent professional interaction with lawyers, public officials, and courts is part of this moving record called reputation. Generally, a psychologist functioning in the role for which he or she is trained, formally appointed, and socially accepted brings into the courtroom an expertise by reputation. Informal communication between judges and attorneys adds to or detracts from this professional reputation, which makes being seated as an expert either increasingly easy or more difficult.

Needless to say, however, reputation is based also upon professional integrity. Judges and lawyers know all too well which "professionals" can be bought as "hired guns," and which can be depended upon for expert opinions based upon professional and personal integrity.

History as an Expert Witness

Now, for the Catch-22 of being an expert witness: Under the law, precedent is a strong determinant. Finding that a witness has testified as an expert many times at all levels of the court system, judges are unlikely to deny seating that person as an expert in their courtroom. However, there obviously has to be a first time.

Again, there are good reasons for getting one's expert feet wet in local lower courts, gradually working up to urban county courts and federal courts. Federal courts are more pressured. Federal judges, with lifetime appointments, often are less accommodating, running tighter ships than local juvenile court or family court judges. Local judges, with more collegial relationships with the professions within their community, are far more willing to inform, to coach, to explain, and even to teach the neophyte in expert witnessing. The best advice, then, is to start at the lower levels of the court system.

THE SEATING OF THE EXPERT WITNESS

First, expert status often is contested, sometimes with the jury present, sometimes with the jury excused and waiting. The process can be tedious and sometimes is even demeaning, but it is necessary. At this point, the psychologist is certainly not in charge. A pleasant, passive demeanor and a helpful attitude toward providing credentials and a clear statement of the nature of the expected contribution to the issue at hand are professional assets.

Second, the psychologist often is seated only tentatively and incompletely as an expert. Often the judge tentatively will agree to allow the psychologist to testify, and then the judge will carefully circumscribe what the psychologist may answer. For example, a judge may allow an expert psychologist to testify as to his or her examination of the child in a custody issue. The psychologist may be asked to answer the questions regarding whether the child expressed an opinion to the psychologist as to where he or she would prefer to live, whether this opinion seemed firmly made, whether it seemed rational and logical, and whether it appeared to be the child's opinion rather than that of the current custodial parent. At the same time, the judge may forbid the psychologist to report the actual choice of the child; the child is the best witness. With a jury in the room, psychologists so restricted can bring about a mistrial and bring down upon their heads the wrath of the judge, should they stray from the fine-line boundary the judge has put into place. The courtroom is no place for subtleties or cuteness; only for a concerted effort to stay within the boundaries prescribed by the judge.

THE OPINION OF THE EXPERT WITNESS

Once seated, the psychologist is now ready to offer expert opinion. This professional opinion is based first upon professional data and then upon professional conclusions.

Professional Data

Expert psychological opinion can be based on firsthand data gathered by the psychologist, or on secondhand data gathered by some other competent source and made available to the psychologist. These latter data differ from hearsay, which is inadmissible, in that they are of recognized quality, such as service records, school records, national examinations, or even previous psychological evaluations for which the protocol is available. The purpose of secondhand data is to establish the premorbid level of functioning upon which to base an expert opinion of change.

FIRSTHAND DATA

Firsthand data come from clinical observations and formal and informal test results. In preparing reports as the basis of depositions and later testimony, precision is important. Use common English; avoid complex, professional jargon. To be effective with judges and juries, the expert opinion needs to be in precise, plain English; so the preliminary report should be written carefully in precise, plain English.

Clinical Observations

Clinical observations most frequently used in expert testimony to lay the groundwork for later conclusions and opinions concern (1) affect, (2) language style, (3) mannerisms, (4) interactive style, and (5) stigmata.

Affect is related to many issues requiring expert testimony, such as competency to stand trial; defense of insanity; mental competence with respect to various legally relevant functions such as making a will, entering into a binding contract, or a marriage; or in regard to major mental dysfunction arising from trauma. Unfortunately, psychologists tend to communicate with each other in a language bewildering to laymen, which includes judges as well as juries. Professional jargon has no place in a court report or in court testimony. A flat affect, for instance, can be described in plain English:

> I found Mr. Jones unusual in his lack of emotional expression. He spoke with no expression on his face and a droning quality to his speech, which had no variation in rhythm or expression. In fact, his words were evenly spaced, as though from a computer. He lacked animation or interest.

Language style can be described, including structure, grammar, dialect, literacy, and vocabulary level. Clinical observation of language style should note present speech and language characteristics to determine consistency with the premorbid language style or with a disputed example of the person's language style. Individuals have highly distinctive manners of speaking. Age equivalency, grammar complexity, and vocabulary are critical identifying characteristics. For example, an alleged confession often can be severely questioned or even dismissed because of obvious differences in language style between the defendant and the detectives who received and reported on the alleged confession.

Mannerisms, as with affect and language style, can afford expert interpretation and conclusion. Again, the expert should describe the specific mannerisms in clear, precise English rather than in technical jargon, considering carefully their relevance to the issue at hand. Mannerism in this sense refers to the overt behavior of an individual recognizable as a consistent pattern. Common and ambiguous mannerisms are less helpful in reaching conclusions than are characteristic patterns of behavior. Spasticity is an example of a mannerism, as is belligerence.

Interactive style, similar to mannerisms but more stereotypic in character, refers to the total impression of social interaction. Expert testimony on interactive style evaluates for the judge or jury behavior with implications for the issue at hand. Interactive style statements can be useful in establishing potential for rehabilitation, an insanity defense, or custody recommendations.

Stigmata, the final clinical observation, concerns particular behavior patterns that in and of themselves present nearly certain conclusions and interpretations. For example, the identifying features of Down's syndrome, cerebral palsy, delirium tremens (DTs), heroin withdrawal, profound mental retardation, and Alzheimer's disease all provide easily identifiable sequelae that add precision to the ultimate certainty of the conclusion the psychologist offers on the witness stand.

Formal Clinical Assessment

The second set of firsthand data is collected by the psychologist from professional psychological test batteries. In many ways these data are superior to clinical observations, because they are nonsubjective, standardized data that are related directly to the general superiority of psychological over psychiatric testimony. Formal psychological testing carries clearly established norms, standard error estimates, and robust probability estimates. Formal testing provides the strongest testimony of psychologists and has the broadest acceptance by the courts and by the public. Generally, it concerns six areas of human performance: (1) social maturity, (2) academic achievement, (3) memory, (4) intelligence, (5) perceptual acuity, and (6) personality. In each of these, the psychologist has access to professional tests with high credibility. A seventh area, neuropsychology, requires significant subspecialty training, including far more comprehensive knowledge of neuroanatomy and neurophysiology than the average clinical psychologist possesses. (See also chapter 7.)

Social maturity can be described accurately by the psychologist with the aid of several tests, including the Vineland Social Maturity Scale,[1] the Adaptive Behavior Scale of the American Association on Mental Deficiency[2] and the Denver Developmental Screening Test,[3] each of which converts to a developmental age useful in defining social competence to laymen. Describing a person as having the maturity of a 5-year-old is understood more easily by a jury than a broad behavioral description of immaturity.

Academic achievement, although often evaluated by quick and simple tests, should be taken quite seriously in court. Choosing the Wide Range Achievement Test (WRAT),[4] for example, is a dangerous decision in a case headed for trial. A psychologist may prefer to defer to a reading specialist, a mathematics specialist, or a learning disability specialist; but if not, by all means assess academic achievement with the best tools available.

At the very least, when commenting on achievement, speak with the authority of a formal, large-battery test, such as the Woodcock-Johnson Psycho-Educational Battery,[5-7] the Peabody Individual Achievement Test (PIAT),[8] or a paper-and-pencil test, such as the California Achievement Tests.[9] A vigorous cross-examination of a psychologist who relied on the Wide Range Achievement Test is pitiful to behold. Such a test may be adequate merely as a check of reading recognition, to allow some certainty that the person possesses the literacy required to complete another test. Even in that instance, however, a reading comprehension test would be more informative and valid.

Memory is evaluated both by free-standing memory scales, such as the Wechsler Memory Scale,[10] and by memory scales embedded in achievement tests, such as the Woodcock-Johnson Psycho-Educational. When a defect or decline in immediate memory is a key element of the expert's testimony, both are helpful. Memory also can be inferred from subscale presentation on the intelligence tests, but again, when the psychologist speaks about memory problems, standardized, professionally accepted memory scales are the only appropriate avenue.

Intelligence evaluation is the strongest and easiest assessment to defend. With the single exception of cross-cultural use of intelligence tests outside specific prediction of academic potential, in which cultural bias does come into play, few opposing counsel will attack the concepts of intelligence quotient (IQ) and mental age.

When properly introduced, the concept of mental age is more useful than IQ, because mental age is so easy to understand. The only problem is in dealing with incompetence in adults, which is difficult to translate to the layman. For instance, a psychologist might proclaim a severely retarded adult "insane" because he was unable to tell the difference between right and wrong when he made a sexual assault upon a young girl. In the first place, this is a legal definition of insanity, **not** a psychological one. In the second place, describing an adult with a 35 IQ as having the mental age of a 6-year-old does not explain to the average layman his being unable to tell the difference between right and wrong in this instance: "What 6-year-old would think a sexual assault right?"

To explain adequately to the jury, the expert must talk about the difference between a 6-year-old body and 6-year-old emotions, as well as 6-year-old intellect. A 6-year-old boy may have an impulse to cry when severely provoked and apparently does not comprehend this as a wrong thing to do. His sexual impulse, however, would be extremely low. His 6-year-old intellect does not control his 6-year-old impulse to cry, just as the adult's 6-year-old intellect does not control his adult impulse toward sexuality. The psychologist in the courtroom must constantly be alert to explain his or her findings in a fashion comprehensible, logical, and understandable to the judge and jury.

Expert analysis of intelligence has many uses in the courtroom. In fact, so pervasive is the implication of intelligence, it is inconceivable that any psychological evaluation for any reason would not include a test of intelligence.

Perceptual acuity, or assessment of perceptual-motor development, often is underprepared by clinical psychologists, who thereby open themselves to severe cross-examination. The psychological measures of fine-motor/visual-motor performance are adequate, with excellent objective criteria and age-specific norms. The Graham-Kendall Memory-for-Designs test,[11, 12] the Beery Developmental Test of Visual-Motor Integration,[13, 14] the Bender Motor Gestalt test,[15-17] each yield reliable scores and objective interpretation and are useful in making predictions regarding the improvement to be expected following trauma or developmental lag. As a general rule, the more confirming data, the sounder and more credible the testimony.

Personality assessment is not as easily acceptable in court as psychological testimony on social maturity, academic achievement, memory, intelligence, and perceptual acuity. The mind-body issue, the tradition of mental condition or mental status as the province of medicine and psychiatry, and the regretfully conflicted opinions regarding personality and mental disorders all suggest a highly cautious, highly systematic, and very conservative approach to psychological testimony concerning personality. Three major testing procedures relate to personality assessment: (1) objective, (2) subjective, and (3) behavioral. (See also chapter 5 on the general subject of psychological testing.)

Objective personality assessment should be a part of every expert psychological testimony on personality. However weak the reliability or validity of an objective test, it is at least known. Data from the Minnesota Multiphasic Personality Inventory (MMPI),[18, 19] Clinical Analysis Questionnaire (CAQ),[20] Personality Inventory for Children (PIC),[21] and the Sixteen Personality Factors Questionnaire (16 PF)[22] allow the psychologist to deal with a known distribution and to place this particular person within that distribution. Not only is objective personality assessment more reliable, valid, and normalized, but it sounds so to laymen.

To know the commonsense underpinnings of these objective personality inventories is important, even though these measures are of empirical validity. Although the standardization of the depression (D Scale) scale of the MMPI[18, 19] does not depend upon the face validity of the questions and answers, psychologists using the instrument should know, and have in their notes, specific examples of the scale that demonstrate its highest face validity. That is, when asked to explain the nature of the D Scale of the MMPI, the psychologist should be able to give samples of questions and answers and be able to say, "People high on the D Scale tend to answer like this, and tend to have the following characteristics."

Thorough familiarity with the construction, standardization, and limitations of the professional instruments used is essential for the psychological expert. As a basic practice, the psychological expert should be at least five studies deep on reliability and validity of the objective personality tests used, but particularly, he or she should be up to date on the standard references.[23-26]

Subjective projective personality tests are amenable to both formal scoring and overall clinical impression. When going into court, the psychologist should have both available. To have both tightly documented norms, such as provided by Exner in his three-volume series on the Rorschach system,[27-29] and sharp examples with high face validity is the key to successful use of projective tests in court.

Projective tests generally are helpful in incompetency proceedings, whether incompetent to stand trial or insane at commission of a criminal act. Remember, the task is not to provide a *DSM III* diagnosis substantiation, but rather to provide answers to issues directly related to the point of law. I believe that projective and objective personality test performance results should be used in the courtroom by the psychological expert primarily to provide confirming evidence of impressions gained from the history and general psychological evaluation. To provide evidence for an insanity defense on the basis of projective personality tests alone is extremely weak expert testimony. The same holds in torts, in which the mental condition of the individual is part of the damage claim. To be effective in court, projective tests should be at the end of a long string of consistent evidence. The projectives, then, fill in the picture and extend it, but they do not define it.[25, 30, 31]

Behavioral, standardized rating scales of personality are useful in court testimony because of high face validity and ease of communication. Ratings of depression, anxiety, and social isolation have the advantage of national norms, reasonably objective language, and consistency with lay belief systems. Even when the scale is not standardized, presenting data in scale format is useful: "On a scale of 1 to 10, when compared with all the depressed people I have evaluated over the past 5 years, I place this person at 7, with 8 and 9 requiring medication, and 10, hospitalization."

Some common examples of behavioral rating scales are the Devereux Child Behavior Rating Scale,[32, 33] the American Association of Mental Deficiency

Adaptive Behavior Scale,[2] the Vineland Social Maturity Scale,[1] the Burks' Behavior Rating Scale,[34] and the Personality Inventory for Children.[21]

Neuropsychological testimony is most effective when related to the rehabilitation aspects of known traumas, least effective when asserting the presence or absence of brain lesions or brain malformations. Both the Luria-Nebraska[35] and the Reitan[36, 37] neuropsychological batteries require clinical interpretation above the specific norms of the instrument, which still are open to inconsistent interpretation. Obviously, use of the instruments requires understanding the current literature on their validity and reliability. The fact that the Reitan, to some extent, is based on instruments with general use outside neurological assessment makes it easier to defend on cross-examination.

For example, a child's brain damage may be associated with a closed head injury, appear to be massive, but may be basically undetectable by current neurological techniques, including all forms of computer-enhanced scanning. The psychologist finds, however, that the child has lost 40 IQ points (from 140 down to 100); has regressed two grade levels in basic study skills; is hyperactive, fearful, and self-destructive; and tends to have some language difficulties with basic syntax. By assessing the precondition and postcondition through measurement and comparison with existing records, the psychologist can determine the magnitude of the loss, predict long-range limitations, and prescribe optimal treatment programming needed for his or her best rehabilitation.

Trying to identify the area of the brain that is most affected and speculations as to the precise area in which the most severe damage is located has great scientific and academic interest, but it has no meaning regarding the **specific task of the jury.** It is particularly unfortunate for the psychologist to testify in the face of a neurologist, who can display in another case highly credible x-ray photographs, echoencephalography, and other enhanced computer scans, which enable him or her with almost total certainty to indicate the size, angle, depth, and mass of a lesion. In this case the neuropsychologist has little to offer regarding the location of the brain damage but much to offer regarding psychological, vocational, and lifestyle consequences of that lesion.

Looking at court testimony over the years, neuropsychological assessment is obviously an all-or-none pursuit: The psychologist is either fully prepared by course work, study, research, and detailed clinical work, or he or she should stay out of the area completely. Even with the most prepared expert, the strongest testimony remains in matters of rehabilitation, not localization of the suggested brain damage. As medical technology in scanning processes improves, the specific contribution of psychological testimony toward localization is likely to diminish. In any event, in court, the issue is functional rather than organic, and the psychologist can make a major contribution toward defining neuropsychological functioning.

Informal Clinical Assessment

In addition to using the many formally standardized tests, psychologists also conduct informal examinations. Their particular advantage is high face validity and ease of communication. By informal is meant practical, commonsense, assessment of an individual as to his or her ability to function at certain tasks for which there are no standardized assessment instruments available. These are the kinds of examinations that are conducted by psychologists with particular experience with a practical requirement. For example, the requirements in most states for competency to stand trial are not defined in specific psychological terms, inasmuch as IQ, diagnosis, and literacy are not specifically required. One such requirement is "the capacity to disclose to attorney pertinent facts surrounding the alleged offense." An informal test involving the psychologist's determination of the capacity is conducted by replicating conditions similar to those of attorney-client interactions, **not** by administering the Stanford-Binet Intelligence Scale.[38] (See also chapter 7.) These informal tests generally are tailored to resemble the realities of the situation in which the behavior is to be predicted. Four informal evaluations frequently are used in expert testimony: (1) orientation, (2) memory, (3) specific content, and (4) specific skill.

Orientation concerns basic awareness at a specific time. In issues such as competency to stand trial, criminal responsibility, or fitness to be a parent, the individual's basic understanding of where he or she is, why he or she is there, and what is going on is critical. Detailed verbatim assessment of this understanding is valuable. An important aspect of the evaluation process, which ultimately will end in court, is how the person answered questions such as, "Do you know who I am?" "Do you know why you are here?" "Do you know what my job is?" The sharper the verbatim material, the more convincing the testimony.

Without a vivid description of the orientation of the person during the assessment process, the basic credibility of the examination can be called into dispute. Often the civil rights of an individual depend upon a proper orientation; psychologists who do not evaluate orientation can do great harm.

Memory can be measured on informal scales helpful in developing claims of specific memory loss. Unlike their formal counterparts, informal memory tests can be related specifically to the characteristics of the person's vocation, family role, or life task. For example, in the case of disability in an air controller, a memory evaluation related to on-the-job performance would be helpful in describing the problem, along with a specific score on a formal test, such as the Wechsler Memory Scale.[9]

Specific content often predicates adequate job performance; for example, parenting requires some knowledge of a specific content related to child rearing. An informal evaluation of that content carries significance in court. A person suing for reinstatement in a specific position in industry can be evaluated best not by a formal intelligence scale but by a test of specific, critical content related directly to on-the-job performance. A person deemed unqualified to run a press because of low IQ or low academic achievement can be evaluated better on an informal content test that taps the specific demands of the job. Probably no specific IQ or achievement level is required for parenting, but adequate parenting does require some specific content. In setting reasonable grounds for removing a child from the parents' care, the cornerstone is the parents' specific content knowledge related to raising children.

Specific skill evaluation is most helpful in testimony, for example, concerning the disability of a welder. An on-site evaluation of the specific behaviors required of welders, the minimum performance demands for employment, is far more important than determining that he lost a specified number of IQ points as a result of his head injury.

SECONDHAND DATA

Because much of a psychologist's testimony relates to a change in behavior, capacity, or function following a particular event, and because the psychologist is unlikely to have been involved prior to this event, a competent expert reconstructs the pre-event condition of the client. This usually can be established by secondhand data available to the industrious expert witness. Highly acceptable secondhand data are (1) personal history, (2) public record, and (3) previous clinical reports.

Personal History

The courts generally accept that a history taken by doctors, including psychologists, is not hearsay but an examination result of the same standing as other measures the doctor employs, whether test, field observation, or physical examination. The professional expert, however, should be aware of the difference between a self-serving history and a verified history. Obviously the latter is preferable and more reliable when brought into court. The quality of a personal history provided by the client or interested parties can be measured and defended by its internal consistency, candidness, plausibility, and objectivity. Its admissibility is dependent upon the skill and reputation of the expert, but self-report should be used only when all attempts to obtain a verified history have failed.

A verified history comes from the client with confirmation from disinterested parties, credible public and private agencies, and sometimes by community reputation. An educational history taken from a client, verified by teachers, parents, and school administrators, is the best foundation for presenting a plunge in academic ability following an accident.

Public Record

We increasingly are becoming a nation of records. Almost everyone now has a cumulative record at school. Our courts keep relatively complete records. Industry keeps cumulative records, as do the Armed Forces, landlords, tax assessors, and the like. Given proper releases, most of this recorded information can be used by the expert who is aggressive and assertive in pursuit of public records, which carry high credibility with jurors.

Previous Clinical Reports

Previous clinical reports at times are part of a public record. Given the relatively high level of standardization of psychological tests, these are usable even when the specific qualification of the examiner is unknown, but the previous examiner should be identified as to qualification whenever possible. These previous clinical reports are even more plausible when raw test data are available. Their consistency with the public record and the verified personal history is important. The job of the expert is to weave the fabric of credibility into a clear picture of the pre-event status of the client.

THE ACQUIRED CHARACTERISTICS OF THE EXPERT WITNESS

Six characteristics of effective expert witnesses result from acquired behavior patterns, each of which is essential. These can be expressed as adjectives that describe the effective expert witness: (1) prepared, (2) exact, (3) brief, (4) coherent, (5) responsiveness, and (6) controlled.

The Prepared Witness

Expert psychological testimony in court can be compared to a single-performance play: Although there can and should be rehearsals, the drama itself happens only once; thus one should be fully prepared. Preparation means not only going over in fine detail the clinical work and conscientious reviewing of the pertinent literature, but it means careful conferences with the attorney, such that proper questions can be formulated and the answers anticipated.

Not at all unusual are 40 to 50 billable hours spent in preparation for trial. Time management, such that each step of the preparation is given proper consideration, is important in functioning as an effective expert witness. An excellent technique is the completion of all preparation for trial several days before the court date, and then, in the final few hours, total immersion in the case.

In addition to performing the clinical work correctly, the expert witness should correctly lay out a chart for courtroom use. This chart (Fig. 21-1) should include all pertinent data, such as family tree; key test results; and time, content, and place of each session with the client. This should be typed if one's handwriting is not impeccable.

Remember that opposing counsel can have complete access to your records, including the chart you take to the stand. Nothing in the chart should cause embarrassment; no cute or private remarks, no suggestion regarding weaknesses in the case; it is the task of the opposition to find the weaknesses. The chart taken to the stand should be brimful of important data, key references, key statistics on standardizations, percentiles, standard errors. It should be neatly organized and carefully stapled in place.

Exactitude

As a result of preparation, an effective expert witness is able to give exact, precise statements, rather than general, vague answers. Having the factual data ready enables an expert to convey to the jury the degree of precision available in psychology. Knowing where one is going, or intends to go, in presenting expert testimony enables the competent witness to have multiple measures of issues under dispute, exact probabilities, precise averages, and crisp linear extensions. Knowing exact, data-based facts about a given person enables the expert to make statements such as, "Given his vocabulary, which is at the 4-year-old level; his grammar, which is at the preschool level; and his mental age, which is at the 5-year-old level; Mr. Edwards could not possibly have given or even understood the confession he is alleged to have dictated."

Brevity

Unfortunately, a great many psychologists come out of the lecture tradition, accustomed to uninterrupted statements running 10 or more minutes. They have great difficulty gearing answers to be brief, concise, and informative. An expert is not confined to yes or no answers, but time is critical. Well-prepared answers responsive to the issues are essential. To be brief is easier when one is prepared and exact. Lead with a sentence such as, "There are three reasons

DATE	WORK	RESULTS	TIME
6-11-83	Reviewed accident report, hospital record, physician's report and deposition, and Plaintiff's deposition	Abstract	5
6-13-83	Interviewed Plaintiff, administered		1
	WAIS	V: 105, P: 100, FS: 103	1
	WRAT	R: 11-0	½
	MMPI	217 Valid	1
6-30-83	Interviewed Plaintiff, administered		1
	ZUNG	70 Severe	½
	TAT	Severely depressed	1
	CAQ	Severely depressed	1
7-5-83	Interviewed Plaintiff, administered		1
	Rotter Adult I.S.B.	Severely depressed	½
	Rorschach	Severely depressed	1
7-9-83	Chart Review and Narrative Report		5
12-12-83	Trial Conference (Sloan)		2
12-19-83	Deposition (Anderson)		2
1-9-84	Trial: Courtroom One, Judge Smith—9:00 AM		

KEY DATES

9-1-28	BN
6-1-46	HS
6-1-49	BA (accelerated)
1949	Married (childhood sweetheart, only date)
6-1-50	BN Angie (33) M—2 children
9-1-51	BN Martha (32) M—4 children
9-16-52	BN Pete (31) M—4 children
6-1-54	BN Walter (29) M—3 children
1-1-82	No other hospitalizations, no prior remarkable illness, no prior mental distress
1-8-82	Accident—8:00 PM Hatcher Road
1-8-82	Ralph and she upside down in car 10 hours. Ralph died in middle of night.
1-12-82	In fugue state in hospital 4 days.
1-12-82	Told by Pete of Ralph's death—10:00 AM
1-20-82	Discharged from hospital
6-20-82	Treated by internist Dr. Smith for depression
8-20-82	Hospitalized for 10 days for workup, negative
Current	Continued with Dr. Smith on follow-up treatment with antidepressants

FIGURE 21-1 This is a sample Work Scope Chart.

why Mrs. Garrison is an unlikely suspect in this matter." Then follow with the enumerated reasons and stop. For an opposing attorney to interrupt such a foray is difficult because to do so would emphasize in the jury's mind that there were two more points.

Coherence

A critical dimension in expert testimony is time management on the stand. Recognizing that only a limited amount of time is yours to inform the jury requires a plan of communication. Being coherent means translating all jargon into plain English; using analogies, examples, critical observations; and having it all geared to a systematic, one-two-three presentation highly organized and pitched at about the ninth-grade vocabulary level. The greatest single complaint of jurors against expert psychological testimony is its incomprehensibility. No one ever failed to communicate on the basis of underestimating the obviousness of a concept.

Responsiveness

Although an expert witness may raise an occasional laugh from a jury by being quick and flippant with an opposing attorney, juries typically consider their business seriously and feel that the job of the expert is to inform them, not to entertain them.

Sometimes psychologists have an answer in mind that would be useful in making a particular point with the jury, but that answer cannot be given if the question is not asked. Judges become severely vexed when an expert tries to control the dialogue by being nonresponsive. An expert witness can lead to an expensive mistrial by making statements not properly predicated upon the question at hand.

In being responsive, the expert must understand the question. The expert should have no hesitation in admitting to not understanding a question or, for that matter, to not remembering a long, drawn-out, complex question.

Controlled Attitude

Psychologists as expert witnesses must recognize that they are strangers in a strange land, that other forces control the flow of the presentation. Unless the expert witness has aided in a meeting of the minds in pretrial conferences, too often the presenting attorney may fail to ask key questions and may be forced to come back during redirect-examination to clarify issues, thereby failing to make the most competent use of the psychological witness. The expert's duty is to follow the rules of the court and to remain under the control of the presenting attorney after the trial has started. It is also his or her duty and obligation to confer with the attorney before the trial.

During testimony, one should remember to provide ample time for the opposing attorney to object to questions and to defend the objection. Unfortunately, whole mornings may be spent determining whether a certain question is proper and whether the expert is permitted to answer that question. This is outside the role of the psychologist as an expert. Blurting out an answer to an improper question prior to the attorney's being able to object could lead to an expensive mistrial, wasting the time of the court and all parties involved. Evenhandedness, deliberate pauses, and careful consideration of each question are the marks of the competent expert. Argumentativeness, bickering, and open hostility are clear marks of the nonprofessional.

THE PITFALLS OF THE EXPERT WITNESS

Expert psychological witnesses can fall into six common pitfalls, if they are not wary: (1) poor scholarship, (2) poor clinical work, (3) poor preparation, (4) poor control, (5) poor grasp of issues, and (6) poor presentation.

Poor Scholarship

Every expert should know, at the rote level, the basic standardization, reliability, validity, and key controversies and issues of every assessment instrument employed as a basis for expert testimony. As a rule of thumb, going into the trial with a tight notation system about five studies deep on all instruments used is the least preparation the competent expert can afford. Keeping an up-to-date ready-reference file for each instrument is critical. An opposing attorney can make even a competent expert look poor if these references are not at the tip of the tongue. Carefully stapled into the file, clearly highlighted and in order, references can turn the tide easily.

In addition, do not claim to know anything you do not know, and do not fall for the bait of the obscure reference who turns out to be a baseball player instead of a key researcher in mental retardation. If you have any doubt at all, in a loud, clear voice, readily admit, "I never heard of him."

Poor Clinical Work

QUICKIES

Under the pressure of time, most of us have fallen short of optimal batteries, but serving as an expert witness does not permit cost cutting or marginal effort. Quickies—such as the WRAT,[4] Kent EGY (Series of Emergency Scales),[39] Slosson's Intellectual Test for Children and Adults,[40] unscored Benders,[15] and card-flashing Rorschach tests[30]—represent the height of folly in an expert. If achievement is at issue, administer a major instrument, such as the Woodcock-Johnson Battery;[5-7] for perceptual-motor functioning, use a carefully scored series of Graham-Kendall,[11, 12] Beery,[13, 14] and Bender[15-17] tests, all with detailed scoring, cross-checking, and careful attention to detail.

SCORING ERRORS

Poor clinical work also results from poor scoring. Under the best of circumstances, computational errors are easy to make. On the witness stand, there is no such thing as a minor clerical error. Rescoring by another clinician is a good check, if the second clinician will take the time to go over every detail. I would never consider going into court without a total review of all scoring, all tabular interpretation, and the basic flow of the report. There is no saving a witness careless in detail.

INTERPRETATION ERRORS

Part of being an expert is giving well-defended interpretations of data at hand. Be aware that other experts probably have access to your data. If alternative interpretations are possible, they must be considered and counterbalanced. Misinterpretation of change scores on test-retest, rather than recognizing them as within the standard error, deservedly makes the psychologist look poor, as does scatter analysis at the chance level.

WORK HISTORY ERRORS

Too often posttraumatic work history is not taken into account by experts in cases involving damages for lost earnings. It can turn out, however, that the work situation actually improved after the accident. The expert must cover all bases in making work predictions. An on-the-job interview and examination may be the key elements in determination of disability. A psychologist who never has been in a modern pressroom, who does not know the work scope of a pressman, can make silly statements easily overturned by the psychologist who took the time to become familiar with the work situation under consideration.

GENERAL HISTORY ERRORS

Often, because of inadequate cross-validation, an expert's history can be flawed by misinformation. Without checking and cross-checking the history against other records, the psychologist is in danger of making a determination while operating under erroneous information. Discovering on the stand that the child was adopted at 3 years of age can bring down the whole case built around attribution of cause in a damage suit.

INSUFFICIENT TIME

Frequently attorneys put off calling the psychologist to the last minute, encouraging just a quick look at the situation. When the usual and customary time is not taken with a case, the psychologist testifies at his or her peril. Always have the time, take the time, and allow the time, or refuse the case. Professional reputation is highly important in expert testimony. Always take sufficient time to do the task at the highest professional level. This could mean dropping everything else, giving up weekends and evenings, but the job still requires so many hours. Take the time or don't take the case.

ERRORS IN PROCEDURE

Over time, psychologists can develop habits in conflict with standardized procedures. Often corners are cut based upon experience that suggests corner cutting makes little difference. On the witness stand, correct procedure makes all the difference. Because the manuals of most professional instruments are so specific, failure to follow their correct procedures is condemned harshly in the writings of test publishers. When they are read in the courtroom, they have a devastating effect upon the effectiveness of the testimony of the expert who ignored their warnings.

Poor Preparation

In addition to poor scholarship and poor clinical work, poor preparation is a common pitfall of the expert witness. Poor preparation is observed frequently in seven areas: (1) poor checking, (2) poor layout, (3) poor review, (4) poor rehearsal, (5) poor timing, (6) poor exhibits, and (7) poor immersion.

POOR CHECKING

Rechecking the basic content of the report; having it cross-checked by a colleague, having it rescored by a technician, and then having it reviewed by another expert are time-consuming, and time is money, but such checking makes the difference. Most serious errors I have seen experts make have emerged from failure to check basic facts, such as birthdays. Going over the details one last time makes the difference between competent and poor expert testimony.

POOR LAYOUT

The file or chart the expert takes to the stand is highly important: It can make or break most experts. The complete test results, findings, interpretations, conclusions, supporting facts, key references, and statistics need to be organized such that the expert can find data without loss of time or dignity. Using the same layout on each court appearance is a useful device. Included should be a Work Scope Chart (see Figure 21-1) indicating the precise examination schedule and basic data collected on each step. Thus, a single sheet stapled in place would list hour, date, instrument, and basic results, as well as time spent on each test. When the testimony deals with an examination extended over several months, the age at each testing should be listed. If the testimony concerns a specific person, a detailed and correct family tree with age and sex of all members back two generations should be included, with a chronology of key events in the history of this individual, noting client's age at each. Fumbling through sheaves of papers, unable to find a key reference or specific test results, is a critical distraction in professional appearance and general effectiveness.

POOR REVIEW

Often the time lapse between evaluation and court appearance may be as long as 3 to 5 years. These data, then, need to be reviewed periodically, assessed for currency and relevancy, and redone systematically. In no case testify from deteriorated data.

In the week prior to the trial, a thorough review of all data, particularly the supporting scientific and professional literature, is mandated. Often their very success spoils some experts, because they do not have time in their active schedules to do systematic and periodic review. Thus they come into trial not thoroughly steeped in the specific case or relevant literature.

POOR REHEARSAL

Expert testimony is, in a real sense, a stage production, with an audience and critics as well. Finely tuning answers to expected questions and rehearsal of essential characteristics of competent witness-stand presentation improve every expert. An unrehearsed presentation, a presentation not reviewed in detail with the presenting attorney, simply is not the best the expert can do. Occasionally, a few attorneys seem not to have time to go over a specific presentation, but unlike psychologists, most attorneys are excellent at last-minute preparation. They often work 20 hours at a stretch over the last few days prior to trial. Thus, they can stand that extra 3 hours to rehearse the presentation of the expert psychologist carefully.

POOR TIMING

Nowhere is Murphy's Law of Time (Everything Takes Longer than It Does) more appropriate than in expert witnessing. The court waits for no one and keeps everyone waiting. Allowing appropriate time for the case, time to examine, time to research, time to prepare, and time to get there is critical to sound expert witnessing.

Not to be stressed, angry, or irritable when going on the stand also is important. One more lie can be added to the three most common lies: "Doc, I know you are busy. We will get you on at 2:00 and on your way by 3:00." A calm, cool, and collected expert, with a good resource book related to the issue at hand, can remain serene in the face of hours of delay if the fee has been set correctly and if the rest of the day has been planned such that a 5-hour delay in getting on the stand and a 3-hour cross-examination are not making a shambles out of other peoples' lives. There simply is no way to estimate accurately the time an expert will testify, and certainly there is no way to estimate when he or she will be dismissed.

POOR EXHIBITS

From time to time, the expert needs to testify from charts or tables. These can range from projections of predicted mental gain over a decade for a brain-damaged child to the observed profile versus the expected profile that leads to the contention of malingering. Such exhibits should be prepared by illustrators and should accommodate to vain, nearsighted jury members who do not wear their glasses. Professionally prepared exhibits can be excellent additions to the craftsmanship of the expert. On the other hand, hand-drawn, inaccurate, sloppy exhibits can be destructive.

An expert good at line drawings can outline the brain in front of the jury with such ease and conviction and can point out exactly where the damage was found and how that relates to the psychological test results as to be utterly spellbinding; but that ability is an unusual talent for a psychologist. It is, however, a talent worth developing if humanly possible, because chalk talk is virtually unstoppable in court and cannot be objected to effectively until it is completed.

POOR IMMERSION

The effective expert witness takes time during the final hours before trial literally to steep in the case, to become totally immersed in it. The information that can be retained for a short period is positively amazing. Reading the file; thinking about the plan, the questions, the answers, the problems; blotting out everything else is important. Securing a driver, arranging a quiet corner in the courthouse, having a cup of coffee, and staying away from others involved in the trial are part of this immersion process. Failure to do this—relying on quick peeps at the chart in the courtroom; running in at the last minute, out of breath, having fought traffic across town and having circled the block twice for a parking place; having difficulty finding the courtroom—tends to blitz the fine details right out of the minds of most experts. Total thought immersion often makes the difference between effective, skilled expert witnessing and strained, inadequate, incompetent expert witnessing.

Poor Control

Few psychologists understand the ebb and flow of the legal process. Not used to a director or orchestrator, psychologists can get out of control during the course of their testimony, mainly by (1) answering too fast, (2) nonresponsive answers, or (3) lack of scientific detachment.

Answering too fast in expert testimony on a contested issue can be hazardous to the entire trial. Nearly every question asked can be properly objected to; the expert should allow time after each question for the opposing attorney to object. This evenhandedness pleases the attorneys and the judge and prevents disruptive arguments and moves for mistrial.

Nonresponsive answers from psychologists can be equally damaging. Often experts don't want to answer a particular question because it is embarrassing, ambiguous, misleading to the jury, or apt to be critical of the expert's performance. Nevertheless, an expert witness must stick to the question and issue at hand, answering as clearly and precisely and to the point as possible, letting the attorneys battle out the rightness or wrongness of the questions. If an expert is asked whether he or she did in fact administer a complete neuropsychological battery, the answer is yes or no, not an elaborate defense of why such a test was not called for. Experts cannot lecture attorneys for their lack of understanding of psychology. They can only answer the question at hand. Occasionally psychologists try inside licks by being nonresponsive. Judges take unkindly to this, jurors get tired of it, and competent experts never practice it.

Lack of scientific detachment is unacceptable in expert testimony. Personal value judgments have no place in the courtroom. Only judgments of the profession are pertinent to the issue. The individual psychologist's attitude toward homosexuality, and thus toward children's being raised by a homosexual single parent, is completely irrelevant. The role of the expert is to provide data to indicate probability of damage to a child and empirical consequences to the child of such parenting, or simply to admit that except for case data and clinical lore, no scientific evidence in psychology is available one way or the other on the long-range consequences of a single homosexual parent raising a child.

Poor Grasp of Issues

Occasionally psychologists attempt court testimony without fully understanding the issues involved. More is at stake in the courtroom than simply the correct reporting of results from appropriate professional instruments. Such misunderstanding can pertain to (1) the law, (2) the purpose, or (3) the disputed issue.

THE LAW

Through reading, discussion, and pretrial conferences, psychologists should develop a thorough understanding of the laws of the state concerning both expert testimony and the specific issue in dispute. For example, in Florida, custody, once adjudicated, cannot be reopened unless substantial change in circumstances can be established.* The psychologist in Florida testifying on custody issues needs to know what the Florida Supreme Court has ruled as substantial change in circumstances* and needs to focus first on that issue exclusively, because unless that hurdle of "substantial change" can be surmounted, the issue of best interest of the child cannot be addressed. No matter what the issue, the specific relevant laws should be understood by the psychologist planning expert testimony. Without such understanding of the law, the expert may never get to the critical issue and thus may serve no purpose.

THE PURPOSE

An effective witness knows why he or she has been brought into the trial, what purpose he or she serves. For example, in an appeal of the firing of an unwed pregnant teacher, the purpose of the expert may be only to determine the effect of her condition on the children in the school. What the mother's unemployment will do to her unborn child is a serious matter, but the school board does not have to deal with that. To get your point across, you must stick to the purpose of your presence.

THE DISPUTED ISSUE

Often in a trial, many matters are not in dispute. Wandering into these undisputed areas not only wastes the time of the court but dilutes the testimony of the expert. For example, in an incest trial, the child in question may be a hypersexual Lolita, highly seductive and manipulative, but that matter is not disputed because it is irrelevant. Whether this crime was committed as a function of the insanity of the father is in dispute. The law does not deal with the seductive nature of a tender-aged daughter. Wandering around trying to explain this misbehavior will only inflame the jury, cause serious objections, and cause the father irreparable harm with a hanging jury.

Poor Presentation

At times, even when the substance of the expert witness's testimony is good, the presentation is so flawed that its effectiveness is spoiled. Flawed presentations can be (1) inaudible, (2) incoherent, (3) too sophisticated, (4) too jargony, (5) too fast, (6) too weak in examples, (7) too lacking in repeatable evidence, or (8) too vague.

Inaudible speech on the witness stand can invalidate completely the effectiveness of an expert witness. For the jury to hear every word is important. Speak up in a loud, firm voice, both to be heard and to imply authority. Speak slowly, distinctly, and clearly. Watch the attorneys and jury to be sure you are being understood.

Incoherent speech is as harmful as inaudible speech. If nervousness makes the expert incoherent, then practice is essential. A "warm-up tape" usually can help the expert over the initial hurdle of courtroom testifying. A warm-up tape is a prepared short talk in response to the prepared question of the attorney

---

* Bennett v. Bennett, 73 So. 2d 274 (Sup. Ct. of Fla., Spec. Div B, 1954)

offering you as a witness and might be as follows: "Good Morning. My name is Wallace A. Kennedy, and I live on route 5 in Tallahassee, Florida. I am a clinical psychologist, a professor of psychology at the Florida State University, and Director of Graduate Studies there. In addition, I am a member of a private practice group. I have both the master's and the doctoral degrees in clinical psychology from the Florida State University. I obtained my doctoral degree in 1956 after having interned at what is now the Hall Institute in Columbia, South Carolina. I was a postgraduate fellow at Harvard Medical School, Massachusetts General Hospital, prior to returning to the faculty at Florida State University in 1957." The tape goes on and describes the vita in considerable detail and as matter-of-factly as possible. By the time the expert has finished this well-practiced self-introduction, he or she should have settled down, adjusted his voice, and made good eye contact with that intelligent friendly face that belongs to the foreman of the jury and that will be the barometer followed for the next several hours. If, however, you do find yourself babbling on the stand, stop talking, organize your thoughts, and make a fresh start. "Let me see if I can express that better" is a good way to turn around an incoherent opening.

Too sophisticated a style of speech in the courtroom also detracts from the witness's presentation. Experience and knowledge tend to make some psychologists speak in a manner too sophisticated, too technical, too complex for the jury to understand fully. Using plain, common language is highly important; taking minute care to make sure that issues are competently but simply stated makes an enormous difference in effective communication on the stand. In interviewing dozens of former jurors, their most frequent complaint against expert psychological testimony was "I couldn't understand him."

Too jargony speech, on the other hand, is worse in a psychological expert. Sophistication can be a problem, but at least it leaves the jury with a good impression of the intellectual level of the expert. His or her conclusions may be followed ultimately, even though he or she muddied the water. But a jargony presentation simply leaves the jury confused and hostile, because jargon implies an "inside" language contemptuous of the intelligence of the jury. No better example of jargon is available than that contained in *DSM III.* Jargon must be avoided as much as possible in expert testimony.

Talking too fast on the stand is a strange thing that happens to personal rhythms and cadences under stress. Juries have serious decisions in their hands—often life-or-death decisions; they want to understand everything a witness has to say. No jury is put off by a slow, deliberate, emphatic cadence. By all means, err in the direction of slowing down too much rather than too little. Many otherwise excellent presentations are seriously flawed by a staccato, rapid-fire cadence that becomes incomprehensible in its speed.

Too weak in providing clear and simple examples is a tendency of most psychologists, perhaps because of their training to deal in abstractions. In jury trials particularly, examples can be everything. In a recent trial, after having described a mother as callous and indifferent to her children, I was asked on cross-examination on what evidence did I base the opinion that this mother was callous and indifferent to her children. "Because she weighs 280 pounds and her children are starving," I answered. For every abstract concept presented by an expert, one or two such examples with high face validity and easy comprehensibility should be readily available.

Coming into court **lacking evidence that can be repeated or verified** is a failure of some psychological experts. The expert should be able to stand aside from the evidence, surrender it, so to speak, to the scrutiny of other witnesses or to the jury itself. Of course the purpose of an expert is to interpret evidence to the jury, but the jury should have reason to believe that evidence to be repeatable and reliable. A single observation of a child in a home setting that "proves," according to the expert, which is the primary parent is highly unrepeatable and unreliable evidence, unless the parenting is so consistent as to be almost common-witness evidence.

Too vague language used in attempting to present key concepts to a jury often results in the psychologist appearing to be incomprehensible, or even incompetent. The statement "This child is now hyperactive, but not motorically so, rather in the sense of an attentional deficit disorder but may have the capacity to flood on a single signal such as a musical modality" may be good seminar language, but it is highly distracting to the layman. On the other hand, the statement that follows says the same things but in a more comprehensible manner: "Now, since the accident, Tommy has a serious problem that has a negative effect on his thinking in school and out of school. He has lost the ability to concentrate; he has a mental disease that the books call an Attention Deficit Disorder. But what that actually means is that he flits from one idea to another in the classroom, can't focus on the teacher's words, on the meaning of paragraphs, or on the material on the board. He gets halfway through a page and loses the whole thing. And the mystery of this flightiness is that sometimes, particularly when listening to a powerful sound—say, rock music or a loud cartoon program—he can become totally lost in it and cannot pick up what is going on around him at all. His problem is severe, has a very negative effect on his grades, and is probably permanent."

CONCLUSION

In the final analysis, of course, the secret of effective expert witnessing is a meeting of the minds. The combination of empathy for the solemn tasks of those involved in judicial decision and willingness to translate patiently and clearly complex, scientific, and artful psychological findings into clear and pertinent meaning for these individuals is the essential tool for the task. Understanding and appreciating the seriousness with which these individuals take their task greatly assists the expert to communicate effectively and comprehensibly with the attorney, a dialogue interrupted from time to time by the opposing attorney and occasionally by the judge.

If empathy for the task of these players of the great drama called the American judicial system is easy, if the thrilling drama of the Constitution of the United States acted out at its simplest and yet most vital level, the interface between evidence and jury, is captivating, then the task of expert witnessing probably should be pursued. Few activities engaging psychologists today have a more profound effect on the way we live out our lives than that of expert witnessing in the courtroom.

REFERENCES

1. DOLL, EA: *Vineland Social Maturity Scale: Condensed Manual of Directions.* American Guidance Service, Circle Pines, MN, 1965.
2. FOGELMAN, CJ (ED): *AAMD Adaptive Behavior Scale Manual (1975 Revision).* American Association on Mental Deficiency, Washington, DC, 1975.

3. FRANKENBURG, WK, DODDS, JB, FANDAL, AW, KAZUK, E, COHRS, M: *Denver Developmental Screening Test*. LADOCA Project and Publishing Foundation, Denver, CO, 1975.

4. JASTAK, JF AND JASTAK, S: *The Wide Range Achievement Test Manual of Instructions (1978 Revised Edition)*. Jastak Associates, Wilmington, DE, 1978.

5. WOODCOCK, RW AND JOHNSON, MB: *Woodcock-Johnson Psycho-Educational Battery*. Teaching Resources Corporation, Hingham, MA, 1977.

6. WOODCOCK, RW: *Development and Standardization of the Woodcock-Johnson Psycho-Educational Battery*. Teaching Resources Corporation, Hingham, MA, 1978.

7. HESSLER, GL: *Use and Interpretation of the Woodcock-Johnson Psycho-Educational Battery*. Teaching Resources Corporation, Hingham, MA, 1982.

8. DUNN, LM AND MARKWARDT, FC: *Peabody Individual Achievement Test Manual*. American Guidance Service, Circle Pines, MN, 1970.

9. *California Achievement Tests*. CTB/McGraw-Hill, Monterey, CA, 1977.

10. WECHSLER, D AND STONE, CP: *Standardized Memory Scale for Clinical Use*. The Psychological Corporation, New York, NY, 1973.

11. GRAHAM, FK AND KENDALL, BS: *Memory-for-designs test: Revised general manual*. Percept Mot Skills 11:147, 1960.

12. KENDALL, BS: *Orientation errors in the memory-for-designs test: Tentative findings and recommendations*. Percept Mot Skills 22:335, 1966.

13. BEERY, KE: *Visual-Motor Integration Monograph*. Follett, Chicago, IL, 1967.

14. BEERY, KE: *Revised Administration, Scoring and Teaching Manual for the Developmental Test of Visual-Motor Integration*. Follett, Chicago, IL, 1982.

15. BENDER, L: *A Visual Motor Gestalt Test and Its Clinical Use*. American Orthopsychiatric Association, Research Monographs, 1938, No 3.

16. KOPPITZ, EM: *The Bender Gestalt Test for Young Children*. Grune & Stratton, New York, 1963.

17. KOPPITZ, EM: *The Bender Gestalt Test for Young Children*, vol 2. Grune & Stratton, New York, 1975.

18. HATHAWAY, S AND MCKINLEY, J: *The Minnesota Multiphasic Personality Inventory Manual*. Psychological Corporation, New York, 1967.

19. MARKS, P, SEEMAN, W, HALLER, D: *The Actuarial Use of the MMPI with Adolescents and Adults*. Williams & Wilkins, Baltimore, 1974.

20. KRUG, SE: *Clinical Analysis Questionnaire Manual*. Institute for Personality and Ability Testing, Champaign, IL, 1980.

21. WIRT, RD AND KLINEDINST, JK: *Multidimensional Description of Child Personality: A Manual for the Personality Inventory for Children*. Western Psychological Services, Los Angeles, 1977.

22. CATTELL, RB: *Sixteen Personality Factor (16PF) Manual*. Institute for Personality and Ability Testing, Champaign, IL, 1979.

23. MATARAZZO, J: *Wechsler's Measurement and Appraisal of Adult Intelligence*. Williams & Wilkins, Baltimore, 1972.

24. WECHSLER, D: *Wechsler Adult Intelligence Scale-Revised Manual*. Psychological Corporation, New York, 1982.

25. CRONBACH, L: *Essentials of Psychological Testing*. Harper & Row, New York, 1970.

26. BUROS, O (ED): *The Eighth Mental Measurements Yearbook*. Gryphon, Highland Park, NJ, 1978.

27. EXNER, J: *The Rorschach: A Comprehensive System*. John Wiley & Sons, New York, 1974.

28. EXNER, J: *The Rorschach: A Comprehensive System, Vol 2: Current Research and Advanced Interpretation*. John Wiley & Sons, New York, 1978.

29. EXNER, J: *The Rorschach: A Comprehensive System, Vol 3: Assessment of Children and Adolescents.* John Wiley & Sons, New York, 1982.

30. RORSCHACH, H: *Psychodiagnostics: A Diagnostic Test Based on Perception.* Hans-Huber, Berne, Germany, 1942.

31. MURRAY, H: *Manual for the Thematic Apperception Test.* Harvard University Press, Cambridge, MA, 1943.

32. SPIVACK, G AND SPOTTS, J: *Devereux Child Behavior Rating Scale Manual.* The Devereux Foundation, Devon, PA, 1966.

33. SWIFT, M: *Devereux Elementary School Behavior Rating Scale II Manual.* The Devereux Foundation, Devon, PA, 1982.

34. BURKS, HF: *Teacher's Guide to the Interpretation and Application of the Burks' Behavior Rating Scales.* Western Psychological Services, Los Angeles, 1980.

35. GOLDEN, CJ, HAMMEKE, TA, PURISCH, AD: *Luria-Nebraska Neuropsychological Battery: Form 2.* Western Psychological Services, Los Angeles, 1980.

36. REITAN, RM: *Manual for Administration of Neuropsychological Test Batteries for Adults and Children.* Neuropsychology Laboratory, Tucson, AZ, 1979.

37. REITAN, RM: *Problems and prospects in studying the psychological correlates of brain lesions.* Cortex 2:127, 1966.

38. TERMAN, L AND MERRILL, M: *Stanford-Binet Intelligence Scale.* Houghton-Mifflin, Boston, 1973.

39. KENT, GH: *Kent Series of Emergency Scales.* Psychological Corporation, New York, 1946.

40. SLOSSON, RL: *Slosson Intellectual Test for Children and Adults Manual.* Slosson Educational Publications, East Aurora, NY, 1984.

CHAPTER 22

THE PSYCHIATRIST AS EXPERT WITNESS

William J. Curran, J.D., LL.M., S.M.Hyg.
A. Louis McGarry, M.D.

THE PSYCHIATRIST AS FORENSIC EXPERT

It has been only in the past decade or so that a consensus has begun to develop that the psychiatrist offering expert testimony in forensic psychiatric matters should have specialized training and experience. Even leading psychiatrists such as Menninger,[1] Guttmacher,[2] and Zilboorg,[3] each of them a recipient of the American Psychiatric Association's Isaac Ray Award for outstanding contributions to the field of law and psychiatry, did not advocate specialized forensic training or official certification in the field. Even today there is no forensic psychiatric subspecialty certification in the national official certification body, the American Board of Psychiatry and Neurology. However, as pointed out in chapter 1, other organized groups in the forensic field have developed standards for specialization in forensic psychiatry. The American Academy of Psychiatry and Law established in 1979 an accreditation service for forensic psychiatry.[4] Before eligibility to take the examination, an applicant must have had 5 years of experience in forensic psychiatric work. Applicants must also have been certified in general psychiatry by the American Board of Psychiatry and Neurology. As indicated in chapter 1, only a small number of experienced practitioners have been accredited by the board in subsequent years, fewer than 150 to date. The current membership of the academy is approaching 1000, but not all members devote a substantial proportion of their professional time to legal and forensic work and so may not wish to seek accreditation. The academy does not require applicants to complete an approved training program in forensic psychiatry. Currently the academy does not operate a formal system of approval for training programs. There are, however, published standards of the academy for fellowships in the field. These are reprinted in the appendix to chapter 1.

In medicine, the only national accreditation of a subspecialty in the forensic area is that in forensic pathology, which is a subspecialty under the American Board of Pathology.[5] Several other forensic scientific groups in the American Academy of Forensic Sciences conduct their own accreditation services in similar fashion to the American Academy of Psychiatry and Law.

Requirements of specialty accreditation in forensic areas does not automatically mean recognition and enforcement in the courts, however. American courts have been notoriously unwilling to set limitations for qualification (in terms of training and experience) for expert witnesses in any field.[6-10] This reluctance has generally been supported by the leading commentators of evidence law.[11, 12] The practice has been that minimum educational standards are adequate for admissibility, such as a primary academic degree in the field (medicine, psychology, social work, and so forth), without requirements for specialization, such as accreditation by the applicable American Medical Specialty Board.[13-15] Of course, we are concerned here with admissibility, not relative weight of one expert's opinion against another.

Courts have been influenced on admissibility rulings by the view that highly qualified experts are usually available only for high fees and only to financially secure parties. Thus, a restrictive attitude on admissibility would tend to penalize severely the poorer parties in private litigation and also the less affluent public agencies operating under strict budget controls. By not allowing the less qualified expert to testify on opinion matters, the courts would be forced to dismiss entire cases against these poorer litigants, who would thus fail to produce admissible evidence to support required elements in the legal action.

As indicated in chapter 1, in 1984 the American Bar Association (ABA) produced and approved a report on mental health standards in the criminal justice field.[16] The report suggests minimum professional standards for mental health professionals who are selected as court-appointed evaluators and also for any testimony as a mental health expert in court. (These recommendations are described in chapter 1 and will not be repeated here.)

We are in agreement with the ABA in its efforts to improve the quality of mental health testimony in all American courts. The content of the proposals on qualifications are actually quite modest. We believe, however, that there is probably more opportunity for support of their proposals in regard to court-appointed evaluators than for expert testimony in general. The arguments against requiring stricter standards in the latter area were explained earlier. For the former area, however, court-appointed evaluators, the circumstances are quite different. The court itself is not under the same restrictions as most private litigants. The courts in urban areas, at least, usually can contact qualified forensic experts and can pay adequate fees. Also—and this is very important—forensic experts of high reputation are often more willing to make themselves available, and at reasonable fees, because court-appointed evaluations are less partisan and more objective than requests from private lawyer-advocates. There are also other reasons for applying stricter standards for court-appointed evaluations. Lay juries are apt to be more impressed with the testimony of court-appointed experts, if they are told of the court appointment, because they expect the judge to select scientifically and ethically qualified people to fill these roles. A few statutes and court decisions have formally prevented juries from being told of a court appointment because of fear that lay juries will give too much weight to such testimony, even to the point of ignoring all other testimony to the contrary.[17, 18]

We are inclined to predict, however, that the first area in which forensic psychiatric accreditation will be required will not be either of the above. It is most apt to occur in the formal requirements for eligibility to be appointed to leadership positions (executive director, clinical supervisor, and director of training) in forensic psychiatric programs provided by state agencies and universities. Although it is not based upon an official survey, it is our impression that specialty forensic training and experience, up to and often including accreditation by the American Academy of Psychiatry and Law, is currently being required for priority consideration for such positions in many parts of the country.

FORENSIC PSYCHIATRIC CONSULTATION

The scope of consultation roles for forensic psychiatrists, and for forensically and legally trained psychologists as well, has been expanding considerably in recent years in relation to court trials. We are also impressed that experienced trial lawyers in serious litigation are becoming more sophisticated in seeking out highly qualified forensic mental health experts to advise them and to participate in many aspects of such litigation.

The roles of mental health consultants are not circumscribed by actual testimony. The broadened roles for such forensic experts prior to the trial and during the trial (including discussion during recess, lunch, and in late hours after court sessions) can be described in rather colorful terms as including the following:

1. As **educator,** providing knowledge and understanding to the attorneys concerning the meaning and application of scientific and technical aspects of the litigation
2. As **investigator,** conducting interviews and gathering data of potential application to the issues in the trial
3. As **clinical evaluator,** preparing formal reports and evaluating parties and witnesses in preparation, if called, to be a witness at trial
4. As **interpreter,** conveying to the trial attorneys the probable correct meaning, whether expressed or implied, in the statements of parties or witnesses who may not be fully understood by the attorneys owing to cultural differences, stress, or serious mental disturbances found in the parties or witnesses making the statements
5. As **trial-strategy adviser,** providing advice on what to use in evidence and when to use it for the best effect, or least damaging impact, of certain information as testimony in court
6. As **venue and jury selection adviser,** providing advice, based on survey techniques and other research, on whether a particular court community is apt to be favorable or unfavorable to a particular case or client, and whether certain types of persons in a jury panel are apt to be favorable or unfavorable to the case or client
7. As **drama coach,** suggesting and demonstrating for trial counsel the more favorable postures or emotional approaches they may take to produce a favorable impact on the jury or court

8. As **drama critic,** providing after-the-fact evaluations of the probable impact of certain testimony or data supplied to the jury during a given stage of the trial
9. As **rewrite editor,** providing advice and actual editing of text for the wording of hypothetical questions to mental health expert witnesses and for the opening and closing arguments of trial counsel
10. As **personal emotional support and/or therapist,** providing professional clinical advice and suggested therapy, when appropriate, for the trial counsel themselves or for the parties or witnesses, who are experiencing the stresses and emotional traumas of a serious and perhaps extended, drawn-out, trial involving very long hours of work and concentration

Many forensic experts will be uncomfortable performing several of the roles described above. Many will avoid all unnecessary contact with trial counsel and will merely provide a written report and appear in court ready to testify, perhaps spending a short time with counsel just before the appearance on the witness stand. The other roles described above will seem much too partisan, too advocacy-oriented, to the more traditional forensic expert, such as a forensic pathologist who is a state or county official medical examiner or coroner's physician. To perform most of the trial consultation roles, it is perhaps better for the mental health professional of very broad orientation (on items 4 through 10 above) not to appear also as an expert forensic witness providing testimony at the trial itself.

PROBLEMS IN COURT PRACTICES AND LEGAL ATTITUDES

The difficulties for the presentation of expert psychiatric evidence in American courts are aggravated by certain conditions prevalent in court practices and legal attitudes toward psychiatry and other mental health professions. The most significant problems can be described as follows:

1. The judicial rulings that many behavioral, emotional, and mental health issues are susceptible to understanding by **common knowledge** and are not subject to expert evaluation
2. The attitude of judges and lawyers that psychiatry and psychology are "soft sciences" without objective standards and reliable interpretations, highly uncertain, and more intuitive and judgmental in reaching conclusions than the "hard sciences"
3. The unfavorable attitude toward psychiatrists of legal and civil rights groups in recent decades
4. The tendency of courts (now changing somewhat) to assume that any well-trained psychiatrist has knowledge and experience in the forensic and legal aspects of any litigation matter involving mental health questions

The items described above have a cumulative effect and are often applied together in one case or one decision to admit or not to admit some type of mental health expert opinion testimony. American courts have traditionally assumed that lay people of ordinary intelligence can evaluate quite complex issues of personal conduct, intellectual capacity, and emotional distress. Perhaps best known, and most protected, is the assumed common knowledge of lay jurors to evaluate the credibility (reliability and truthfulness) of witness testimony.[19, 20] Courts and legal commentators have frequently expressed the view that lay people, including jurors and judges, are at least as able, and often more able, to form judgments in these areas than psychiatric or psychological experts.[21-23]

The questioning of the general evidentiary value of psychiatric expert opinion often overlaps with distrust of psychiatrists and concern about the "soft science" unreliability of behavioral science conclusions. In a recent federal court decision, an experienced jurist observed, "[P]sychiatry is at best an inexact science, if, indeed, it is a science, lacking the coherence set of proven underlying values necessary for ultimate decisions on knowledge and competence."[24]

In a very significant legal psychiatry case in the Supreme Court of the United States, *O'Connor v. Donaldson*, Chief Justice Berger was even more pointed in his viewpoints. He asserted, quite formally, "The Court appropriately takes notice of the uncertainties of psychiatric diagnosis and therapy and the reported cases are replete with evidence of the divergence of medical opinions in this vexing area."[25]

Concern over "this vexing area" of psychiatry is not new to the courts. One of the best-known examples came in a 1926 opinion by Chief Justice Rugg of Massachusetts, one of the most respected jurists of his day, in a decision upholding a trial judge's determination of a defendant's mental condition based **solely** upon the judge's personal observation of the defendant's demeanor on the witness stand. The chief justice observed,

> The [trial] judge may well have been able to form a judgment as to the legal responsibility of the defendant for the crime, based upon common sense inferences and intelligent observation, **more reliable** as a practical guide to accomplishment of justice than **refined distinctions and technical niceties of alienists and experts in pathological inferiority.**[26] [emphasis supplied]

The attitude that psychiatry is too "soft" a science has led to the view that there is more ground for a courtroom "battle of the experts," adding only confusion upon confusion, in psychiatry than in any other field of litigation.[27] There do not seem to be any reliable survey data to support this view, and it has been disputed.[28] Nevertheless, the mass media have often concentrated attention upon differences of opinion expressed on the witness stand by psychiatrists in such recent trials as that of John W. Hinckley, Jr. and in past trials involving such famous defendants as Sirhan Sirhan, Jack Ruby, and Patty Hearst, thus producing an impression of total confusion and lack of settled principles in behavioral science areas.

The unfavorable attitude toward psychiatry has often been supported, probably not intentionally in all instances, by law school courses in law and psychiatry since the early 1960s. It should be understood that the values emphasized in these courses are not usually related to clinical needs of patients for treatment or emotional support. Their objectives are to teach civil rights issues, freedom of individuals from unnecessary restraint, and the due process of law requirements for involuntary hospitalization. The mental health professionals involved in the mental health system are often depicted as "the heavies" in the legal process that the courses focus attention upon. In addition to case law and statutory materials, these courses generally assign mental health literature as well as law review articles and research studies, many of which are highly critical of the role of psychiatrists and other mental health professionals.[29-32] It cannot be denied that a large part of this criticism has been justified at times. The problem has been that many of these students and later lawyers develop a generally unfavorable, often quite distrustful, attitude toward all psychiatrists unmitigated by experience with the effective application of psychiatric skills and methods with seriously disturbed patients.

These developments in the 1960s and later decades may be contrasted with almost diametrically opposite practices in the American trial courts in the earlier decades of this century. These courts, both in urban and rural areas, placed heavy reliance, without any observable scrutiny, upon the untrained staffs of large, nearby mental hospitals to provide forensic evaluations on patients sent to the hospitals for observation.[33-35] The courts assumed that these hospital-based physicians were well-educated psychiatrists with forensic training and experience. Actually, the majority of these facilities were chronically understaffed with physicians who often had limited psychiatric training, let alone any appreciable knowledge of the legal requirements for the forensic examinations they were requested to perform. These physicians generally resolved any doubts about a patient's condition in favor of treatment and hospitalization. They answered the legal questions in whatever way was suggested that would achieve their desired result of continued hospitalization. An earlier article by one of the authors, William J. Curran, describes this era of overreliance by the courts on hospital-based forensic evaluations resulting in widespread frustration of legal objectives in these evaluations.[36] (See also the section on burden of proof, later in this chapter.)

There is currently an indication in legal circles of greater acceptance of the need to seek out well-trained psychiatrists with formal training and experience in forensic psychiatry. There is still a strong demand, however, in the courts for degrees of certainty and trial advocacy that the best and most ethical of psychiatrists and psychologists are reluctant to provide within the legitimate limits of their personal integrity and convictions. These issues will be examined more fully later.

EXPERT TESTIMONY: GENERAL CONSIDERATIONS

There are excellent general reviews of expert psychiatry testimony and the functions of forensic psychiatrists in the courts.[37-40] There are also useful publications of extracts of forensic psychiatric testimony from actual cases and mock trials involving well-known trial attorneys and expert witnesses.[41, 42]

The professional duty of the expert psychiatric witness is threefold: (1) to provide scientifically and clinically accurate testimony; (2) to provide this testimony in an ethically responsible manner; (3) to provide answers, as complete as possible, to the legal questions asked in the litigation.

Each of these duties will be explored in this chapter. More fully developed aspects of the ethical responsibility noted above will be found in chapters 2 and 3 of this text.

The two most important attributes of the **effective** expert witness are the capacity to produce a high level of **authority** for opinions expressed and the ability to **convince** the fact-finder of the correctness of that opinion. If these two qualities are not displayed during direct examination and sustained throughout cross-examination, the witness is not likely to be called upon again by the attorneys familiar with his or her performance.

Authority is usually conveyed by the review of the expert's background, education, training, and specific experiences in the issues under consideration in the litigation. The person's demeanor, bearing, and appearance also contribute to his or her impression of authoritative expertise. The matter of conviction is more difficult to describe. It is displayed in the manner of answering questions and the detail and completeness of the descriptions and opinions. Often the full dimensions of the conviction of the witness, the persuasiveness of his or her testimony, become evident only after cross-examination and perhaps a brief re-direct examination for purposes of clarification. The challenge of pointed, intelligent cross-examination often produces greater, not less, strength to a witness's performance, owing to the contrast with a direct examination that may often be rather matter-of-fact and somewhat undramatic. In fact, many experienced trial lawyers will purposely avoid asking any cross-examining questions of an expert with a weak or dull performance on direct examination just in order to avoid awakening the aggressive spirit and greater persuasiveness of the witness.

There are other important characteristics of the effective expert witness. These are integrity, impartiality, and objectivity. The expert forensic specialist should avoid overstatement of either qualifications or the degree of certainty in the various elements of the testimony. If some needed information was missing, or if some usual tests were not performed, these matters should be disclosed on direct examination and their significance explained. Witnesses should resist either attorney who tries to push them to conclusions they cannot support or to offer opinions in areas outside their expertise. To maintain impartiality, both attorneys should be treated with the same professional courtesy and distance, avoiding undue familiarity. Effort should be made to avoid verbal sparring or debating with the cross-examiner.

Personal appearance is often stressed in advising novice expert witnesses. It probably isn't as important to effectiveness of testimony as is often claimed. Most trial attorneys advise expert witnesses to avoid garish, flashy, or disheveled dress. This means a rather conservative appearance, avoiding extremes which detract from the testimony itself and make the witness's appearance and personality the focal points of first impressions and later recall at the end of the testimony. The male witness should wear a business suit or plain trousers and a sport jacket (not too flamboyant, please), a shirt and tie, and clean shoes. The female expert should wear a two- or three-piece suit with a skirt (not slacks, please) and a minimum of jewelry. Make-up should be to the taste of the witness. Jurors notice age: Younger witnesses can break dress codes and conduct themselves more casually than the middle-aged and older persons whose credentials take some time to describe. It must be said, however, that the key is to allow witnesses, especially in first appearances, to be themselves; an abrupt change in personal appearance and dress can adversely affect composure and conviction on the witness stand for the expert as well as for the general witness.

REPORTS AND PREPARATION FOR TESTIMONY

There is a substantial array of legal issues for which expert forensic psychiatric testimony is required or requested. Usually, the testimony is preceded by a clinical examination of the party involved and perhaps study of previous history in clinical records and interviews with other significant persons. The forensic evaluator should make maximum use of whatever legal discovery mechanisms are available in the jurisdiction in order to conduct a thorough review of all antecedent data of relevance to the litigation. In criminal matters, for example, not only prior medical and psychological records but investigative reports by detectives and arresting police officers should be sought and reviewed. It is often advisable to use direct quotations from reviewed documents and from interviews with the party and other persons in order to give the full flavor of the events and the impressions they made on the observers, however credible or unreliable these statements may prove to be later.

One of the authors, A. Louis McGarry, currently makes a practice of audiotaping clinical examinations, at least when conducting evaluations for private parties. This practice may not be feasible in a busy, high-volume public agency. As indicated in chapter 3, the forensic expert can expect to be required to tolerate and to adapt to the presence of attorneys, including opposing attorneys, at clinical examinations of the party. Such presence may be required by statute[43] or case law.[44] Also, it should be recalled that the American Psychiatric Association ethical principles (official **annotations** to the AMA Code) hold it unethical for a psychiatrist to conduct a forensic examination of a criminal defendant prior to access to and availability of legal counsel.[45]

Often the forensic expert examiner will prepare the report on the forensic evaluation; furnish it to the attorney, or attorneys, or directly to the court; and will not be called as a witness. Nevertheless, every report should be prepared with the expectation that it may need to be explained and defended in court. (The form and content of reports for the courts were reviewed by Dr. McGarry in chapter 4 of this text.)

PRETRIAL FORENSIC EXAMINATIONS

When preparing to conduct a forensic examination, the expert must be careful to ascertain **what** specific legal (and clinical) **questions** are to be addressed. The mere request to "do a forensic examination" is not enough. The issues differ considerably in a will contest case, a worker's compensation case, or a criminal investigation. Although the retaining lawyer has the clear responsibility to articulate the relevant legal issues to the forensic expert, this often is not done well or completely—either consciously or unconsciously—by attorneys or courts. When this occurs, the examiner should seek out the attorney or court to clarify the issues. It is often necessary, however, for the forensic specialist who handles many cases in different jurisdictions to review the applicable substantive or procedural law so that the proper criteria may be followed. As indicated in chapter 4, the report of the evaluation should, at the outset, indicate the questions addressed, providing legal citation to case or statutory authority wherever advisable.

It is also important to be aware of **who** is requesting a forensic examination. Responsibilities and expectations differ according to which party in the particular litigation is retaining the expert. When the forensic evaluation is being conducted for a private party, it is usually assumed that the content of the evaluation and all that is discussed during the examination is confidential and privileged, available only to the retaining attorney and through that attorney to other parties and the court. The retaining attorney may generally use or suppress the examination results. However, this degree of confidentiality cannot always be legally assured. As indicated in chapter 3, one federal court decision has allowed discovery of the name of an expert who examined the defendant on the issue of criminal responsibility and, when not called by the defense, has allowed the prosecution to call that evaluator as a prosecution witness to reveal the content and conclusions of the examination.[46] The basis for the ruling was that the examination was not confidential because it was not intended for treatment.

It should also be noted that in criminal as well as civil cases the reports of experts who are indicated as trial witnesses may be required to be exchanged with opposing counsel, or the content of their reports described, or the experts themselves may be made available for pretrial deposition (examination under oath) by opposing counsel. The United States Supreme Court has recently ruled, however, that this breadth of availability of the expert's report and evaluation does **not** mean that the attorney's "work product" concerning the strategy for use of the expert at trial must be revealed to opposing counsel.[47]

The nature of the forensic examination, or at least the attitude of the examinee toward the forensic evaluator, may be substantially affected by who the evaluator is seen as identified with in the case.[48, 49] If seen as an ally retained by the examinee's own lawyer, the evaluator must guard against uncritical acceptance of self-serving statements or even outright malingering of symptoms and claims. If seen as the opposition, the evaluator must be prepared for possible evasion or even hostile refusal to cooperate.

In the case of the court-ordered examination, as indicated in chapters 2 and 3, the party should be informed that the interview is not confidential and that the content must be reported to the court along with the opinion of the forensic examiner on the questions asked by the court. (The only exception to this disclosure rule is that in most states the court-ordered examiner evaluating competency to stand trial or criminal responsibility cannot be required to reveal a "confession" of the crime by the examinee. However, even this exception can be relaxed when the examiner finds the person "insane" and not responsible and the examinee, with advice of counsel, waives the requirement of confidentiality in order to utilize the examiner's full testimony.)

The forensic expert in a court-ordered examination should consider himself or herself an agent of the court in conducting the evaluation and in writing the report for the court. This assumption should be applied even though there are decisions denying this capacity to court-appointed experts in some situations. These decisions are examined in chapters 2 and 3. As indicated in chapter 3, a *Miranda*-type warning should be given before the examination begins. Because he or she should act as if an agent of the court, the examiner should avoid becoming involved in too close and too intimate a degree of cooperation in concert with the party who intends to call the examiner as a witness. In order to assure fairness to both sides, the examiner ideally ought to afford opportunity for both counsel to be present at conferences on the case.

There is often an assumption expressed that forensic evaluators conducting pretrial evaluations for a prosecutor, especially when they are employed by state or county agencies, will be biased toward the prosecution and find most or a majority of defendants to be criminally responsible. This is a classic problem of an apparent "double agent"; that is, representing both court and prosecutor, reviewed in chapter 3 of this text. In practice, this type of court-ordered pretrial examination does not inevitably produce the biased effect expected. Quite contrary results are illustrated in Table 22-1, which reflects recent experience in New York State regarding numbers of uses of the insanity defense.[50] As the table indicates, the great majority of cases of uses of the insanity defense resulted in the acceptance of a plea of not guilty on these grounds. These pleas were based on the high percentage of reports by prosecution-retained forensic examiners finding that there was a persuasive basis for such a plea by the defendants examined by them in these years.[51]

Precautions

The pretrial psychiatric examiner should use caution in the application of treatment-oriented interviewing skills or the application of "emotionally seductive" methods[52] which may mislead the party concerning the purposes of the forensic evaluation. The examiner is **not** authorized to offer treatment or to reassure the party about that party's own "proper" motives for previous conduct. We also see it as unethical for the forensic examiner to seek to augment too forcefully the partisan purposes of the advocate attorney who retained the expert's services beyond providing complete answers to the legal and clinical questions asked. Such rigorous pursuit of impartiality and objectivity may on occasion lead to more cautious findings and more ambiguous or circumscribed results in a report than the more aggressive trial attorneys may prefer from their retained experts. There are times when this cannot be avoided if professional integrity is to be retained. One of the authors, William J. Curran, has recently described the all-too-often "shabby" uses of psychiatry in the overly strident application of the adversarial legal system. As he observed,

> It often seems that the more ethical, cautious and professionally skilled the psychiatrist, the less his or her evaluations are welcomed in the courtroom where certainty and a willingness to play the adversarial game are attributes most valued, not only by the competing lawyers, but by the presiding justices, from the lowest to the highest of our courts.[53]

TESTIMONIAL PREPARATION

The preparation of courtroom testimony is quite different from the preparation of a forensic report on a pretrial clinical examination. For courtroom testimony, the attorney and the witness need to go over the actual areas of questions and

TABLE 22-1. Insanity Acquittals, New York State

	1980 (6 MONTHS TO DEC. 31, 1980)	1981	1982	1983	TOTALS
Plea resolution	68%	86%	79%	83%	81%
Verdict	32%	14%	21%	17%	19%
Total number	34	116	113	77	340

Review of percentage of pretrial dismissals of prosecutions on a **plea resolution** basis as not guilty by reason of insanity (NGRI) as compared with verdicts of NGRI by the jury or by the court following trial.

answers that will be presented in court. Most of the serious problems in expert witness testimony are the result of inadequate pretrial consultation on the specific areas that are going to be covered and areas to be avoided in direct examination. It is a cardinal principle that there should be no surprises in either questions or answers in direct examination. This does not mean that the answers of the expert are rehearsed. In fact, the witness should resist such strict, rote repeating of arranged statements. The questions, however, especially any long recitations of scientific or technical terms in general inquiry or hypothetical questions, may need to be prepared in written, draft form.

The length of time needed for pretrial conferences varies, depending on the weight given to the following factors:

1. The familiarity, or lack of it, in working together of the forensic expert and trial counsel
2. The complexity of the scientific, technical, and clinical issues involved in the case and the relative need to educate trial counsel to put these issues into questions and answers understandable to court and jury
3. The novelty of the legal issues in the case, either in the case in chief or the defense, requiring collection of psychiatric-psychological data not usually presented in court
4. The need to anticipate and to prepare for a vigorous cross-examination of the forensic expert

It may be surprising to note the priority given to item 1 above. The pretrial conference on testimony is first and foremost designed to acquaint the forensic expert and the trial counsel with each other and their styles of communication. If the two have worked together frequently on very similar clinical and legal issues, the pretrial preparation can and usually is relatively short and pointed. The less the two principals have met and worked together, the more carefully all aspects of the case and the testimony must be reviewed.

Most expert witnesses expect the second item to be the most significant and time-consuming aspect of pretrial consultation. It is, of course, the major aspect of the substantive part of the testimony. It is usually shaped by the evaluation report of the expert and any pretrial depositions or statements of the witnesses that were exchanged between opposing counsel or sent to the court in a court-ordered examination. Deviations from findings and conclusions of the report should be avoided even in matters of detail, unless justified by the receipt of other data changing these findings or conclusions.

The complexity of the clinical issues in a case can extend the need for pretrial consultation considerably, as was the experience of one of the authors, William J. Curran, in the *Von Bulow* case in Rhode Island, in which he was a medicolegal consultant to the prosecution. A recent book details the preparation of this case and the trial presentation.[54] The case involved criminal charges of attempted murder by the defendant of his wife on two different occasions 1 year apart. It was alleged that insulin was used to attempt to produce an undetectable death in each instance. The case also involved alleged uses of other substances, including tranquilizers and aspirin and the effect of extreme cold on the human body. The case thus turned upon deeply complex medical issues and legal questions in the atmosphere of a televised trial receiving daily coverage by national and international news media. Pretrial consultations with expert medical witnesses and with the physicians who provided emergency treatment to the wife in each incident were extensive. The court required exchange of pretrial statements and names of expert witnesses to avoid unfairness or surprise in the complex aspects of the prosecution and defense. The guilty verdicts on both counts were later reversed by the Rhode Island Supreme Court, primarily on nonmedical issues of search and seizure and failure to obtain search warrants.[55] A second trial has now been held and resulted in a not guilty finding.

The novelty of the legal issues in a case can also prolong pretrial consultation with experts because of the unusual nature of the data that may be needed to support the issues. This was the atmosphere of the famous trial of Patty Hearst in San Francisco on numerous charges of involvement in a series of crimes with a small terrorist group, most of whose members were later killed in a shoot-out with police in Los Angeles. Trial attorney F. Lee Bailey advanced the highly novel defense of psychological and political "brainwashing" by the terrorists to achieve Miss Hearst's cooperation in the crimes after they had admittedly kidnapped her forcibly and held her for ransom. The behind-the-scenes story of the trial by a reporter provides considerable insight into the preparation of the defense and of the prosecution in the case.[56] The jury did not accept the "brainwashing" defense, and Miss Hearst was found guilty.

The last item noted above, the need to prepare for vigorous cross-examination, often concerns the inexperienced expert witness.[37, 38, 42] He or she usually asks the retaining lawyer what to expect on cross-examination. A few lawyers provide effective advice on such matters, but most do not. They are generally too "wrapped up," emotionally as well as intellectually, in their own side of the case and their own theory of the psychiatric issues to be of much help. The expert usually must construct his or her own anticipations concerning the weakness of the formal part of the testimony and the alternative theories of the scientific, technical, and clinical aspects of the case. It is best that the expert explain these to the trial counsel so that the direct examination may deal with these problems as best it can. The lawyer should, however, warn the expert about procedural problems and matters of possible bias or weakness in the expert's qualifications or past professional work that might be explored on cross-examination.

COURTROOM TESTIMONY: STYLE AND SUBSTANCE

General advice on manner and style of testimony by expert witnesses is available in extensive commentary.[35, 40, 41, 57-60] The advice provided by Dr. Kennedy in chapter 21 for psychologists as witnesses is generally applicable to psychiatrists as well.

Expert forensic witnesses should make an effort to study and to improve upon their courtroom performances. It is an essential part of their specialty activity. If they are not effective in their testimony, they will not be called upon by the trial attorneys and judges, no matter how proficient they may be in the scientific and technical aspects of their forensic work. To an appreciable degree, the frequent courtroom expert witness should actually enjoy the experience most of the time. This is the strong position of one of the authors, A. Louis McGarry, who appears in court as a witness fairly regularly.

In order to produce a degree of satisfaction with courtroom performance, the forensic expert should be reasonably articulate and secure in quick-witted exchange with attorneys. Attention to detail in all aspects of forensic work is essential to avoid exposure and discredit in court.

The forensic expert must speak clearly, loudly, distinctly, and slowly enough to be heard and understood by the judge and jury. The witness should be sure that **the jurors** hear the responses, not merely the lawyer asking the questions. Many courts have installed microphones to amplify weak voices and to project them throughout the courtroom. The expert should not hesitate to use the microphone; in fact, it is highly advisable, no matter what the timbre of the unaided vocal cords. A mild foreign accent is usually not a handicap. Actually, it is our experience that judges and jurors often listen more closely and intently to the accented voice than to more familiar speech.

The witness should pause before answering questions, both in direct and cross-examination, in order to respond effectively and to allow time for objection to the question by opposing counsel. Too rapid a response, often before the examiner has finished a question, is one of the most common problems of the ineffective expert witness. This practice creates the impression of a nervous, insecure witness and often presents an appearance of overanxiety to express partisan views. This type of witness is also prone to "volunteer" information and opinion that was not solicited by the question. This is improper testimony and is subject to objection and exclusion from evidence. Highly damaging "volunteered" and unresponsive testimony can result in a mistrial.

If a question is not understood, the witness should ask that it be repeated. Often the repeated question differs from the first. If the difference is significant, the witness should call attention to the discrepancy and ask clarification. Many experts object to answering yes or no to scientific questions. This practice usually occurs only on cross-examination when the witness is pressed on overly wordy evasive responses, or when opposing counsel is challenging the witness with differing theories of the psychiatric-psychological issues involved in the case. Most judges currently will allow the expert witness to resist a short, categorical answer and to provide more depth of response. This is especially true if the witness pauses before answering and turns to the judge and asks, "May I explain my answer, Your Honor?" Only the most unsympathetic, aggravated, impatient jurist can resist this request if put politely and clearly.

USE OF TECHNICAL LANGUAGE IN TESTIMONY

Advice is often given to expert witnesses to avoid technical jargon and to use simple language understandable to the jury. It should be remembered, however, that the expert must appear **authoritative** in his or her presentation and should provide complete and scientifically accurate testimony. This cannot be done without producing technical data. The science of the expert's field should not be avoided. Stress should be placed upon objective data that support the conclusions of the witness. After these data are produced, their meaning and significance to the case at hand should then be explained in terms comprehensible to intelligent lay persons. The questioning counsel should help in this effort to provide adequate understanding. Illustrations or similarities to more common experience can help explain highly technical concepts. Drawings on a blackboard can also be helpful. A. Louis McGarry finds it very effective to use literal quotes from the examined person or from the records to illustrate clinical points made in testimony.

When technical terms are used, they should be current and acceptable within the profession. This means that the classifications and terminology of the 1980 *Diagnostic and Statistical Manual of Mental Disorders (DSM III)* should be used when applicable in reports and testimony. The older clinician or forensic specialist should not use outmoded terminology to display obstinacy with the current "established order" of things. It should be noted, however, that the manual makes a specific point of cautioning against the application of the manual to "nonclinical purposes," such as the determination of "legal responsibility, competency or insanity" without critical examination of the applicability of the terms to that situation within its own "institutional context."[61] This does **not** mean that the proper terminology from *DSM III* should not be used in legal cases. The currently accepted terminology should be used when describing psychiatric clinical entities. The caution provided in the manual is against the use of terminology as a complete substitute for a required legal standard in an area of legal responsibility or competency. (See, for example, discussions in chapters 7 and 8 on competency to stand trial and criminal responsibility, respectively.)

CROSS-EXAMINATION TECHNIQUES

Lawyers and judges have great confidence in intelligent, aggressive cross-examination to expose untruth and exaggeration in direct testimony. Effective cross-examination of an expert witness, especially an experienced forensic specialist, requires the cross-examiner to have mastered the subject area quite well and to be ready with a substantive critique applicable to the issues of the case.[37, 40, 41, 60] Much of cross-examination of the opposing side's expert witnesses will be drawn from the differing clinical or technical theories suggested by the experts retained by the cross-examiner. Also, the cross-examiner will pick up cues to areas of questioning during the direct examination. These may be suggested when the witness has hesitated, or has given weak responses, to points raised on direct examination.

As noted earlier, the witness under cross-questioning should pause before responding in order to give opportunity to the lawyer who called him for direct questioning to object to the inquiry if it is improper. Basically, under the rules of evidence, trial counsel must make its objections in timely fashion to the **question asked,** not to the responsive answer.

One technique of vigorous cross-examination is to ask a series of connected questions in an accelerating rhythm. Often the next query in the series is put to the witness before a prior answer is completed. The result can be to confuse and to upset the witness and to force short, passive answers favorable to the questioner, just to bring the ordeal to a close. The effective expert witness should avoid falling into this trap. He or she should slow down the responses and take the time to answer each separate inquiry one at a time. If the cross-examiner overlaps questions, interrupting an answer, the witness should pause and finish his or her response to the first question and then ask that the next question be repeated. This style of unruffled response should break the rhythm of the questioner and enable the witness to proceed properly. The other counsel will also often object to this rapid-fire method of questioning. The very fact of the objection and the accompanying remarks of the objecting counsel also helps, quite intentionally, to break the rhythm of the cross-examiner, even if the objection is overruled.

Many of the techniques of cross-examination are not direct challenges to the substance of the expert's testimony. They are indirect attacks on areas of possible bias or conflict of interest on the part of the witness or on the extent of his or her qualifications and experience to offer opinion evidence on all or certain aspects of the testimony.[62] As indicated earlier, both the expert and the retaining counsel should explore these potential areas of vulnerability and should be prepared to answer them.

Some cross-examiners are quite skillful in challenging witnesses with published articles, papers, and textbooks taking a different view of the subject than that offered by the witness in direct testimony. The witness should be ready to explain differences with these published materials. It should be noted that most American jurisdictions will **not allow** the expert witness to be challenged with a statement from a published paper, article, or textbook unless the witness agrees that the publication is authoritative on the subject.[63] Although admitting its authoritative nature, the witness can still point out that the quoted statement is now out of date, or is a minority view, or is contradicted by other parts of the same publication and was thus quoted out of context.

LIMITATIONS ON PSYCHIATRIC TESTIMONY

An important area of concern that we should explore is the suggested limitation on mental health testimony in the report of the American Bar Association (ABA) on standards for the mental health aspects of criminal justice.[16] The ABA House of Delegates adopted all of the recommendations by voice vote at the annual meeting in August 1984. The recommendations were noted briefly in chapter 2 of this text because of their relationship to ethical responsibility, but their basis and implications were not explored. The testimonial limitations would totally bar admission into evidence of opinion testimony on the following matters:

1. Concerning an "ultimate question" of law, or a moral or social value properly reserved to the court or jury
2. Concerning a prediction that a particular person will, or will not, engage in dangerous behavior in the future
3. Concerning the mental condition of a person that the expert witness has not personally interviewed or examined

All the above are significant restrictions on current practice in the courts. The draftsmen admit that all three of these areas are presently allowable areas of testimony under the Federal Rules of Evidence.

The report defends these limitations on psychiatric-psychological testimony essentially on the grounds that they are outside the area of expertise of these professions.

The first limitation, avoidance of "ultimate questions," has long been an area of contention in American law. It was supported in several forms in past decades but has largely been disparaged in more recent years.[64, 65] Earlier, the conclusion was considered an improper invasion of "the province of the jury."[66] For example, the expert witness was allowed to provide an opinion on each element of the legal requirements for making a valid will but could not add them up and offer a conclusion personally that the person was or was not of "sound mind" or legally competent.[67, 68] Obviously, in opening and closing arguments, the trial counsel pointed out to the jury that these "elements" automatically added up to the proper legal answer.

In other fields, the application of the "ultimate question" exclusion resulted in much less rational results than in mental health matters. For example, expert witnesses were not allowed to become **too certain** in their conclusions about scientific causal relationships.[66, 69] Witnesses were allowed to conclude that an event "could have" caused an injury, but not that it "did" cause the injury. The current formula acceptable to most courts before stating a conclusion on causality, and on most other scientific or clinical matters, is for the questioning counsel to ask if the witness has an opinion "within reasonable scientific certainty" or "within reasonable medical certainty." When explored, the degree of certainty in this formulation is usually stated as "probability," or "more likely than not."[70, 71]

The most noted of the legal scholars on evidence law, Dean John Wigmore, always pungent in his comments on evidentiary rules he did not favor, was highly critical of the "ultimate issue" exclusionary rule. He asserted that it was "so misleading as well as unsound" that it should be repudiated.[72] McCormack, another leading authority in the field, also believed the rule unnecessarily restrictive.[73] Many psychiatrists and psychologists, however, have favored the limitation, perhaps because of their own discomfort in providing testimony using the technical terms of the law rather than confining themselves to their own areas of professional expertise.

The other aspect of the first limitation, that of preventing mental health experts from testifying upon "moral and social values properly reserved to the jury" should present no particular problem as long as the proper reservations are within the modern rules of evidence law. The areas of reservation are perhaps more correctly stated as "within rules of law" rather than the "province of the jury" exclusionary rule. For example, the witness ought not to describe antisocial behavior based solely on the witness's personal standards of acceptable behavior. The principle behind this ABA recommendation can be applied to civil law areas as well as criminal law. For example, the expert testifying about the suitability of a parent to have custody of a child should limit the opinion to the legal grounds of the jurisdiction for such custody, not apply his or her own social or moral standards as to the propriety of granting custody to that parent.

The second limitation should be familiar to any reader of the quite voluminous literature of the questionable ability of psychiatrists and psychologists to predict potential for dangerous or violent conduct in particular individuals. It would not be feasible to cite all the papers and articles in the field, but a few of the most recent and leading commentaries and research efforts may be noted herein.[74-77] The bar association's position does contain its own qualifications, which circumscribe the scope of the primary recommendation. The standards would allow testimony on potential for violence when confined to general observations on such matters as the clinical significance of past medical or psychiatric history or criminal record. The witness could also testify on the probable effects of efforts at treatment of a mentally disturbed person or habilitation of a retarded person upon those factors tending to enhance or to diminish the likelihood of such a person's dangerous behavior in the future. The expert would also be allowed to testify regarding general scientific studies bearing upon the subject of predicting potential for violence in persons with problems similar to those of the defendant.

The movement to exclude psychiatric-psychological testimony on the dangerousness of specific individuals suffered a severe blow recently when the U.S. Supreme Court in *Barefoot v. Estelle*[78] rejected the argument of the defendant and of an amicus brief of the American Psychiatric Association on this basis. The majority opinion would not exclude such testimony but would clearly allow questioning of its weight and persuasiveness in given cases.

The Supreme Court in the *Barefoot* decision also rejected the ABA's last-listed limitation. The Court refused to rule that psychiatrists could not testify on the potential for violent conduct of a person they had not personally examined for that purpose.

The draftsmen of the ABA report admitted that this last limitation had perhaps the least support in law of any of the recommendations and was "a major departure from existing practice."[79] Testimony based upon clinical-record review ("chart review") and on controlled hypothetical questions without personal examination of the patient has traditionally been allowed in all American courts for many decades.[80, 81] The report cited two annotations to the AMA Ethical Code prepared by the American Psychiatric Association to support the ABA's contention that no psychiatrist should be allowed to testify in court on the mental condition of a party not personally examined. (These annotations were examined in chapter 2, "Ethical Perspectives: Formal Codes and Standards.")

Neither of the annotations cited are directly in point. The first annotation (to Section 7) states that a psychiatrist should not offer to provide a diagnosis on a public figure who is exposed to public attention in the mass media without having examined the person. The draftsmen argued that this ethical principle should be applied to **courtroom testimony** because of the public nature of the courtroom. Actually, the argument has no support in the history of the annotation. It arose out of the presidential campaign of 1964 when many psychiatrists answered an unsolicited, politically motivated mail inquiry about the mental status of the Republican Party candidate, Senator Barry Goldwater. Many of the respondents willingly gave diagnoses of mental disturbance and thus publicly labeled the senator as mentally ill. The APA's annotation was clearly aimed at such situations of public diagnosis by newspaper and television observation. It was not addressed to judicially controlled conditions in a court of law under the rules of evidence. The ABA draftsmen did not display a knowledge of this history of the annotation.

The other annotation cited by the ABA was closer to the point. It provides that a psychiatrist should not certify a patient as mentally ill for purposes of involuntary commitment unless a personal examination has been conducted (also a note to Section 7). It should be pointed out, however, that civil commitment certification is an out-of-court statement uncontrolled at that time by a judge. As pointed out in chapter 2, virtually all American jurisdictions already require by statute or regulation that all such certifications be made based on personal examinations conducted within 3 to 10 days of the certification.

The above critical discussion of the ABA mental health standard is not intended to argue against the relatively greater weight of an opinion based upon a personal interview and clinical evaluation of the person concerned. Such a practice is always clinically appropriate when the interview is allowed. However, there are circumstances in which an examination is either not possible because of death, disappearance, or flight from justice or is not feasible legally because the person has refused to cooperate in the examination. When these circumstances occur, it seems reasonable for a court to allow testimony based upon clinical records and past history and hypothetical questions, based upon credible evidence to support the questions. Nevertheless, even in such cases, when commenting on the evidence, the courts will traditionally point out the generally greater reliability of personally conducted clinical examinations of the person.

Rather than condemn outright all testimonial opinions without personal examinations in all possible situations, we would prefer to point to some particularly objectionable practices. The first is that of offering an opinion based solely on observing a party or witness in the courtroom and in testimony. This limited observation should not support diagnostic impressions or opinions about testimonial credibility.

The second questionable practice is that of "traveling circuit" forensic experts who go from state to state testifying in cases of choice in their own forensic specialty. Because of lack of time, or reluctance of retaining legal counsel to pay for such services, these experts often forego lengthy personal interviews and other investigations and provide only courtroom testimony based on chart review and evaluation of available investigative material.[82] It seems ethically advisable for these specialists, or any other forensic specialist, to insist on the time to conduct personal clinical evaluations whenever feasible.

The other ethically objectionable practice is found in child custody litigation. As examined by Dr. McGarry in chapter 11, this involves the offering of an opinion, without examination, on the appropriateness (or, more frequently, the inappropriateness) of a parent to be awarded full custody of a child or several children in a separation or divorce action. The witness will usually have been retained by one parent whom the witness has had in therapy or has evaluated for purposes of the litigation, but the witness will not have seen or clinically evaluated the opposing parent. Despite this, the mental health professional willingly comes into court and testifies that the unseen spouse is an unsuitable parent to have custody. (There would be nothing improper, of course, if the witness were to limit the testimonial opinion to the general suitability for custody of the parent who was clinically evaluated, saying nothing at all about the other parent.)

CERTAINTY AND BURDENS OF PROOF

The last issue we would explore in this chapter is another "vexing area," that of degrees of certainty (or doubt) in scientific, technical, and clinical matters. Many inexperienced expert witnesses assume that law courts regularly require very high degrees of certainty in scientific and clinical areas. This assumption is often linked to the belief that courts always require categorical answers of yes or no to all questions, no matter how difficult the issues.

Actually, the courts rarely require extremely high levels of certainty. The objective of the court system is not to find truth; the objective is to **settle disputes** fairly and finally.[83, 84] The settlement is effected by one party winning the lawsuit and the other losing, not by proving one or the other to have truth on his or her side. The settlement of the lawsuit is achieved by placing the burden of proof upon one side or the other.[85, 86] If that party does not produce enough admissible evidence to sustain that burden, then the other side wins the lawsuit. The party having the burden of proof is usually the party making the claim (the claimant or plaintiff). In civil litigation, the burden is generally not stated in degrees of certainty or truth. It is stated as preponderance (somewhat greater weight) of the evidence produced by both parties. Increased weight of evidence in civil cases is often placed on certain elements in a case by various means. For example, in negligence actions, a very important part of civil litigation, the burden may be increased by requiring a party to "prove" (sustain the weight of preponderance) that the defendant was **grossly negligent** rather than only ordinarily negligent in a particular accident. Such a burden is required when a fellow passenger is suing the driver of a motor vehicle in a negligence case. Conversely, in a civil action against a pharmacist for negligently filling a prescription improperly, the suing plaintiff need prove only a **slight degree of negligence,** because pharmacists are held to a very high standard of care in filling medical prescriptions.

It is in the criminal area that we find the burden of proof increased to "beyond reasonable doubt." Even this burden does not require absolute certainty. The doubt remaining must be reasonable and of substance, not merely an uneasiness or unreasonable prejudice or superstition.

Complexity is introduced into burdens of proof when the courts place separate burdens on defendants to "prove" certain affirmative defenses in the case. For example, in medical malpractice cases, the burden of proof (by preponderance of evidence produced) on "informed consent" may be placed on the defendant doctor rather than on the suing patient.

Recent decisions and statutory changes have affected matters of burden of proof in the field of mental health law. Several states have imposed the burden of "beyond reasonable doubt" in cases of involuntary commitment to a mental hospital. Others have increased the burden by requiring that the jury find the person mentally ill and committable on the basis of "clear and convincing" evidence. The latter is considered a lesser burden than the former, but both are considered greater burdens than a merely general preponderance of the evidence. In a significant decision[87] the United States Supreme Court ruled that the Constitution requires only "clear and convincing evidence" for involuntary commitment.

Chapter 8 of this text reviews the statutory changes in several states concerning the burden of proof in criminal cases on the insanity plea. The changes are mainly in the direction of placing the burden of proof (in differing degrees in different legislation) on the **defendant** as an affirmative defense rather than on the prosecution to prove the sanity of the defendant beyond reasonable doubt as part of the prosecution's case in chief.

As noted earlier, one of the common errors of the past among inexperienced mental health expert witnesses was the assumption on the part of a clinical evaluator that all doubts should be resolved in favor of psychiatric treatment when the clinician thought that the person might benefit from such treatment. Also, the clinician was inclined to believe the allegations made against the person by family members or others seeking an involuntary commitment, or the allegations against a criminal defendant in a police report. When the person denied these allegations, the clinician often considered this a sign of delusion or lack of cooperation in the examination. On the contrary, the law of this country sets up two **presumptions** which should apply to these situations. The first is the presumption of **sanity,** or sound mind, unless rebutted by clear and credible evidence. The second is the presumption of **innocence of crime.** In perhaps an unconscious way, the inexperienced (in forensic psychiatry) clinicians of past decades violated both of the presumptions regularly.

We end this review by noting again the practice of most courts in requiring psychiatric-psychological (and all other scientific) expert testimony to be provided "within reasonable scientific (or medical or psychological) certainty."[70, 71, 86] This common formula avoids application of **degrees of certainty,** which can put severe strain on the ethically responsible professional witness.[88] The jury may need to go beyond the statement of the expert witness to achieve a higher degree of certainty such as "beyond reasonable doubt." It should be pointed out that an expert's opinion that a conclusion is only a **possibility** will not satisfy the civil burden of proof, let alone the criminal burden of proof. An equivocal type of conclusion is the assertion that one condition is (or is not) "consistent with" another condition or set of facts. In causal relationship, for example, the statement might be that a condition (epilepsy, behavior change) is "consistent with" an injury (blow to the head). This form of conclusion is often utilized as a rebuttal or cross-examination question in order to shake the confidence level of an expert's conclusion in direct examination. In a recent important case, the California Supreme Court ruled that an expert could not testify, on the basis of finding that a person was suffering from "rape trauma syndrome," that the person was actually raped.[89] The court found that the syndrome was not adequately accepted scientifically to support the burden of proof of a criminal charge. Nevertheless, the court found that such testimony could be used to rebut an inference of rape when the person's condition was found "not consistent" with rape trauma syndrome.

When a witness is cross-examined and asked to admit that a situation might have reached a level of consistency with an alleged event, the expert can accept that it is "consistent with" the happening of the alleged event but can point out that it had not reached the level of probability or reasonable scientific certainty.

The discussion in this section should underscore a persistent theme recited throughout this text: The forensic mental health expert who is going to appear as a courtroom witness on a regular basis must have legal training as well as forensic clinical skills and knowledge to enjoy a successful and satisfying career in the interdisciplinary field of law and mental health.

REFERENCES

1. MENNINGER, KA: *The Crime of Punishment.* Viking Press, New York, 1968.
2. GUTTMACHER, MS: *The Mind of the Murderer.* Farrar, Stans & Cudahy, New York, 1960.
3. ZILBOORG, G: *The Psychology of the Criminal Act and Punishment.* Harcourt, Brace, New York, 1954.
4. DIETZ, PE: *Educating the forensic psychiatrist.* J Forensic Sci 24:880, 1979.
5. SAGALL, E: *Courtroom qualification of medical witnesses.* Trial 6:56, 1970.
6. State v. Carter, 217 La. 547, 1950.
7. Katsetos v. Nolan, 170 Conn. 637, 1976.
8. Steinberg v. Indemnity Ins. Co., 364 F. 2d 266 (5th Cir, 1966).
9. ENNIS BJ AND LITWACK, TR: *Psychiatry and the presumption of expertise: Flipping coins in the courtroom.* California Law Review 25:37, 1978.

10. Slovenko, R: *Reflections on the criticisms of psychiatric expert testimony.* Wayne Law Review 25:37, 1978.

11. Ladd, M: *Expert testimony.* Vanderbilt Law Review 5:414, 1952.

12. Cleary, EW: *McCormack's Handbook of the Law of Evidence,* ed 2. West Publishing, St Paul, MN, 1972, p 216.

13. Oleinick, R: *Expert witnesses under rule 702: Circuit court attitudes toward qualifications of experts during the period 1971-1977.* Environmental Law Review 8:753, 1978.

14. Swan v. Lamb, 584 P. 2d 814 (Utah, 1978).

15. Martinez v. Equitable Equip. Co., 330 So. 2d 634 (La. App., 1976).

16. *First Tentative Draft, Criminal Justice Mental Health Standards.* American Bar Association, Washington, DC, 1983.

17. Wick, J and Knightlinger, SJ: *Impartial medical testimony under the federal rules: A tale of three doctors.* Insurance Counsel Journal 34:115, 1967.

18. Van Dusen, H: *The impartial medical expert system: The judicial point of view.* Temple Law Quarterly 34:386, 1961.

19. People v. Barbara, 400 Mich. 352, 1977.

20. Walter v. O'Connell, 339 N.Y.S. 2d 386, 1973.

21. Slovenko, R: *The developing law on competency to stand trial.* Journal of Psychiatry and Law 5:165, 1977.

22. Trovcak v. Hafliger, 7 Ill. App. 3d 495, 1972.

23. On English law reaching similar conclusions, see R. vs. Turner, (1975) Q. B. 834.

24. Suggs v. LaVallee, 570 F. 2d 1092 at 1120, 1978 (Kaufman, J.).

25. 422 U.S. 563 at 579, 1975.

26. Comm. v. Devereaux, 257 Mass. 391, 1926.

27. Beis, EB: *Mental Health and the Law.* Aspen, Rockville, MD, 1984.

28. Diamond, BL and Louisell, DW: *The psychiatrist as an expert witness: Some ruminations and speculations.* Michigan Law Review 63:1335, 1965.

29. See materials collected in Katz, J, Goldstein, J, Dershowitz, A: *Psychoanalysis, Psychiatry and Law.* Free Press, New York, 1967.

30. See materials collected in Brooks, AD: *Law, Psychiatry and the Mental Health System.* Little, Brown & Co, 1974.

31. Szasz, TS: *Law, Liberty and Psychiatry.* Macmillan, New York, 1963.

32. Gleuck: *Law and Psychiatry: Cold War or Entente Cordiale?* Johns Hopkins University Press, Baltimore, 1962.

33. McGarry, AL: *The holy war against state hospital psychiatry.* N Engl J Med 294:318, 1976.

34. *Misuse of Psychiatry in the Criminal Courts,* Publication No 89. Group for the Advancement of Psychiatry, New York, 1974.

35. Halpern, AL: *Use and misuse of psychiatry in competency examination of criminal defendants.* Psychiatric Annuls 5:4, 1975.

36. Curran, WJ: *Community mental health and the commitment laws: A radical new approach is needed.* Am J Public Health 57:110, 1967.

37. Rothblatt, HB: *The preparation of the psychiatric defense and the direct and cross-examination of the psychiatric witness.* Leg Med Annu 1971, p 801.

38. Watson, A: *On the preparation and use of psychiatric expert testimony: Some suggestions in an ongoing controversy.* Bull Am Acad Psychiatry Law 6:226, 1978.

39. MacDonald, JM: *Psychiatry and the Criminal: A Guide to Psychiatric Examinations for the Criminal Courts,* ed 3. Charles C Thomas, Springfield, IL, 1976.

40. Ziskin, J: *Coping With Psychiatric and Psychological Testimony,* ed 3. Law and Psychology Press, Venice, CA, 1981.

41. *Effective Utilization of Psychiatric Evidence.* Practicing Law Institute, New York, 1970.

42. WATSON, AS: *Untying the knots: The cross-examination of the psychiatric witness.* In *Examination of Medical Experts.* Matthew Bender, New York, 1968.

43. See, for example, N.Y. Crim. Procedure Law, Section 250.10 (3).

44. Lee v. County Court, 267 N.E. 2d 452, 1971.

45. *Principles of Medical Ethics with Annotations Especially Applicable to Psychiatry.* American Psychiatric Association, Washington, DC, 1981.

46. U.S. v. Smith, 425 F. Supp. 1038 (U.S.D.C., E.D., N.Y. 1976).

47. *Bogosian v. Gulf Oil Corporation.* United States Law Week 53:2026, 1984.

48. WEBSTER, CD, MENZIES, RJ, JACKSON, MA: *Clinical Assessment Before Trial: Legal Issues and Mental Disorder.* Butterworths, Toronto, 1982.

49. ROSENBERG, AH: *Competency for trial: A problem of interdisciplinary communication.* Judicature 53:316, 1970.

50. Personal communication to A. Louis McGarry from C.L.J. Stokman, August 1984.

51. ROGERS, JL, BLOOM, JD, MANSON, SM: *Insanity defenses: Contested or conceded?* Am J Psychiatry 141:885, 1984.

52. STONE, AA: *Law, Psychiatry and Morality.* American Psychiatric Association Press, Washington, DC, 1984, pp 69-71.

53. CURRAN, WJ: *Uncertainty in prognosis of violent conduct: The supreme court lays down the law.* N Engl J Med 310:1651, 1984.

54. WRIGHT, W: *The Von Bulow Affair.* Delacourt Press, New York, 1983.

55. State v. Von Bulow, 475 A.2d 995, 1984.

56. ALEXANDER, S: *Anyone's Daughter: The Times and Trials of Patty Hearst.* Viking Press, New York, 1979.

57. WALLACE, W: *Demonstrative evidence—some practical pointers.* Trial 12:50, 1976.

58. SHAPIRO, DL: *Psychological Evaluation and Expert Testimony—A Practical Guide for Forensic Work.* Von Nostrand Reinhold, New York, 1984.

59. For an older view, see this classic paper by FOSTER, F: *Expert testimony—prevalent complaints and proposed remedies.* Harvard Law Review 11:169, 1897.

60. CURRAN, WJ: *Tracy's The Doctor as a Witness,* ed 2. WB Saunders, Philadelphia, 1965.

61. *Diagnostic and Statistical Manual of Mental Disorders,* ed 3. American Psychiatric Association, Washington, DC, 1980.

62. See analysis and citations on qualifications and collateral attack collected in CURRAN, WJ AND SHAPIRO, ED: *Law, Medicine and Forensic Science,* ed 3. Little, Brown & Co, Boston, 1980, pp 252-259.

63. See, for example, Kansas Stat. Ann. 60-460(c); interpreted in State v. McDonald, 222 Kan. 494, 1977.

64. The rule is rejected in the federal courts; see Fed. Rules of Evidence, Rule 704.

65. *The Demise of the Ultimate Fact Rule in Indiana.* Indiana Law Journal, 53:365, 1978.

66. NORVELL, RJ: *Invasion of the province of the jury.* Texas Law Review, 31:731, 1953.

67. Gillmore v. Atwell, 283 S.W. 2d 636, Mo., 1955.

68. SLOUGH, MC: *Testamentary capacity—evidentiary aspects.* Texas Law Review 1:11, 1957.

69. Buchler v. Beadia, 343 Mich. 692, 1955.

70. FIRESTONE, M: *With reasonable medical certainty (probability).* Legal Aspects Medical Practice 12(6):1, 1984.

71. MARKUS, RE: *Semantics of traumatic causation.* Cleve-Mar. Law Review 12:233, 1963.

72. WIGMORE, JH: *Evidence* (CHADBOURNE, CE) rev ed. Little, Brown & Co, Boston, 1970, § 898.

73. CLEARY, EW: *McCormack's Handbook of the Law of Evidence*. West Publishing, St Paul, MN, 1972, p 27.

74. EWING, CP: *"Dr. Death" and the case for an ethical ban on psychiatric and psychological predictions of dangerousness in capital sentencing cases*. Am J Law Med 8:407, 1983.

75. MONAHAN, J: *The Clinical Prediction of Violent Behavior*. US Department of Health and Human Services, Monograph Series, Crime and Delinquency Issues, Washington, DC, 1981.

76. COCOZZA, R AND STEADMAN, HJ: *The failure of psychiatric prediction of dangerousness— clear and convincing evidence*. Rutgers Law Review 29:1084, 1976.

77. SHAH, SA: *Dangerousness: A paradigm for exploring some issues in law and psychology*. American Psychologist 33:224, 1978.

78. Estelle vs. Barefoot, 104 S.Ct. 209, 1983.

79. Tentative Draft Report, sup ref 16, p 152.

80. See for example, Langerfelder v. Thompson, 179 Md. 502, 1974.

81. VOGEL, JE: *Hypothetical questions on cross-examination of medical experts*. De Paul Law Review 7:149, 1958.

82. This practice of the "traveling circuit" forensic expert was suggested in a recent paper. See MILLIER, RD: *The Treating Psychiatrist as Forensic Expert*. J Forensic Sci 29:825, 1984.

83. HOLMES, OW, JR: *The Common Law*. Little, Brown & Co, Boston, 1881.

84. CARDOZO, BN: *The Nature of the Judicial Process*. Yale University Press, New Haven, CT, 1921.

85. CLEARY, EW: *McCormack's Handbook of the Law of Evidence*, sup ref 73, p 136.

86. EGGLESTON, R: *Evidence, Proof and Probability*, ed 2. Weidenfeld & Nicolson, London, 1978.

87. Addington vs. Texas, 435 U.S. 39, 1979.

88. WALLS, HJ: *What is "reasonable doubt"?—a forensic scientist looks at the law*. Criminal Law Review 458, 1971.

89. People v. Bledsoe, 681 P.2d 291, 1984.

INDEX

A "t" following a page number indicates a table. A page number in *italics* indicates a figure.

kleptomania
clinical features of, 417
diagnosis of, 417-418
etiology, pathogenesis, dynamics of, 418
treatment of, 418
pathological gambling
clinical features of, 419
diagnosis of, 419
etiology, pathogenesis, dynamics of, 419-420
treatment of, 420
pyromania
clinical features of, 415
diagnosis of, 415-416
etiology, pathogenesis, dynamics of, 416-417
treatment of, 417
terminological difficulties of, 410-411
Diversion, treatment, and recidivism of juvenile delinquency, 271-275
"Double agent," therapist as, 70, 70-71
DSM III
forensic psychiatric reports and, 85-87
Dual-purpose court orders, competency assessment and, 159-160
Durham insanity test, 177

Education, training, licensure, and certification
psychologist as expert witness and, 488-489
Environmental factors, juvenile delinquency and, 268-270
Environmental measures, tools of psychological assessment and, 121
Ethical codes in forensic areas, 52
code of forensic scientists, 52-54
cruelty, torture, and inhuman treatment and, 54-56
unethical advertising and publicity, 56-57
Ethical codes in medicine and psychiatry, 47-50
Ethical issues of interdisciplinary cooperation, 61-71
Ethical principles for psychologists, 50-52
Ethical standards, importance of, 46-47
Etiologic perspectives, antisocial personality and, 398-402
Evaluation mechanisms and procedures for pretrial competency cases, variations in, 152
Exhibitionism, 292-293

Experience, psychologist's
expert witness and, 489
Expert testimony
general considerations for, 518-519
reports and preparation for, 519-520
Expert witness
consultation functions of, 45
opinion of, 491-498
psychiatrist as
certainty and burdens of proof and, 530-532
cross-examination techniques and, 526-527
forensic psychiatric consultation and, 515-516
general considerations for expert testimony and, 518-519
limitations on psychiatric testimony and, 527-530
pretrial forensic examinations and, 520-522
insanity defense use and, 522, 522t
precautions for, 522
problems in court practices and legal attitudes and, 516-518
psychiatrist as forensic expert and, 513-515
reports and preparation for testimony and, 519-520
style and substance of courtroom testimony and, 524-525
technical language in testimony and, 525-526
testimonial preparation and, 522-524
psychologist as, 498
brevity and, 499-500
coherence and, 500-501
controlled attitude and, 501
exactitude and, 499
preparedness and, 499
responsiveness and, 501
aptitude in the courtroom of, 490
education, training, licensure, and certification of, 488-489
experience and, 489
history of, 490-491
opinion of, 491
professional data and, 491-492
firsthand, 492-497
secondhand, 497-498
pitfalls of, 501
poor clinical work and, 502-503
errors in procedure and, 503
general history errors and, 503
insufficient time and, 503
interpretation errors and, 502

Seating of expert witness, 491
Secondary gain, worker's compensation claims and, 477-478
Sentencing, classification, and parole correctional psychiatrist and, 456-458
developmentally disabled persons and, 215-217
Sex, juvenile delinquency and, 266-267
Sexual inhibition, posttraumatic stress disorder and, 471
Sexually abused child
behavior of, 320-322
characteristics of, 320
criminal justice process and
legal issues and concerns in, 329-330
prevention and amelioration of stress and trauma and, 331
victim as witness and, 320
extrafamilial abuse, procedures in cases of, 325-326
impact of victimization on
long-term effects of, 327-328
short-term effects of, 326-327
incidence and prevalence of, 317-320
interviewing of, 322-324
intrafamilial abuse, procedures in cases of, 324-325
legal definitions of, 315-317
psychiatric definitions and, 317
treatment of, 331-334
Sexually aggressive behavior, 289-310
Sexual molestation, rape, mental health legal problems and, 480
Sexual psychopath statutes, male genital exhibitionism and, 378-379
Shoplifting, 418
Situational determinants of behavior
situational context in legal settings and, 112
situational context of legal questions and, 111
Social and treatment goals of pretrial competency cases, 153
Social control, juvenile delinquency and, 265
Social environmental factors, increasing predictive accuracy and, 133-134
Social learning, juvenile delinquency and, 265
Social skills deficits, paraphiliac offender and, 304-305
Social withdrawal
posttraumatic stress disorder and, 471-472
Social work, programs in law and, 24-25

Sociological and psychiatric variables, antisocial personality and, 399-402
Sociopathic personality. *See* Antisocial personality
Sociopathy, mentally ill prisoner and, 440
Somatiform disorder, civil law and psychiatric testimony and, 472-473
Special issues in forensic psychiatry, curriculum for, 38
Specialized forensic measures, tools of psychological assessment and, 118-120
Standards for fellowship programs in forensic psychiatry, academic affiliation for, 36
Statutory and case law, child custody and, 249-250
Statutory penalties, male genital exhibitionism and, 377-378
Stress, rape as cause of, 347-349
Subculture, juvenile delinquency and, 265-266
Suicides in prisons and jails, 447-449
Supervised clinical experiences
civil forensic psychiatry and, 39
correctional psychiatry and, 39
criminal forensic psychiatry and, 38-39
legal regulation of psychiatry and, 39
special issues in forensic psychiatry and, 39

Tactical misuse of competency procedures, 152
Testifying about legal competency, 161-162
Testamentary capacity, mental health legal problems and, 482
Testimony, practical considerations for, 124
Theoretical models for male genital exhibitionism, 367-371, *370*
Therapeutic identity, preservation of, role of correctional psychiatrist and, 458-461
Therapist as "double agent," *70,* 70-71
Thioridazine, treatment of male genital exhibitionism and, 375
Tools of psychological assessment
aids to problem analysis as, 112
base rate information, 113-114
behavioral observation methods as, 113
demographic and archival data as, 113